A

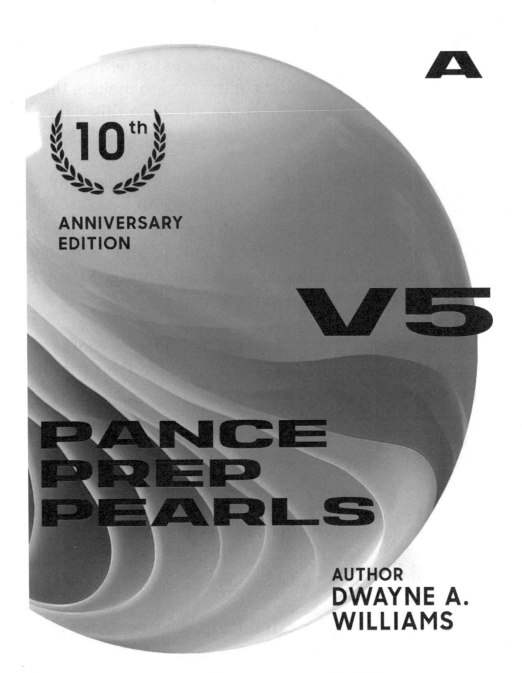

10th
ANNIVERSARY EDITION

V5

PANCE PREP PEARLS

AUTHOR
DWAYNE A. WILLIAMS

ISBN: 9798322874775
Imprint: Independently published
Printed by Kindle Direct Publishing Platform
Cover design: Eli Ofel: support@applocal.co

DEDICATION

Thanks to my foundation teachers Marion Masterson, Medea Valdez, Gerard Marciano. A very special thanks to Stacey Hughes (words can't describe my gratitude to you), Sharon Verity and William Ameres for being my inspirational teachers as a student. To all those who contributed to making this profession great and to all my fellow educators who contribute to this field on so many levels.

Thanks to all of the owners of the photos. Your images helped to make this book a visual experience. Your contribution is invaluable. An extra special thanks to **Ian Baker**, the illustrator of most of the pictures in the book. You added a special touch to this project. Thanks Dr. Frank Gaillard and Jason Davis for your help during the process. Special thanks to **Kevin Young, Xiana Flowers & Kristen Risom** (the best illustrators I know!)

Special thanks to my parents Winifred & Robert Williams. Xiomara & Froylan Flowers (my second parents), Mercedes Avalon, Gilda Cain (the best nurse I know!) and my big brother Danilo Avalon.

To my gurus: Stacey Hughes, Tse-Hwa Yao, Ingrid Voigt, Dr. Antonio Dajer, & Dr. Kenneth Rose you guys have helped shaped the PA I became.

Thanks to Isaak Yakubov (my Akim) for the Ultimate Mnemonic Comic Book and the amazing journey we have embarked on together.

Pamela Bodley, the world's best manager. You are the real boss lady!

To Eli Ofel. Thank you for your friendship, partnership, and amazing covers.

Last but not least a very special thank you to my PPP warriors for rocking with me for 10 years! This book would have been nothing without the support of each and every one you! Thanks for being always being there!!!! YOU ARE PPP WARRIORS.....WARRIORS WIN!

PREFACE

STUDENTS
This book is designed for use in both didactic and clinical education. It is formatted to make you a rockstar on clinical rotations! It is a **review book**, which means **it is not meant to replace textbook-based education** but as an additional study tool to enhance your knowledge base. Textbooks provide the foundation for understanding and learning medicine.

PRACTITIONERS
This book is purposed to increase your knowledge & retention of important clinical information and for use as a quick resource that is not time consuming.

THE STYLE OF PPP
Pance Prep Pearls is not written in the traditional style of a textbook but rather to feel like a collection of notes, drafts, charts, mnemonics and clinical pearls to make learning effective while entertaining. The use of bold and asterisks are to help you to organize the information and stress the importance of certain aspects of the disease states. The charts are designed for you to compare and contrast commonly grouped diseases and high-yield information. It is loaded with helpful algorithms to help you see the big picture on how to approach the disease.

I personally recommend that you use what I call the 6 P's of the **Patient-Centered Learning Model** as you study the different diseases:

1. **Pathophysiology:** imagine explaining the pathophysiology of a disease to your patient in 1 sentence (2 sentences maximum) in simple terms. Understanding the pathophysiology will often explain the clinical manifestations, physical examination findings, why certain tests are used and usually the treatment reverses the pathophysiology. This step is often skipped but is probably the most important (in terms of knowledge retention).
2. **People** be comfortable knowing the epidemiology of the diseases.
3. **Present** – based on the pathophysiology, how would this patient present? Know both the classic and the common findings and presentations (they aren't always the same).
4. **Pick it up**? – How would you diagnose the disease. Make sure to understand what is usually first line vs. gold standard (definitive diagnosis). Understand the indications and contraindications for each test.
5. **Palliate** – how do you treat (palliate) the disorder. Many people can list out the treatments but fail to remember first line treatments vs. alternative treatments. Make sure to understand the indications and contraindications of each treatment.
6. **Pharmacology** – understand the mechanism of action and understand why a medication is used for that disease. This helps to reinforce the pathophysiology as well as the presentation of the disease since the pharmacology often reverses the problem or treats the symptoms. A very important point is that if you see a medication that is used for different disorders, try to understand what connects the use of that drug to the different disorders.

PANCE PREP APP AVAILABLE ON IPHONE PLATFORMS!

EARN 20 CATEGORY 1 SELF-ASSESSMENT CME CREDITS

Go to Panceprepapp.io for more information

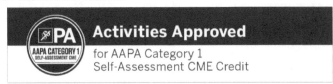

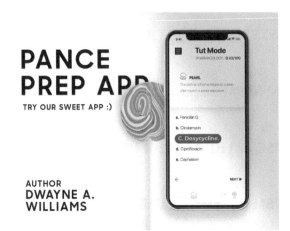

Over 15,000 clinically-based practice examination questions specifically formulated to enhance clinical skills and improve performance on examinations, such as the PANCE, PANRE, OSCES, USMLE, end of rotation examinations and comprehensive medical examinations.

PANCE PREP QUESTION BOOK

EARN 20 CATEGORY 1 SELF-ASSESSMENT CME CREDITS

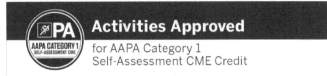

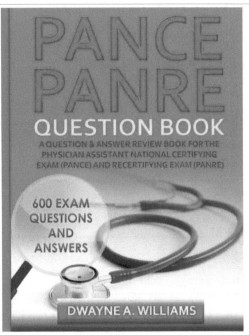

TABLE OF CONTENTS

CHAPTER 1 – CARDIOVASCULAR DISORDERS

ECG CHEAT SHEET

STEP 1: DETERMINE THE RHYTHM

Regular or Irregular?
☑ **Use Rhythm strip.** Check R-R intervals: if <0.12 second difference, consider it a regular rhythm.

STEP 2: DETERMINE THE RATE

If **Regular** rhythm ⇨ 1500/# of small squares **OR** 300-150-100-75-60-50 method between an R-R interval.
If **Irregular** rhythm ⇨ count the number of R waves in a 6 second strip & multiply that number by 10.

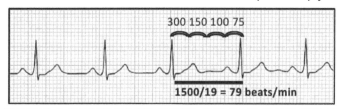

STEP 3: DETERMINE THE QRS AXIS

	Normal	LAD	RAD
Lead I	+	+	-
aVF	+	-	+

*If Left Axis Deviation (LAD) based on I and aVF ⇨ check lead II.
- If QRS is predominantly positive in lead II ⇨ normal axis (0° to -30°)
- If QRS is predominantly negative in lead II ⇨ LAD (<-30°)

STEP 4: EVALUATE THE P WAVES/PR INTERVAL

(Look in Lead II and V_1 for P wave morphology)
☑ **Sinus?** If positive/upright in I, II, avF, & negative in avR. Each P wave followed by QRS complex.
☑ **PR interval normal?** Normal PRI = 0.12–0.20 sec (or 3-5 boxes). Prolonged (>.20s); shortened (<.12s)
☑ **Atrial enlargement?**

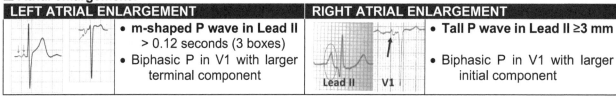

LEFT ATRIAL ENLARGEMENT	RIGHT ATRIAL ENLARGEMENT
• **m-shaped P wave in Lead II** > 0.12 seconds (3 boxes) • Biphasic P in V1 with larger terminal component	• **Tall P wave in Lead II ≥3 mm** • Biphasic P in V1 with larger initial component

STEP 5: EVALUATE THE QRS COMPLEX

☑ **Narrow v. Wide** (normal <0.12 seconds). If QRS is narrow, skip looking for bundle branch blocks.

☑ **Bundle Branch Blocks?**

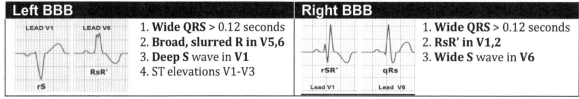

Left BBB	Right BBB
1. **Wide QRS** > 0.12 seconds 2. **Broad, slurred R in V5,6** 3. **Deep S** wave in **V1** 4. ST elevations V1-V3	1. **Wide QRS** > 0.12 seconds 2. **RsR'** in **V1,2** 3. **Wide S** wave in **V6**

☑ **Ventricular Hypertrophy**
RIGHT VENTRICULAR HYPERTROPHY: look at V1: R>S in V1 or R >7 mm in height in V1

LEFT VENTRICULAR HYPERTROPHY:
Sokolow-Lyon criteria: S in V1 + R in V5 (or V6) >35 mm in men; >30 mm in women.
Cornell Criteria: R in aVL + S in V3 >28 mm in men; >20 mm in women.

☑ **Pathological Q waves?** Q wave >1 small box in depth or width.

STEP 6: EVALUATE ST SEGMENT

☑ ST depression or elevation >1 mm in depth/height?

STEP 7: EVALUATE T WAVES

☑ Any T wave inversions (TWI); T wave flattening? Is the QT interval prolonged?

QRS AXIS DETERMINATION

Axis is the general direction of the impulse through the heart.
Normal axis is usually directed to the bottom left (-30° to +90°).

To determine QRS axis:
Step 1: look at lead I and aVF.
- **Normal axis:** positive in lead I & positive in aVF
- **Left axis deviation:** positive in lead I & negative in aVF & lead II.
- **Right axis deviation:** negative in lead I & positive in aVF.

Step 2: (only performed if left axis is determined by step 1). Confirm with lead II.
- If the QRS is predominantly negative in lead II, then it is true left axis.
- If QRS is predominantly positive then it is normal axis (falls in between -30° and 0°).

Useful tip: your left thumb represents lead I and your right thumb represents lead avF.
- Two thumbs up (good thing) = normal axis.
- Left thumb up right thumb down, left axis.
- Right thumb up, left thumb down, right axis.

PERPENDICULAR METHOD

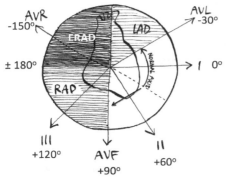

1. Look for the most isoelectric trace.
2. The axis will be perpendicular to that lead orientation (in this case +71 degrees).

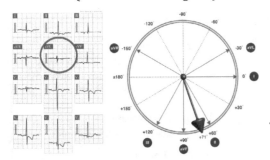

QUADRANT METHOD

Lead I	Lead aVF	QUADRANT	QRS electrical axis
Left hand.	Right hand		

Normal electric axis
0° – 90°

Positive	Positive

Positive	Negative

Possible Left axis deviation
Check lead II

If QRS is + In lead II Normal	If QRS is - In lead II LAD

Negative	Positive

Right axis deviation
-90° – +180°

QUADRANT METHOD: If LAD (based on I and aVF) ⇨ check lead II. If QRS is predominantly negative in lead II ⇨ LAD

AXIS	Lead I	aVF	ETIOLOGIES OF LEFT & RIGHT AXIS DEVIATION
Normal	⊕	⊕	Normal
LAD	⊕	-ve	LBBB, LVH, inferior MI, elevated diaphragm, L anterior hemiblock, WPW
RAD	-ve	⊕	RVH, lateral MI, COPD, Left posterior hemiblock
ERAD	-ve	-ve	

LAD – vectors move towards hypertrophy (LVH) or away from infarction (inferior MI ± cause LAD).
RAD – vectors move towards hypertrophy (RVH) or away from infarction (lateral MI ± cause RAD).

TACHYCARDIA ALGORITHM

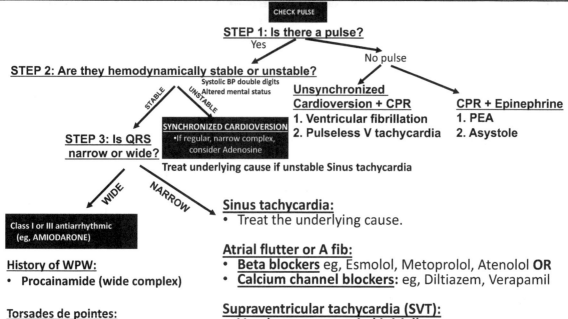

CHECK PULSE

STEP 1: Is there a pulse?

Yes / No pulse

STEP 2: Are they hemodynamically stable or unstable?
Systolic BP double digits
Altered mental status

STABLE / UNSTABLE

SYNCHRONIZED CARDIOVERSION
• If regular, narrow complex, consider Adenosine

Unsynchronized Cardioversion + CPR
1. Ventricular fibrillation
2. Pulseless V tachycardia

CPR + Epinephrine
1. PEA
2. Asystole

STEP 3: Is QRS narrow or wide?

Treat underlying cause if unstable Sinus tachycardia

WIDE / NARROW

Class I or III antiarrhythmic (eg, AMIODARONE)

History of WPW:
• Procainamide (wide complex)

Torsades de pointes:
• Magnesium sulfate

Sinus tachycardia:
• Treat the underlying cause.

Atrial flutter or A fib:
• **Beta blockers** eg, Esmolol, Metoprolol, Atenolol **OR**
• **Calcium channel blockers:** eg, Diltiazem, Verapamil

Supraventricular tachycardia (SVT):
• **Vagal maneuvers tried initially**
• **Adenosine first-line medical treatment**
• Beta blockers of Calcium channel blockers 2nd line.

BRADYCARDIA ALGORITHM

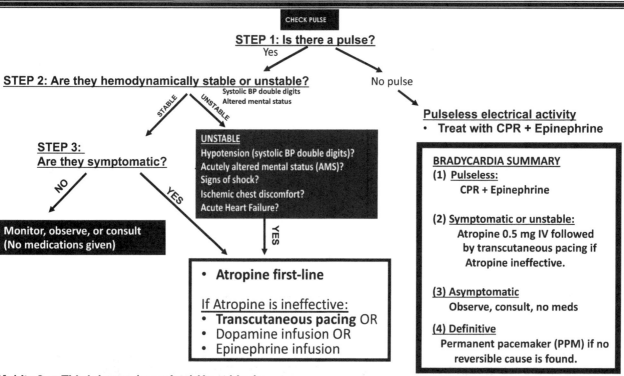

CHECK PULSE

STEP 1: Is there a pulse?

Yes / No pulse

STEP 2: Are they hemodynamically stable or unstable?
Systolic BP double digits
Altered mental status

STABLE / UNSTABLE

Pulseless electrical activity
• **Treat with CPR + Epinephrine**

STEP 3: Are they symptomatic?

NO / YES

Monitor, observe, or consult (No medications given)

UNSTABLE
Hypotension (systolic BP double digits)?
Acutely altered mental status (AMS)?
Signs of shock?
Ischemic chest discomfort?
Acute Heart Failure?

YES

• **Atropine first-line**

If Atropine is ineffective:
• **Transcutaneous pacing** OR
• Dopamine infusion OR
• Epinephrine infusion

BRADYCARDIA SUMMARY
(1) Pulseless:
  CPR + Epinephrine

(2) Symptomatic or unstable:
  Atropine 0.5 mg IV followed by transcutaneous pacing if Atropine ineffective.

(3) Asymptomatic
  Observe, consult, no meds

(4) Definitive
  Permanent pacemaker (PPM) if no reversible cause is found.

Mobitz 2 or Third-degree (complete) Heart block:

• Unstable or symptomatic: **Transcutaneous pacing for stabilization is the most effective treatment for symptomatic or unstable patients, especially if block is below the AV node.** Transvenous pacing is an alternative if normal blood pressure & no Heart failure.

• Atropine may be tried as per the ACLS algorithm if source is thought to be above the AV node; if the source is thought to be below the AV node, Atropine may worsen infranodal blocks.

• If patients remain unstable after pacing, IV Dopamine if low blood pressure may be used; IV Dobutamine if Heart failure.

SINUS ARRHYTHMIA

- **Regularly irregular rhythm** originating from the sinus node with **variations in the rhythm associated with changes of the respiratory cycle.**
- **Normal variation of normal sinus rhythm — meets the same criteria for Normal sinus rhythm except that the rhythm is irregular.**

EPIDEMIOLOGY
- More commonly seen in children, young adults, healthy individuals, & with Sinus bradycardia.

PHYSIOLOGY
Respiratory-phasic:
- **Beat to beat variations with respiration — rhythm increases with inspiration and decreases with expiration, reflecting changes in stroke volume during respiration. Most common.**
- During inspiration, blood shunts to the right side to get oxygenated, leaving less blood volume on the left side during inspiration. Because cardiac output = heart rate x stroke volume (CO = HR x SV), during inspiration, the left side of the heart compensates for the physiologic decrease in stroke volume by increasing heart rate to maintain the same cardiac output.

Non-respiratory Sinus arrhythmia:
- ECG will appear similar to the respiratory type; the difference is that it is not associated with the respiratory cycle. Although it may occur in healthy individuals, it may be indicative of an underlying pathology.

CLINICAL MANIFESTATIONS
- **The majority of patients with Sinus arrhythmia are asymptomatic (considered a normal variant).** It is rare for patients to develop symptoms.
- In patients with significant bradycardia, symptoms such as fatigue, exercise intolerance, lightheadedness, dizziness, syncope or presyncope, altered mental status changes, or anginal symptoms may occur.

DIAGNOSIS
ECG:
- **Regularly irregular rhythm: regularly occurring beat to beat variation of the P-P interval (>0.12 sec), shorter intervals during inspiration (increased rate), and longer P-P intervals during expiration (decreased heart rate).**
- Normal-appearing P waves that are monoform in appearance and consistent with origination from the sinus node — the P wave is upright in leads I and II, P wave is biphasic in V1. The maximum height of a P wave is less than or equal to 2.5 mm in leads II and III.

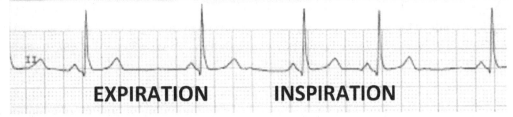

EXPIRATION   **INSPIRATION**

MANAGEMENT:
- **No treatment needed in most cases as it is considered a normal variant in young healthy adults.**
Symptomatic:
- If symptomatic bradycardia occurs, Atropine is the first-line management.
- Transcutaneous pacing, Epinephrine and Dopamine are second-line options.

SINUS TACHYCARDIA

- **Regular cardiac rhythm originating from the sinus node with an increased heart rate >100 bpm in adults** (normal resting heat rate for adults is 60-100 bpm).
- **Can be a normal variant but the presence of tachycardia at rest could be an early indication of a serious underlying condition.**

ETIOLOGIES
- **Physiologic:** <u>Catecholaminergic triggers</u> — eg, exercise, stress, pain, and anxiety; Young children/infants; Postural orthostatic tachycardia syndrome is also often seen in young females and after stress (eg, sepsis, pregnancy, surgery, or trauma).

- **Pathologic:** <u>Infectious:</u> fever, infection, sepsis; <u>Hypovolemia:</u> dehydration, shock, hemorrhage; <u>Cardiac etiologies:</u> Myocarditis, Cardiac tamponade, Acute coronary syndrome; <u>Respiratory:</u> Hypoxia, Pneumonia, Pulmonary emboli, Pneumothorax; <u>Metabolic:</u> hypoglycemia, hyperthyroidism, electrolyte disorders (eg, calcium, potassium, magnesium disorders), anemia, pregnancy. Clonidine, alcohol, benzodiazepine, or opioid withdrawal; <u>Sympathomimetics</u> eg, decongestants, cocaine use.

CLINICAL MANIFESTATIONS
- **Most patients with Sinus tachycardia are commonly asymptomatic from the rhythm itself.**
- Depending on the underlying etiology, Sinus tachycardia may present with dyspnea, chest pain, lightheadedness, dizziness, syncope, and presyncope.

PHYSICAL EXAMINATION
- Evaluation of the patient's hemodynamic status is crucial to stabilization of the patient, particularly to ensure that the patient is not on the verge of cardiovascular collapse due to shock.

DIAGNOSIS:
ECG:
- **Regular, rapid rhythm (>100 bpm).** Normal-appearing P wave; every P followed by a QRS complex.

Workup:
- Depending on the suspected etiology, workup may include electrocardiogram, echocardiogram, 24-hour Holter recording (can confirm the presence of inappropriate sinus tachycardia), arterial blood gas, lactic acid level, chest radiograph, D-dimer, chest CT angiography, ventilation-perfusion scan, cardiac enzymes levels, glucose level, electrolytes, complete blood count, and/or a toxicology screen.

MANAGEMENT
- **Identifying and treating the underlying cause of Sinus tachycardia is the cornerstone of management, even in hemodynamically unstable patients.**
- Benign causes (eg, physical activity or stress) often do not require any specific cardiac treatment.
- If Sinus tachycardia is due to a medical condition or the patient is at risk for worsening of clinical status (eg, sepsis, shock, hypoxia, metabolic acidosis, Acute coronary syndrome), admission and urgent evaluation is recommended with treatment of the underlying cause.
- Beta blockers (eg, Metoprolol) used in the management of persistent Sinus tachycardia in the setting of Acute coronary artery syndrome.

SINUS BRADYCARDIA

- **Regular cardiac rhythm originating from the sinus node with a decreased heart rate <60 beats per minute (bpm) in adults.** Normal resting heat rate for adults 60-100 bpm.

PATHOPHYSIOLOGY:
- **Sinus Bradycardia is caused by different intrinsic and extrinsic factors which may increase vagal tone or compromise the integrity of the sinus node.**

ETIOLOGIES:
- **Physiologic: Healthy young adults and athletes often have an increased vagal tone which keeps them in Sinus bradycardia at rest,** patients >65 years often have Sinus bradycardia secondary to aging of the sino-atrial node; Vasovagal reaction, vasovagal stimulation (eg, endotracheal suctioning), carotid sinus sensitivity; Increased intracranial pressure; Sleep; nausea and/or vomiting, Carotid massage.
- Pathologic: Medications: Beta blockers, Calcium channel blockers, Digoxin, Adenosine, Narcotics. Ischemic heart disease: sinoatrial node ischemia, inferior or posterior wall Myocardial infarction. Infection: Gram-negative sepsis, Lyme disease. Sick sinus syndrome, Hypothyroidism, hypoxia.

CLINICAL MANIFESTATIONS
- **The majority of patients with Sinus bradycardia are asymptomatic.**
- Symptoms: fatigue, exercise intolerance, lightheadedness, dizziness, syncope or presyncope, altered mental status changes, anginal symptoms.

DIAGNOSIS:
ECG: Regular, slow rhythm (<60 bpm). Normal-appearing P wave; every P followed by a QRS complex.

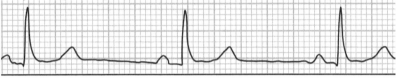

Workup:
- **History and physical examination are the most significant components of evaluation of a patient presenting with signs and symptoms of Sinus bradycardia** — vital signs (respiratory rate, blood pressure, temperature, and heart rate) and an electrocardiogram. **Hemodynamically unstable patients may develop hypotension, altered mental status, dyspnea, or angina.**
- Laboratory workup: may include basic metabolic panel (including calcium and magnesium), glucose levels, thyroid function testing, cardiac enzymes (eg, Troponin &/or CK-MB), and toxicology drug screen.

MANAGEMENT:
[1] Symptomatic or hemodynamically unstable:
- **Atropine first-line treatment.** Atropine is an anticholinergic drug that decreases vagal tone (increased vagal tone due to a variety of reasons is the most common cause of Sinus bradycardia). Intravenous (IV) Atropine 0.5 mg push every 3-5 minutes up to 3 mg total. Treat any underlying causes.
- **Second-line Temporary cardiac pacing &/or IV Dopamine or Epinephrine infusion if the patient's symptoms and heart rate fail to improve with Atropine.** Epinephrine directly stimulates the adrenergic beta-1 receptor, leading to increased heart rate and contractility.
- Permanent pacemaker: definitive management.
- Hypothermic patients are warmed to normothermia before making definitive determinations on treatment.
[2] Asymptomatic:
- **No medical treatment or specific cardiac medications are needed if asymptomatic** — observation, cardiac consult, further workup, or cardiology follow up may be needed if pathologic.
- In older individuals, Sinus bradycardia may be due to sinus node abnormalities or underlying ischemic heart disease so further workup is often warranted.

SINUS NODE DYSFUNCTION [SND (SICK SINUS SYNDROME)]

- **The inability of the SA node to generate a heart rate that meets the physiologic needs.**

ETIOLOGIES:

- <u>Intrinsic causes</u> **include Degenerative fibrosis — The most common cause of sinus node dysfunction is the replacement of sinus node tissue by fibrous tissue (age-related)**, which is often associated with degeneration and fibrosis of other components of the conduction system.
- <u>Extrinsic</u>: <u>Medications</u> — Non-dihydropyridine Calcium channel blockers, Beta blockers, Digoxin, Antiarrhythmics, Acetylcholinesterase inhibitors (eg, Rivastigmine). Parasympathomimetics, sympatholytics (eg, Clonidine, Methyldopa), Ivabradine. <u>Metabolic</u> — hypothyroidism, hyperkalemia, hypokalemia, hypocalcemia, hypoxia, and hypothermia can lead to depression of pacing or autonomic instability. Inflammatory disease, trauma. <u>Abnormally increased vagal tone</u> — carotid sinus hypersensitivity, autonomic dysfunction. Infiltrative disease (Amyloidosis, sarcoidosis, scleroderma).

CLINICAL MANIFESTATIONS

- <u>Hypoperfusion:</u> When symptoms do develop, they are usually attributed to hypoperfusion to vital organs with high oxygen demand. Cerebral hypoperfusion (syncope or near-fainting).
- <u>Nonspecific symptoms</u>: **fatigue, exercise intolerance, lightheadedness, palpitations, presyncope, syncope, dyspnea on exertion, or chest discomfort.**

WORKUP

- Prior to any testing beyond an ECG, the first step in evaluating Sinus node dysfunction is to exclude reversible causes — eg, electrolyte or metabolic abnormalities, uncontrolled sleep apnea, medications (eg, Beta-blockers, Calcium channel blockers, Digoxin), MI, systemic illness (eg, hypothyroidism).
- **Because of the transient episodic nature of SND, diagnosis on 12 lead ECG is uncommon and prolonged monitoring (eg, 24-48 hour Holter) to detect and document bradycardic episodes is often indicated.**

Electrocardiogram:

- **Alternating bradycardia (eg, sinus pauses, sinus arrest) and atrial tachyarrhythmias in >50% of cases.** Atrial fibrillation is most common, Atrial flutter, Paroxysmal supraventricular tachycardia.

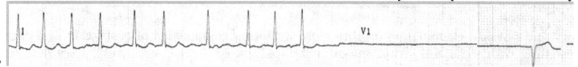

MANAGEMENT

- The initial step is identifying and correcting reversible factors, removing extrinsic factors, symptom control, when possible, and permanent pacemaker placement (definitive management) for patients without an identifiable reversible etiology.

Hemodynamically unstable patients:

- **Management options include IV Atropine (first-line), IV Dopamine or Epinephrine infusion, as well as temporary cardiac pacing (either with transcutaneous or, if immediately available, transvenous pacing)** to increase heart rate and cardiac output.
- Signs and symptoms of hemodynamic instability include hypotension, altered mental status, signs of shock, ongoing ischemic chest pain, and evidence of acute pulmonary edema.

Hemodynamically stable patients:

- **Monitoring, evaluation, and treatment of reversible causes of SA nodal depression,** such as drugs (eg, Beta blockers, Calcium channel blockers, Digoxin), ischemia, and autonomic imbalance.

Asymptomatic patients:

- **Persons with bradycardia and no symptoms due to the bradycardia are treated with intermittent examinations.**

Patients with persistent symptoms:

- Pacemaker placement is indicated if documented correlation between symptoms and sinus bradycardia or sinus pauses to relieve symptoms.

ATRIOVENTRICULAR CONDUCTION BLOCKS

AV BLOCK: interruption of the normal impulse from the SA node to the AV node (AV node dysfunction).
- **PR interval most helpful in determining the presence of an AV conduction block.**
- **Blocks occur either [1] in the AV node (first-degree & second-degree Mobitz type I) or [2] below the AV node (second-degree Mobitz type II & third degree).**

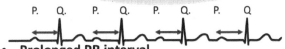

- **Prolonged PR interval**
- **Every P followed by QRS** (all atrial impulses conducted to ventricles)

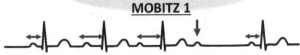

- **Progressive PRI interval lengthening** until
- **occasionally non-conducted atrial beats** (one or more P waves without corresponding QRS complexes)

Mobitz II
- **Constant PRI interval length**
- **occasionally non-conducted atrial beats**

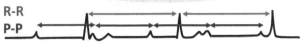

- **AV dissociation –** Normal P-P and R-R intervals that (the atrial beats are not related to the ventricular beats)

SECOND DEGREE AV BLOCK

- 2nd = not all of the atrial impulses are conducted to the ventricles.
  This leads to some P waves that are not followed by QRS complexes ('dropped QRS').

MOBITZ I – WENCKEBACH

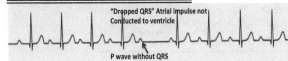

- <u>PROGRESSIVE</u> <u>PRI LENGTHENING</u> ⇨ **dropped QRS.**
  Shortened R-R interval

MANAGEMENT
<u>Asymptomatic</u> ⇨ observation. ± Cardiac consult.
<u>Symptomatic</u> ⇨**Atropine**. Epinephrine, ± pacemaker.

MOBITZ II

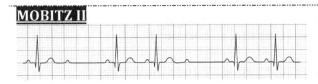

MOBITZ II: block commonly in the bundle of HIS.
- <u>CONSTANT/PROLONGED PRI</u> ⇨ **dropped QRS.**

MANAGEMENT: Temporary pacing (Atropine can be used but may worsen infranodal blocks).
Progression to 3rd degree AV block common so Permanent pacemaker is the definitive treatment if a reversible cause cannot be found.

FIRST-DEGREE ATRIOVENTRICULAR BLOCK (AVB)

- **Prolonged AV conduction** characterized by a longer than normal delay in conduction from the atria to the ventricles (prolonged PR interval >0.20 seconds at resting heart rates) without interruption in atrial to ventricular conduction (**delayed but 1:1 conducted impulses**).

PATHOPHYSIOLOGY
- The AV node normally delays the conduction from the atria to the ventricles briefly to allow for full ventricular filling before contraction, represented by a normal PR interval of 0.12-0.20 seconds.
- In First degree AVB, the **conduction delay is most frequent in the AV node** but may also be in the His-Purkinje system. Morphology and size of the QRS complex will reflect the site of conduction delay.
- **It is not a true "block" because all of the atrial impulses are conducted to the ventricles; it is more appropriately characterized as a prolonged delay in AV conduction.**

ETIOLOGIES
The two most common etiologies of First-degree AVB are result of [1] increased vagal tone (eg, endurance athletes or patients with lower resting heart rates) **or [2] AV node-blocking medications.**
- **[1] Increased vagal tone without structural heart disease (eg, well-conditioned endurance athletes) & patients with a slow resting heart rate** may develop a First-degree AVB as a result of increased vagal tone & baseline lower resting heart rate. **Often a normal variant.**
- **[2] AV nodal blocking drugs eg, Digoxin, Beta blockers, Non-dihydropyridine Calcium channel blockers, antiarrhythmic agents.** Fibrosis in the conduction system in older patients, intrinsic AV node disease, vagal tone increase, Acute MI, electrolyte disturbances (eg, hyperkalemia).
- Infiltrative diseases: eg, Amyloidosis, Sarcoidosis, Systemic sclerosis. Myocarditis (eg, Lyme disease).

CLINICAL MANIFESTATIONS
- **Asymptomatic in most cases and is most commonly benign in nature.** It is uncommon for patients to develop symptoms directly related to First degree AV block.
- It is rarely symptomatic, but if symptomatic, bradycardia-related decreased perfusion produces symptoms — fatigue, dizziness, dyspnea, chest pain, and syncope.

DIAGNOSIS
- ECG: all atrial impulses are delayed but conducted to the ventricles — **prolonged PR interval (>0.20 seconds)** at resting heart rates + **all P waves are followed by QRS complexes (1:1 conduction).**

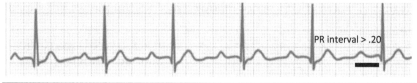

PR interval > .20

MANAGEMENT
Asymptomatic:
- **Asymptomatic patients with first degree AV block do not require any specific therapy** beyond potential observation, surveillance, or cardiac consult if there is concern for underlying pathology.
- Any reversible causes of AV block (eg, prior use of AV nodal blocking agents, ischemia) should be determined and managed (ischemia) or withdrawn (causative medications).
Symptomatic:
- **Atropine** first-line. Atropine's vagolytic properties can improve AV node conduction.
Definitive:
Permanent pacemaker:
- Most cases of First-degree AV block do not require pacemaker placement but may be needed if severe.

MOBITZ I SECOND-DEGREE ATRIOVENTRICULAR (AV) BLOCK (Wenckebach)

- **Interruption of electrical impulse at the AV node**, resulting in occasional non-conducted impulses.
- PATHOPHYSIOLOGY: AV node dysfunction (commonly above the bundle of HIS).

ETIOLOGIES
- **Often a normal variant** in individuals with high vagal tone without structural heart disease.
- **Inferior wall MI** (AV node ischemia), **AV nodal blocking agents** (eg, Beta blockers, Digoxin, Calcium channel blockers), myocarditis due to Lyme, Hyperkalemia, cardiac surgery.

CLINICAL MANIFESTATIONS
- Asymptomatic in most cases.
- Bradycardia-related decreased perfusion — eg, fatigue, dizziness, dyspnea, chest pain, syncope, or in severe cases, hypotension &/or altered mental status.

DIAGNOSIS
- ECG: **progressive lengthening of the PR interval** until occasional non-conducted atrial impulses (dropped QRS complexes).

MANAGEMENT
- **Asymptomatic: observation & no initial treatment**. Cardiac consultation in some cases.
- **Symptomatic or Hemodynamically unstable: IV Atropine first-line**; Epinephrine.
- Permanent pacemaker definitive management in persistent cases (rarely needed).

MOBITZ II SECOND-DEGREE ATRIOVENTRICULAR (AV) BLOCK

- Interruption of electrical impulse resulting in occasional non-conducted impulses.
- Pathophysiology: **often occurs below the AV node (infranodal)** at His-Purkinje system.

ETIOLOGIES
- **Most occur in the presence of structural heart disease: eg, myocardial ischemia, myocardial fibrosis**, myocarditis (eg, Lyme disease), endocarditis, infiltrative disease (eg, Amyloid, Sarcoidosis).
- Hyperkalemia, Increased vagal tone, iatrogenic (eg, AV nodal blockers, post-cardiac surgery/ablation).

CLINICAL MANIFESTATIONS
- Asymptomatic in most cases, especially if there are infrequent non-conducted P waves.
- Symptomatic: due to bradycardia-related decreased perfusion — fatigue, dizziness, dyspnea, chest pain, syncope, or in severe cases, hypotension or altered mental status.

DIAGNOSIS
- ECG: **constant PR interval before & after the non-conducted atrial beats** (dropped QRS complexes).
- If ischemia is suspected based on clinical picture, cardiac biomarkers, chest radiograph, and electrolytes should be ordered.

MANAGEMENT
[1] Asymptomatic:
- **Mobitz type II second-degree AV block is by nature unstable and frequently progresses to Third degree (complete) AV block**, so patients should be continuously monitored with Transcutaneous pacing pads in place in the event of clinical deterioration.

[2] Symptomatic or Hemodynamically unstable:
- **Beta-adrenergic agent (eg, Isoproterenol, Dopamine, Dobutamine, Epinephrine) and/or temporary cardiac pacing** (either with transcutaneous or, if immediately available, transvenous pacing). Atropine may be used but may worsen infranodal block.
- **Definitive: symptomatic block below the AV node without reversible cause usually warrants permanent pacemaker placement** (Mobitz II often progresses to Third-degree AVB).

THIRD-DEGREE (COMPLETE) ATRIOVENTRICULAR (AV) BLOCK

- **AV dissociation:** complete absence of AV conduction where no atrial impulses conduct to the ventricles, so the atrial activity and ventricular activity are independent of each other.

ETIOLOGIES
- **Secondary or Primary (idiopathic) progressive cardiac conduction disease with myocardial fibrosis and/or sclerosis that affects the conduction system** — eg, **myocardial ischemia** involving the conduction system (acute or chronic), myocardial fibrosis, myocarditis (eg, **Lyme disease**), Restrictive cardiomyopathy leading to infiltrative disease involving the conduction system (eg, **Amyloidosis, Sarcoidosis**), or Infective endocarditis associated with abscess formation. Increased vagal tone, hypothyroidism, hyperkalemia, and myocarditis.
- **Inferior wall MI:** the right coronary artery supplies the AV node in ~90% of the population. Anterior myocardial infarctions may involve infranodal tissues.
- **Hyperkalemia**, Hypothyroidism, increased vagal tone.
- **Autoimmunity:** eg, Systemic lupus erythematosus, Rheumatic fever, Systemic sclerosis.
- **Iatrogenic — AV nodal blockers (eg Beta blockers, Non-dihydropyridine Calcium channel blockers, Digoxin),** Amiodarone, post-catheter ablation, post-cardiac surgery, post-transcatheter aortic valve implantation, surgery near the septum (eg, mitral valve repair).

CLINICAL MANIFESTATIONS
- **Patients are infrequently asymptomatic; most patients present with some degree of symptoms.**
- **If symptomatic, it is due to bradycardia-related decreased perfusion**, especially during exertion — fatigue, dyspnea, dizziness, chest pain, near syncope, syncope.
- Signs of hemodynamic instability include hypotension, altered mental status, signs of shock, ongoing ischemic chest pain, and evidence of acute pulmonary edema.

DIAGNOSIS
- ECG: **AV dissociation:** evidence of atrial (P waves) and ventricular (QRS complexes) activity which are independent of each other and an atrial rate faster than the ventricular rate. **Regular P-P intervals & regular R-R intervals independent of each other.** Patients are often bradycardic.

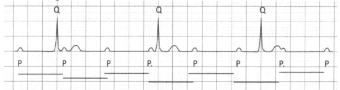

MANAGEMENT
Asymptomatic:
- **Continuous monitoring, transcutaneous pacer pads are placed in case of clinical deterioration,** and assessment for reversible causes should be sought and corrected, with observation for improvement after correction. Urgent use of Atropine not needed if asymptomatic.

Symptomatic & stable:
- **Atropine** first-line if clinically symptomatic bradycardia occurs as per ACLS. **However, Atropine is rarely effective in raising the heart rate in complete heart block, so pacing is often needed.** Atropine is 0.5 mg IV may be repeated every 3-5 minutes to a total dose of 3 mg.

Hemodynamically unstable:
- **Urgently treated with Atropine, and in most cases, temporary cardiac pacing to increase heart rate and cardiac output,** either with transcutaneous or, if immediately available, transvenous pacing.
- **Treatment with Atropine should not delay intervention with temporary pacing (transcutaneous or transvenous) for stabilization &/or a chronotropic medication [eg, Dopamine (if hypotensive) or Epinephrine].**

Definitive management:
- **Permanent pacemaker** indicated in most patients when there is no reversible etiology present.

ATRIAL FLUTTER

- **Characterized by rapid, regular atrial depolarizations at a characteristic rate ~300 beats/min (240–400) due to 1 single irritable atrial focus firing at a fast rate** with some degree of AV node conduction block [often with a regular ventricular rate of ~150 beats/min (2:1 conduction)].
- **Similar to Atrial fibrillation, Atrial flutter is associated with an increased risk of atrial thrombus formation that can lead to cerebral &/or systemic embolization (eg, Stroke).**

EPIDEMIOLOGY
- Atrial flutter & Atrial fibrillation are more common in men than in women; increased risk with age.

PATHOPHYSIOLOGY
- Typical (classic) Atrial flutter involves a single reentrant circuit in the right atrium around the tricuspid valve annulus. The electrical wavefront often propagates in a counterclockwise direction.

ETIOLOGIES:
- **~60% of patients with Atrial flutter have Coronary artery disease or hypertensive heart disease**; 30% have no underlying cardiac disease.
- Rheumatic heart disease, Congenital heart disease, Pericarditis, Cardiomyopathy, open heart surgery.
- Alcohol consumption, Pulmonary embolism, hypoxia, Hyperthyroidism, Pheochromocytoma, electrolyte imbalance, obesity, Digitalis toxicity.

CLINICAL MANIFESTATIONS
- **Symptomatic: palpitations, dizziness, fatigue, poor exercise tolerance, mild dyspnea, and presyncope** due to decreased cardiac output as a result of rapid ventricular rate.
- **Unstable:** symptoms are due to hypoperfusion and can include **hypotension** (eg, systolic BP in double digits), **altered mental status, or refractory chest pain.**

DIAGNOSIS
- **ECG: Identical flutter ("sawtooth") atrial waves usually ~250-300 beats per minute with no discernable P waves**, often with regular ventricular rate of ~125-150 beats/min (2:1 conduction).

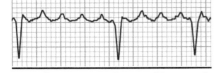

- **Transthoracic echocardiography: preferred initial imaging modality for evaluating Atrial flutter.** Echocardiogram can evaluate right and left atrial size, the size and function of the right and left ventricles, and assess for valvular heart disease, LVH, and pericardial disease.

MANAGEMENT
- **Stable:** rate control with non-dihydropyridine **Calcium channel blockers (eg, Diltiazem, Verapamil) or Beta blockers (eg, Esmolol, Metoprolol, Atenolol).** Digoxin is another option for rate control but is usually reserved for patients in whom Beta blockers or CCBs are contraindicated [eg, severe heart failure (New York Heart Association class III or IV), hypotension)] due to its adverse effects and toxicity.
- **Unstable: Direct current (synchronized) cardioversion.**
- Anticoagulation: similar criteria (eg, CHA_2DS_2-VASc) for nonvalvular Atrial fibrillation in patients at risk for embolization to decrease thromboembolic complications.

- Reversion to normal sinus rhythm:
  - **Radiofrequency catheter ablation (definitive management) & superior to antiarrhythmics.**
  - Direct current cardioversion (electrical cardioversion) 50-100 Joules.
  - Pharmacological reversion: Class IA, IC, or III antiarrhythmics (eg, Ibutilide drug of choice).

ATRIAL FIBRILLATION (AF)

- **Multiple irritable atrial foci fire at fast rates.**
- Atrial fibrillation is the most common chronic arrhythmia.
- **Atrial fibrillation is associated with an increased risk of atrial thrombus formation that can lead to cerebral &/or systemic embolization (eg, acute ischemic stroke).**

TYPES
- <u>Paroxysmal:</u> self-terminating within 7 days (usually <24 hours). ±Recurrent.
- <u>Persistent:</u> fails to self-terminate within 7 days. Requires termination (medical or electrical).
- <u>Permanent:</u> persistent AF >12 months refractory to cardioversion or cardioversion never tried.
- <u>Lone:</u> paroxysmal, persistent or permanent *without evidence of heart disease.*

RISK FACTORS
- <u>Cardiac disease:</u> eg, hypertension, valvular heart disease, Heart failure ischemia. Advanced age, <u>Pulmonary disease</u> eg, Obstructive sleep apnea, PE. <u>Metabolic:</u> obesity (BMI >30 kg/m^2), Chronic kidney disease, electrolyte imbalance (eg, Hypomagnesemia, Hypokalemia), <u>Endocrine:</u> Diabetes mellitus, Hyperthyroidism, Pheochromocytoma. Alcohol consumption. Omega-3 fatty acid use.

CLINICAL MANIFESTATIONS
- Up to 90% of Atrial fibrillation episodes are asymptomatic.
- **<u>Symptomatic:</u> palpitations, dizziness, fatigue, generalized weakness, poor exercise tolerance, mild dyspnea, and presyncope** due to decreased cardiac output as a result of rapid ventricular rate.
- **<u>Hemodynamically unstable:</u>** symptoms are due to hypoperfusion and can include **significant hypotension** (eg, systolic BP in double digits), **altered mental status, refractory chest pain** (uncontrolled angina or ischemia), and Acute decompensated (congestive) heart failure.

DIAGNOSIS
- <u>ECG:</u> **Irregularly irregular rhythm with fibrillatory waves & no discrete (discernable) P waves.**

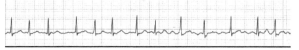

  - Often atrial rate >250 beats per minute.
  - The AV nodal refractory period determines the ventricular rate.
- <u>Cardiac monitoring:</u> a Holter monitor or telemetry can be used if Atrial fibrillation is not seen on an ECG but is suspected.

MANAGEMENT
Hemodynamically stable:
- **<u>Rate control:</u> Non-dihydropyridine Calcium channel blockers [CCBs (eg, Diltiazem, Verapamil)] OR Beta blockers (eg, Esmolol, Metoprolol, or Atenolol)** to slow AV node conduction. **Beta blockers preferred in the setting of Heart failure and post MI; CCBs (or Esmolol) preferred in setting of severe reactive airway disease (Asthma) or cocaine-induced Myocardial infarction.**
- Digoxin is another option for rate control but is usually reserved for patients in whom Beta blockers or CCBs are contraindicated [eg, severe heart failure (NYHA class III or IV), hypotension].

Hemodynamically unstable:
- **Direct current (synchronized) cardioversion.**

<u>Long-term:</u>
- Rate control usually preferred over rhythm control for long-term management.
- Direct current (synchronized cardioversion) or pharmacologic cardioversion.
- Radiofrequency catheter ablation or surgical "MAZE" procedure.
- CHA2DS2-VASc criteria for nonvalvular Atrial fibrillation to determine the patient's yearly thromboembolic risk, in order to select the appropriate anticoagulation regimen. **In patients with AF and elevated CHA$_2$DS$_2$-VASc score of ≥2, oral anticoagulation is recommended.**

CARDIOVERSION
- Direct current (synchronized cardioversion) or pharmacologic cardioversion (eg, Flecainide, Dofetilide, Propafenone, Amiodarone, Ibutilide). Cardioversion is most successful when performed within 7 days after the onset of Atrial fibrillation.
- **Transesophageal echocardiogram** **done prior to cardioversion** to ensure there are no atrial clots.
- AF >48 hours: **initiate anticoagulation therapy for at least 3 weeks before & at least 4 weeks after cardioversion**. If cardioversion is required sooner, anticoagulate with IV Heparin & perform TEE as close to the time of cardioversion as possible. If thrombus is observed or suspected based on TEE, delay cardioversion. Rate control & therapeutic anticoagulation required for 4 week minimum.
- AF <48 hours cardioversion may be attempted as soon as possible often with anticoagulation.
- **Anticoagulation must be continued for 4 weeks after cardioversion.** With effective anticoagulation, the stroke risk is decreased 3-fold after 4 weeks of anticoagulation.

CANDIDATES FOR ANTICOAGULATION WITH NONVALVULAR ATRIAL FIBRILLATION OR FLUTTER
- CHA_2DS_2-VASc score for nonvalvular Atrial fibrillation and A flutter assesses patients' risk for embolization. **Chronic oral anticoagulation (eg, Direct oral anticoagulants or Warfarin) is recommended for moderate to high risk (score of ≥2).**
- The use of anticoagulant therapy has been shown to reduce embolic risk by 70%.

ANTICOAGULATION RISK STRATIFICATION IN NONVALVULAR ATRIAL FIBRILLATION		
CHA_2DS_2- VASc CRITERIA	**POINTS**	**RECOMMENDED THERAPY**
Congestive Heart Failure	1	**≥ 2 = Moderate to high risk:** **chronic oral anticoagulation recommended.**
Hypertension	1	
A₂ge ≥ 75y	2	
Diabetes Mellitus	1	**1 = low risk:**
S₂: Stroke, TIA, thrombus	2	Based on clinical judgment, consideration of risk to benefit assessment & discussion with patient.
Vascular disease (prior MI, aortic plaque, peripheral arterial disease)	1	Anticoagulation may be recommended in some cases.
Age 65 – 74y	1	**0 = very low risk:**
Sex (female)	1	No anticoagulation needed.
MAXIMUM SCORE	**9**	May be recommended in some (based on clinical judgment & consideration of risk to benefit ratio).

ANTICOAGULANT AGENTS:
1. **Direct oral anticoagulants (DOACs): are recommended over Warfarin in most cases** due to similar or lower rates of major bleeding as well as lower risk of ischemic stroke, convenience of not having to monitor via the INR, & less drug interactions.
   - **Direct thrombin inhibitors: (eg, Dabigatran)** bind & inhibit thrombin.
   - **Factor Xa inhibitors: Rivaroxaban, Apixaban, Edoxaban.**

2. **Warfarin:**
   Indications: may be preferred in some of the following patients — some with severe chronic kidney disease, contraindications to the DOAC (eg, HIV patients on protease inhibitor-based therapy, on CP450-inducing antiepileptic medications such as Carbamazepine, Phenytoin etc.), patients already on Warfarin who prefer not to change, cost issues (Warfarin is less expensive). Warfarin usually bridged with Heparin until Warfarin is therapeutic.
   Monitoring: International Normalized Ratio **(INR) goal of 2-3.** Prothrombin Time (PT).

3. Dual antiplatelet therapy: (eg, Aspirin + Clopidogrel). Anticoagulant monotherapy is superior to dual antiplatelet therapy. Dual antiplatelet therapy may be reserved for patients who cannot be treated with anticoagulation (for reasons OTHER than bleeding risk).

PAROXYSMAL SUPRAVENTRICULAR TACHYCARDIA (PSVT)

- **SVT is an umbrella term when a more specific term can't be applied to a tachyarrhythmia originating above the ventricles** (atrial or AV nodal source); usually regular ventricular response.

PATHOPHYSIOLOGY:
- **Reentry is the most common cause of narrow QRS complex tachycardia** — AV nodal reentry (most common type) and AV reciprocating tachycardia. In reentry, there exists 2 distinct electrical conduction tissues or pathways with different electrophysiologic attributes that are connected both proximally and distally, creating a functional or anatomical circuit.
- **AV node re-entrant tachycardia: (AVNRT) two pathways both located within the AV node or perinodal tissue (1 normal & 1 accessory pathway). Most common type.**
- AV reciprocating tachycardia: (AVRT) two pathways with one being an extranodal accessory pathway (1 normal and 1 accessory pathway outside of the AV node).
- **A narrow QRS complex (<120 milliseconds) indicates rapid activation of the ventricles via the normal His-Purkinje system** (origination above or within the His bundle). Orthodromic.
- **A widened QRS** (≥120 milliseconds) occurs when ventricular activation is abnormally slow due to **[1] origination below the His bundle** in the bundle branches, Purkinje fibers, or ventricular myocardium (eg, ventricular tachycardia); **[2] aberrant conduction of the supraventricular tachycardia, or [3] conduction occurs over an accessory pathway** (eg, antidromic conduction).

CLINICAL MANIFESTATIONS
- Symptomatic: palpitations (most common), anxiety, exercise intolerance, dizziness, lightheadedness, diaphoresis, fatigue, dyspnea, presyncope, syncope (rare), chest pain or discomfort.
- Unstable: symptoms are due to hypoperfusion and can include hypotension (eg, systolic BP in double digits), altered mental status, refractory chest pain, signs of Heart failure (eg, pulmonary edema).

ECG
- **Orthodromic (95%): regular, narrow-complex tachycardia (>100 bpm + QRS <120 milliseconds) + no discernable P waves** due to the rapid rate.
- **Antidromic (5%): regular, wide-complex tachycardia (>100 bpm + QRS ≥120 milliseconds)** that mimics Ventricular tachycardia.

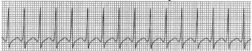

- Heart rate >100 bpm.
- **Rhythm usually regular with narrow QRS complexes.**
- P waves hard to discern due to the rapid rate.

MANAGEMENT
[1] Hemodynamically stable + regular, narrow QRS complexes:
If no severe symptoms or hemodynamic collapse or asymptomatic patients, the sequential approach is Vagal maneuvers, followed by IV Adenosine if Vagal maneuvers are ineffective.
- **Vagal maneuvers: bearing down, breath holding, carotid massage; cold to the forehead in infants.** Carotid sinus pressure can be performed but *should be avoided if the patient has a carotid bruit.*
- **IV Adenosine: first-line medical management if Vagal maneuvers are ineffective.**
- Second-line: AV nodal-blocking agents — IV Non-dihydropyridine Calcium channel blockers (eg, Diltiazem, Verapamil) or IV Beta blockers (eg, Esmolol, Metoprolol, Atenolol); Digoxin.
[2] Hemodynamically stable + wide QRS complexes:
- **Antiarrhythmics: Class I or Class III — eg, IV Amiodarone or IV Procainamide.**
- **IV Procainamide if WPW or antidromic rhythm is suspected.**
[3] Hemodynamically unstable:
- **Direct current (synchronized) cardioversion should be performed urgently in most.**
[4] Definitive:
- **Radiofrequency catheter ablation** is an option if an accessory pathway is identifiable in patients with recurrent or refractory SVT.

WOLFF-PARKINSON-WHITE (WPW) SYNDROME

- **A ventricular preexcitation syndrome resulting in an abnormal aberrant conduction through an accessory pathway (bundle of Kent) that bypasses the atrioventricular (AV) node.**
- WPW is a type of AV reciprocating tachycardia (AVRT).

PATHOPHYSIOLOGY
- **Antegrade conduction through the fast accessory pathway outside of the AV node (bundle of Kent) bypasses the slower-conducting AV node, "preexciting" the ventricles** (depolarization & activation of the ventricles earlier than normal via direct connection between the atria & ventricles), leading to aberrant conduction and the characteristic delta wave (slurred and widened QRS).

CLINICAL MANIFESTATIONS
- Most patients with WPW pattern are asymptomatic but are prone to developing tachyarrhythmias.
- <u>Symptomatic</u>: palpitations (most common), anxiety, exercise intolerance, dizziness, lightheadedness, diaphoresis, fatigue, dyspnea, presyncope, syncope (rare), chest pain or discomfort.

DIAGNOSIS: ECG: 3 components "WPW"
- <u>W</u>ave — **delta wave** (initial slurred upstroke of the QRS)
- <u>P</u>R interval that is short — <0.12 seconds
- <u>W</u>ide QRS complexes — >0.12 seconds

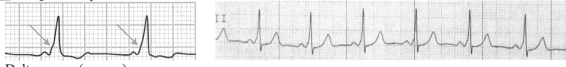

Delta waves (arrows)

MANAGEMENT
[1] Hemodynamically stable + wide QRS complexes:
- **Procainamide preferred in hemodynamically stable WPW with wide complex tachycardia** (including known or suspected antidromic AVRT) **or Atrial fibrillation due to WPW syndrome.** Synchronized cardioversion if Procainamide is ineffective or not available.
- **Atrial fibrillation due to WPW: IV Procainamide preferred.** IV Ibutilide is an alternative.
- **Avoid AV nodal blocking agents ABCD (Adenosine, Beta blockers, Calcium channel blockers, Digoxin) in wide complex WPW and Atrial fibrillation due to WPW** because AV nodal blockade can lead to preferential conduction down the aberrant tract, worsening the tachycardia.

[2] Hemodynamically stable + narrow QRS complexes:
- **Treated similar to SVT: Initial treatment of acute symptomatic orthodromic AVRT with one or more vagal maneuvers**: eg, Valsalva maneuvers or carotid sinus pressure (if no carotid bruits).
- **If vagal maneuvers are ineffective, AV nodal blocking agents — Adenosine, usually preferred.**
- IV Non-dihydropyridine Calcium channel blockers (eg, Diltiazem, Verapamil) often used second-line to Adenosine. IV Beta blockers (eg, Metoprolol, Esmolol, Atenolol). Procainamide.

[3] Hemodynamically unstable:
- **Direct current (synchronized) cardioversion should be performed urgently in hemodynamically unstable patients with tachyarrhythmias when the rhythm is not sinus tachycardia** (preferred management in most).
- Signs of instability include hypotension, hypoxia, altered mental status, signs of shock or poor end-organ perfusion, ongoing ischemic chest pain, and evidence of acute pulmonary edema.

CHRONIC PREVENTION:
- **Radiofrequency catheter ablation of the accessory pathway is the long-term definitive management of SVT due to its high success rate and low complication rates.** Indicated for the long-term management of symptomatic tachyarrhythmias associated with WPW, occupations in which the development of symptoms would put themselves or others at risk (eg, truck drivers, bus and train operators, airline pilots), and some selected asymptomatic patients.

WANDERING ATRIAL PACEMAKER (WAP) & MULTIFOCAL ATRIAL TACHYCARDIA (MAT)

WANDERING ATRIAL PACEMAKER (WAP):

- Multiple ectopic atrial foci generate impulses that are conducted to the ventricles.
- **ECG: heart rate <100 bpm & ≥ 3 P wave morphologies.**

MULTIFOCAL ATRIAL TACHYCARDIA (MAT):

- Same as Wandering atrial pacemaker except the heart rate is >100 bpm.
- **ECG: atrial rate >100 bpm & ≥3 P wave morphologies.**
- **MAT classically associated with severe COPD** (Chronic obstructive pulmonary disease).
  Difficult to treat: Calcium channel blocker (eg, **Verapamil)** or β-blocker used if LV function is preserved.

PATHOPHYSIOLOGY

- Organized atrial activity with multiple atrial foci competing, including the sinus node, resulting in multiple P waves on the ECG and irregular atrial rhythms.

RISK FACTORS

- **Pulmonary disease: seen in ~60% of patients — COPD most common pulmonary disorder associated with MAT.** Pneumonia, Pulmonary embolism, Pulmonary HTN, Pulmonary failure, hypoxemia, hypercarbia.
- **Cardiac disease**: structural heart damage, Heart failure, acute MI.
- Chronic renal disease
- Medications: eg, Aminophylline, Theophylline, Isoproterenol.
- Electrolyte abnormalities — eg, Hypomagnesemia, Hypokalemia.

CLINICAL MANIFESTATIONS

- Usually asymptomatic until patients develop Multifocal atrial tachycardia.
- Symptomatic: palpitations, dizziness, fatigue, dyspnea, & chest pain.
- Symptoms predominantly relate to the underlying associated illness rather than tachycardia.

PHYSICAL EXAMINATION:

- Irregular pulse, may be rapid if MAT

DIAGNOSIS:
ECG:

- **Irregularly, irregular rhythm + 3 or more identifiable P wave morphologies** (including the normal sinus P wave).
- **Heart rate <100 bpm = WAP; Heart rate >100 bpm = MAT.**

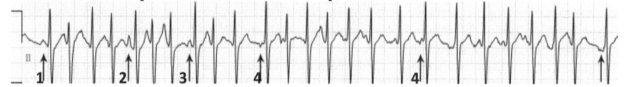

MANAGEMENT:
MAT:

- **Non-dihydropyridine Calcium channel blocker first-line (eg, Diltiazem, Verapamil).** They decrease atrial activity and slow atrioventricular node conduction.
- Beta blockers are an option if no underlying lung disease. **Avoid Beta blockers if underlying pulmonary disease** (can cause bronchoconstriction).
- In patients with Hypomagnesemia or Hypokalemia, magnesium and potassium repletion is paramount.

SUPRAVENTRICULAR PREMATURE BEATS

- **Supraventricular premature beats represent premature activation of the atria from a site other than the sinus node.**
- **Most originate from the atria (premature atrial complexes [PACs])** but less commonly originate from the atrioventricular node (premature junctional beats [PJBs]).

PATHOPHYSIOLOGY
- PACs are very common, in all ages and in those with and without significant heart disease.
- PJBs are uncommonly seen, especially compared to both PACs and Premature ventricular complexes/contractions (PVCs).

CLINICAL MANIFESTATIONS
- PACs and PJBs are asymptomatic in most patients but may produce symptoms such as palpitations, sensation of "skipping or racing", or dizziness.
- Physical examination may reveal an irregular pulse.

DIAGNOSIS
- The evaluation of patients with suspected PACs or PJBs may include ECG or ambulatory cardiac monitoring.
- Further testing is indicated only when this initial evaluation reveals significant structural cardiac abnormalities that require further workup.

ECG:
- **PACs: P waves that occur earlier than the anticipated next sinus P wave and has a different morphology** (eg, inverted, biphasic, different shape) from the sinus P wave. Often the PR interval is different from that during sinus rhythm.

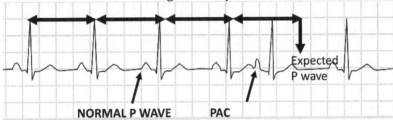

- **PJBs:** a narrow QRS complex with inverted P waves or no preceding P wave in leads where they should be upright, with the P wave occurring too soon before the QRS to be considered to be conducted through the AV node.

MANAGEMENT
[1] Asymptomatic PACs or PJBs:
- **No treatment needed in most cases:** PACs and PJBs are usually a benign finding requiring no treatment in the absence of symptoms.

[2] Symptomatic PACs or PJBs:
- **Minimize potential PAC or PJB triggers: For patients with symptomatic PACs, education & reassurance of the benign nature of PACs is often sufficient to alleviate symptoms.** Patients should be educated to avoid or minimize potential PAC precipitants (eg, smoking, alcohol intake, caffeine intake, stress, obesity, low physical activity).
- Persistent symptomatic PACs: Beta blockers (eg, Metoprolol) may be indicated for patients with persistent symptomatic PACs despite efforts to minimize potential PAC precipitants.

[3] Definitive management:
- Catheter ablation may be indicated in persistent or frequent PACs that are symptomatic and documented to trigger atrial arrhythmias (eg, SVT, Atrial fibrillation) or persist despite medical management.

AV JUNCTIONAL DYSRHYTHMIAS

- AV node/junction becomes the dominant pacemaker of the heart in AV junctional rhythms.

ECG:
- Regular rhythm. **P waves are not seen or are inverted (negative) if present** in leads where they are normally positive (I, II, aVF). **Classically associated with a narrow QRS** (±wide).
  Junctional Rhythm: heart rate is usually 40-60 bpm (reflecting the intrinsic rate of the AV junction).
  Accelerated Junctional: heart rate 60-100 bpm.
  Junctional Tachycardia: heart rate >100 bpm.

Junctional rhythm with inverted P waves   Junctional rhythm with absent P waves (note the narrow complexes)

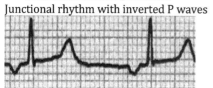 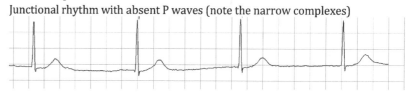

VENTRICULAR DYSRHYTHMIAS

PREMATURE VENTRICULAR COMPLEXES (PVCs)

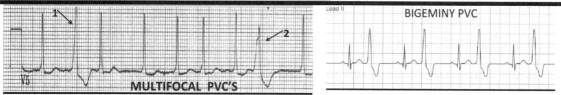

Unifocal (one morphology)   Multifocal (>1 morphology)   **Bigeminy** (every other beat is a PVC)   **Couplet** (two PVCs in a row)

- **PVC:** premature beat originating from the ventricle ⇨ **wide, bizarre QRS occurring earlier than expected.** With a PVC, **the T wave is usually in the opposite direction of the QRS.** Associated with a **compensatory pause** = overall rhythm is unchanged (AV node prevents retrograde conduction).

MANAGEMENT
[1] Low risk for heart disease:
- **No treatment is needed for PVCs in patients with low risk of heart disease. PVCs are typically self-limiting, rarely life-threatening, and in most cases do not require treatment.**
- Low-risk patients include overall good health with no personal or family history of heart disease (structural or electrical), minimal to no symptoms due to PVCs, no symptoms of heart disease, normal physical examination, and normal-appearing ECG (other than PVCs).

[2] Asymptomatic PVCs:
- **Observation and reassurance alone are the initial management of choice for low PVC burden (<10%) and without apparent underlying structural heart disease, and no symptoms.**
- In asymptomatic patients with structural heart disease, management centers on providing appropriate management of the specific underlying condition. In many cases, treatment for the underlying condition (eg, Beta blockers) may reduce the occurrence of PVCs.

[3] Symptomatic patients:
- **Beta-blockers are often first-line medical therapy for patients with significant symptoms due to PVCs in addition to reduction, correction, or elimination of underlying triggers.** Non-dihydropyridine Calcium channel blocker may be used.
- **Radiofrequency catheter ablation may be indicated in cases refractory to medical therapy, if adverse effects due to medical therapy occurs, or for those who do not prefer to be on long-term antiarrhythmic therapy.** Successful treatment may reverse PVC-induced cardiomyopathy
- Class I antiarrhythmics: eg, Flecainide or Amiodarone are suitable alternatives for patients <u>without</u> apparent structural heart disease in whom catheter ablation is not performed.

VENTRICULAR TACHYCARDIA (VT)

- **Defined as ≥3 consecutive PVCs (wide complex QRS duration >120 ms) at a rate >100 beats per minute (usually between 120-300 beats per minute).**
- If sustained Ventricular tachycardia (VT) is not managed, it can result in Ventricular fibrillation (VF).

CLASSIFICATION
- **Sustained VT = duration ≥30 seconds or causes hemodynamic collapse in <30 seconds.** Regular wide QRS complex (≥120 ms) at a rate >100 bpm with uniform consecutive beats.
- Monomorphic (same QRS morphology); Polymorphic (different morphologies).

ETIOLOGIES
- **Underlying heart disease: ischemic heart disease most common cause (eg, post MI) 70%,** structural heart defects, Cardiomyopathies.
- **Prolonged QT interval.** Electrolyte abnormalities (eg, **Hypomagnesemia,** Hypokalemia, Hypocalcemia), Digoxin toxicity. Medications: Digoxin toxicity.

CLINICAL MANIFESTATIONS
- Symptomatic: palpitations, dizziness, fatigue, dyspnea, & chest pain.
- **Unstable: hypoperfusion can cause hypotension (eg, systolic BP in double digits), altered mental status, refractory chest pain, or acute pulmonary edema.**

ECG:
- **Regular, wide complex tachycardia (uniform & stable QRS morphology);** no discernable P waves.

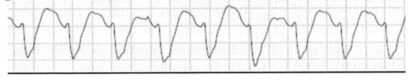

MANAGEMENT OF MONOMORPHIC VENTRICULAR TACHYCARDIA (VT)
[1] Hemodynamically stable VT:
- **Antiarrhythmics: Class I or III** — eg, **IV Amiodarone (often first-line) or Procainamide.** Lidocaine may be helpful in the setting of acute myocardial ischemia or infarction. Sotalol can be used in patients without structural heart disease.

[2] Hemodynamically unstable VT:
- **Direct current (synchronized) cardioversion initial management of choice.** Initial recommended dose for wide regular: 100 J. Consider sedation prior to cardioversion.

[3] Pulseless VT:
- **Unsynchronized cardioversion (defibrillation) + CPR.**

[4] Non-sustained VT:
- Asymptomatic patients with non-sustained Ventricular tachycardia (VT) and no underlying cardiac comorbidities require no additional therapy.

CHRONIC THERAPY OF VT
- **Beta blockers — unless contraindicated, nearly all patients who experience sustained monomorphic VT should be placed on Beta-blocker therapy,** including patients with a prior MI, patients with HF and reduced LV systolic function. **Beta blockers reduce the risk of recurrent ventricular tachyarrhythmias and sudden cardiac death as well as improve survival** most likely due to their blockade of sympathetic activity to the heart.
- Implantable cardioverter defibrillator (ICD) therapy: indicated in patients with ischemic heart disease that survive sudden cardiac arrest due to Ventricular tachycardia or experience hemodynamically unstable or stable VT if estimated survival >1 year.

TORSADES DE POINTES (TdP)

- **A variant of <u>Polymorphic Ventricular tachycardia</u>.**

PATHOPHYSIOLOGY:
- **<u>QTc prolongation:</u> TdP is a result of QTc prolongation >450 ms in males and >460 ms in females** (heart rate adjusted lengthening of the QT interval). A QTc >500 ms has been associated with a 2-fold to 3-fold increase in risk for TdP. May be either be congenital or acquired.
- **Acquired QTc prolongation is most often medication related** — antimicrobials, antiarrhythmics, antipsychotics, antiemetics, and antifungals.
- **<u>Prolonged repolarization</u> phase** due to inhibition of the delayed rectifier potassium current, leading to an excess of positive ions within the cellular membrane.
- **<u>R-on-T phenomenon</u> is the most common ECG phenomenon during ventricular arrhythmia initiation in long QT syndrome.** "R on T" phenomenon — a premature ventricular contraction (PVC) or other ectopic beat causes a ventricular depolarization so early in the cardiac cycle it falls on the relative refractory period (apex of the T wave) or during the prolonged repolarization phase, possibly triggering Ventricular tachycardia (VT) or Ventricular fibrillation (VF).
- **Prolonged repolarization and early afterdepolarization + triggered activity** [long-QT-related ventricular ectopic beats (eg, PVC occurring on the preceding T wave] can trigger TdP. Bradycardia is a risk factor for this type.

CLINICAL MANIFESTATIONS
- Up to 50% of patients are asymptomatic. May terminate spontaneously or degenerate to VF.
- <u>Symptomatic:</u> **palpitations, dizziness, and syncope.** Sudden cardiac death in up to 10%.

DIAGNOSIS
- <u>ECG:</u> **<u>Polymorphic Ventricular tachycardia</u> — cyclic alterations, twisting, & oscillations of the QRS amplitude around the isoelectric line** (aka sinusoidal waveform).

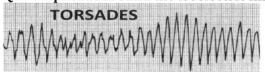

- <u>Labs:</u> rule out causes, such as Hypomagnesemia, Hypokalemia, and Hypocalcemia.

MANAGEMENT
[1] Hemodynamically stable TdP:
- **IV Magnesium sulfate first line and highly effective treatment for persistent Torsades de pointes.** IV Magnesium suppresses early afterdepolarizations, terminating the arrhythmia. Correct any electrolyte abnormalities and discontinue all QT prolonging drugs.
- **<u>Second-line:</u> Isoproterenol or Transvenous overdrive pacing if refractory to IV Magnesium. Isoproterenol increases the heart rate & shortens the QT**, reducing TdP in patients with prolonged QT refractory to Magnesium & patients with TdP triggered by pauses or bradycardia.

Congenital long QT syndrome:
- **Beta blockers** may be used to reduce the frequency of premature ventricular contractions and shorten the QT interval. **Avoid Isoproterenol in Congenital long QT syndrome.**

[2] Hemodynamically unstable TdP:
- **Synchronized cardioversion** should be performed on hemodynamically unstable patients in Torsades with a pulse — 100J monophasic; 50J Biphasic.

[3] Pulseless TdP:
- **Prompt defibrillation (unsynchronized) cardioversion + CPR** is indicated in patients in cardiac arrest (remember that TdP is a variant of VT and pulseless VT is treated with defibrillation).

VENTRICULAR FIBRILLATION (VF)

- **A type of sudden cardiac arrest (SCA) or sudden cardiac death (SCD) with ineffective ventricular contraction.** Without treatment, the chances of survival decline by ~2-10% per minute. For those who survive, anoxic brain damage and neurological deficits are common.

ETIOLOGIES:
- **Ischemic heart disease most common — 65-70% of all SCDs are attributable to Coronary heart disease (CHD) if >35 years of age.** Among patients hospitalized with acute MI, 5%-10% have VF or VT, and another 5% will have VF or VT within 48 hours of admission. Heart failure.
- Structural heart defects, Cardiomyopathies, Brugada syndrome. Congenital QT abnormalities.
- Sustained Ventricular tachycardia (VT) may transition to VF. Myocarditis, Hypothermia.
- Electrolyte abnormalities: Hypokalemia, Hyperkalemia, Hypomagnesemia; Acidosis, hypoxia.

CLINICAL MANIFESTATIONS:
- **Sudden collapse with the patient becoming unconscious, unresponsive, and without palpable pulse (pulseless)** due to low cardiac output as a result of ineffective ventricular contraction.
- Patients may demonstrate signs of acute MI before the event (eg, chest pain or discomfort, shortness of breath, diaphoresis, nausea, and vomiting).

DIAGNOSIS:
- Electrocardiogram: **Disorganized high frequency undulations with erratic pattern of electrical impulses, fibrillation waves of varying amplitude, shape, and periodicity, occurring at a rate >320/minute** with no identifiable P waves, QRS complexes, or T waves.

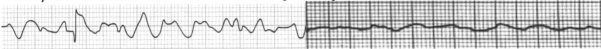

Coarse ventricular fibrillation   Fine ventricular fibrillation

MANAGEMENT
- **Unsynchronized cardioversion (Defibrillation) early + prompt, high-quality Cardiopulmonary resuscitation (CPR) instituted while awaiting arrival of a defibrillator.**
- Prompt defibrillation is essential once a defibrillator arrives. The chest compressions should cease, and the rhythm analyzed as soon as the defibrillator or AED becomes available. The CPR should be interrupted for the application of paddles and delivery of the shock.
- **If the rhythm is shockable, defibrillation at 120-200 Joules on a biphasic defibrillator or 360 Joules using a monophasic is recommended**; otherwise, CPR should be continued.
- CPR should be resumed immediately after defibrillation, and rhythm analysis should be conducted after 5 cycles of chest compressions or 2 minutes.
- Pharmacological intervention should not delay or replace prompt and early defibrillation in shockable cardiac rhythms.
- **Administer Epinephrine and Amiodarone as per ACLS protocol in patients sustaining VF rhythm regardless of receiving 3 shocks.** Amiodarone significantly improves survival to hospital admission without affecting survival to hospital discharge.

PREVENTATIVE MANAGEMENT:
Implantable cardioverter-defibrillator (ICD) placement: due to high recurrence rate.
- Secondary prevention: **Implantable cardioverter-defibrillator (ICD) placement is indicated for secondary prevention of SCD in patients with prior episodes of VF and sustained VT.** ICDs improve long-term survival status-post VF when compared to patients receiving only medications.
- **Primary prevention: ICD placement** is recommended for primary prevention of SCD in patients at increased risk of life-threatening VF/VT (eg, **left ventricular ejection fraction ≤35%**).

PULSELESS ELECTRICAL ACTIVITY (PEA) & ASYSTOLE

- **Pulseless electrical activity** (PEA): the presence of coordinated (organized) rhythms on ECG (other than VT or VF) without sufficient mechanical cardiac contraction to produce a palpable pulse or measurable blood pressure (electrical activity is not coupled with sufficient mechanical cardiac contraction).
- **Asystole** complete absence of demonstrable electrical and mechanical cardiac activity.

ETIOLOGIES:
- **6 "H"s: H**ypovolemia, **H**ypoxia, **H**ydrogen ions (Acidosis), **H**yper/**H**ypokalemia, **H**ypothermia
- **6 T"s: "T**oxins, Cardiac **T**amponade, **T**ension Pneumothorax, **T**hrombosis (MI, PE), **T**achycardia, **T**rauma (hypovolemia).
- **Narrow-complex PEA may be the result of mechanical problems** — eg, cardiac tamponade, pneumothorax, mechanical hyperinflation, pulmonary embolism, or myocardial rupture.
- **Wide-complex PEA may be the result from a metabolic problem** — eg, hyperkalemia, drug toxicity (eg, sodium channel–blocker toxicity), cardiac ischemia (acute MI with pump failure), or left ventricular failure and should be treated as appropriate.

MANAGEMENT OF ASYSTOLE & PEA
- **High quality CPR + IV Epinephrine administered as soon as possible after CPR has been initiated, rapid identification & reversal of underlying causes & checks for shockable rhythms every 2 minutes.** Epinephrine (1mg IV every 3-5 minutes). Institute the secondary ABCDs.
- Vasopressin alone or in combination with Epinephrine is no more effective than Epinephrine alone but Vasopressin may be used to replace the first or second dose of Epinephrine.
- **Neither asystole nor PEA respond to Unsynchronized cardioversion (defibrillation).**

Narrow-complex PEA:
In addition to above, consider mechanical causes:
- Cardiac tamponade — treat with bedside Pericardiocentesis.
- Tension Pneumothorax — treat with Needle decompression, followed by chest tube thoracotomy.
- Pulmonary embolism — treat with Thrombolysis (if not contraindicated).
- Hypovolemia/bleeding — treat with resuscitation (eg, fluids and blood products).

Wide-complex PEA
In addition to above, consider metabolic cause:
- Hyperkalemia — IV Calcium gluconate, Insulin/glucose, sodium bicarbonate bolus.
- Sodium channel blocker overdose — treat with IV Sodium bicarbonate boluses.
- Cardiac ischemia, or left ventricular failure and should be treated as appropriate.
- Hypoxia — assess for correct placement of the airway adjunct and check breath sounds to rule out slippage of the endotracheal tube or that a tension Pneumothorax is not present.
- Hydrogen ion (acidosis) — Respiratory acidosis managed by early endotracheal intubation and alveolar ventilation. Metabolic acidosis may be partially managed with good-quality CPR. Continuous endovenous hemodialysis may be required for severe acidosis. Sodium bicarbonate may be needed for severe metabolic acidosis (not used routinely).
- Hypothermia — treat with gradual rewarming with blankets and warm IV fluids. If there is no recovery of consciousness in the hypothermic patient following ROSC, maintain a body core temperature of 33°C until further assessment and decisions can be determined.
- Beta-blocker or Calcium channel–blocker overdose may require high-dose Insulin therapy and lipid emulsion infusion.

PROGNOSIS:
- Survival is low if patients in asystole do not achieve return of spontaneous circulation (ROSC) in the field or convert to a shockable rhythm.

EARLY REPOLARIZATION ABNORMALITIES

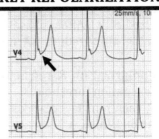

- Usually a normal variant.
- May be seen in thin, healthy males.

EARLY REPOLARIZATION ABNORMALITIES
- **Diffuse CONCAVE ST elevations >2 mm with large T waves** (especially precordial).
- **Tall QRS voltage.**
- Fishhook (slurring/notching) at the J point (arrow).

LVH with Left Ventricular STRAIN

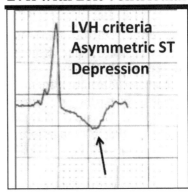

LVH criteria
Asymmetric ST Depression

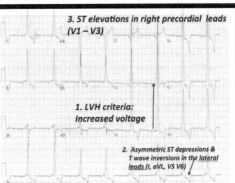

3. ST elevations in right precordial leads (V1 – V3)

1. LVH criteria: Increased voltage

2. Asymmetric ST depressions & T wave inversions in the lateral leads (I, aVL, V5 V6)

Often seen in patients with left ventricular hypertrophy (LVH) who also suffer from ischemic disease.

The coronary artery supply is "strained" trying to supply the excess hypertrophic cardiac muscle.

BRUGADA SYNDROME

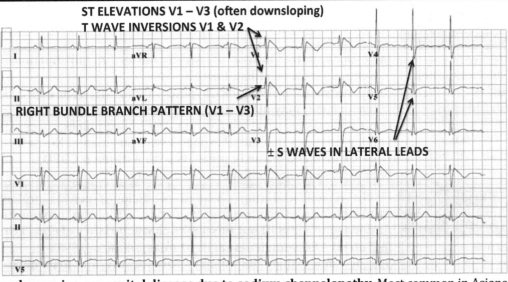

ST ELEVATIONS V1 – V3 (often downsloping)
T WAVE INVERSIONS V1 & V2
RIGHT BUNDLE BRANCH PATTERN (V1 – V3)
± S WAVES IN LATERAL LEADS

Brugada syndrome: is a congenital disease due to sodium channelopathy. Most common in Asians.
ECG (Brugada pattern):
- **(1) Right bundle branch block (RBB) pattern** (often incomplete).
- **(2) ST elevation V$_1$-V$_3$** (often downsloping or coved pattern).
- T wave inversions in **V$_1$ & V$_2$, ±S waves in the lateral leads.**

Treatment: placement of an Implantable cardioverter defibrillator (ICD) to reduce the risk of sudden cardiac death.

ANTI-ARRHYTHMIC AGENTS

CLASS I **NA+ CHANNEL BLOCKERS**	Decrease sodium conduction (especially depolarized cells). Affect phase 4 of depolarization (by blocking Na+ channel opening, they reduce SA node automaticity & cause membrane stabilization).
Class IA: **Procainamide** Quinidine Disopyramide	MOA: decrease conduction velocity, **prolong repolarization & refractory period. Prolong action potential** & increase excitation threshold. Ind: atrial AND ventricular arrhythmias (eg, SVT, reentrant tachycardias, VT especially if resistant to other meds). **Wolff-Parkinson White.** S/E: Torsades de pointes, hypotension, tachycardia, tinnitus. Caution if kidney disease. **Procainamide & Quinidine associated with drug-induced lupus-like syndrome.** Quinidine may enhance Digoxin toxicity.
Class IB: **Lidocaine** Tocainide	MOA: **decreases conduction velocity & shortens repolarization,** shortens action potential (affects ischemic as well as depolarized ventricular tissue – **most useful in abnormal ventricular tissue as seen post MI**). Indications: stable Ventricular arrhythmias (VT, VF) as an alternative agent. Contraindications: Narrow complex supraventricular tachycardia
Class IC: **Flecainide** Propafenone Encainide	MOA: decreases conduction velocity significantly (↑QRS prolongation). Affects ventricular tissue in healthy cells. No effect on action potential duration. Rarely used. Indications: Ventricular tachycardia (last line management). A. fibrillation. **Contraindication: proarrhythmic in patients with structural disease & increases mortality in patients with a history of Myocardial infarction.**
CLASS II **BETA- BLOCKERS**	Antagonizes beta adrenergic receptors to different degrees by decreasing slope of phase 4 (decreased calcium currents – **decreased SA & AV node conduction.**
Cardio selective (β₁): **Atenolol, Metoprolol, Esmolol** Nonselective (β₁, β₂): Propranolol, Sotalol Nonselective α & β₁,₂: Labetalol, Carvedilol	Indications: **rate control of Atrial flutter, Atrial fibrillation,** PSVT, Ventricular tachycardias. Post MI. S/E: **Bradycardia, AV blocks,** hypotension, CNS (fatigue, depression, sexual dysfunction) **may mask the symptoms of hypoglycemia.** Contraindications: sinus bradycardia, 2nd/3rd heart block, shock, ADHF. Caution: Diabetes mellitus, Peripheral vascular disease. **Nonselectives may cause bronchospasm in patients with Asthma & COPD.** Glucagon is antidote for Beta-blocker toxicity.
CLASS III **K+ CHANNEL BLOCKERS**	Blocks K+ efflux during phase 3 ⇨ action potential prolongation & prolongation of effective refractory period, QT interval prolongation. **Amiodarone: class III but possesses characteristics of class I through IV.**
Amiodarone Ibutilide Dofetilide **Sotalol**	Ind: **atrial AND ventricular arrhythmias;** refractory SVT. S/E of Amiodarone: **pulmonary fibrosis, thyroid disorders** (contains iodine so can cause hyperthyroidism or hypothyroidism), corneal deposits (>6 months use), **hepatotoxicity,** blue-green skin discoloration, hypotension. Monitor TFTs, PFTs, & LFTs in patients on long-term Amiodarone.
CLASS IV **Ca+2 CHANNEL BLOCKERS**	**Slows SA node & AV node conduction** (decreases L-type Ca+2 channels ⇨ decreased conduction speed, ↑PR interval, prolonged refractory period).
Verapamil **Diltiazem**	Ind: **atrial arrhythmias:** atrial flutter, atrial fibrillation, PSVT Adverse effects: **peripheral edema,** bradycardia, AV blocks. Antimuscarinic S/E with **Verapamil (constipation,** dizziness, flushing).
Class V (Other)	Digoxin (cardiac glycoside). Indications: **Atrial fibrillation, Heart failure.** MOA: inhibit ATP-ase ⇨ positive inotrope, negative chronotrope/dromotrope.

Nets play in **B K** for the **C**hampionship (Useful mnemonic to help remember the classes).
Also note: Class I and III used primarily for rhythm control. Class II & IV primarily for rate control.

ADENOSINE

INDICATIONS

- **[1] Paroxysmal supraventricular tachycardia (PSVT): Adenosine slows the sinus rate, slows AV node conduction time, and blocks AV nodal reentry pathways.** Adenosine can be both therapeutic and diagnostic (Adenosine can slow down the heart rate long enough to determine if the cause of the tachycardia is due to a different narrow complex tachycardia — eg, Atrial fibrillation or Atrial flutter). **Because it has a short half-life (<10 seconds), each dose of Adenosine needs to be flushed rapidly with 10-20 mL of Normal saline.**
- **[2] Pharmacologic cardiac stress testing in patients unable to exercise**: activates adenosine receptors (A1 & A2). **Adenosine A2A receptor activation causes vasodilation of normal coronary arteries (excluding diseased coronary arteries). This leads to a shunting effect to mimic increased demand.** Adenosine is usually used with thallium-201 stress testing.

ADVERSE EFFECTS

- **Common & short-lived — chest discomfort, dyspnea, flushing, lightheadedness, & headache.**
- Serious — **bronchospasm,** hypertension, arrhythmias, myocardial infarction, asystole.

CAUTIONS/CONTRAINDICATIONS

- Use in patients with second and Third-degree atrioventricular block (without a pacemaker), WPW, wide complex tachycardias.
- Clinically active bronchospastic disorders (severe asthma/COPD), acute myocardial ischemia.
- **Hypotension** due to A2A activation-related vasodilatation.
- **AV blocks** — A1 receptor activation causes atrioventricular conduction delay. Not used in patients with second or third-degree Heart block without a pacemaker.

AMIODARONE

MECHANISM OF ACTION

- **Class III antiarrhythmic (K+ channel blocker) with class I through IV properties.**
- Prolongs the action potential.

INDICATIONS

- **Most commonly used for stable wide-complex tachycardias** but useful for both atrial and ventricular arrhythmias, including refractory SVT.
- May be used for rate control in the setting of concomitant Atrial fibrillation + Decompensated heart failure (in this setting both Calcium channel blockers and Beta blockers are contraindicated).

ADVERSE EFFECTS

- IV use: **hypotension most common** (due to vasodilation), bradycardia, heart block, polymorphic ventricular tachycardia, phlebitis.
- Long-term use: **corneal deposition with >6 months use** (most common adverse effect), **thyroid disorders: hypo- or hyperthyroidism** (Amiodarone contains iodine), **pulmonary fibrosis, increased LFTs,** blue-green discoloration of the skin. **Monitoring: chest radiographs annually and PFTs as needed, TFTs every 6 months, and LFTs every 6 months.**

CAUTION

- Procainamide and Amiodarone are not generally used together.
- Amiodarone is a cytochrome p450 inhibitor.

CONTRAINDICATIONS

- Second or third-degree heart block who do not have pacemakers
- Wolff-Parkinson-White with concurrent Atrial fibrillation.

BETA BLOCKER TOXICITY

- <u>Lipophilicity</u> – **Beta blockers with high lipid solubility (eg, Propranolol)** most commonly associated with severe poisoning.

<u>Physical examination</u>:
- **Hypotension, bradycardia, heart block, bronchospasms.**
- **Mental status changes,** including delirium, coma, and seizures (lipophilic beta blockers rapidly cross the blood brain barrier causing neurologic sequelae). Severe hypotension can cause hypotension.

<u>Laboratory evaluation</u>:
- **<u>Labs</u>: may show hypoglycemia.**
- **<u>Electrocardiogram (ECG)</u>:** decreased conduction velocity of the AV node, resulting in prolonged PR & possibly AV block. Bradycardia (decreased SA node automaticity).

<u>Management</u>:
- **Hemodynamic support, IV isotonic fluid for hypotension; Atropine for symptomatic bradycardia; IV Dextrose for hypoglycemia.**
- **Additional treatment may include <u>IV Glucagon</u> to increase cAMP, increasing contraction,** IV calcium salts, IV vasopressor (eg, Epinephrine), IV high-dose insulin and glucose, IV lipid emulsion therapy for poisoning involving lipophilic medications (eg, Propranolol, Metoprolol, Labetalol).

<u>DIFFERENTIAL DIAGNOSIS</u>

Calcium channel blocker poisoning:
- **Less likely than Beta blockers to produce alterations in mental status,** and frequently do not do so unless the patient is in profound shock.
- **Hyperglycemia occurs more often with Calcium channel blocker toxicity, while Beta blockers are associated with hypoglycemia.**

Digoxin poisoning:
- Nausea and vomiting occur more often with Digoxin toxicity than beta blocker toxicity.
- Digoxin may cause characteristic changes in an electrocardiogram, such as scooped ST segment depressions.
- Digoxin is more likely to produce rhythms of increased automaticity, such as atrial tachycardia with atrioventricular block, premature ventricular contractions, or ventricular arrhythmias.

Clonidine poisoning:
- **Clonidine produces a constellation of signs that can resemble opioid overdose, including somnolence and miosis,** but are accompanied by hypotension and bradycardia.

Cholinergic drug poisoning:
- Cholinergic poisoning may occur with **insecticides (eg, Organophosphates), Medications, and Sarin gas.**
  - **<u>Increased SLUDD-C</u>: increased <u>S</u>alivation and <u>S</u>weating, <u>L</u>acrimation, <u>U</u>rination, Digestion (eg, vomiting, GI cramps), <u>D</u>efecation (diarrhea), <u>C</u>onstriction of the pupil (pupillary miosis).** The most common cause of death is respiratory failure.
  - **<u>Beta receptors (muscarinic)</u>: bradycardia, bronchorrhea, bronchospasm,** muscle fasciculations.
  - **<u>Nicotinic effects</u>: fasciculations, muscle weakness, paralysis due to neuromuscular blockade** (similar to succinylcholine), seizures, **tachycardia,** hypertension.
  - <u>CNS</u>: Nicotinic & muscarinic effects — central respiratory depression, lethargy, seizures, and coma.

DYSLIPIDEMIA

ETIOLOGIES
- Hypercholesterolemia: hypothyroidism, pregnancy, kidney failure.
- Hypertriglyceridemia: Diabetes Mellitus, ETOH, obesity, steroids, estrogen.

CLINICAL MANIFESTATIONS OF DYSLIPIDEMIA
- Most patients are asymptomatic. Hypertriglyceridemia may cause pancreatitis.
- May develop Xanthomas (eg, Achilles tendon) or Xanthelasma (lipid plaques on the eyelids).

SCREENING FOR DYSLIPIDEMIA
Based on risks: sex, age, cardiac risk factors such as smoking, hypertension, family history of coronary heart disease (first-degree male relative with CHD before age 55; first-degree female relative with CHD before age 65).

1. American College of Cardiology/American Heart Association: (2019): in adults between the ages 20 to 39 who are free of cardiovascular disease (CVD) it is "reasonable" to assess risk factors every 4–6 years to calculate their 10-year CVD risk.

There is considerable controversy regarding the optimal age for initiating screening.
- Higher risk = >1 risk factor (hypertension, smoking, family history) or 1 severe risk factor. initiate screening at age 20-25 for males; 30-35 for females.
- Lower risk: initiate screening at age 35 for males; 45 for females.

The U.S. Preventive Services Task Force (USPSTF) strongly recommends that clinicians routinely screen men aged 35 years and older and women aged 45 years and older for lipid disorders and treatment in people who are at increased risk of Coronary heart disease.

LIPID GUIDELINES FOR THE INITIATION OF STATIN THERAPY
Determined by calculation of 10-year and lifetime risk for having a heart attack or stroke instead of strict numbers only. Risk factors include gender, age, race, smoking, blood pressure, blood cholesterol levels & Diabetes mellitus. It recommends treatment in the following patients:

1. **Patients with type 1 or 2 Diabetes Mellitus between the ages 40-75 years of age.**

2. **Based on 10-year estimated CVD risk group if LDL-C 100 to <190 mg/dL:**
   - **Very high risk patients (≥20% 10-year risk)** and LDL-C in the range of 100 to <190 mg/dL (2.6 to <4.9 mmol/L), **high-dose Statin therapy is usually initiated**.

   - **High risk patients (≥7.5-19% 10 year risk): Patients without cardiovascular disease ages 40-75 years of age &, especially if** LDL-C 100 to <190 mg/dL (or 2.6 to <4.9 mmol/L), **moderate intensity Statin often initiated**.

   - **Intermediate-risk patients (5-7.4% 10-year risk of CVD)**: For patients with a 5-7.4% 10-year risk of CVD & LDL-C in the range of 100 to <190 mg/dL, discuss the potential benefits and costs/risks to patients (shared decision-making); if there are very high LDL-C levels (eg, >160 mg/dL [>4.14 mmol/L]), **statin therapy is usually suggested**.

   - **Low-risk patients (<5% 10-year risk)**: For most patients with a low CVD risk, further risk stratification is used with repeat screening as per follow-up recommendations. **Statin therapy is not usually indicated**.

3. People ≥21 years of age with LDL levels ≥190 mg/dL.
4. Any patient with any form of clinical atherosclerotic cardiovascular disease.
5. Patients <19 years of age with familial hypercholesterolemia.

HMG-COA REDUCTASE INHIBITORS (STATINS)

- **High intensity:** **Rosuvastatin most potent statin followed by Atorvastatin.** Reduce LDLC by 50%.
- **Moderate intensity:** **Pitavastatin, Simvastatin.** They reduce LDLC by 30-50%.
- **Low intensity:** **Fluvastatin is the least potent Statin** (<30% LDL reduction).

MECHANISM OF ACTION

- **They prevent synthesis of mevalonate, a cholesterol precursor, via inhibition of the enzyme Hydroxymethylglutaryl-CoA (HMG-CoA) reductase, the first & rate-limiting step in hepatic cholesterol synthesis.**
- **Decrease LDL:** a reduction in intrahepatic cholesterol leads to liver compensation by increasing low-density lipoprotein (LDL) receptor turnover that results from an enhanced rate of hepatic LDL receptor cycling, which clears LDL and VLDL remnants from the blood.
- Lower total cholesterol, (LDL-C), apo-B, and triglycerides concentrations (TG by 20-40%) while moderately increasing high-density lipoprotein cholesterol (HDL-C) concentration (~5%).
- **Cardiovascular protection:** direct anti-atherosclerotic effects & anti-inflammatory effects: Statins stabilize coronary artery plaques, reduces inflammation associated with atherosclerotic plaques by reducing the level of pro-inflammatory cytokines (TNF-a, IL-6, IL-8) and decrease the level of CRP. Statins have been shown to prevent bone loss.

BENEFITS

- **Aside from proprotein convertase subtilisin/kexin type 9 (PCSK9) inhibitors, Statins are the most powerful drugs for lowering low-density lipoprotein (LDL) cholesterol.**
- **Cardiovascular benefits:** Treatment and/or prevention of primary and secondary prevention clinical atherosclerotic cardiovascular disease [eg, Acute coronary syndrome (ACS), Myocardial infarction, Stroke] — decreased mortality in patients with Coronary artery disease and with ACS.

INDICATIONS

- People 21 years of age or with LDL levels ≥190 mg/dL.
- Any patient with any form of clinical atherosclerotic cardiovascular disease (ASCVD).
- **Based on 10-year atherosclerotic cardiovascular disease (ASCVD) risk.**
- **The most effective and best tolerated agents to treat dyslipidemias, especially elevated LDL-C.**

ADVERSE EFFECTS

Musculoskeletal:

- **Myopathy (eg, myalgia) is common adverse effect of Statins** (up 10%).
- **Myositis** (increased creatine kinase), **Rhabdomyolysis** (rare), especially with Fibrates or Niacin.
- **Rosuvastatin & Pravastatin safest in patients with history of Myopathy** once symptoms resolve. In patients who develop muscle adverse effects on Pravastatin or Fluvastatin, decrease the dose.

Hepatotoxicity:

- Increased LFTs: Mild elevations of serum aminotransferases are common but are not often associated with hepatic damage. Patients with preexisting liver disease may have more severe reactions. **If an individual on a Statin develops serum transaminases three times the upper limit of normal, reduce the dose of Statin, alternate day therapy, change to a different Statin (preferably Pravastatin), or change to a different class of lipid-lowering drugs.** Monitor lipid profile, liver function tests, and creatine kinase in individuals initiated on Statins. Gastrointestinal symptoms.

Other adverse effects:

- **Renal impairment:** Statins used with caution in patients with renal impairment. Atorvastatin is often the statin of choice for severe renal dysfunction, as it does not require dose adjustment.
- **Hyperglycemia:** increased risk of developing Diabetes mellitus. Statins inhibit the biosynthesis of cholesterol, essential for the production of GLUT-1, which mediates glucose uptake into the cell.
- Contraindications: **Statins are contraindicated during pregnancy** & should be discontinued prior to conception. Data regarding Statin while breastfeeding are limited, & use should be discouraged.

EZETIMIBE
MECHANISM OF ACTION:
- **Inhibits intestinal cholesterol absorption** — inhibits sterol transporter at small intestine's brush border, preventing the absorption of cholesterol. This decreases the liver's stores of cholesterol & increases LDL receptors with removal of LDL lipoproteins from the blood.

INDICATIONS:
- **Often used in combination with a Statin to reduce LDL levels.**
- As monotherapy, ezetimibe reduces LDL cholesterol by about 20%.

ADVERSE EFFECTS:
- Headache, GI upset, Diarrhea
- **Increased liver transaminase levels** and Hepatotoxicity rare (increased risk with concomitant Statin use).
- Bile acid sequestrants inhibit absorption of Ezetimibe; avoid concurrent use.

BILE ACID SEQUESTRANTS
Cholestyramine, Colestipol, Colesevelam
MECHANISM OF ACTION:
- **Bile acid sequestrant large cationic exchange resin polymer that binds bile acids in the intestine, blocking enterohepatic reabsorption of bile acids** and increasing fecal bile acid secretion. Because normally, 90% of bile acids are reabsorbed for reuse, **Resins reduce cholesterol pool, lowers intrahepatic cholesterol.**
- **Because the liver has to make new bile acids, it increases its LDL receptors, decreasing serum LDL levels.** They are relatively safe because they are not absorbed from the intestine.
- The resins cause a modest reduction in LDL cholesterol but have little effect on HDL cholesterol or triglycerides.

INDICATIONS:
- **Primarily used to decrease LDL levels, often used in combination with a Statin.** If mild to moderate increases in HDL needed.
- **Safe in pregnancy and safest lipid-lowering medications** (not systemically absorbed).
- **Cholestatic pruritus:** They have also been used to **reduce pruritus in patients with cholestasis and bile salt accumulation.**
- Cholestyramine has been shown to decrease cardiovascular mortality and morbidity by 19% compared to placebo in patients with Hypercholesterolemia.

ADVERSE EFFECTS:
- **GI adverse effects: most common** — constipation, nausea, vomiting, bloating, flatulence, crampy abdominal pain, dyspepsia. Absorption of vitamins (especially of fat-soluble vitamins A, D, E, & K, dietary folates) & drugs (eg, thiazide diuretics, Warfarin, Pravastatin, Fluvastatin, antibiotics) are impaired by the resins. Patients may require supplementation of fat-soluble vitamins.
- Increased liver transaminases. Osteoporosis with long-term use.
- **Prolonged PT/INR:** because Bile acid sequestrants interfere with the absorption of fat-soluble vitamins such as vitamin K, they can lead to derangements in vitamin K-dependent clotting factors.
- Cholestyramine and Colestipol bind and interfere with absorption of many drugs; administer all other drugs either 1 hour before or 3–4 hours after dose of a bile acid resin
- **Increased triglyceride levels:** Severe hypertriglyceridemia is a contraindication to its use.

CONTRAINDICATIONS:
- Severe Hypertriglyceridemia, Complete biliary obstruction.

NICOTINIC ACID (NIACIN, VITAMIN B3)

MECHANISM OF ACTION:

- In adipose tissue, niacin activates a signaling pathway that reduces hormone sensitive lipase activity and thus decreases plasma fatty acid and triglyceride levels. Consequently, LDL formation is reduced, and there is a decrease in LDL cholesterol.
- Favorably affects all lipid parameters. **Niacin is the most effective agent for increasing HDL-C.**
- **Increases HDL availability** by decreasing HDL uptake in the liver, delaying hepatic HDL clearance.
- Niacin speeds up the intracellular degradation of Apolipoprotein B (ApoB) containing lipoproteins, such as VLDL and LDL by inhibiting triglyceride synthesis — **decreases hepatic production of LDL & its precursor VLDL and decreases triglyceride synthesis.**
- Inhibits peripheral mobilization of fatty acids.

ADVERSE EFFECTS

Increased prostaglandins:

- **May cause cutaneous flushing, warm (burning) sensation usually limited to the face and chest generalized pruritus, paresthesias, & headache for 20-30 minutes**, especially if taken with hot beverages and alcohol.
- Flushing minimization: Low-dose Aspirin or NSAIDs greatly reduces pruritus & flushing if taken 30 minutes before Niacin. Flushing also minimized if therapy is initiated with low doses (250–500 mg qd) and if taken after a meal. Tolerance to flushing reaction usually develops within days to 2 weeks.

Other adverse effects:

- **GI symptoms: nausea, vomiting, dyspepsia, Peptic ulcer disease — GI symptoms reduced if taken with meals**.
- Liver abnormalities: ↑serum transaminases; severe hepatotoxicity. Hyperuricemia ~20% of patients.
- Hyperglycemia: carbohydrate tolerance may be moderately impaired, If Niacin is given in diabetics, monitor blood glucose weekly until stable. Hypotension.
- Concurrent use of Niacin and statins increase risk for myopathy. Arrhythmias, macular edema.
- Contraindicated in pregnancy, peptic ulcer disease, concurrent use of statins, gout.

OMEGA 3 FATTY ACIDS [EPA, DHA, ICOSAPENT ETHYL]

MECHANISM OF ACTION:

- Omega3 fatty acids, commonly eicosapentaenoic acid (EPA) and docosahexaenoic acid (DHA) ethyl esters, reduce VLDL triglycerides and are used as an adjunct to diet for treatment of adult patients with severe hypertriglyceridemia.
- The AHA recommends that consumers eat a variety of fish at least twice a week.
- Icosapent ethyl, a highly purified ethyl ester of EPA available in 1 and 0.5g capsules, is FDA approved as adjunctive therapy for patients with hypertriglyceridemia. Daily oral dosing for adults is 4 g/day, dosed twice daily with food.

INDICATIONS

- Adjunct for treating severe hypertriglyceridemia (triglycerides >1,000 mg/dL)
- Icosapent ethyl: Adjunct to maximally tolerated statin therapy to reduce risk of cardiovascular events in adults with triglyceride levels ≥150 mg/dL
- Adjunct to diet in adults with severe hypertriglyceridemia (triglycerides ≥500 mg/dL).

ADVERSE EFFECTS

- Arthralgia, nausea, fishy burps, dyspepsia, and increased LDL.
- Since omega3 fatty acids may prolong bleeding time, patients taking anticoagulants should be monitored.

PCSK9 INHIBITORS Alirocumab and Evolocumab, antibodies to PCSK9

MECHANISM OF ACTION:

- Evolocumab & Alirocumab are fully humanized monoclonal antibodies that bind free PCSK9, thereby interfering with its binding to the LDL receptor, leading to reduced degradation of the LDL receptor and increased liver clearance of LDL from the circulation, thereby lowering serum LDLC levels.
- PCSK9 inhibition lowers LDL-C and cardiovascular risk.

BENEFITS

- **PCSK9 inhibition significantly lowers LDL-C and cardiovascular risk.** Their use is associated with lower rates of myocardial infarction and stroke. Alirocumab in addition to intensive statin therapy may lead to reduced overall mortality risk after acute coronary syndrome in the long term.
- **Most effective agents at reducing LDLC.**

INDICATIONS:

Used in addition to maximally tolerated statin doses (complementary mechanism)

- (1) to lower risk of myocardial infarction, stroke, and unstable angina requiring hospitalization in patients with established cardiovascular disease,
- (2) to lower LDLC as adjunctive therapy alone or in combination with other LDLC–lowering medication in adult patients with HeFH.
- Unlike other medications used to treat dyslipidemias, PCSK9 inhibitors do NOT appear to substantially increase the risk of myopathies when used as monotherapy or in combination with statins.

ADVERSE EFFECTS

- Injection site reactions are the most frequent adverse effect of the antibodies
- Neurocognitive effects: Several clinical trials have identified a small (<1%) risk of neurocognitive effects in patients treated with PCSK9 antibody inhibitors compared to placebo.
- Similar to other monoclonal antibodies, risk of infections, including nasopharyngitis, urinary tract infections, or upper respiratory infections, is slightly increased.

FIBRATES

Gemfibrozil, Fenofibrate

MECHANISM OF ACTION:

- Fibrates activate peroxisome proliferator-activated receptors alpha (PPAR-alpha), which upregulate & increase the activity lipoprotein lipase (stimulating catabolism of triglyceride-rich lipoproteins and affect expression of the gene products that mediate metabolism of TG and HDL).
- They reduce the availability of substrates needed for hepatic triglyceride and very-low-density lipoproteins (VLDL) synthesis and enhance the clearance of triglyceride-rich particles.

Indications:

- Because these drugs have only a modest ability to reduce LDL cholesterol and can increase LDL cholesterol in some patients, they might be combined with other cholesterol lowering drugs for treatment of patients with elevated LDL.

Adverse effects:

- GI symptoms (5%): nausea most common adverse effect, diarrhea, dyspepsia, hepatitis.
- **Increased lithogenicity of bile: increased risk of cholesterol gallstones.**
- **Myopathy:** When used in combination with reductase inhibitors, the fibrates significantly increase the risk of myopathy.
- Contraindications: Renal dysfunction, hepatic dysfunction, and gallbladder disease are relative contraindications. Contraindicated in children and pregnancy.

SALICYLATE (ACETYLSALICYLIC ACID, ASPIRIN)

MECHANISM OF ACTION
- **Non-selectively and irreversibly inhibits cyclooxygenase (COX-1 & COX-2), decreasing prostaglandin and thromboxane A2 synthesis, producing anti-inflammatory, analgesic, antipyretic effects, and reduces platelet aggregation.**

INDICATIONS
- Pain, fever arthritis (anti-inflammatory at high doses), anti-platelet aggregation (eg, ACS, MI, TIA, thromboembolic stroke prevention, Rheumatic fever, or Kawasaki disease.

ADVERSE EFFECTS
- **GI upset: is the most common adverse effect from therapeutic anti-inflammatory doses of Aspirin due to COX1 inhibition. Chronic use can result in gastric ulceration**, upper gastrointestinal bleeding. Pill-induced esophagitis.
- **Renal effects: eg, acute kidney injury** (due to afferent arteriole constriction) & interstitial nephritis.
- Asthma exacerbation: when thromboxane and prostaglandin synthesis is inhibited by even small doses of Aspirin, persons with Aspirin hypersensitivity (especially associated with nasal polyps) may develop Asthma exacerbation from the increased synthesis of leukotrienes. Arachidonic acid is converted to leukotrienes, leading to bronchoconstriction.
- At very high doses, metabolic acidosis, dehydration, hyperthermia, collapse, coma, and death may occur.
- Reye syndrome: in children with infections (especially viral) who are treated with Aspirin have an increased risk for developing Reye syndrome, a rare but serious syndrome of rapid liver degeneration and encephalopathy.
- **Increased bleeding.** Decreased uric acid excretion (cautious use in patients with Gout).
- Medication interactions: Aspirin enhances the effect of Lithium, Warfarin, Heparin, and Digoxin.

CONTRAINDICATIONS/CAUTIONS
- **Renal injury** (eg, acute renal failure, interstitial nephritis) **or gastric mucosal injury (eg, gastritis, gastric ulcer, GI bleed) due to loss of the protective effect of prostaglandins**.
- Possible hemolytic anemia in patients with G6PD deficiency.
- Contraindicated in hemophiliacs; increased bleeding with Von Willebrand disease because Aspirin increases the bleeding time.

ACUTE TOXICITY OR OVERDOSE
- Neurologic symptoms: **Hyperthermia, hyperpnea, & tachycardia.** Altered mental status changes, lethargy, seizures. **Ototoxicity: hearing loss, tinnitus, vertigo, cranial nerve VIII (8) toxicity.**
- GI symptoms: **nausea, vomiting, diarrhea, and tinnitus are early symptoms of toxicity.**
- Noncardiogenic pulmonary edema (ARDS)
- **Respiratory alkalosis** (early on from respiratory center stimulation, leading to hyperventilation) **followed by high anion-gap Metabolic acidosis** (inhibits oxidative phosphorylation & Krebs cycle, leading to accumulation of lactic acid). Renal insufficiency, hypokalemia, and liver injury.

MANAGEMENT OF TOXICITY OR OVERDOSE
- **Supportive care & IV hydration as there is no antidote for ASA toxicity. Avoid endotracheal intubation, if possible.**
- **Alkalinization of the urine and serum with IV Sodium bicarbonate to increase salicylate excretion and decrease CNS toxicity.**
- GI decontamination: Activated charcoal to block salicylate absorption in those who ingested salicylate within the past 2 hours (used in those who are alert with a secured airway).
- Dialysis in severe cases: eg, salicylate concentration >100 mg/dL, pH <7.2 or <7.3 with treatment.

CHRONIC STABLE ANGINA PECTORIS (CHRONIC CORONARY SYNDROME)

- **Chest discomfort** due to myocardial ischemia as a result of fixed epicardial coronary artery obstruction (insufficient blood flow to the cardiac muscle as a result of ischemic heart disease).
- **Symptoms are a complication of Coronary artery disease (CAD) usually due to Atherosclerosis** (hardening and narrowing of the coronary arteries).

RISK FACTORS
- **Major: Diabetes mellitus: worst risk factor, considered a CAD equivalent; Smoking most important modifiable risk factor.** Hyperlipidemia, Hypertension, male sex, age >45 years in men or >55 years in women, family history of Coronary artery disease.
- Minor: obesity, elevated homocysteine, increased C-reactive protein, & lack of estrogen.
- Coronary artery disease equivalents include Diabetes mellitus, Carotid artery disease, Abdominal aortic aneurysm, Peripheral arterial disease, or 10-year risk of MI ≥20%.

PATHOPHYSIOLOGY
- **Myocardial ischemia: inadequate myocardial tissue perfusion due to imbalance between (1) increased myocardial oxygen demand & (2) decreased coronary artery blood supply, leading to chest pain or pressure or its equivalent.**
- Increased myocardial oxygen demand: with increased heart rate, systolic blood pressure (afterload), myocardial contractility, and myocardial wall tension or stress.

CLINICAL MANIFESTATIONS
- **Chest pain or discomfort: classic** — although there is significant variation, the pain is classically **substernal, poorly localized, exertional, short in duration (<30 minutes** but often resolves within 5 minutes of cessation of activity), exacerbated with activity or stress, **relieved with rest &/or Nitroglycerin,** & may radiate to the arm, teeth, lower jaw, back, epigastrium, or shoulders.
- Associated symptoms: dyspnea, fatigue, nausea, vomiting, numbness, or diaphoresis.
- Anginal equivalent: instead of chest pain, patients may develop dyspnea, epigastric, or shoulder pain. This is especially seen in women, elderly, diabetics, and obese patients.
- Physical examination is usually normal.

DIAGNOSIS
- Stable angina is usually a clinical diagnosis along with testing.
- **ECG: initial test of choice** — **ST depression (horizontal or downsloping) classic,** T wave inversion, poor R wave progression, & T wave pseudonormalization. **The resting ECG is normal in 50%.**
- **Stress testing: most important noninvasive testing.** Options include stress ECG, Myocardial perfusion imaging, or Stress echocardiography.
- **Coronary angiography: definitive diagnostic test.** Defines location and extent of CAD.

MANAGEMENT
- **Typical outpatient regimen for Stable Angina includes 4 drugs: [1] Beta blockers daily (most important drug to decrease mortality), [2] sublingual short-acting Nitroglycerin as needed for immediate symptom relief, [3] daily Aspirin** (mortality benefit), and **[4] a daily Statin.**
- Calcium channel blockers & long-acting Nitrates can be used in lieu of Beta blockers if Beta blockers are contraindicated or have adverse effects, or in Vasospastic disorders (eg, Prinzmetal angina).
- Reduction of risk factors: hypertension and DM control, exercise, diet, smoking cessation.
Revascularization: definitive management.
- **Percutaneous transluminal coronary angioplasty** — 1 or 2 vessel disease in nondiabetics not involving the left main coronary artery, with normal or near-normal ejection fraction.
- **Coronary artery bypass graft** — **left main coronary artery stenosis, 3 vessel disease (2 vessel disease in diabetics),** or decreased left ventricular ejection fraction <40%.

> Class I: angina only with *unusually strenuous activity.* No limitations of activity.
> Class II: angina with *more prolonged or rigorous activity.* Slight limitation of physical activity.
> Class III: angina with usual daily activity. Marked limitation of physical activity.
> Class IV: *angina at rest.* Often unable to carry out any physical activity.

STRESS TESTING IN CAD

- **Most useful noninvasive test in the diagnosis of Coronary artery disease.**

[1] Stress ECG

- <u>Indications:</u> **most commonly used stress test. Useful only if baseline ECG is normal.**
- Positive findings include ECG changes (eg, ST depressions, T wave inversions, poor R wave progression) or reproduction of symptoms or signs.
- <u>Limitations:</u> does not locate the area of ischemia.

[2] Myocardial perfusion imaging:

- **Uses Thallium or Technetium for imaging.**
- <u>Indications:</u> can be used if baseline ECG is abnormal. Gives information regarding the location & extent of ischemia.
- Can be performed either with (1) exercise or (2) with a pharmacologic agent if the patient cannot exercise — vasodilators (eg, **Adenosine or Dipyridamole**).
- Theophylline and caffeine should be stopped 48 hours and 12 hours respectively.
- <u>Contraindications to vasodilators:</u> **bronchospastic disease, hypotension, or AV blocks.**

[3] Stress echocardiogram:

- <u>Indications:</u> can be used if baseline ECG is abnormal. Similar to Myocardial perfusion imaging, Stress echocardiogram gives information regarding the location & assess the extent of ischemia.
- Can be performed with (1) exercise or (2) a pharmacologic if patient cannot exercise **[positive inotropes (eg, Dopamine or Dobutamine)].**
- <u>Contraindications to positive inotropes:</u> severe LV outflow obstruction (eg, **Aortic stenosis**), ventricular arrhythmias, recent MI (1-3 days), or severe systemic Hypertension.

Other considerations:

- During stress testing in patients <u>without</u> a history of Coronary artery disease, antianginal medications (Nitrates, Beta blockers & Calcium channel blockers) should be withheld 48 hours prior to stress testing.
- Patients <u>with known history of coronary artery disease</u> should continue their antianginal medications prior to stress testing. This allows for the evaluation of the efficacy of the patient's current treatment regimen and also to determine the appropriate level of exercise that is safe for the patient.

CORONARY ANGIOGRAPHY

- **Definitive diagnosis/gold standard.** "Cath" outlines the coronary artery anatomy. Angiography also defines location & extent of coronary artery disease (CAD).

  <u>Indications:</u>
  1. Confirm/exclude CAD in patients with symptoms consistent with CAD.
  2. Confirm/exclude CAD in patients with negative noninvasive testing for CAD.
  3. Patients who may possibly need revascularization (PTCA or CABG).

MEDICATIONS USED IN THE MANAGEMENT OF STABLE ANGINA PECTORIS

- **Typical outpatient regimen for Stable Angina includes 4 drugs: [1] Beta blockers daily (most important drug to decrease mortality), [2] sublingual short-acting Nitroglycerin as needed for immediate symptom relief, [3] daily Aspirin** (mortality benefit), **and [4] a daily Statin.**
- Calcium channel blockers can be used in lieu of Beta blockers if Beta blockers are contraindicated or in Vasospastic disorders (eg, Prinzmetal) but does not reduce mortality. Long-acting Nitroglycerin.

BETA BLOCKERS

Indication: **First-line long-term therapy to reduce anginal episodes & improve exercise tolerance.**
Benefits:
- **Reduce mortality,* prevent ischemic occurrences, and improve symptoms by reducing myocardial oxygen demand via decrease in heart rate and myocardial contractility.**

Mechanism of action:
- **Increase myocardial blood supply** — increase coronary artery filling time (coronary arteries fill during diastole), improving coronary circulation.
- **Decrease myocardial oxygen demand** — reduce myocardial O_2 requirements during stress & exercise (negative chronotropes & inotropes that decrease heart rate and contractility), as well as decrease blood pressure.
- Because Beta blockers reduce the heart rate-blood pressure product during exercise, the onset of angina or the ischemic threshold during exercise is delayed or prevented.

Contraindications:
- **Vasospastic (Variant, Prinzmetal) angina** — Beta blockers may increase the tendency to induce coronary vasospasm from unopposed alpha-receptor activity (vasoconstriction).

SHORT-ACTING NITROGLYCERIN

Indications:
- **First-line therapy for immediate relief of acute anginal symptoms** (acts in 1-2 minutes). No mortality benefit. Short-acting Nitrates in the sublingual form most commonly used.

Mechanism of action:
- **Increases myocardial blood supply** — increases coronary artery blood flow & collateral circulation as well as reduces coronary artery vasospasm.
- **Decreases myocardial oxygen demand** — venodilation (decreases preload) & vasodilation of arteries (decreases afterload).

Administration:
- Administered sublingual if chest pain occurs. Given up to 3 doses 5 minutes apart.
- Can be used prophylactically 5 minutes before activities likely to cause ischemia.

Adverse effects:
- **Vasodilation: headache, flushing of the skin, hypotension, and peripheral edema.**
- **Tolerance:** tachyphylaxis after 24 hours (allow for nitrate-free period for 8 hours).
- Deteriorates with exposure to light, moisture, and air.

Contraindications:
- **Hypotension: Systolic blood pressure <90 mmHg**
- **Use of phosphodiesterase-5 inhibitors** (eg, Sildenafil, Tadalafil). Phosphodiesterase-5 inhibitors when coadministered with Nitrates can cause significant hypotension.
- **Acute right ventricular infarction:** eg, inferior or posterior wall Myocardial infarction.

ASPIRIN

Indications:
- **In the absence of a contraindication, all patients with established Cardiovascular disease (CVD) should be treated with daily Aspirin** (81–325 mg orally daily).

Benefits:
- Reduces in the risk of subsequent myocardial infarction (MI), stroke, and vascular death among a wide range of patients who have survived an occlusive cardiovascular disease (CVD) event.

Considerations:
- <u>Risk stratification</u> is important as the use of Aspirin comes with an increased risk of major bleeding.

Adverse effects:
- **Increased risk of major bleeding** — extracranial (upper GI bleeding most common) and intracranial hemorrhage.
- **In patients who are unable to take Aspirin, or those with a history of gastrointestinal bleeding, Clopidogrel is a reasonable alternative.**
- **The most common adverse effect from therapeutic Anti-inflammatory doses of Aspirin is gastric upset due to COX1 inhibition. Chronic use can result in gastric ulceration.**
- **Renal injury** including Acute kidney injury and Interstitial nephritis.
- <u>Aspirin hypersensitivity</u>: When thromboxane and prostaglandin synthesis is inhibited by even small doses of Aspirin, individuals with Aspirin hypersensitivity (especially associated with nasal polyps) can experience Asthma from the increased synthesis of leukotrienes.
- At higher doses of Aspirin, tinnitus, vertigo, hyperventilation, and respiratory alkalosis may occur. At very high doses, the drug causes metabolic acidosis, dehydration, hyperthermia, collapse, coma, and death.
- Children with viral infections who are treated with Aspirin have an increased risk for developing Reye syndrome, a rare but serious syndrome of rapid liver degeneration and encephalopathy.

CALCIUM CHANNEL BLOCKERS

- <u>LONG-acting Non-dihydropyridines</u>: Diltiazem or Verapamil
- <u>LONG-acting Dihydropyridines</u>: Amlodipine or Felodipine. <u>Other CCBs</u>: Nifedipine, Nicardipine.

Indications:
- Calcium channel blockers and long-acting Nitrates are alternatives if Beta blockers are contraindicated or cause adverse effects.
- They can also be added as combination therapy if monotherapy is unsuccessful.
- Long-acting Diltiazem or Verapamil or a second-generation Dihydropyridine (Amlodipine or Felodipine) are preferred.

Caution:
- Short-acting dihydropyridines, especially Nifedipine, should be avoided unless used in conjunction with a Beta blocker in the management of CCS because of evidence of an increase in mortality after a myocardial infarction and an increase in acute myocardial infarction in hypertensive patients
- Unlike the Beta-blockers, Calcium channel blockers have not been shown to reduce mortality postinfarction and in some cases have increased ischemia and mortality rates. This appears to be the case with some short-acting dihydropyridines (eg, Nifedipine) and with Diltiazem and Verapamil in patients with clinical heart failure or moderate-severe LV dysfunction.

LONG-ACTING NITROGLYCERIN

Administration:

- Oral Isosorbide dinitrate, isosorbide mononitrate, Nitroglycerin ointment, 2% ointment, and transdermal nitroglycerin patches.
- Patches should be taken off after 12–14 hours of use for a 10–12-hour patch-free interval daily.

Indications:

- Calcium channel blockers and long-acting Nitrates are alternatives if Beta blockers are contraindicated or cause adverse effects.
- They can also be added as combination therapy if monotherapy is not successful.

Adverse effects:

- Tachyphylaxis: The main limitation to long-term Nitrate therapy is tolerance, which can be limited by a regimen that includes a minimum 8-10 hour period per day without Nitrates (overnight).
- Vasodilation: headache (Nitrate therapy is often limited by headache), flushing, hypotension, light-headedness, or peripheral edema.

Contraindications:

- Phosphodiesterase inhibitors commonly used for erectile dysfunction should not be taken within 24 hours of Nitrate use (eg, Sildenafil, Tadalafil).

RANOLAZINE

Mechanism of action:

- **Late sodium channel blocker: Reduces oxygen requirements of cardiac muscle (reduced tension in the heart wall)** by reducing intracellular calcium overload and the subsequent increase in diastolic tension via its inhibition of late inward sodium channel in myocardial diseased states (eg, ischemia and hypertrophy).
- It does not exert a significant effect on the normal myocardium at usual dosages.

Indications:

- **Ranolazine is effective at reducing anginal symptoms and improving exercise capacity when added to conventional medical therapy, especially in patients refractory to conventional therapy.**
- **Ranolazine has no effect on heart rate and blood pressure, and it has been shown in clinical trials to prolong exercise duration and time to angina,** both as monotherapy and when administered with conventional antianginal therapy.
- Ranolazine is safe to use with erectile dysfunction medications.
- Ranolazine decreases the occurrence of Atrial fibrillation and results in a small decrease in HbA1c. In spite of the QT prolongation, there is a significantly lower rate of ventricular arrhythmias with its use following acute coronary syndromes.

Important note:

- **Ranolazine is not to be used for treatment of acute anginal episodes.**

Contraindications:

- **Because Ranolazine can cause QT prolongation, it is contraindicated in patients with existing QT prolongation**; in patients taking QT prolonging medications, such as class I or III antiarrhythmics (eg, Quinidine, Dofetilide, Sotalol); and in those taking potent and moderate CYP450 3A inhibitors (eg, Clarithromycin, Rifampin).
- Significant liver and kidney disease.

ACUTE CORONARY SYNDROME (ACS)

- Symptoms of acute myocardial ischemia secondary to <u>acute plaque rupture</u> & varying degrees of <u>coronary artery thrombosis (occlusion).</u>

SPECTRUM OF ACUTE CORONARY SYNDROMES			
	UA	NSTEMI	STEMI
HISTORY	Angina that is new in onset, crescendo, or at rest (usually >30 minutes). >90% occlusion can cause symptoms at rest		
CORONARY THROMBOSIS	Subtotal artery occlusion		Total arterial occlusion
ECG	ST DEPRESSIONS &/or T WAVE INVERSIONS		ST ELEVATIONS
CARDIAC ENZYMES	Negative	Positive (cell death) seen in both NSTEM & STEMI	

ETIOLOGIES
- **Atherosclerosis: most common cause of MI.** Plaque rupture ⇨ acute coronary artery thrombosis with platelet adhesion/activation/aggregation along with fibrin formation. Vasculitis, embolism.
- **Coronary artery vasospasm** (2%): **cocaine-induced MI or Variant (Prinzmetal) angina.**

CLINICAL MANIFESTATIONS
- **Chest pain:** retrosternal pressure **not relieved with rest or nitroglycerin, pain at rest**, often lasting **> 30 minutes;** may radiate to the lower jaw & teeth, left arm, epigastrium, back or shoulders; or **change from typical pattern.** Pain at rest usually indicates >90% coronary artery occlusion.
- Sympathetic stimulation: anxiety, diaphoresis, tachycardia, palpitations, nausea, vomiting, dizziness.
- Silent MI: **~25% are atypical/silent: eg, women, elderly, diabetics & obese** patients. **Atypical symptoms include abdominal pain, jaw pain, or dyspnea, often <u>without</u> chest pain.**

PHYSICAL EXAMINATION
- No specific findings due to acute cardiac ischemia. Patients may be tachycardic.
- **Inferior wall MI: may be associated with bradycardia or atrioventricular heart blocks** (the RCA supplies the AV node in 90%). **May have an S4 gallop (especially with inferior MI).**
- **Triad of right ventricular infarction: increased JVP + clear lungs + positive Kussmaul sign.**

DIAGNOSTIC STUDIES
- 12 lead ECG
- Cardiac enzymes

•**STEMI:** ST elevations >1mm in ≥ 2 anatomically contiguous leads with reciprocal changes in the opposite leads.

ECG progression: **Hyperacute T waves first change ⇨ ST elevations ⇨ Q waves**

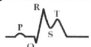 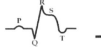 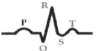

A new Left bundle branch considered an STEMI equivalent

AREA OF INFARCTION	ST ELEVATIONS/Q WAVES	ARTERY MOST LIKELY INVOLVED
ANTERIOR WALL	V1, V2, V3, V4	Left anterior descending (LAD)
Septal	V1 and V2	Proximal LAD
LATERAL WALL	I, aVL, V5, & V6	Circumflex (CFX)
ANTEROLATERAL WALL	I, aVL, V4, V5, & V6	Mid LAD, CFX, or Left main coronary
INFERIOR WALL	II, III, AVF	Right coronary artery (RCA)
POSTERIOR WALL	ST DEPRESSIONS V1, V2	RCA or CFX

^Troponin may be falsely elevated in patients with renal failure, advanced heart failure, acute PE, CVA.

Cardiac markers 3 sets 8 hours apart. **CK-MB & Troponin most commonly ordered.**

	Appears	Peaks	Returns to baseline
CK, CK-MB	4-6 hours	12-24 hours	3-4 days
Troponin I & T	4-6 hours	12-24 hours	7-10 days
Myoglobin	2-4h (fastest)	4-6 hours	1 day

OVERVIEW OF THE MANAGEMENT OF ACUTE CORONARY SYNDROME (ACS)

Perform brief history & physical examination
Obtain cardiac markers

- **Obtain ECG**: within first 10 minutes of arrival to the Emergency department (ED).
- **Aspirin 325 mg nonenteric coated chewed for faster absorption.**
- **Nitroglycerin** sublingual (0.4 mg) or spray every 5 minutes x 3 doses **if** persistent chest discomfort, hypertension, or signs of Heart failure **and** there is no sign of hemodynamic compromise (eg, right ventricular infarction) and no use of phosphodiesterase inhibitors (eg, for erectile dysfunction); add IV Nitroglycerin for persistent symptoms despite SL NTG.
- **Oxygen** given only if hypoxic to maintain SaO2 >90%.
- Morphine: may consider if pain is refractory not relieved with IV Nitroglycerin.

Patients with Unstable angina (UA) or acute NSTEMI should be treated with an early medical regimen similar to that used in an acute STEMI with one major exception: There is no evidence of benefit (and possible harm) from Fibrinolysis.

NORMAL ECG	UA/NSTEMI	STEMI	Inferior & Posterior STEMI
Initial:	**Initial:**	**Initial:**	**Initial: OA:**
• **Aspirin, Nitroglycerin,** Oxygen (if hypoxemic), Morphine.	• **Aspirin, Nitroglycerin,** Oxygen (if hypoxemic), Morphine.	• **Aspirin, Nitroglycerin,** Oxygen (if hypoxemic), Morphine.	• **Aspirin,** Oxygen, **Fluids***
Serial ECG & Enzymes:	• **Anticoagulant:** eg, **Unfractionated Heparin** (if undergoing invasive strategy), **Enoxaparin or Fondaparinux** (if treated conservatively)]	• **Anticoagulant:** eg, **Unfractionated Heparin** (if undergoing invasive strategy), **Enoxaparin or Fondaparinux** (if treated conservatively)]	• **Anticoagulant: Unfractionated Heparin, Enoxaparin**
• Repeat ECG every 10-15 minutes if initial ECG is nondiagnostic.			
	• **Beta blocker (Metoprolol, Atenolol).**	• **Beta blocker** (cardioselective)	
• If ST-segment depressions or deep T-wave inversions without Q waves develop + negative enzymes -> UA.	• High intensity statin: 80 mg Atorvastatin; Rosuvastatin	• High intensity statin: Atorvastatin, Rosuvastatin	• High intensity statin: Atorvastatin, Rosuvastatin
	• **Dual antiplatelet therapy: Aspirin + P2Y12 receptor antagonist (Clopidogrel, Ticagrelor)**	• **Dual antiplatelet therapy: Aspirin plus a P2Y12 receptor** antagonist (eg, Clopidogrel, Ticagrelor)	• **Dual antiplatelet therapy: Aspirin plus a P2Y12 receptor** antagonist (eg, Clopidogrel, Ticagrelor)
• If ST-segment depressions or deep T-wave inversions without Q waves develop + positive enzymes -> NSTEMI.	• **Risk assessment**: to determine if PCI is needed (TIMI, GRACE, HEART scores).	• **GIIb/IIIa** if PCI performed.	• **REPERFUSION* (PCI or CABG; fibrinolytics** if PCI cannot performed)
		• **REPERFUSION* (PCI or CABG; fibrinolytics** if PCI cannot be performed.	
	• **NO FIBRINOLYTICS.**	• **ACE inhibitors** long term.*	• **NO Nitroglycerin, Morphine, CCBs**

NOTABLE DIFFERENCES:

[1] Cocaine-related ACS:

- **Benzodiazepines** (eg, Lorazepam 2-4 mg IV every 15 minutes or as needed) to relieve symptoms. Give standard therapies (eg, Aspirin, Nitroglycerin, Heparin), but **DON'T give Beta blockers (can cause unopposed alpha-1 mediated vasoconstriction, worsening the ischemia).**

[2] Right ventricular (inferior or posterior wall) MI:

- **Give IV fluids to increase preload.**
- **CAUTIOUS use of IV Nitroglycerin or Morphine use** (may cause unsafe drop in preload); Inferior and Posterior wall MIs are more preload dependent to maintain cardiac output.
- Although Beta blockers may be used cautiously in some patients, Calcium channel blockers usually avoided due to their negative impact on contractility.

[3] Avoid Nitrates if recent Phosphodiesterase 5 inhibitor use (can cause Hypotension).

UNSTABLE ANGINA (UA)

- A type of ACS associated with critical coronary artery stenosis <u>without</u> myocardial cell death.
- **UA is characterized by: (1) ischemic symptoms suggestive of Acute coronary syndrome, (2) <u>negative cardiac biomarkers</u> Troponin and CK-MB, (3) <u>with or without ECG changes</u> indicative of ischemia (eg, ST segment depression &/or new T wave inversion).**

PATHOPHYSIOLOGY:
- **<u>Plaque rupture</u>: The most common cause is plaque rupture** of a previous nonsevere lesion with subsequent thrombus formation, leading to critical coronary artery stenosis that is not fully occlusive (so no myocardial cell death).
- Unstable plaques (eg, thin fibrous cap, large lipid core, & increased macrophages) are more prone to rupture than more stable plaques (eg, thick fibrous cap, small lipid core, & less macrophages).
- **<u>Coronary artery vasospasm</u>:** Less common cause — eg, Variant (Prinzmetal) angina or Cocaine use.

CLINICAL MANIFESTATIONS:
- **Angina is considered unstable if it presents in any of the following 3 ways: [1] rest Angina, generally lasting longer >20-30 minutes; [2] new-onset Angina,** especially if it significantly limits physical activity, or **[3] <u>change in Angina pattern</u>:** — increasing Angina that is more frequent, lasts longer, or occurs with less exertion than previous episodes of Stable angina.
- **<u>Chest discomfort</u>:** Chest discomfort (eg, pain, pressure, tightness, constriction, heaviness, or burning) in the center or the left of the chest is classically substernal, diffuse and poorly localized, exertional, **not relieved with rest &/or nitroglycerin, pain at rest, >30 minutes, or change from typical pattern** (eg, longer to resolve, increase in severity).
- May radiate to the lower jaw & teeth, left arm, epigastric area, or shoulders.

DIAGNOSIS:
- **<u>Electrocardiogram:</u> with or without ECG changes indicative of ischemia — eg, ST segment depression, new deep T wave inversions or flattening,** poor R wave progression, pseudonormalization of the T wave, or hyperacute T-waves.
- Cardiac enzymes: **Negative CK and Troponin, reflecting ischemia <u>without</u> cell death.**

MANAGEMENT OF UA/NSTEMI:
The management of UA/NSTEMI include simultaneous management consisting of:
- **<u>relief of ischemic pain</u>** — eg, Aspirin, Beta blocker, and Oxygen **(only if hypoxic)** to prevent recurrent ischemia and life-threatening ventricular arrhythmias. Morphine in select cases.
- **<u>initiation of antithrombotics</u> — dual antiplatelet therapy (Aspirin + P2Y12 receptor blocker) and anticoagulant therapies (eg, Unfractionated Heparin, Enoxaparin, Fondaparinux, Bivalirudin)** to prevent further thrombosis. **High-intensity statin.**
- **<u>risk factor assessment</u>** — long-term risk stratification with assessment of left ventricular function and either diagnostic coronary arteriography or pre-discharge stress testing. TIMI, GRACE, and PURSUIT scores are used to identify patients at highest risk for further cardiac events who may benefit from a more aggressive therapeutic approach (eg, immediate coronary arteriography and revascularization). A majority of other patients without extremely high risk undergo early coronary revascularization (eg, within 24 hours).
<u>Acute management of UA/NSTEMI:</u>
- **<u>Dual antiplatelet therapy</u> P2Y12 receptor antagonist (eg, Ticagrelor, Prasugrel, Clopidogrel) in addition to Aspirin to all patients.** Consider adding a GP IIb/IIIa inhibitor (either Eptifibatide or Tirofiban) in patients not treated with an invasive approach.
- **<u>Anticoagulant therapy</u> in all patients: eg, Unfractionated Heparin, Enoxaparin, Bivalirudin, Fondaparinux.**
- **Fibrinolytic therapy (eg, Alteplase) is harmful in UA & NSTEMI** (unlike in STEMI).

NON-ST ELEVATION MYOCARDIAL INFARCTION (NSTEMI)

- A type of ACS with **critical coronary artery stenosis <u>with</u> myocardial cell injury or death**.

CHARACTERISTICS
- **NSTEMI is characterized by: [1] ischemic symptoms suggestive of Acute coronary syndrome (ACS), [2] <u>positive cardiac biomarkers</u> elevated troponin levels** and/or CK-MB reflecting some cell death/injury, **[3] <u>with or without ECG changes</u> indicative of ischemia** (eg, new horizontal or downsloping ST-depression ≥0.5 mm in ≥2 contiguous leads and/or T wave inversion >1 mm in two contiguous leads with prominent R wave or R/S ratio >1).

PATHOPHYSIOLOGY:
- **<u>Plaque rupture</u>: The most common cause is plaque rupture** of a previous nonsevere lesion with subsequent thrombus formation, leading to critical coronary artery stenosis with some myocardial injury or cell death.
- Unstable plaques (eg, thin fibrous cap, large lipid core, increased macrophages) are more prone to rupture than more stable plaques (eg, thick fibrous cap, small lipid core, decreased amounts of macrophages).
- **<u>Coronary artery vasospasm</u>:** Less common cause: eg, Variant (Prinzmetal) angina or Cocaine use.

CLINICAL MANIFESTATIONS
- **<u>Chest discomfort</u>:** eg, pain, pressure, tightness, constriction, heaviness, or burning in the center or the left side of the chest. The pain is classically substernal, diffuse and poorly localized, exertional, **not relieved with rest &/or nitroglycerin, pain at rest, >30 minutes, or change from typical pattern** (eg, longer to resolve, increase in severity, additional symptoms).
- May radiate to the lower jaw & teeth, left arm, epigastric area, shoulders.
- <u>Levine sign:</u> clenched fist over the chest.

DIAGNOSIS:
- **<u>Electrocardiogram</u>: with or without ECG changes indicative of ischemia — eg, ST segment depression, new deep T wave inversions or flattening,** poor R wave progression, pseudonormalization of the T wave, or hyperacute T-waves.
- **<u>Cardiac biomarkers</u>: Positive (reflecting cell injury/death).** May be normal early on. Cardiac-specific troponins (eg, Troponin I and T) are the preferred cardiac biomarker because they are highly specific for detecting cardiac myocyte injury & are also more sensitive than CK-MB for myocardial necrosis, improving early detection of small myocardial infarctions.
- Although blood Troponin levels increase simultaneously with CK-MB levels (within 6 hours after the onset of infarction), they remain elevated for as long as 2 weeks. As a result, Troponin values cannot be used reliably to diagnose reinfarction (CK-MB may be more helpful to diagnose reinfarction).

MANAGEMENT
- The management of UA/NSTEMI are the same (see previous page).
- **Fibrinolytic therapy (eg, Alteplase) is harmful in UA & NSTEMI (unlike the beneficial effects of fibrinolytic use in STEMI).**

ANTERIOR AND LATERAL WALL MI

- **Complete occlusion of the left anterior descending artery (anterior) or left circumflex (lateral).**

ECG

- **Anterior MI: ST elevations >1 mm in at least 2 contiguous anterior leads (V1 through V4)** with or without reciprocal changes (ST depressions) in the inferior leads (II, III, aVF).
- **Lateral MI: ST elevations >1 mm in at least 2 contiguous lateral leads (I, aVL, V5, V6)** with or without reciprocal changes (ST depressions) in the inferior leads (II, III, aVF).
- Left bundle branch block (LBBB): **Left bundle branch block, especially when new (or not known to be old), in a patient with symptoms of an acute MI is considered to be a "STEMI equivalent" and should be treated as a STEMI.** Patients with a pre-existing LBBB can be further evaluated using Sgarbossa's criteria: ST-segment elevation of ≥1 mm that is concordant with (in the same direction as) the QRS complex; ST-segment depression of ≥1 mm in lead V1, V2, or V3; ST-segment elevation of ≥5 mm discordant with (in the opposite direction) the QRS complex.

Cardiac enzymes: **positive CK-MB &/or Troponin.**

MANAGEMENT

- **Aspirin 325 mg (non-enteric coated) to be chewed and swallowed for faster absorption.**
- **Nitroglycerin:** 3 sublingual NTG tablets (0.4 mg) one at a time, spaced 5 minutes apart, or one aerosol spray under the tongue every 5 minutes for 3 doses **if** patient has persistent chest discomfort, hypertension, or signs of heart failure **and there is no sign of hemodynamic compromise (eg, right ventricular infarction) and no use of phosphodiesterase inhibitors [eg, for erectile dysfunction (eg, Sildenafil)]; add IV Nitroglycerin for persistent symptoms.**
- Oxygen as needed if hypoxic to maintain O_2 saturation >90%. Establish IV access.
- Morphine for unacceptable, continued discomfort or anxiety related to myocardial ischemia after IV Nitrate administration when Nitrates fail to relieve the pain. Morphine is rarely used.
- **High-intensity statin (eg, Atorvastatin 80 mg daily or Rosuvastatin 20-40 mg daily)** should be initiated as early as possible in all patients with STEMI.
- Risk stratification — those with high-risk factors (eg, new Mitral regurgitation) should undergo immediate coronary angiography and revascularization because they are at extremely high risk of an adverse cardiovascular event in the short term.

Additional acute management of STEMI:

- **Beta blockers** (eg, Metoprolol 25 mg PO) to prevent further ischemia or life-threatening arrhythmias if no contraindications (eg, hypotension, cardiogenic shock, bradycardia, severe airway disease).
- **Dual antiplatelet therapy P2Y12 receptor antagonist (eg, Ticagrelor, Prasugrel, Clopidogrel) in addition to Aspirin to all patients.** Clopidogrel in patients treated with fibrinolytics; Ticagrelor if no reperfusion therapy administered or if treated with primary PCI. Consider adding a GP IIb/IIIa inhibitor (either Eptifibatide or Tirofiban) in patients not treated with an invasive approach.
- **Anticoagulant therapy:** eg, **Unfractionated Heparin or** Bivalirudin if undergoing primary PCI; **Enoxaparin** if treated with fibrinolysis; **Fondaparinux** for those at high bleeding risk.
- **ACE inhibitors** indicated for all patients following STEMI who do not have contraindications.

Reperfusion therapy:

- **Percutaneous coronary intervention (strongly preferred) or Fibrinolytics most important component of therapy and should be done as soon as possible, with certain exceptions.**
- **Percutaneous coronary intervention (PCI) ideally within 90 minutes of ED presentation of PCI-capable hospital (or transfer to a PCI capable hospital within the first 120 minutes), within 12 hours of chest pain onset, and no contraindications.** Reperfusion allows for restoration of blood flow for myocardial salvage & reduces mortality.
- **Thrombolytics within 30 minutes of ED presentation is an alternative to catheterization if PCI is not possible & within 12 hours of chest pain onset.**

RIGHT VENTRICULAR MI (INFERIOR or POSTERIOR WALL MI)

- **Acute coronary syndrome with complete occlusion of the right coronary artery (RCA) through the RV marginal branches in 80%.** 20% from posterior descending artery, a branch of the LCA.

PHYSICAL EXAMINATION
- **Bradycardia or atrioventricular heart blocks** the RCA supplies the AV node in 90% so bradycardia may be due to AV nodal dysfunction (less commonly sinoatrial dysfunction) due to ischemia, activation of cardioinhibitory reflexes, or both. Tachycardia may be seen due to increased sympathetic activity from decreased cardiac output or anxiety.
- **Fourth heart sound: may have an S4 gallop** (especially with inferior wall MI).
- **Hypotension is commonly seen with large RVMI** (may be accompanied by shock).
- **Triad of right ventricular infarction: [1] increased JVD (jugular venous distention) + [2] clear lungs + [3] positive Kussmaul sign.**

ELECTROCARDIOGRAM
- **Inferior MI: ST elevations >1 mm in ≥2 contiguous inferior leads (II, III, aVF)** with or without reciprocal changes (ST depressions) in the lateral leads (I and aVL).
- **Posterior MI: ST depressions: often horizontal ST depressions in ≥2 contiguous anterior leads (V1 through V4), tall broad R waves (>30 ms), or dominant R wave (R/S ratio >1) in V2.** Because the standard ECG does not look directly at the posterior heart, these changes occur because the standard ECG sees the "ST elevation MI" backwards (ST depressions) and the "Q waves" backwards (as tall broad R waves).
- **Right-sided ECGs may increase the diagnosis if visualization of ST elevations in V4R-V6R (ST elevation >1 mm in lead V4R** has a sensitivity & specificity for >90%).

MANAGEMENT
- Treated in a manner similar to those with acute left ventricular ST-elevation MI, including Aspirin, oxygen (if hypoxic), reperfusion therapy (PCI preferred or thrombolytics), dual oral antiplatelet therapy (Aspirin plus a platelet P2Y12 receptor blocker), statin therapy, and an anticoagulant.
- Although Beta blockers can be used in some patients, **medications to improve chest pain (eg, Nitrates, Opioids, and Beta blockers) should be used with caution due to their potential to negatively impact preload, leading to hypotension (Opioids and Nitrates) or decreased heart rate and contractility (Beta blockers and Calcium channel blockers).** This is because Inferior and Posterior wall MIs are more preload dependent to maintain cardiac output.
- **Volume loading: Because the right heart is more dependent on preload, IV fluids (eg, Normal saline) improve preload and forward flow out of the right ventricle.** IV fluids should be given to patients with evidence of low cardiac output [eg, hypotension, hypoperfusion, and a low or normal jugular venous pressure (JVP)] who do not have pulmonary congestion or evidence of right heart failure. In most cases, a carefully monitored volume challenge is initiated by infusing small amounts (200-300 mL) of Normal saline with continuing assessment of JVP and blood pressure.

Other considerations:
- Correct any electrolyte abnormalities, especially hypokalemia and hypomagnesemia, which often occur simultaneously. Maintain the serum potassium concentration >4.0 mEq/L and a serum magnesium concentration >2.0 mEq/L (2.4 mg/dL or 1 mmol/L) during the acute phase.

MEDICATIONS TO AVOID
- **NSAIDs (except Aspirin) should be discontinued immediately if possible** due to an increased risk of cardiovascular events associated with their use.
- Although Beta blockers can be used in some patients, **medications to improve chest pain (eg, Nitrates, Opioids, and Beta blockers) should be used with caution due to their potential to negatively impact preload, leading to hypotension (Opioids and Nitrates) or heart rate and contractility (Beta blockers and Calcium channel blockers).** This is because Inferior and Posterior wall MIs are more preload dependent to maintain cardiac output.

CONSERVATIVE MANAGEMENT

- Used in patients whose chest pain began >12 hours (without current/active chest pain) or low TIMI:
  - **Aspirin (± Clopidogrel** x 9 months), **statin, beta blocker, ACE Inhibitor. Nitroglycerin** as needed.
- For patients with symptoms of >12 hours, fibrinolytic therapy is not indicated, but emergent PCI may be considered, especially for patients with evidence of ongoing ischemia or high-risk features.

COMPLICATIONS OF MYOCARDIAL INFARCTION

- **Arrhythmias (eg, ventricular fibrillation), ventricular aneurysm/rupture,** cardiogenic shock, papillary muscle dysfunction, heart failure, left ventricular wall rupture.
- **Dressler syndrome: post-MI pericarditis + fever + pulmonary infiltrates.**

ADJUNCTIVE THERAPY	
Drug	**Comment**
ß-blockers _Cardioselective: • **Metoprolol** • **Atenolol**	Mechanism of action: • Beta-receptor blockade leads to decrease in cardiac output, myocardial oxygen demand, blood pressure, heart rate, & contractility (except those with intrinsic sympathetic activity); decreased renin secretion, decreased post myocardial infarction-induced ventricular remodeling. Often titrated to pulse <70 beats per minute. Indications: • Stable angina, ACS (eg, Unstable angina, non-ST elevation MI, ST elevation MI) • STEMI: **15% ↓in mortality in STEMI** (decrease wall tension & prevent MI complications). Adverse effects: • Fatigue, depression, erectile dysfunction, bronchospasm. Contraindications: • **Decompensated (congestive) heart failure, bradycardia (HR <50 bpm), heart block (2ⁿᵈ/3ʳᵈ), hypotension (SBP <100 mmHg), severe reactive airway disease** (severe Asthma/COPD), **shock, cocaine-induced MI** (causes unopposed ↑alpha-1 mediated vasoconstriction).
Nitrates	Mechanism of action: • **Increased myocardial blood supply** – increase coronary artery blood flow & collateral circulation as well as reduces coronary artery vasospasm. Vasodilatation occurs due to stimulation of guanylate cyclase, which increases cGMP. • Decreased cardiac demand – **decreases preload & afterload.** Routes: • Sublingual, translingual, transdermal, transmucosal, ointment, IV, oral sustained-release. Indications: • **Stable angina, Acute coronary syndrome, Pulmonary edema, Heart failure, Decompensated heart failure,** hypertensive emergencies, vasospastic disorders (eg, Prinzmetal angina), Esophageal varices (prophylaxis). • Administration: administered sublingual if chest pain occurs. Given up to 3 doses 5 minutes apart. Can be used prophylactically 5 minutes before an activity likely to cause ischemia. Adverse effects: • **Headache, flushing, tolerance, hypotension, peripheral edema, tachyphylaxis** after 24 hours (allow for nitrate-free period for 8 hours), reflex tachycardia. Deteriorates with light, moisture, and air. **Contraindications for IV Nitrates:** • **Hypotension (systolic blood pressure <90 mm Hg), RV infarction** (inferior or posterior wall MI), **& use of phosphodiesterase-5 inhibitors (eg, Sildenafil, Tadalafil).**
ACE Inhibitors	Indications: • **STEMI: slows progression of CHF during & after STEMI by ↓ventricular remodeling,** (↓mortality) especially in patients with HF, STEMI, LBBB, ejection fraction <40%. • Given within the first 12-24 hours, after the patient is stabilized. • Adverse effects: **angioedema & cough (due to ↑bradykinin, a potent vasodilator),** renal failure, **Hyperkalemia.** • Contraindications: severe hypotension (SBP <100 mmHg), renal failure, pregnancy.
Morphine	Relieves pain, ↓anxiety, and venodilation ⇨ ↓preload.

ANTITHROMBOTIC & ANTIPLATET TREATMENT

ANTI-PLATELET DRUGS	
Aspirin	**Prevents platelet activation/aggregation.** Inhibits cyclooxygenase ⇨ ↓thromboxane A$_2$. **Chewed for faster absorption.** 20% reduction in death from MI.
ADP INHIBITORS **Clopidogrel** Prasugrel Ticlopidine	Indications: **Good in patients with Aspirin allergy.** Give if conservative strategy or if PCI planned. 20% ↓in death/MI/stroke. Mechanism of action: **inhibits ADP-mediated platelet aggregation.** Caution if CABG planned within 7 days, hepatic/renal impairment, bleeding.
GP IIb/IIIa Inhibitors Eptifibatide, Tirofiban Abciximab	MOA: inhibits the final pathway for platelet aggregation. Indication: good for UA, NSTEMI, patients undergoing PCI. CI: internal bleeding within 30 days; major trauma/surgery, thrombocytopenia.
ANTICOAGULANTS	
UNFRACTIONATED HEPARIN	MOA: **binds to & potentiates antithrombin III's ability to inactivate Factor Xa, inactivates thrombin (Factor IIa),** inhibiting fibrin formation. Prevents new clot formation (however, does not dissolve existing clots). Ind: **ACS patients with ECG changes or ⊕ cardiac markers** (↓ in death/MI).
LOW MOLECULAR WEIGHT HEPARIN **Enoxaparin** Dalteparin	MOA: **binds to & potentiates antithrombin III's ability to inactivate Factor Xa.** LMWH more specific to Factor Xa than UFH. Ind: **Same as UFH.** LMWH superior to UFH: longer ½ life (~12 hours) no need for IV infusion or PTT monitoring, ↓incidence of Heparin-induced thrombocytopenia, more reliable dosing. Long ½ life may be an issue for CABG. S/E: **thrombocytopenia** (obtain CBC prior to use). Obtain serum creatinine level (must be renally dosed if renal impairment to prevent complications).
Fondaparinux	Direct factor Xa inhibitor (binds to & enhances antithrombin). No direct effect on thrombin.

To form a clot, Factor Xa converts prothrombin (II) ⇨ thrombin (Factor IIa). Thrombin activates fibrinogen ⇨ fibrin clot.

REPERFUSION IN ST ELEVATION MI (STEMI)

- **Mainstay of treatment — done within 12 hours of symptom onset or if ongoing chest pain.**
- **Either [1] PCI** (percutaneous transluminal coronary angioplasty) **or [2] thrombolytics.**

PCI (Percutaneous Coronary Intervention):

- **Best within 3 hours of symptom onset (especially within 90 minutes). PCI superior to thrombolytics.**
- Useful especially for cardiogenic shock, large anterior MI, prior CABG, and if thrombolytics are contraindicated.
- Coronary Artery Bypass Graft: 3-vessel disease, L main coronary artery, ↓left ventricle EF <40%.

THROMBOLYTIC (FIBRINOLYTIC) THERAPY: Used if PCI is not an option/unable to get PCI early (90-120 m).

THROMBOLYTIC (FIBRINOLYTIC) THERAPY	
Drug	**Comments**
Tissue Plasminogen Activators:	MOA: **dissolves clot by activating tissue plasminogen ⇨ plasmin.** Plasmin is a proteolytic enzyme that degrades fibrin.
• **Alteplase (rTPA)**	Ind: **STEMI (earlier patency of coronary artery, shorter half-life),** thrombotic strokes, pulmonary embolism. S/E: **higher rebleed risk.** Expensive.
• Reteplase (RPA)	↑ potency. Used in STEMI, pulmonary embolism.
• Tenecteplase (TNK)	Long ½ life. Used in STEMI.
Streptokinase	MOA: binds to plasminogen, activating it into plasmin. Derived from streptococcus. Ind: Less effective than TPA so only used in patients in whom PCI is contraindicated & patient has a high risk of intracerebral hemorrhage **(least chance of intracranial bleeding with streptokinase), less expensive.** S/E: derived from streptococcus so usually only given once (tolerance develops).

Unlike antithrombotic drugs that prevents new clots, thrombolytics (fibrinolytics) dissolve existing clots.

VASOSPASTIC (VARIANT, PRINZMETAL) ANGINA

- Spontaneous episodes of transient ischemia (angina) accompanied by transient ischemic ST changes on ECG due to <u>epicardial coronary artery vasospasm (vasoconstriction).</u>

PATHOPHYSIOLOGY

- **<u>Coronary artery vasospasm:</u>** diffuse or segmental spasm of the smooth muscle layer of the epicardial coronary arterial wall may result in transient ST segment elevation & transmural ischemia.
- <u>Endothelial dysfunction</u> and vascular smooth muscle hyperreactivity.

TRIGGERS

- **Cold weather, vasoconstrictors, or <u>alpha agonists</u>** [eg, Pseudoephedrine, Oxymetazoline, Amphetamines, cocaine use (especially with cigarette smoking history), and Sumatriptan].
- **Hyperventilation;** Coronary manipulation through cardiac catheterization, Marijuana, Alcohol. **Although exercise is a potential trigger, exercise doesn't usually provoke episodes.**

RISK FACTORS

- Females, smoking, **other vasospastic disorders** (eg, Raynaud phenomenon, Migraine). **Compared to Stable angina, patients with Vasospastic angina are often younger (<50 years) and exhibit fewer classic cardiovascular risk factors (except for cigarette smoking).** Magnesium deficiency.

CLINICAL MANIFESTATIONS

- **<u>Chest pain:</u> mainly at rest (especially midnight to early morning), usually not triggered by exertion nor relieved with rest as is typical Angina.** Often, the patient is younger with few or no classical cardiovascular risk factors. Episodes last between 5-15 minutes but may be persistent.

DIAGNOSIS

- <u>ECG:</u> **transient <u>ST elevations</u> in the pattern of the affected artery that resolve with symptom resolution (<u>ST elevations may resolve with Nitroglycerin</u> or Calcium channel blockers).** May have ST depressions. The ECG is usually normal between anginal episodes.
- **<u>Angiography:</u>** rules out coronary artery disease: **[1] <u>No significant obstruction of major coronary artery vessels</u> (no evidence of high-grade stenosis)** and **[2] <u>coronary vasospasm</u> during angiography** (>90% constriction), **especially with the use of Ergonovine,** hyperventilation, or Acetylcholine; spasms responsive to intracoronary Nitroglycerin or Calcium channel blockers.

MANAGEMENT

- Initial therapy includes cessation of smoking and pharmacologic therapy with Calcium channel blockers and sublingual Nitroglycerin as needed for symptoms of Angina.
- **<u>Calcium channel blockers</u> mainstay of therapy — eg, Diltiazem, Amlodipine, long-acting Nifedipine** cause vasodilation effect in the coronary vasculature and prevent vasoconstriction, alleviating symptoms. The use of a long-acting calcium antagonist is recommended to be given at night as the episodes of vasospasm are more frequent at midnight and early in the morning.
- **<u>Short-acting nitrates:</u> sublingual Nitroglycerin with the onset of anginal episodes can be used to decrease both the duration of symptoms and ischemia.**
- **<u>Long-acting Nitrates:</u> second-line** due to the occurrence of tolerance with chronic use. Long-acting Nitrates can be added in patients on CCBs without an adequate response to treatment. Nitrates produce direct endothelium vasodilatation, prevent vasospasm, & reduce preload.
- Nicorandil, a nitrate and K-channel activator also suppress vasospastic attacks.
- <u>During an acute chest pain episode</u> prior to the diagnosis of Variant angina, Aspirin and Heparin may be given until atherosclerotic disease is ruled out.

<u>Medications to avoid:</u>

- **<u>Beta blockers</u> (especially non-selective Beta blockers) are usually avoided** as they may lead to unopposed alpha-mediated vasoconstriction and vasospasm. Aspirin should be used with caution.

COCAINE-INDUCED MYOCARDIAL ISCHEMIA OR INFARCTION

PATHOPHYSIOLOGY
- **Coronary artery vasospasm** due to cocaine's activation of the sympathetic nervous system & alpha-1 receptors ⇨ vasoconstriction of the coronary arteries. Ischemia is also caused by a prothrombotic state in the coronary circulation, and increases in heart rate and blood pressure, which increase myocardial demand for oxygen consumption.
- Myocardial infarction may occur if vasoconstriction is prolonged (due to decreased blood flow).

CLINICAL MANIFESTATIONS
- **Chest pain or discomfort:** Cocaine-induced myocardial ischemia symptoms are **indistinguishable from other causes of myocardial ischemia.**
- Associated symptoms: The chest pain is often accompanied by anxiety, dyspnea, palpitations, and nausea.
- Focal neurological & extremity symptoms may suggest vascular complications (eg, Aortic dissection).

PHYSICAL EXAMINATION
- Vital signs: Hypertension and tachycardia almost universal; hyperthermia may occur.
- CNS: agitation common; focal signs suggest cerebrovascular accident (CVA).
- Pupils: Mydriasis common.
- Lungs: Decreased breath sounds after smoking crack suggest Pneumothorax.
- Extremities: Decreased pulses suggest vascular complications (eg, Aortic dissection).

DIAGNOSIS
- **ECG: transient ST elevations classic.** May induce Myocardial infarction if prolonged constriction.
- Laboratory evaluation: fingerstick glucose, Acetaminophen and salicylate levels, and urine pregnancy test in women of childbearing age. Urine toxicology screening & cardiac enzymes.

MANAGEMENT
Cocaine-associated Myocardial ischemia:
- **Calcium channel blockers & Nitrates are the drugs of choice to reverse the vasospasm.**
- **Often treated with Aspirin, Heparin, & Benzodiazepines until atherosclerotic disease is ruled out.**
- **Aspirin** 325 mg oral (nonenteric coated) should be given to the patient to chew and swallow (assuming Aortic dissection not suspected).
- **Nitroglycerin** 0.4 mg sublingual up to 3 doses every 5 minutes, with or without continuous infusion.
- Phentolamine 1-5 mg IV, repeat as necessary; hold for SBP <100 mmHg.
- **Avoid nonselective β-blockers in cocaine-induced MI — increased risk of vasospasm (unopposed alpha-1 mediated constriction).** If Beta blockers are to be used, mixed alpha/beta blockers (eg, Labetalol and Carvedilol) should be used rather than nonselective beta blockers.

Psychomotor agitation:
- **Benzodiazepine:** Administer Diazepam (5 mg IV) or lorazepam (1 mg IV) every 3 to 5 minutes until agitation is controlled. Also helpful for Hypertension; may repeat as necessary.

STEMI & recent cocaine use
- In addition to above, patients with STEMI and recent cocaine use should proceed to reperfusion via either (1) coronary angiography and primary percutaneous coronary intervention (if indicated, usually preferred over fibrinolysis) or (2) fibrinolytic therapy is an alternative when timely coronary angiography is not feasible.

HEART FAILURE (HF)

- Inability of the heart to pump sufficient blood to meet the metabolic demands of the body at normal filling pressures.

TYPES
- **Left-sided: Coronary artery disease most common cause. Hypertension** (due to increased afterload), **valvular disease** [Aortic stenosis causes pressure overload (increased afterload) and regurgitant valve disease causes volume overload], Cardiomyopathies.
- **Right-sided: Left-sided Heart failure most common cause. Pulmonary disease** (eg, COPD, Pulmonary hypertension); Mitral stenosis.

- **HF with reduced ejection fraction (HFrEF) due to systolic dysfunction. Post myocardial infarction most common etiology,** myocarditis, dilated cardiomyopathy. HFrEF is associated with **decreased ejection fraction and S3 gallop.**
- **Heart failure with preserved ejection fraction (HFpEF) characterized by diastolic dysfunction & normal or increased ejection fraction. Etiologies include longstanding Hypertension (eg, in the elderly),** Left ventricular hypertrophy (LVH), & valvular heart disease.

PATHOPHYSIOLOGY
- **[1] Initial injury:** an initial injury to the heart leads to (1) pathologic increase in preload, (2) increase in afterload, and/or (3) decrease in contractility, subsequently decreasing cardiac output (CO).
- **[2] Compensatory responses:** After a Myocardial infarction and other pathological insults, compensatory responses, such as activation of the Renin angiotensin aldosterone system, increased sympathetic activity, and ventricular remodeling confer short-term benefit.
- **[3] Decompensation:** However, long-term activation of these compensatory responses are maladaptive, leading to sodium, water, and volume overload (continued RAAS activation), and pathological ventricular remodeling (dilatation of the ventricular walls and systolic dysfunction). Lower cardiac output results in reduction of renal blood flow and glomerular filtration rate, which leads to further sodium and fluid retention.

CLINICAL MANIFESTATIONS
Left-sided Heart failure:
- **Pulmonary symptoms:** increased pulmonary venous pressure from **fluid backing up into the lungs** (Think **L for Lungs and L-sided**).
- **Dyspnea: progressive dyspnea most common symptom** — includes exertional dyspnea, which may progress to orthopnea (on lying flat), paroxysmal nocturnal dyspnea, or dyspnea at rest. **May have exercise intolerance or fatigue.** Fluid retention may contribute to the symptoms.
- **Cough:** chronic, nonproductive cough or productive with pink, frothy sputum, worse in the supine position or at night. **Rales may be heard on examination.**

Right-sided Heart failure:
- **Systemic symptoms of peripheral and abdominal congestion** due to increased systemic venous pressure from fluid backing up into the "roads" **[R for R-sided and 3 Roads to the heart = inferior vena cava (IVC), Superior vena cava (SVC), & hepatic circulation].**
- **Peripheral edema:** pitting edema of the legs, cyanosis. May have increased body weight.
- **Jugular venous distention** due to increased jugular venous pressure.
- **GI & hepatic congestion:** anorexia, loss of appetite, nausea, vomiting, hepatojugular reflux (increased JVP with liver palpation), hepatosplenomegaly, ascites.

Noncardiac symptoms:
- Anorexia, nausea, fatigue, weakness, nocturia, and memory impairment.

PHYSICAL EXAMINATION

Signs due to congestion (eg, dyspnea, fatigue, and fluid retention):

Lungs:

- **Crackles (rales) due to fluid in the alveoli; rhonchi, or expiratory wheezing.**
- Diminished air entry at the lung bases if a Pleural effusion is present (more common on the right side).
- Tachypnea (rapid, shallow breathing).
- Advanced disease: **Cheyne-Stokes breathing** — deeper, faster breathing with gradual decrease & periods of apnea. Cyanosis.

Peripheral:

- **Lower extremity edema (especially in the pretibial region and ankles in ambulatory patients** with sacral edema in bedridden patients), elevated jugular venous pressure.
- Pulsus alternans.
- Dusky pale skin, diaphoresis, and cool lower extremities may be suggestive of worsened cardiac output "cold and wet".
- Abdomen: Epigastric tenderness, positive hepatojugular reflex (sustained moderate pressure on the liver may increase jugular venous pressure); tender and enlarged liver. Ascites or hepatomegaly may be seen.

Cardiac examination:

- **S3 gallop: advanced systolic dysfunction associated with a third heart sound (S3 gallop) due to rapid filling of a dilated ventricle;** laterally displaced apex beat.
- A murmur of Mitral regurgitation is often audible when the left ventricle (LV) is markedly enlarged, or a Tricuspid regurgitation murmur is present when the right ventricle is volume or pressure overloaded.
- **S4 gallop: with diastolic dysfunction** due to atrial contraction into a stiff noncompliant ventricle.

DIAGNOSIS:

Echocardiogram:

- Indications: **diagnostic test of choice in an outpatient setting to make the diagnosis of Heart failure.** Doppler echocardiography is helpful in the diagnosis and classification of HF, enables evaluation of ventricular size, global and regional systolic function, diastolic function, valvular disease, & pericardial disease. It measures ejection fraction, assesses ventricular function, and may reveal the cause **(ejection fraction most important determinant of prognosis).**
- **Heart failure with reduced ejection fraction:** (HFrEF) — **decreased ejection fraction, thin ventricular walls, and dilated LV chamber cavity due to systolic dysfunction.**
- **Heart failure with preserved ejection fraction:** (HFpEF) — **normal or increased ejection fraction, thick ventricular walls, and small LV chamber cavity due to diastolic dysfunction.**

Electrocardiogram (ECG):

- Assesses for evidence of ACS (myocardial ischemia or MI) and dysrhythmias (eg, Atrial fibrillation).
- The ECG may also identify other predisposing or precipitating conditions for HF such (eg, ventricular hypertrophy or left atrial abnormalities). ECG findings often nonspecific.

Labs:

- Serum electrolytes, renal tests (eg, BUN, creatinine, urinalysis), CBC, lipid levels, LFTs, TSH, cardiac markers if there is a concern for cardiac injury,

NEW YORK HEART ASSOCIATION FUNCTIONAL CLASS
Class I — No symptoms, no limitation during ordinary physical activity.
Class II — Mild symptoms (dyspnea &/or angina), slight limitation during ordinary activity.
Class III —Symptoms cause marked limitation in activity (even with minimal exertion) comfortable only at rest.
Class IV — Symptoms even while at rest, severe limitations, & inability to carry out physical activity.

MANAGEMENT OF HEART FAILURE WITH REDUCED EJECTION FRACTION (HFrEF)
LIFESTYLE MODIFICATION
- <u>Self-management:</u> includes daily monitoring of signs and symptoms (including daily weight monitoring to detect fluid accumulation) and lifestyle modifications.
- **<u>Sodium restriction:</u>** 3 g/day with avoidance of excessive intake >6 g/day.
- **<u>Fluid restriction:</u>** 1.5-2 L/day only in patients with refractory (stage D, class IV) HF or symptomatic or severe Hyponatremia (serum sodium <120 mEq/L).
- Smoking cessation, alcohol abstinence or restriction. <u>Weight management</u> avoidance of obesity.

<u>Guideline-directed medical therapy</u> (GDMT) for Heart failure (HF) with reduced ejection fraction (HFrEF) who have New York Heart Association (NYHA) class 2-4 **now includes <u>4 medication classes</u>:**
- **[1] <u>Angiotensin system blocker</u> — <u>Angiotensin receptor neprilysin inhibitor</u> (Sacubitril-Valsartan) most effective. ACE inhibitors alternative.** Angiotensin receptor blocker (ARB).

- **[2] <u>Beta-blockers</u> eg, Carvedilol, Carvedilol CR, Bisoprolol, Metoprolol succinate CR.**

- **[3] <u>Mineralocorticoid receptor antagonist (MRA):</u> eg, Eplerenone, Spironolactone.**

- **[4] <u>Sodium glucose cotransporter-2 inhibitors (SGL2i):</u> eg, Dapagliflozin or Empagliflozin preferred;** Canagliflozin an alternative.

SECONDARY THERAPY
- **[1] <u>Isosorbide dinitrate plus Hydralazine</u>: alternative to ARNI, ACE inhibitor, ARB; additional therapy for persistent symptoms; antihypertensive.**
- **[2] <u>Ivabradine</u>:** Additional therapy for persistent symptoms; most appropriate for patients in sinus rhythm with HR ≥70 bpm despite maximal Beta blocker therapy.
- [3] <u>Vericiguat</u>: Additional therapy for persistent symptoms; rarely used.
- [4] <u>Digoxin</u>: Additional therapy for persistent symptoms; rarely used.

OTHER THERAPIES
- **An implantable cardioverter-defibrillator (ICD) for primary or secondary prevention of SCD in patients with an ejection fraction (EF) ≤35% and clinical Heart failure is well established** (an arrhythmia can be lethal in these patients).
- <u>Biventricular pacing</u> (resynchronization) if EF ≤35% & QRS duration of 120 msec or more, in addition to optimal medical therapy, reduces mortality & hospitalization from any cause by ~20%.

THERAPIES THAT SHOULD BE AVOIDED:
- **<u>Thiazolidinediones</u>** (glitazones) can worsen or precipitate Heart failure.
- **<u>Most Calcium channel blockers</u> (with the exception of Amlodipine and Felodipine) because there is no mortality benefit from non-Dihydropyridine Calcium channel blockers with negative inotropy (Diltiazem, Verapamil) in the management of HFrEF and there may be a possible deleterious effect** of the use of non-Dihydropyridines. Amlodipine appears to be safe in HF and may be used if a CCB is necessary for a concomitant disease, such as Hypertension or Angina.
- **<u>NSAIDs:</u>** Nonsteroidal anti-inflammatory medications, and Cyclooxygenase-2 inhibitors (eg, Celecoxib) can lead to sodium and water retention as well as renal impairment.
- Combination of an ACE inhibitors, ARB, and aldosterone blocker - increases the risk of hyperkalemia.

ANGIOTENSIN RECEPTOR-NEPRILYSIN INHIBITOR (SACUBITRIL-VALSARTAN)

Mechanism of action:
- **Combined increased BNP + ARB effects:** Sacubitril is an angiotensin receptor neprilysin inhibitor ⇨ inhibiting neprilysin reduces breakdown of beneficial peptides (eg, **inhibits metabolism of natriuretic peptides, such as BNP).**

Indications:
- NYHA class II-III symptoms and LVEF ≤40% who are appropriately treated for volume overload and who are otherwise clinically well-compensated.
- **Most effective drug for HFrEF & superior to ACE inhibitors.** Improving outcomes: **strongest for ARNI,** intermediate for ACE inhibitor, weakest for Angiotensin receptor blocker (ARB). ARNI became the preferred agent for patients in whom there is no history of angioedema due to a 20% reduction of death & hospitalization (PARADIGM-HF trial).
- **Patients who have a systolic blood pressure ≥100 mmHg and who can reliably afford the drug.** Other vasodilator therapies, except for vasodilating Beta blockers and Mineralocorticoid receptor antagonists (MRAs), should be discontinued to allow for therapy with Sacubitril-Valsartan.

Adverse effects:
- **Higher rates of hypotension & non-serious angioedema** (especially in Blacks) compared to Enalapril.
- Sacubitril-Valsartan inhibits the breakdown of BNP. Therefore, BNP will typically be elevated in patients being treated with Sacubitril-Valsartan, and BNP may not be a reliable marker of Heart failure exacerbation in these patients.

Contraindications:
- Pregnancy (risk of fetal toxicity & death), history of angioedema (of any cause), severe hepatic impairment (Child-Pugh C classification), and chronic kidney disease.
- Not used concomitantly with ACEIs (increased risk of angioedema), Aliskiren in patients with Diabetes mellitus, or another Angiotensin II receptor blocker (ARB) to avoid dual ARB therapy.
- Hypotension or decompensated heart failure. Use of ACE inhibitor within the past 36 hours.

MINERALOCORTICOID RECEPTOR ANTAGONIST (MRA)

Eplerenone, Spironolactone

Rationale:
- **Reduced mortality** due to aldosterone antagonism: Mortality benefit: Mediates some of the major effects of Renin–angiotensin–aldosterone system (RAAS) activation, such as myocardial remodeling and fibrosis, as well as sodium retention and potassium loss at the distal tubules.

Indications:
- **HFrEF:** part of the 4 pillars of treatment of HFrEF.
- **HFpEF: used in combination with SGLT2 inhibitors in HFpEF.**

Sequence of therapy:
- **MRA therapy soon after initiation of a RAAS-neprilysin inhibitor and a Beta blocker,** while allowing enough time to assess the effect of these other agents on renal function, Hyperkalemia, and overall clinical stability.

Adverse effects:
- **Hyperkalemia** due to aldosterone antagonism (normally aldosterone causes sodium retention at the expense of increased potassium and hydrogen ion renal secretion; by blocking aldosterone, the opposite occurs).
- **Blockage of testosterone & progesterone: gynecomastia, breast pain, menstrual irregularities, erectile dysfunction, decreased libido.**
- **Eplerenone may be preferred due to lower risk of endocrine adverse effects** (eg, gynecomastia, erectile dysfunction in males). However, Spironolactone is cheaper if cost is a barrier to treatment with Eplerenone. Eplerenone has similar adverse effect profile but greater specificity for the mineralocorticoid receptor.

DRUG/INTERVENTION	COMMENTS
ACE INHIBITORS **"PRILS"** Captopril Enalapril Ramipril Benazepril Lisinopril Quinapril Trandolapril	Mechanism of action (MOA): • Reduce preload, afterload, ventricular remodeling, aldosterone secretion, salt and water retention, and vascular resistance. Indications: • **Most effective <u>singular</u> medication for mortality benefit in HFrEF,** decreased rehospitalization. • **<u>Reduced mortality</u>**: Improved survival in patients with LV systolic dysfunction (LVEF ≤40%). Prevent or slow progression of HF, lower MI rate. Adverse effects: • **Hyperkalemia. Nonproductive cough & angioedema (due to increased bradykinin),** first-dose hypotension, azotemia, renal insufficiency in occasional patients with preexisting renal vascular disease (**although ACE inhibitors generally *protect* the diabetic and proteinuric kidney**). Contraindications: • **Pregnancy** (teratogenic), hypotension, severe renal insufficiency, bilateral renal artery stenosis. History of angioedema. • Although there has been some concern about their effectiveness in Blacks, the available evidence is **not** sufficient to support a difference in ACE inhibitor use based on race.
BETA-BLOCKERS Nonselective ($\beta_{1,2}, \alpha_1$) - **Carvedilol** - **Carvedilol CR** Cardioselective (β_1 only) - **Metoprolol succinate** - **Bisoprolol**	Mechanism of action: • Decrease harmful effects of sustained sympathetic & renin activation, **reduce ventricular size & remodeling,** increase ejection fraction (EF) long-term (after initial transient decrease in EF for the first 1- 10 weeks), & prevent arrhythmias. Start at low doses and titrate upwards. • **<u>Reduction of excessive sympathetic stimulation</u>: Anti-ischemic & antiarrhythmic effect** (decreased O_2 consumption). Indications: • **Heart failure with reduced ejection fraction with no or minimal current evidence of fluid retention** (especially class II –III HF). • **<u>Decreased mortality</u>**: 35% (increase EF average ~10% over time and reduces ventricular size/mass. Decrease afterload. • Beta blockers commonly initiated after optimal treatment for volume overload & soon after the patient has started an ARNI, ACE inhibitor, or ARB. Adverse effects: • **<u>Decompensated HF</u>: discontinue or reduce beta-blocker dose in decompensated HF.** Caution if NYHA class IV (4) HF or Stage D HF. • **<u>Second- or third-degree AV blocks</u>** in the absence of a pacemaker. • **<u>Bradycardia</u>: Heart rate <50 bpm** (unless pacemaker is present). • **<u>Hypotension</u>: SBP <90 mmHg** or symptomatic hypotension.
ANGIOTENSIN II RECEPTOR BLOCKERS (ARB) Losartan Valsartan Candesartan Irbesartan	Mechanism of action • **Blocks effects of angiotensin II** (not its production, so there is no increase in bradykinin ⇨ no cough or angioedema). Indications: • **Patients unable to tolerate ACE inhibitors.** Adverse effects: Hyperkalemia. Contraindicated in pregnancy (teratogenic).
HYDRALAZINE + NITRATES COMBINED	Mechanism of action: • Nitroglycerin decreases preload & afterload, Hydralazine decreases afterload. Indications: • **<u>Isosorbide dinitrate plus Hydralazine</u>: Alternative to ARNI, ACE inhibitor, ARB; additional therapy for persistent symptoms; antihypertensive.** • **The combination is associated with decreased mortality in HFrEF.** Adverse effects: • Dizziness, headache, tachyphylaxis (8 hour nitrate-free period to prevent it).

DIURETICS **POTASSIUM SPARING DIURETICS** 　**Spironolactone** 　**Eplerenone**	Mechanism of action: • **Decreased mortality** due to aldosterone antagonism. • Mediates some of the major effects of Renin–angiotensin–aldosterone system (RAAS) activation (eg, myocardial remodeling and fibrosis, as well as sodium retention and potassium loss at the distal tubules). Indications: • **MRA therapy soon after initiation of a RAAS-neprilysin inhibitor and a Beta blocker,** while allowing enough time to assess the effect of these other agents on renal function, Hyperkalemia, and overall clinical stability. Adverse effects: • **Hyperkalemia** due to aldosterone antagonism (normally aldosterone causes sodium retention at the expense of increased potassium and hydrogen ion renal secretion; by blocking aldosterone, the opposite occurs). • **Blockage of testosterone & progesterone**: gynecomastia, breast pain, menstrual irregularities, erectile dysfunction, decreased libido. • **Eplerenone may be preferred due to lower risk of endocrine adverse effects** (eg, gynecomastia, erectile dysfunction in males). However, Spironolactone is cheaper if cost is a barrier to treatment with Eplerenone. Eplerenone has similar adverse effect profile but greater specificity for the mineralocorticoid receptor.
LOOP DIURETICS 　**Furosemide** (Lasix) 　**Bumetanide** 　**Torsemide**	Mechanism of action: • Inhibits water transport across Loop of Henle ⇨ ↑excretion of H_2O, Cl^-, Na^+, K^+. Indications: • **Most effective treatment for symptoms for mild-moderate ADHF (CHF).** Adverse effects: • Volume depletion decreased electrolytes (Cl^-, Na^+, K^+), **hyperglycemia, hyperuricemia**, sulfa allergies, hypochloremic metabolic alkalosis. Contraindications: • Renal failure, hyponatremia.
Hydrochlorothiazide **Metolazone**	Adverse effects: • **Increased "GLUC":** <u>G</u>lucose (Hyperglycemia), <u>L</u>ipids (Dyslipidemia), <u>U</u>ric acid (Hyperuricemia), and <u>C</u>alcium (Hypercalcemia). • Hyponatremia, Hypokalemia, hypochloremic metabolic alkalosis. • Sulfa allergies

↓PRELOAD

SYMPATHOMIMETICS **(Positive Inotropes)** **DIGOXIN**	Mechanism of action: • Cardiac glycoside that is a **positive inotrope** (increased contraction), negative chronotrope (decreases heart rate by increasing vagal tone), and **negative dromotrope** (slows conduction velocity). Its positive inotropic effects are due to Na^+/K^+ pump inhibition, increasing calcium-mediated contraction. Indications: • **HFrEF (Systolic heart failure)** — **decreases rate of hospitalization in advanced HF but does not decrease mortality.** • **Atrial fibrillation** (eg, patients in whom Beta blockers and/or Calcium channel blockers are contraindicated, such as hypotension or ADHF). Adverse effects: • <u>CNS:</u> seizures, dizziness. • <u>GI:</u> anorexia common early finding, nausea, vomiting, diarrhea. • Gynecomastia. • <u>Digitalis effect on ECG:</u> PVCs most common, **downsloping of the ST segment.** • Visual: double/blurred vision green/yellow disturbances, halos around lights. • Arrhythmias (especially with hypokalemia or myocardial ischemia present; typically supraventricular arrhythmias with heart block or atrial or ventricular extrasystole. <u>Digitalis toxicity</u> • **Digitalis toxicity directly causes Hyperkalemia but Hypokalemia predisposes to Digoxin toxicity.** • <u>Clinical manifestations:</u> **GI symptoms most common** (nausea, vomiting, abdominal pain), **visual changes (yellow/green color changes**, double vision, halos around lights), Arrhythmias (eg, **bradycardia** > tachycardia, atrial fibrillation with a slow ventricular response), headache, confusion. • <u>Management:</u> Digoxin-specific antibody (DSFab), Magnesium.
Dobutamine	↑contractility (β_1 agonist), produces peripheral vasodilation.
Dopamine	High doses acts as β/α agonist. at low doses, acts as a diuretic by ↑renal blood flow.

(left margin vertical text: POSITIVE INOTROPES)

Nesiritide | <u>MOA:</u> **synthetic BNP** (↓'es RAAS activity, ↑'es Na^+ excretion). Only used in ER or inpatient settings.

SILENT ISCHEMIA	STABLE ANGINA	STEMI	HEART FAILURE
• **Beta blockers** • **Nitroglycerin** • **Aspirin** • **Statins**	• **Beta blockers** (↓ mortality) • **Nitroglycerin** (as needed for symptoms) • **Aspirin** • **Statins**	• **Beta blockers** • **Nitroglycerin** • **Aspirin** • Statins • **ACE inhibitors**	**GDMT 4 pillar therapy:** **(1) Angiotensin blockers:** • ARNI, ACEI, ARB **(2) Beta blockers:** • if chronic stable HF **(3) MRAs:** • **Spironolactone, Eplerenone** **(4) SGLT2 inhibitors:** • "flozins" eg, Dapagliflozin
• **Calcium channel blockers** (alternative to beta blockers)	• **Calcium channel blockers** (alternative to beta blockers)		
<u>Angiotensin-converting enzyme (ACE) inhibitors</u> and Angiotensin receptor blockers (ARBs) have known benefits for only a subset of patients with Chronic coronary syndrome (CCS), such as those with • Hypertension • Diabetes mellitus • Decreased left ventricular ejection fraction (<40%), or • Chronic kidney disease.			**Secondary therapy:** • NTG + Hydralazine
		Drugs not used: • **Calcium channel blockers NOT** used.	**Drugs not used:** • **Calcium channel blockers NOT** used.

SODIUM GLUCOSE TRANSPORT 2 (SGLT2) INHIBITORS

- **Dapagliflozin or Empagliflozin preferred;** Canagliflozin an alternative.

Mechanism of action:
- **Inhibit the reabsorption of sodium as well as glucose in the proximal tubule of the nephron. They also reduce preload & afterload.**

Rationale:
SGLT2 inhibitors reduce blood glucose, lower blood pressure, & reduce weight.
- **SGLT2 inhibitors substantially reduce the risk of cardiovascular death & hospitalization for HFrEF or HFpEF, with or without diabetes.**
- **Decreased mortality:** Dapagliflozin also reduced all-cause mortality.
- **SGLT2 inhibitors also reduce kidney disease progression.**
- SGLT2 inhibitors have an added benefit of reducing hyperglycemia and **reducing the progression of diabetic kidney disease.**

Adverse effects:
- **Thirst, nausea, abdominal pain**
- **Urinary tract infections, yeast infections.**
- **Hypotension** may occur in patients on hypertension meds (cause mild diuresis)
- Acute kidney injury, bone fractures. Dyslipidemia. Euglycemic DKA.

Contraindications and precautions — SGLT2 inhibitors should be avoided in the following clinical settings
- **Presence of type 1 DM** (increased risk for Diabetic ketoacidosis).
- **Presence of type 2 DM with prior diabetic ketoacidosis (DKA)** or a condition predisposing to DKA (including pancreatic insufficiency or drug or alcohol addiction). Temporary discontinuation of SGLT2 inhibitors and monitoring for ketoacidosis are recommended in situations known to predispose to ketoacidosis (such as prolonged fasting due to illness or perioperative state).
- **Volume depletion or symptomatic hypotension.**
- Severely impaired or rapidly declining kidney function: eGFR <20 mL/min per 1.73 m^2, end-stage kidney disease, or rapidly declining renal function.
- **History of complicated urinary tract infections or genitourinary infections.**
- Presence of risk factors for foot amputation (including those with neuropathy, foot deformity, vascular disease, and/or history of previous foot ulceration). **Patients taking SGLT2 inhibitors should be monitored for signs and symptoms of foot ulceration.**

DIURETICS

- Thiazides: when fluid retention is mild, thiazide or related diuretics (eg, Hydrochlorothiazide, Metolazone, Chlorthalidone) may be sufficient and can offer improved control of Hypertension.
- Loop diuretics: may be indicated for more severe Heart failure (eg, Furosemide, Bumetanide, Torsemide).
- The oral Mineralocorticoid receptor antagonists (potassium-sparing agents) are often useful in combination with the Loop diuretics and Thiazide diuretics.

IVABRADINE

Mechanism of action:
- Selective sinus node inhibitor which slows the sinus rate.

Indications:
- Associated with ↓hospitalization & ↓mortality.
- Used in symptomatic chronic stable heart failure with LVEF ≤35%, in sinus rhythm with a resting pulse of ≥70 bpm & already maxed out on the Beta-blocker dose or are unable to take Beta-blockers.

IMPORTANT PRINCIPLES IN THE MANAGEMENT OF HEART FAILURE WITH REDUCED EF (HFrEF):

- **ACE inhibitors are the <u>single</u> most effective medications for mortality benefit in Heart failure with reduced ejection fraction (systolic heart failure). However, ARNI is the most effective medication.**
- Beta-blockers (Carvedilol, Metoprolol, Bisoprolol) are often added to ACE inhibitors for additional mortality benefit.

Medications & interventions that decrease mortality:

- ACE inhibitors, Beta blockers, Angiotensin receptor blockers, Angiotensin receptor-neprilysin inhibitors, Hydralazine plus Nitrate, and mineralocorticoid receptor antagonists.
- Automated Implantable Cardioverter Defibrillator in patients with EF <35% (because these patients tolerate arrhythmias poorly).

Medications with no mortality benefit

- **There is no mortality benefit of non-Dihydropyridine Calcium channel blockers** (Verapamil, Diltiazem) **in the management of Heart failure with reduced ejection fraction and there may be a possible deleterious effect** (they have a greater depressive effect on cardiac conduction and contractility and are somewhat less potent dilators in comparison to the Dihydropyridines).
- Digoxin is associated with decreased hospitalization but no mortality benefit.

HEART FAILURE REVIEW LIST

CHRONIC HFrEF:

- **Angiotensin blockers:** ARNI, ACEI, ARB

- **Beta blockers:** if chronic **stable** HF

- **MRAs:** Spironolactone, Eplerenone

- **SGLT2 inhibitors:** "flozins"

- **Oral diuretics: Thiazides, Loop**

- **Vasodilators: NTG + Hydralazine**

- **Oral positive inotrope: Digoxin** (Na+/K+ ATPase inhibitor)

Acute Decompensated HFrEF (CHF) :

- **IV Loop diuretics: Furosemide***

- **IV Vasodilators: Nitrates, Nitroprusside**

- **Natriuretic peptide: Nesiritide**

If SBP <85 mm Hg or evidence of shock:

- **IV Positive inotropes: Beta-1 agonists (eg, Dopamine, Dobutamine), PDE inhibitors (Milrinone)**

- **Vasopressors: Norepinephrine**

HEART FAILURE WITH PRESERVED EJECTION FRACTION (HFpEF)

MANAGEMENT

General management:

- For patients with HFpEF, the goals of treatment are to reduce HF symptoms, increase functional status, and reduce the risk of hospital admission.
- **Healthy lifestyle:** **Prescribed exercise training when possible;** sodium restriction, caloric restriction. **Cardiac rehabilitation.**
- **Management of associated conditions** — conditions commonly associated with HFpEF include Hypertension, Atrial fibrillation (AF), Coronary artery disease, Dyslipidemia, obesity, anemia, Diabetes mellitus, Chronic kidney disease, and sleep-disordered breathing.

Medical management:

The mainstays of treating Heart failure with preserved EF are (1) SGLT2 inhibitors, (2) Mineralocorticoid receptor antagonists, (3) treatment of underlying comorbid conditions, and (4) treatment of volume overload with diuretics).

- **[1] SGLT2 inhibitors (eg, Empagliflozin) with or without a [2] Mineralocorticoid receptor antagonist (MRA), [eg, Spironolactone, Eplerenone]** added later (eg, 2 weeks later) if the patient tolerates initial therapy with SGLT2i. **The only therapy shown to reduce cardiovascular death or heart failure hospitalization in this population is Empagliflozin.**
- **[3] Treat comorbidities** like hypertension, diabetes, and arrhythmias.
- **[4] Diuretic therapy: fluid management to avoid or treat volume overload (eg, Loop diuretics).**

Patients with volume overload:

- **Diuretic therapy:** patients with HFpEF and suspected or documented volume overload require diuretic therapy (eg, Loop diuretics, such as Furosemide) before initiating other pharmacologic therapies.

Patients with HF symptoms and elevated BNP:

- **Combination SGLT2 inhibitors and Mineralocorticoid receptor antagonists (MRAs): first-line therapies for patients with HFpEF as they reduce the risk of hospitalization.**
- For most patients with HFpEF who have New York Heart Association (NYHA) class II to III symptoms and an elevated B-type natriuretic peptide (BNP; eg, BNP >100 pg/dL or N-terminal pro-BNP [NT-proBNP] >300 pg/dL), treatment with both a sodium-glucose co-transporter 2 (SGLT2) inhibitor and a Mineralocorticoid receptor antagonist (MRA) rather than no HFpEF-specific therapy is recommended.
- Both agents are preferred, rather than either drug alone or treatment with other agents (eg, Sacubitril-Valsartan, Angiotensin II receptor blockers [ARBs], Angiotensin converting enzyme [ACE] inhibitors, or Calcium channel blockers [CCBs]).

Secondary pharmacotherapies:

Clinical trials evaluating other agents (Sacubitril-Valsartan), ARBs, ACE inhibitors, CCBs in HFpEF have not demonstrated a clinically significant benefit, and these drugs are not routinely used in this setting except in the following circumstances:

- For patients with HFpEF who have poorly controlled Hypertension & persistent HF symptoms despite optimal SGLT2 inhibitor & MRA therapy, Sacubitril-Valsartan may be added.
- For patients with comorbid diabetes and chronic kidney disease (CKD), ACE inhibitors and ARBs may be used as first-line therapy.

ACUTE DECOMPENSATED HEART FAILURE (ADHF, CONGESTIVE HEART FAILURE)

- **Acute decompensated heart failure (ADHF) is a clinical syndrome of new or worsening signs and symptoms of Heart failure, often leading to hospitalization or an ED visit.**

TRIGGERS:

The most frequent causes of decompensation if previously compensated include
- **(1) Inappropriate reduction in the intensity of treatment: eg, dietary sodium indiscretion, physical activity reduction, or inappropriate drug treatment.**
- **(2) Uncontrolled hypertension**, which is closely followed by
- **(3) Cardiac arrhythmias** (usually Atrial fibrillation).
- (4) Combination of Heart disease: eg, someone with LVH develops an acute Myocardial infarction.

CLINICAL MANIFESTATIONS
- **Left-sided:** pulmonary symptoms — **progressive dyspnea most common complaint. Cough, pulmonary rales, expiratory wheezing.** Think **L for L-sided and Lungs.**
- **Right-sided:** systemic symptoms of peripheral and abdominal congestion — **eg, increased JVP, lower extremity edema, hepatojugular reflux, GI symptoms).** Think **R for R-sided and 3 roads to the heart (IVC, SVC, portal vessels).**
- **Other symptoms include nocturia** and neurologic symptoms (eg, confusion, headaches, insomnia, anxiety, disorientation, and impaired memory).
- Cardiogenic shock: systolic blood pressure <90 mmHg with symptoms and signs of decreased end-organ perfusion — fatigue, altered mental status, tachycardia, diaphoresis, cold and cyanotic periphery with poor capillary refill and cold mottled skin; diminished pulse pressure, or signs of organ hypoperfusion (eg, prerenal azotemia or abnormal hepatic enzymes).

PHYSICAL EXAMINATION

Signs are due to congestion:
- **Lungs: crackles (rales), rhonchi, or wheezing.** Diminished air entry at the lung bases if a Pleural effusion is present (more common on the right side).
- **Peripheral: lower extremity edema (especially in the pretibial region and ankles in ambulatory patients** with sacral edema in bedridden patients), elevated jugular venous pressure. Pulsus alternans. Cool lower extremities may be suggestive of worse cardiac output.
- Abdomen: epigastric tenderness, positive hepatojugular reflex; tender and enlarged liver. Ascites or hepatomegaly may be seen.
- Cardiac examination: — **advanced systolic dysfunction associated with a third heart sound (S3) and a laterally displaced apex beat**. A murmur of Mitral regurgitation is often audible when the left ventricle (LV) is markedly enlarged, or a tricuspid regurgitation murmur is present when the right ventricle is volume or pressure overloaded.

DIAGNOSIS:
- **The diagnosis of ADHF is based primarily on signs and symptoms (eg, exertional dyspnea and fluid retention) and supported by biomarkers (B-type natriuretic peptide [BNP] or N-terminal proBNP [NT-proBNP]), chest radiograph**, ECG, and Doppler echocardiography.

Chest radiograph:
- Indications: important to assess for signs of pulmonary congestion or edema in acute decompensated heart failure.
- Findings: **cephalization of flow** (redistribution of blood flow from bases to the upper lobes) followed by **Kerley B lines (thin septal lucent horizontal lines in the peripheral lung fields), butterfly (bat wing) appearance** (bilateral perihilar alveolar edema), followed by **cardiomegaly, pleural effusions, and alveolar or pulmonary interstitial edema** (bilateral interstitial markings).
- Up to 20% of ADHF may have normal chest radiographs.

Kerley B Lines (PCWP 18-25 mmHg)

Short linear markings @ lung periphery

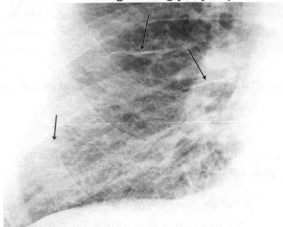

Butterfly (Batwing) Pattern (PCWP >25mmHg)

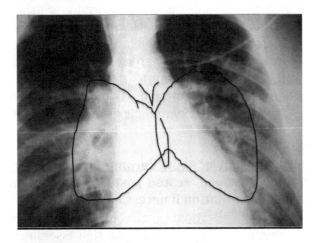

CONGESTIVE HEART FAILURE SIGNS

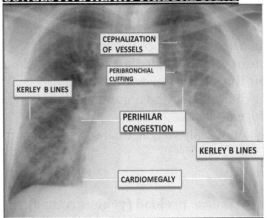

PULMONARY EDEMA

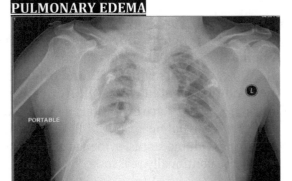

Brain natriuretic peptide:

- **Brain natriuretic peptide levels (BNP) >100 or N-terminal proBNP >125 pg/mL makes CHF likely** (increases in BNP levels may be caused by intrinsic cardiac dysfunction).
- Indications: **A BNP or NT-proBNP level is obtained when the diagnosis of ADHF is uncertain.** The high negative predictive value of BNP tests is particularly helpful for ruling out Heart failure as BNP is an objective measure of cardiac function.
- BNP levels increase with age & with renal insufficiency; May be decreased on chronic treatment.

Electrocardiogram (ECG):

- Indications: assesses for evidence of ACS (myocardial ischemia or MI) and arrhythmias (eg, Atrial fibrillation). The ECG may also identify other predisposing or precipitating conditions for HF such (eg, ventricular hypertrophy, left atrial abnormalities).
- Findings: often nonspecific ST & T changes.

Other labs:

- Serum electrolytes, bicarbonate, CBC, blood urea nitrogen (BUN), and serum creatinine.
- Lactic acid level in patients in shock as well as in those with marked weakness and/or uncertain peripheral perfusion. Serum troponin (T or I) levels are obtained in any patient with possible ACS.

Echocardiogram
- Indications: particularly helpful if first presentation of HF or if there has been abrupt deterioration in the patient's baseline.
- Benefits: Doppler echocardiography is helpful in the diagnosis and classification of HF. Doppler echocardiography enables evaluation of ventricular size, global and regional systolic function, diastolic function, valvular disease, & pericardial disease. Also aids in estimation of right atrial pressure, pulmonary artery pressures, and pulmonary capillary wedge pressure.

Swan-Ganz catheterization
- Generally, not required but helpful when the diagnosis is uncertain and for management of patients with persistent symptoms despite treatment of HF.

MANAGEMENT
Initial therapy of Acute decompensated Heart failure: includes early IV loop diuretic therapy for volume overload, seated posture, supplemental oxygen to treat hypoxemia (SpO2 <90%), and assisted ventilation if necessary.
- Initial stabilization: eg, airway assessment, continuous pulse oximetry, supplemental oxygen and ventilatory support, and vital sign assessment, as well as cardiac and urine output monitoring.

Loop diuretic (eg, Furosemide, Bumetanide):
- Mechanism of action: **IV diuretics decrease dyspnea, symptoms of fluid overload, and peripheral edema** (removes fluid off of the lungs). Have venodilation and anti-vasoconstrictor effects.
- Indications: **patients with ADHF and evidence of volume overload, regardless of etiology, should be promptly treated with IV diuretics as part of their initial therapy without delay.**
- Contraindications: Rare exceptions in which some delay in diuresis may be required include patients with severe hypotension (eg, SBP < 85 mmHg) or cardiogenic shock.
- Monitoring: volume status, evidence of congestion, oxygenation, daily weight, fluid intake, and output should be continually reassessed.

Position:
- Posture: **Seated posture with legs dangling over bed to decrease preload (venous return).**
- **Positive pressure ventilation — Continuous Positive Airway Pressure (CPAP) & Bilevel Positive Airway Pressure (BiPAP)** are noninvasive methods of respiratory support for respiratory insufficiency secondary to pulmonary vascular congestion & pulmonary edema. CPAP & BIBAP reduce the need for intubation & mechanical ventilation in HF with respiratory decompensation.

Oxygen (O2):
- Mechanism of action: relieves the sensation of dyspnea.
- Indications: **hypoxemia (eg, SpO2 <90%).** O2 supplementation can be titrated to keep the patient comfortable and arterial oxygen saturation consistently >90% (88-92% in patients with COPD). Oxygen not recommended as routine therapy without hypoxemia as it may cause vasoconstriction and reduction in cardiac output.
- **Non-rebreather facemask (high-flow 100% oxygen) preferred route of oxygen delivery because the concentration of oxygen delivered is greater than with nasal cannula.**
- Noninvasive ventilation (NIV) indicated if respiratory distress, respiratory acidosis, and/or hypoxia persist on oxygen therapy, as long as emergent intubation is not indicated.
- Endotracheal intubation & mechanical ventilation if severe/no response to NIV (within 30 mins–2 h).

Morphine (opiates):
- Mechanism of action: decreases dyspnea and anxiety. Venodilator (decreased preload).
- Given the limited evidence of benefits and potential risks of opiates (eg, CO2 retention reducing the respiratory drive), opiate therapy is not generally indicated in the routine management of ADHF.

Nitrates: Sublingual Nitroglycerin or Isosorbide dinitrate, topical Nitroglycerin, or IV nitrates

- Mechanism of action: **Nitrates reduce LV filling pressure primarily via venodilation** (venous > arterial vasodilation). At higher doses, Nitrates lower systemic vascular resistance & LV afterload (blood pressure reduction), increasing stroke volume & cardiac output. Anxiolytic & analgesic.
- Indications: **In ADHF, early use of a vasodilator that decreases venous tone (eg, Nitroglycerin) & improves dyspnea when response to diuretics is not sufficient for respiratory distress**.
- Administration: IV route is used for faster onset, reliability of delivery, and ease of titration. An initial dose of 5-10 mcg/min with the dose increased in increments of 5-10 mcg/min every 3-5 minutes as required and tolerated (dose range 10-200 mcg/min).
- Adverse effects: headache, Hypotension. Should be avoided or used with caution in settings in which Hypotension is likely or could result in serious decompensation (eg, RV infarction or aortic stenosis).
- **Contraindications: after the use of PDE-5 inhibitors (eg, Sildenafil) — concomitant use of both can cause profound vasodilatation & hypotension.**

Nitroprusside:

- Mechanism: vasodilator that lowers arterial tone.
- Indications: IV Sodium nitroprusside may be used in selected patients with ADHF who require a rapid decrease in systemic vascular resistance and LV afterload (eg, severe Hypertension, acute Mitral regurgitation, or acute Aortic regurgitation).

MANAGEMENT OF HYPOTENSION

- **The management of ADHF with hypotension may include positive Inotropic agents (eg, Dopamine, Dobutamine, Milrinone) &/or Vasopressor therapy (eg, Norepinephrine).**

Dopamine, Dobutamine, & Milrinone:

- Mechanism of action: positive inotropes that increase contractility to increase cardiac output.
- Indications: **temporary (short-term) positive inotrope for severe decompensated Heart failure with hypotension to maintain systemic perfusion to vital organs. Indicated if systolic blood pressure is <85 mmHg or there is evidence of shock** (eg, cool extremities, narrow pulse pressure, low urine output, confusion) and severe LV dysfunction.
- May be needed until definitive therapy (eg, coronary revascularization, mechanical circulatory support, or heart transplantation) is instituted or resolution of the acute precipitating problem.
- Dobutamine is preferable for Beta-blocker naive patients, while Milrinone is preferred for patients previously taking oral Beta blockers who experience an acute decompensation.
- Contraindications: Not generally used as long-term therapy (long-term use can increase mortality). Inotropes are not indicated for ADHF treatment with preserved systolic function.

Vasopressor therapy: Norepinephrine or high-dose Dopamine.

- Indications: **vasopressor use is limited to patients with persistent hypotension with symptoms or evidence of consequent end-organ hypoperfusion despite optimization of filling pressures and use of inotropic agents as appropriate.** Used as a temporizing measure to preserve BP.

CAUTION

- **Beta blockers (BB) reduce mortality when used in the long-term management of patients with HFrEF, but should be used cautiously in patients with Acute decompensated HFrEF because of the potential to worsen acute HF.** For patients already on BBs with severe decompensation (eg, severe volume overload and/or requiring inotropic support), BBs are usually temporarily withheld. For patients who are already taking a BB with moderate-to-severe decompensation or hypotension, decreasing or withholding Beta blocker therapy is recommended.
- **Non-Dihydropyridine CCBs: There is no mortality benefit of non-Dihydropyridine Calcium channel blockers in the management of Heart failure with reduced ejection fraction (HFrEF) and there may be a possible deleterious effect** of the use of non-Dihydropyridines.
- Amlodipine & Felodipine are Dihydropyridine CCBs that appear to be safe in HF and may be used if CCB is necessary for a concomitant disease, such as Hypertension or Angina.

DILATED CARDIOMYOPATHY (DCMP)

- Disease of the heart muscle characterized by [1] <u>systolic dysfunction</u> (impaired contraction) and [2] <u>dilation</u> of one or both ventricles (a dilated, weak heart).

PATHOPHYSIOLOGY
- **[1] Impaired systolic function impaired contraction & decreased left ventricular ejection fraction (LVEF) <40%.** Reduction in systolic function is thought to be secondary to myocardial remodeling that results in an increase in both end-systolic and end-diastolic volumes.
- **[2] Cardiac chamber dilation** leading to progressive enlargement of one or both ventricles. Ventricular dilation results in decreased contractility, tricuspid and mitral valve insufficiency, and decreased ejection fraction leads to systolic dysfunction.

EPIDEMIOLOGY
- **Most common type of Cardiomyopathy** — represents 90% of all Cardiomyopathies.
- Most present between 20-60 years of age. Male gender associated with higher incidence.

ETIOLOGIES
Excludes heart disease secondary to coronary artery disease, valvular, or congenital heart disease.
- **Idiopathic most common cause of Dilated cardiomyopathy (50%).** Genetic disease.
- **Infectious myocarditis eg, viral infection most common cause of Myocarditis (eg, Coxsackievirus B and Echovirus),** Parvovirus B19, Human herpesvirus 6, Influenza virus, adenovirus, echovirus, cytomegalovirus, and HIV. **Chagas disease.** Lyme disease.
- Infiltrative diseases: Hemochromatosis & Sarcoidosis can also cause Restrictive cardiomyopathy but Dilated cardiomyopathy is a more common complication. Autoimmune diseases.
- **Peripartum & pregnancy:** occurs in late pregnancy and the early postpartum period.
- **Toxic: chronic alcohol use, cocaine,** amphetamines, & radiation lead to toxic cardiac damage.
- Metabolic: eg, thyroid disorders, **vitamin B1 (Thiamine) deficiency.** Tachycardia-mediated.
- Medications: **Anthracyclines (eg, Doxorubicin); Trastuzumab.**

CLINICAL MANIFESTATIONS
Systolic heart failure:
- **Left-sided failure symptoms (pulmonary) — dyspnea on exertion (most common symptom), fatigue, & impaired exercise capacity.** Orthopnea, paroxysmal nocturnal dyspnea.
- **Right-sided failure symptoms (systemic) — peripheral edema** (leg swelling), **jugular venous distention,** hepatomegaly, GI symptoms.
- Nonspecific symptoms: fatigue, malaise, weakness, anorexia, nausea, nocturia, and memory impairment.

Other symptoms:
- Thromboembolic complications. Atrial and/or ventricular arrhythmias, and sudden death can occur at any stage of the disease; conduction disturbances. Many patients are asymptomatic.

PHYSICAL EXAMINATION
- **S3 gallop hallmark of DCMP* and represents rapid filling of a dilated ventricle.** S3 heart sounds can be normal in some populations, including pregnant women and young athletes.
- **Lateral displacement of the point of maximal impulse (PMI)** due to cardiac enlargement.
- Mitral or Tricuspid regurgitation (due to ventricular enlargement and annular dilation).
- **Left-sided failure crackles (rales)** due to pulmonary edema.
- **Right-sided failure peripheral edema, jugular venous distention,** positive hepatojugular reflux with inspiration, ascites.

DIAGNOSTIC STUDIES

Echocardiogram:

- **Echocardiogram is the most useful noninvasive test of DCMP** — provides an objective assessment of ventricular size, function, and any associated valvular abnormalities, help to determine the type and possible etiology of the cardiomyopathy, & assess for ejection fraction.
- **Systolic dysfunction: decreased left ventricular ejection fraction <40%** or fractional shortening **<25%. Global ventricular hypokinesis.**
- **Ventricular dilation**: dilated ventricular chambers & thin-walled ventricles.

Chest radiograph:

- **Cardiomegaly**, pulmonary edema, venous congestion, and pleural effusion.

ECG: may show sinus tachycardia, nonspecific ST & T wave changes, or arrhythmias (eg, A. fib).

MRI: increasingly used to provide further information on myocardial tissue characterization.

Laboratory testing:

- Thyroid function tests, HIV serology, electrolytes, CBC (rule out anemia), and iron studies (to rule out Hemochromatosis). Urine toxicology screen and alcohol if substance abuse is suspected. Genetic testing considered if familial. Serum B-type natriuretic peptide (BNP) levels when diagnosis is unclear. Low levels of BNP are helpful in excluding CHF and are useful for prognosis.

Coronary angiography:

- Should be performed in those without a known history of CAD to further define coronary anatomy and rule out occult ischemic disease as the cause of DCM.

Myocardial biopsy:

- Rarely used and reserved for evaluation of storage diseases or infiltrative causes when suspected.

MEDICAL MANAGEMENT

- **Standard systolic heart failure treatment: mortality reduction with Angiotensin system blockers (eg, Sacubitril-Valsartan, ACE inhibitors, or ARBs), Beta blockers** (eg, long-acting Metoprolol, Carvedilol, Bisoprolol), **& Mineralocorticoid receptor antagonists (Spironolactone or Eplerenone). Symptom control with diuretics** (to achieve a euvolemic state). Isosorbide dinitrate plus Hydralazine also have been shown to increase survival amongst those with advanced disease. Digoxin.
- Treating any identifiable and reversible underlying causes. Alcohol cessation.
- Anticoagulation in patients with artificial valves, Atrial fibrillation, and known mural thrombus. Oral anticoagulants can reduce the risk of stroke at the risk of increased bleeding complications.

Medications to avoid:

- **NSAIDs Nonsteroidal anti-inflammatory drugs (NSAIDs) may exacerbate Heart failure** — NSAIDs can cause sodium retention and peripheral vasoconstriction and can attenuate the efficacy and enhance the toxicity of diuretics and ACE inhibitors.
- **Calcium channel blockers — There is no mortality benefit of non-Dihydropyridine Calcium channel blockers in the management of Heart failure with reduced ejection fraction and there may be a possible deleterious effect** of the use of non-Dihydropyridines. Amlodipine, a Dihydropyridine CCB, appears to be safe in HF and may be used if CCB is necessary for a concomitant disease, such as Hypertension or Angina.
- Most antiarrhythmic agents may exacerbate heart failure and should be avoided in most patients.

OPERATIVE MANAGEMENT

- Implantable AICD: Automated implantable cardioverter/defibrillator if ejection fraction ≤35-30% for primary prevention of sudden cardiac death due to arrhythmias.
- Cardiac resynchronization therapy: Biventricular pacemaker indicated if QRS >120 ms (with a widened QRS, the ventricles are not in synchrony).
- Patients with disease refractory to maximum medical therapy should be considered for cardiac transplantation and left ventricular assistance device (LVAD) as a bridge or for "destination" therapy in those who are not candidates for transplantation.

MYOCARDITIS

- **Inflammation of the heart muscle resulting in myocardial necrosis & degeneration that may lead to Dilated cardiomyopathy (DCMP).**

ETIOLOGIES:
- **Idiopathic:** **50% of cases.** In some, viral particles may be found in biopsy specimens.
- **Infectious:** Viral **most common infectious cause, especially the Enteroviruses [Echoviruses & Coxsackieviruses (Coxsackie B most common viral cause)];** Parvovirus B-19, Adenoviruses, Herpes viruses (eg, CMV, Epstein-Barr virus, HHV 6), Influenza virus, HCV, HIV, SARS-CoV-2. Bacterial: *Borrelia burgdorferi* (Lyme disease), *Mycoplasma pneumoniae, Corynebacterium diphtheriae.* Parasitic: *Trypanosoma cruzi* (Chagas disease), *Toxoplasma gondii, Trichinella spiralis.*
- Autoimmune: SLE, RA, Wegener's granulomatosis, Kawasaki disease, Giant cell arteritis.
- Medications: **Clozapine,** Methyldopa, antibiotics, Isoniazid, Cyclophosphamide, Indomethacin, Phenytoin, sulfonamides, Lithium, TCA antidepressants, **Doxorubicin.**
- Other: Cocaine, alcohol, and uremia.

EPIDEMIOLOGY
- **Most common in young previously healthy adults, typically between 20-50 years.**

CLINICAL MANIFESTATIONS
Clinical presentation of Myocarditis is highly variable and may include any of the following:
- **Viral prodrome** — flu-like illness that may consist of fever, myalgias, malaise, vomiting, and/or diarrhea for 7-14 days.
- **New onset or worsening HF: syndrome of Heart failure and Dilated cardiomyopathy** in the absence of CAD and known causes of HF **(most common in adults) — over 2 weeks to 3 months after respiratory or GI infection, with symptoms including dyspnea, fatigue, exercise intolerance, peripheral edema, chest discomfort, and arrhythmias (sinus tachycardia most common)** with echocardiographic evidence of global or regional LV and/or RV dysfunction.
- **ACS-like: patients present similar to Acute coronary syndrome with acute chest pain 1-4 weeks after respiratory or GI infection** (may be recurrent), with ST/T changes (including ST segment elevation or depression and T wave inversions), elevated cardiac biomarkers (eg, Troponin), echocardiographic evidence of global or regional LV and/or RV dysfunction, with no evidence of significant coronary artery disease on angiography.
- **Pericarditis:** at least two of the following — typical chest pain (eg, pleuritic, postural), pericardial friction rub, classic ECG changes (widespread ST segment elevation), and/or new or worsening pericardial effusion.
- **Myopericarditis:** diagnosis of Acute pericarditis **PLUS** suggestive symptoms (eg, palpitations, dyspnea, chest pain) & **certain ECG features more than normal variants not documented previously** [ST/T abnormalities, atypical ECG changes such as localized ST-elevation (inferolateral or anterolateral) and T-wave inversion before ST-segment normalization, **cardiac arrhythmias —** supraventricular or ventricular tachycardia or frequent ectopy, atrioventricular block]] **OR focal or diffuse decreased LV function** of undetermined age by an imaging study); 1 of the following features: elevated cardiac biomarkers (creatine kinase-MB fraction, or troponin I or T), **OR** new onset of focal or diffuse decreased LV function by an imaging study, **OR abnormal imaging consistent with myocarditis** (MRI with gadolinium, gallium-67 scanning, anti-myosin antibody scanning); absence of any other cause.
- **Life-threatening condition:** in the absence of CAD and known causes of HF with one or more of the following — life-threatening arrhythmias, cardiogenic shock occurring around 2 weeks after a distinct viral prodrome.
- Children will often present with grunting respirations and intercostal retractions.
- Other: **Megacolon.**

PHYSICAL EXAMINATION:
- **Vital signs** are often abnormal — eg, fever, tachycardia, tachypnea, and occasionally hypotension.
- Heart failure: signs of fluid overload (eg, peripheral edema, elevated jugular venous pressure, and pulmonary crackles), **S3 gallop** (third heart sound reflecting filling of a dilated ventricle). If left or RV dilation is severe, functional mitral or tricuspid regurgitation may occur.
- Pericarditis: pericardial friction rub and/or effusion (muffled heart sounds).

DIAGNOSIS:
- **Acute myocarditis should be in the differential diagnosis in a patient with new onset of Heart failure or chest pain or arrhythmia, positive cardiac biomarkers, absence of traditional coronary risk factors, and a history of preceding viral illness or infection.**

Chest radiograph: **cardiomegaly classic.**

ECG:
- Nonspecific — **sinus tachycardia most common**, normal, or may show Pericarditis (eg, diffuse ST elevations and PR depressions in precordial leads), widened QRS patterns, low voltage, prolonged QT, or variable atrioventricular (AV) blocks. An acute myocardial infarction pattern may be seen.

Labs:
- **Cardiac biomarkers may be positive (eg, Troponin)** due to myocardial damage & myonecrosis.
- Erythrocyte sedimentation rate (ESR), C-reactive protein (CRP), and WBC count may be elevated.
- Viral antibody titers include coxsackievirus B, HIV, CMV, Epstein-Barr virus, Hepatitis, and Influenza.

Echocardiogram:
- **Should be ordered in all patients with Myocarditis and is also helpful to rule out other causes.**
- **Nonspecific** findings include ventricular systolic dysfunction — eg, decreased left ventricular function, decreased ejection fraction, global hypokinesis, and regional wall motion abnormalities.

Endomyocardial biopsy:
- **Definitive diagnosis gold standard — histopathologic evidence of myocardial tissue necrosis and increased inflammatory cellular infiltrates** (eg, histiocytic, lymphocytic, mononuclear, eosinophilic, granulomatous, or giant cells).
- Indications: **usually reserved for severe or refractory cases** after other causes have been excluded.

MANAGEMENT
Supportive management
- **Mainstay of treatment** — including supplemental oxygen and fluid status optimization.
- Management goals are to preserve left ventricular function and may include limitation of activity up to standard Heart failure treatment.
- **Patients with mild symptoms do improve spontaneously but recovery may take months.**
- All patients with Myocarditis should receive routine follow-up, including serial echocardiography or other cardiac imaging.

Standard Heart failure treatment:
- **HF with reduced EF treatment — eg, triple therapy with Angiotensin system blocker (eg, Sacubitril-Valsartan, ACE inhibitor, or Angiotensin receptor blocker), evidence-based Beta blocker (eg, Carvedilol, Bisoprolol, extended-release Metoprolol), and diuretics** for symptom control as well as to decrease preload and volume overload.
- Mineralocorticoid receptor antagonist (eg, Spironolactone, Eplerenone) in patients with persistent symptomatic HF with left ventricular ejection fraction (EF) ≤35%.

Things to avoid:
- **Patients with Myocarditis should avoid NSAIDs, cardiotoxic medications, heavy alcohol consumption, and exercise;** physical activity should be restricted during the acute phase.
- NSAIDs should be withheld as they impede healing of the myocardium and exacerbate the inflammatory process.
- **Digoxin should be avoided** acutely (may increase proinflammatory cytokines, worsening the injury).

STRESS (TAKOTSUBO) CARDIOMYOPATHY

- **Transient regional systolic dysfunction of the left ventricle that can imitate Myocardial infarction but is associated with the <u>absence</u> of significant obstructive coronary artery disease or evidence of acute plaque rupture.** A form of non-ischemic dilated cardiomyopathy.

RISK FACTORS
- <u>**Postmenopausal women**</u> **exposed to physical or emotional stress** (eg, death of a relative, catastrophic medical diagnoses) — aka "broken heart syndrome". Loss of estrogen's protective effects & increased catecholamines directly injure the myocardium (eg, myocardial stunning).

PATHOPHYSIOLOGY:
- **Thought to be multifactorial, including <u>catecholamine surge</u> during physical or emotional stress**, microvascular dysfunction, and coronary artery spasm.
- <u>**Transient apical ballooning:**</u> transient regional systolic dysfunction of the left ventricle and systolic apical ballooning appearance.

CLINICAL MANIFESTATIONS:
- **Similar to Acute coronary syndrome (ACS) - eg, substernal chest pain, dyspnea, & syncope.** May be triggered by intense emotional or physical stress. May have symptoms or signs of Heart failure.

DIAGNOSIS:
- **Takotsubo cardiomyopathy is a diagnosis of exclusion that can only be made <u>after</u> coronary angiography** because of the indistinguishable features from Acute coronary syndrome.
- <u>Labs:</u> **cardiac biomarkers often positive** as is B natriuretic peptide (BNP) or N-terminal pro-BNP.
In addition to the absence of Pheochromocytoma, all 3 must be present as part of the Mayo criteria:
- **[1] ECG: ST elevations most common,** especially in the anterior leads similar to anterior STEMI. May have ST depressions. The classic pattern is stage I: ST-segment elevation followed by; stage II: normalization of the ST segment followed by stage III: T wave inversions, followed by stage IV: complete normalization of the T waves (T wave inversions rarely persist).
- **[2] Coronary angiography: absence of acute plaque rupture or obstructive coronary disease;** normal coronary anatomy or mild to moderate coronary atherosclerosis.
- **[3] Echocardiogram: transient regional LV systolic dysfunction (hypokinesis, akinesis, or dyskinesis), especially systolic apical ballooning of the left ventricle (most common).** Mid-ventricular type hypokinesis second most common variant.

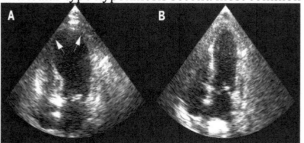

(A) Echocardiograph showing dilatation of the left ventricle in the acute phase.

(B) Resolution of left ventricular function on repeat echocardiograph 6 days later.

Photo credit: Tara C Gangadhar, Elisabeth Von der Lohe, Stephen G Sawada and Paul R Helft [CC BY 2.0 (https://creativecommons.org/licenses/by/2.0)]

INITIAL MANAGEMENT
- Because the initial presentation of Takotsubo cardiomyopathy presents similar to Acute coronary syndrome (ACS), patients are treated initially as ACS with Aspirin, Nitroglycerin, Beta blockers, Heparin, statins, and coronary angiography to rule out obstructive coronary artery disease.

SHORT-TERM MANAGEMENT
- **Because Takotsubo cardiomyopathy is a transient condition, conservative and supportive care is the mainstay of treatment** — eg, Beta blockers (especially cardioselective agents), ACE inhibitors for short period (eg, 3-6 months), and serial imaging to assess for improvement.

CARDIOMYOPATHY: disease of the heart muscle (myocardial tissue) with cardiac dysfunction NOT due to cardiac causes.

	DILATED CARDIOMYOPATHY (95%)	RESTRICTIVE CARDIOMYOPATHY (1%)	HYPERTROPHIC CARDIOMYOPATHY (4%)
DEFINITION	SYSTOLIC DYSFUNCTION • (1) ventricular dilation and • (2) impaired contraction of one or both ventricles, resulting in a "dilated weak heart".	• DIASTOLIC DYSFUNCTION ventricular rigidity impedes diastolic LV filling (decreased LV compliance). • Preserved contractility in early disease.	• DIASTOLIC DYSFUNCTION due to impaired LV relaxation & filling. Subaortic outflow obstruction: • Hypertrophied septum • Systolic anterior motion of mitral v.
ETIOLOGIES	• Idiopathic: most common cause of DCM • Viral myocarditis: eg, enteroviruses • Toxic: Alcohol, Cocaine, Autoimmune • Medications: Doxorubicin, Trastuzumab • B1 deficiency, pregnancy, genetics	Infiltrative disease: • Amyloidosis most common cause. • Sarcoidosis • Hemochromatosis • Fibrosis	Inherited genetic disorder: • Inappropriate LV &/or RV hypertrophy (especially septal)
CLINICAL MANIFESTATIONS	• Heart failure: dyspnea, edema, increased JVD, rales (crackles), chest pain, syncope • Embolic phenomenon, arrhythmia	• Right-sided Heart failure: peripheral edema, increased JVD, hepatomegaly > Left-sided Heart failure (eg, pulmonary rales). • Dyspnea most common symptom.	Harsh systolic murmur best heard at the let lower sternal border • ↓ murmur intensity: ↑venous return (eg, squatting, lying supine, leg raise). Handgrip increases afterload. • ↑murmur intensity: ↓venous return (Valsalva, standing). Amyl nitrate.
PHYSICAL EXAMINATION	• Third heart sound: S3 gallop • Left-sided HF: crackles, rales, cough, pleural effusion • Right-sided HF: peripheral edema, increased JVD, hepatic congestion	• Kussmaul sign: ↑JVD with inspiration. • R-sided HF: ↑JVD, peripheral edema, hepatic congestion. • L-sided HF: pulmonary crackles (rales)	• Fourth heart sound (S4 gallop) • Pulsus bisferiens (biphasic pulse) • Increased risk of sudden death from ventricular arrhythmias.
DIAGNOSIS	Echocardiogram: • (1) LV dilatation and thin ventricular walls • (2) decreased ejection fraction (EF) • (3) hypokinesis (regional or global) Chest radiographs: • Cardiomegaly, pulmonary edema	Echocardiogram: • (1) Diastolic dysfunction • (2) Biatrial enlargement* • (3) Ventricles with normal wall thickness. Endomyocardial biopsy: • Criterion standard (definitive diagnosis)	Echocardiogram: • (1) Diastolic dysfunction • (2) Asymmetric wall thickness >1.5 cm • (3) SAM of the mitral valve ECG • Q waves in inferolateral leads, LVH
MANAGEMENT	Standard HF treatment: • Angiotensin blockers (eg, ACE inhibitors), Beta blockers, Mineralocorticoid antagonists (eg, Eplerenone). • Symptom control (eg, diuretics) • AICD placement if ejection fraction <35%	No specific treatment: • Treat the underlying cause.	• Beta blockers first-line • Calcium channel blockers • Myectomy, Alcohol septal ablation • Cautious use of diuretics, nitrates, digoxin, and overexertion

RESTRICTIVE CARDIOMYOPATHY (RCM)

- **Diastolic dysfunction** in a non-dilated, rigid (stiff) ventricle, which impedes diastolic ventricular filling.

ETIOLOGIES
Infiltrative diseases: "osis"
- **Amyloidosis most common cause of RCM in the US.** It affects the elderly more often; however, it is seen in people as young as 40 years old. >95% of clinical presentations of cardiac Amyloidosis are due to transthyretin Amyloidosis (ATTR) or light chain amyloidosis (AL).
- **Sarcoidosis:** suspect in younger patients presenting with unexplained syncope and heart blocks. More common in women, with the highest prevalence among Black women. Northern Europeans.
- **Hemochromatosis** causes Dilated cardiomyopathy but can also cause Restrictive cardiomyopathy.
- **Fibrosis:** post-radiation therapy, Scleroderma, Metastatic disease, chemotherapy.

PATHOPHYSIOLOGY
- **The 3 leading causes of RCM: [1] cardiac Amyloidosis, [2] Sarcoidosis, & [3] Hemochromatosis** lead to a build-up of a substance (amyloid fibril deposition, granulomas, & iron respectively) in the myocardium, making the ventricles stiff (decreased compliance & diastolic dysfunction).
- **The stiff myocardium leads to decreased compliance, restrictive filling** (increased effort to fill the ventricles causes **elevated ventricular filling pressures & subsequent dilation of the atria**).

CLINICAL MANIFESTATIONS
- **Right-sided failure (systemic)** — **peripheral edema** (leg swelling), **jugular venous distention,** hepatomegaly, GI symptoms. **Right-sided failure symptoms more common than left-sided.**
- **Left-sided failure symptoms (pulmonary)** — **dyspnea on exertion, orthopnea, paroxysmal nocturnal dyspnea, fatigue, cough, & exercise intolerance.**
- Amyloidosis may present with HF, syncope, proteinuria, peripheral neuropathy, carpal tunnel syndrome, and gastrointestinal symptoms (eg, malabsorption).

PHYSICAL EXAMINATION
- **Right-sided failure peripheral edema, jugular venous distention,** elevated jugular venous pressure with prominent rapid y descents, positive hepatojugular reflux with inspiration, ascites. Elevated central venous pressure (hepatosplenomegaly) & pulmonary HTN in advanced disease.
- **Left-sided failure crackles** due to pulmonary edema. Dullness to percussion (pleural effusion).
- **Kussmaul's sign: either the lack of an inspiratory decline or an increase in jugular venous pressure with inspiration** (due to increased resistance to atrial filling during inspiration).
- **A fourth heart sound (S4) is more common than S3 in sinus rhythm. Palpitations.**
- Features in Amyloidosis: periorbital purpura, thickened tongue, and hepatomegaly. Kidney impairment, proteinuria, peripheral neuropathy (eg, Carpal tunnel syndrome), malabsorption.

DIAGNOSIS
Chest radiograph:
- Normal ventricular chamber size, cardiomegaly due to enlarged atria, pulmonary venous congestion, pleural effusions.
ECG:
- **Nonspecific: diffuse low-normal voltage QRS complex** (especially in the limb leads), prolonged PR interval, arrhythmias (eg, Atrial fibrillation, premature beats), ST-T wave abnormalities.
- B-type natriuretic peptide (BNP) level may help distinguish Restrictive cardiomyopathy from Constrictive pericarditis. **Higher levels of BNP (eg, ≥400 pg/mL) are suggestive of Restrictive cardiomyopathy rather than Constrictive pericarditis** (limited diagnostic value in patients with renal failure). Biomarkers such as troponin T, B-type natriuretic peptide (BNP), and pro-BNP are also useful diagnostic and prognostic factors of RCM.

Echocardiogram:

Primary diagnostic imaging test of choice for identifying patients with RCM. 3 key features:

- **[1] Diastolic dysfunction & restrictive filling pattern.** Systolic function preserved in early disease.
- **[2] Biatrial enlargement marked dilation of one or both atria is a key feature of RCM.***
- **[3] Non-dilated ventricles with normal thickness (may be slightly thick with infiltrative diseases, such as Amyloidosis) with normal or small ventricular cavity.** "Square root" sign.
- Sarcoid cardiac disease: global or regional (typically basal posterior and lateral) left ventricular wall motion abnormalities may be seen and a left ventricular aneurysm may be seen.
- **Amyloidosis**: **bilateral ventricular wall and interventricular septal thickness often seen (normal wall thickness may also be seen)** with granular appearance of the myocardium **('speckled or sparkling' appearance).**

Endomyocardial biopsy:

- **Definitive diagnosis (criterion standard).** Often reserved for selected patients with RCM to identify or rule out specific etiologies (eg, Sarcoidosis, Amyloidosis, Hemochromatosis).
- **Amyloidosis associated with apple-green birefringence with Congo red stain under polarized light microscopy.**
- Sarcoidosis is associated with noncaseating granulomas.

DIFFERENTIAL DIAGNOSIS

Restrictive cardiomyopathy (RCM) vs. Constrictive pericarditis (CP):

- Constrictive pericarditis (CP) and Restrictive cardiomyopathy (RCM) present almost identically, except for a few hallmark signs and symptoms.
- Seen in both CP and RCM: diastolic dysfunction with normal (or near normal) systolic function, characteristically abnormal ventricular filling, right-sided heart failure symptoms (eg, jugular venous distension, Kussmaul sign, ascites, hepatomegaly), diastolic sounds, pulsus paradoxus.
- **RCM: third heart sound (S3), elevated BNP, elevated capillary wedge pressure and pulmonary arterial pressure, and biatrial enlargement are far more common in RCM.** Ventricular interaction is absent in RCM and accentuated with respiration in CP.
- CP: a pericardial knock, pericardial calcifications on chest radiographs, pericardial thickening on imaging, and BNP levels <100 pg/mL are more likely seen in CP. Ventricular dependence seen only in CP (increased filling of one of the ventricles only, with a reciprocal decreased filling of the other ventricle).

MANAGEMENT

- **No specific treatment** specific treatment options are limited.
- **Treat the underlying disorder** — **eg, therapeutic phlebotomy for Hemochromatosis, Glucocorticoids for Sarcoidosis.**
- Heart transplant is the only definitive treatment of Restrictive cardiomyopathy.

Heart failure:

- **Low- to medium-dose diuretics are the mainstay of treatment of Heart failure to reduce volume overload but must be monitored closely to prevent excessive diuresis as patients with RCM require high filling pressures to maintain cardiac output.**
- Calcium channel blockers rate reducing CCBs (eg, Diltiazem, Verapamil) improve diastolic dysfunction by myocyte relaxation and increase filling times by rate control.
- Beta blockers decrease the deleterious consequences of long-term compensatory sympathetic activation on the function of cardiac myocytes.
- Angiotensin-converting enzyme (ACE) inhibitors and/or Angiotensin II receptor blockers may improve diastolic filling by counteracting the compensatory neurohormonal changes.

HYPERTROPHIC CARDIOMYOPATY (HCM)

- **Autosomal dominant genetic disorder of inappropriate LV and/or RV hypertrophy resulting in left ventricular outflow obstruction, diastolic dysfunction, and myocardial ischemia.**

ETIOLOGY
- Familial Hypertrophic cardiomyopathy most common ~50% of cases. Associated with autosomal dominant mutations on chromosome 14 (the genes encoding for sarcomere proteins).

PATHOPHYSIOLOGY
- Concentric hypertrophy (especially septal) from sarcomeres added in parallel without chamber dilation.
- **Diastolic dysfunction:** ventricular hypertrophy results in impaired left ventricular relaxation (decreased LV compliance). The ventricles are hypercontractile.
- **Subaortic outflow obstruction** left ventricular outflow tract (LVOT) obstruction due to [1] asymmetrical septal hypertrophy and [2] systolic anterior motion (SAM) of the mitral valve.
- **The obstruction worsens with [1] increased contractility (eg, exercise, Digoxin, beta agonists) & [2] decreased LV volume** (eg, dehydration, decreased venous return, Valsalva maneuver).
Histology:
- Myocyte hypertrophy with a gross disarray of the myofibrils & disorganization of the muscle architecture with varying amount of interstitial fibrosis. Abnormal internal coronary vessels.

CLINICAL MANIFESTATIONS:
- **Many patients with HCM are asymptomatic** and are diagnosed during family screening, by auscultation of a murmur during routine examination, or incidentally after an abnormal ECG.
- **Symptomatic patients usually present with left ventricular outflow tract (LVOT) symptoms of dyspnea on exertion (most common 90%), fatigue, chest pain, and syncope.**
- **Chest pain anginal or atypical.** Typical exertional chest pain (angina) seen in 25-30% of patients with HCM, usually in the setting of a normal coronary arteriogram.
- **Pre syncope, syncope, or dizziness especially during or immediately after exertion.** Palpitations.
- **Sudden cardiac death especially in adolescent or preadolescent children especially during times of extreme exertion often due to Ventricular arrhythmias** (eg, Ventricular fibrillation).
- May have a family history of Sudden cardiac death.

PHYSICAL EXAMINATION:
- **Loud fourth heart sound (S4)** occurs during left ventricular (LV) filling when atrial contraction forces blood into a noncompliant (stiff/hypertrophic) LV. Double apical impulse (noncompliant LV).
- **Pulsus bisferiens: biphasic pulse** — aortic waveform with two peaks per cardiac cycle, a small one followed by a strong and broad one). Due to sudden deceleration of blood due to the development of midsystolic obstruction to blood flow and partial closure of the aortic valve.

Systolic murmur
- **Harsh crescendo-decrescendo systolic murmur that begins slightly after S1 and is heard best at the apex and lower left sternal border.** Usually no carotid radiation (unlike Aortic stenosis & AS is best heard at the right upper sternal border).
- **Increased murmur intensity with ↓ preload & ↓ afterload — decreased venous return (eg, Valsalva, standing, or assuming an upright posture** from a squatting, sitting, or supine position) **due to decreased preload; decreased afterload (eg, vasodilators like Amyl nitrate)** due to increased forward flow through the LV outflow tract.
- **Decreased murmur intensity: with ↑ preload & ↑ afterload — increased venous return (eg, after going from a standing to squatting or supine position, leg raise) due to increased preload; increased afterload (eg, handgrip** decreases forward flow through LV outflow tract).

DIAGNOSIS

- A cardiac history, physical examination, ECG, and cardiac imaging (eg, echocardiogram or cardiac MR) to identify left ventricular hypertrophy should be performed in all patients with suspected HCM.

ECG:

- **ECG testing is the most sensitive routinely performed diagnostic test for HCM.** Because the ECG abnormalities are not specific to HCM, echocardiography often also performed.
- **LVH: left ventricular hypertrophy** associated with left axis deviation.
- **Prominent abnormal Q waves — pseudo q waves in the anterolateral (l, aVL, V4-V6) and inferior leads (II, III, aVF)** due to septal depolarization of the hypertrophied myocytes.

Echocardiography:

Key diagnostic test for HCM:

- **Diastolic dysfunction & hypertrophy: asymmetric ventricular wall thickness ≥15 mm (especially interventricular septum), systolic anterior motion of the mitral valve, small LV chamber size, and diastolic dysfunction.**

Genetic testing: for patients or their first-degree relatives to look for disease-causing mutation.

MANAGEMENT

Focused on early detection, medical management, surgical management, and/or ICD placement.

- **Pharmacological therapy is the first-line approach to symptomatic HCM. The best initial medications include negative inotropic agents, including [1] Beta blockers (preferred in most), [2] nondihydropyridine Calcium channel blockers (Verapamil), or [3] Disopyramide.**

Medical management:

- **Beta blockers first-line medical management for symptomatic patients.** Beta blockers are negative inotropes that increase LV outflow and improve anginal symptoms by improving diastolic ventricular filling by decreasing heart rate, increase LV compliance, and reduce diastolic dysfunction since HCM is associated with poor relaxation.
- **Calcium channel blockers: Non-dihydropyridine Calcium channel blockers (eg, Verapamil) are alternatives to Beta blockers when there are contraindications to Beta blockers (eg, reactive airway disease)** or if unable to tolerate Beta blockers due to adverse effects. They should not be used in HCM and LVOT obstruction with volume overload, severe dyspnea, or hypotension at rest.
- **Disopyramide: may be added onto BBs or CCBs** — negative inotrope that increases LV outflow.

Surgical:

- **Myectomy septal reduction therapy usually performed in young patients with persistent symptoms despite maximal dual medical therapy**, patients with symptoms + severe LVOT obstruction (≥50 mmHg at rest or with provocation), persistent NYHA III/IV class Heart failure despite optimal medical therapy, or syncope related to LVOT obstruction.
- **Alcohol septal ablation: a minimally invasive procedure that is an alternative to surgical myectomy or if myectomy is contraindicated.** Alcohol septal ablation reduces LVOT obstruction, improves symptoms, increases exercise capacity, and may improve long-term survival. Alcohol is injected via the septal artery to obliterate obstructing muscle tissue.
- Implantable cardioverter defibrillator recommended for secondary prevention of Sudden cardiac death when there is any personal history of Ventricular fibrillation or sustained Ventricular tachycardia, in patients with a history of syncope or events seen on Holter monitor.

CAUTIONS

- **Patients should avoid dehydration, extreme exertion, and strenuous exercise, especially athletic activities.** Low-level physical activity is not a risk factor for Sudden cardiac death.
- **Cautious use of Digoxin in HCM because Digoxin increases contractility.**
- Medications that decrease left ventricular preload or systemic vascular resistance should be avoided, as they can decrease the diastolic volume in the LV and increase left ventricular tract outflow obstruction — vasodilators (eg, Dihydropyridine Calcium channel blockers), diuretics, ACE inhibitors, Nitrates, or Angiotensin receptor blockers.

HYPERTENSION

2017 ACC/AHA GUIDELINES				
Classification	Systolic BP		Diastolic BP	
Normal BP	<120	and	<80	
Elevated BP	120–129	and	<80	**Lifestyle changes**
Stage 1 Hypertension	130–139	or	80-89	**Lifestyle changes, ±1 antihypertensive** **1 antihypertensive if comorbid DM, CKD, ASCVD**
Stage 2 Hypertension	≥ 140	or	≥90	**Lifestyle changes + 1-2 antihypertensives** **2 drug combo if ≥20/10 mmHg above target**

- **Systolic blood pressure of ≥130 mmHg and/or diastolic blood pressure ≥80 mmHg.**
- The elevations must be **at least 2 different readings on at least 2 different visits.**

ETIOLOGIES
Primary (essential):
- **Most common cause (95%) — due to idiopathic etiology.**
- Associated with increased salt sensitivity, increases sympathetic activity, and increased mineralocorticoid activity.

Secondary: 5% — due to an underlying, often correctable cause:
- **Renovascular most common cause of secondary HTN (4%) — eg, renal artery stenosis.**
- Endocrine (0.5%): Cushing syndrome, Hyperaldosteronism, & Pheochromocytoma.
- Coarctation of the aorta, sleep apnea, alcohol use, oral contraceptives, COX-2 inhibitors.

COMPLICATIONS
- **Cardiovascular:** coronary artery disease, heart failure, myocardial infarction, left ventricular hypertrophy, aortic dissection, aortic aneurysm, peripheral vascular disease.
- **Neurologic:** TIA, stroke (CVA), ruptured aneurysms, encephalopathy.
- **Nephropathy:** renal stenosis & sclerosis. **Hypertension is the second most common cause of end-stage renal disease in the US (after Diabetes mellitus).**
- **Optic:** retinal hemorrhage, blindness, retinopathy.

WORKUP
In addition to funduscopy for retinopathy, laboratory evaluation in a newly hypertensive:
- Renal function tests: serum electrolytes: eg, Na+, K+, Ca+2; serum creatinine, Urinalysis, Urine albumin/creatinine ratio (optional).
- Endocrine tests: fasting plasma glucose, lipid profile, TSH, CBC
- Cardiac tests: ECG (document LVH), Echocardiography

MANAGEMENT
Lifestyle management:
Initial management of choice of a newly diagnosed hypertensive:
- Weight loss: achieve BMI 18.5-24.9. Weight reduction may lower BP 5-20 mmHg per 10 kg of weight loss in a patient whose weight is >10% of ideal body weight.
- Exercise: ≥30 minutes of exercise/day for most of the week. Smoking cessation.
- Dash Diet: ↑ fruits & vegetables with ↓ saturated/total fats & low sodium (≤2.4 g of sodium/day).
- Intake of dietary potassium, calcium, and magnesium consumption is recommended as they have been shown to have an inverse effect on BP.
- Decreased alcohol intake adult men and women with hypertension should be advised to drink no more than two and one standard drinks per day, respectively.
- **Blood pressure target is <140/90 mmHg** (<150/90 mmHg in adults 60 years of age or older).
- **Medical management in patients who fail a trial of diet and exercise.**
- Treatment results in 50% ↓ of heart failure; 40% ↓ of strokes, 20-25% ↓ of myocardial infarctions.

PHARMACOLOGIC MANAGEMENT OF HYPERTENSION

INITIAL HYPERTENSIVE THERAPY IN UNCOMPLICATED HTN (NON-BLACK/AFRICAN AMERICANS)

Any 1 of the 4 classes:
1. Thiazide-type diuretics
2. ACE inhibitors
3. Calcium channel blockers
4. Angiotensin II receptor blockers

HYPERTENSIVE THERAPY WITH COEXISTING CONDITIONS OR CONSIDERATIONS

COMORBID DISEASE	OPTIMAL THERAPY
Angina	β-blockers or Calcium channel blockers (CCBs)
Post Myocardial Infarction	ACE Inhibitors or β-blockers
Heart Failure with reduced EF	ACEI, ARB, β-blockers, or diuretics
Diabetes mellitus, Chronic kidney disease	ACE inhibitors, Angiotensin receptor blockers (ARBs)
Isolated systolic HTN in elderly	Diuretics, Calcium channel blockers
Osteoporosis	Thiazide diuretics
BPH	α₁ blockers
Blacks & African Americans	Thiazides, Calcium channel blockers
Young, Caucasian males	Thiazides, ACEIs, ARBs
Gout	Calcium Channel Blockers Losartan is the only ARB that doesn't cause hyperuricemia.

COMORBID DISEASE	LIKELY TO HELP
Atrial flutter or fibrillation	β-blockers, Calcium channel blockers (CCB)
Raynaud phenomenon	Dihydropyridine, Calcium channel blockers
Hyperthyroidism	Beta blockers (eg, Propranolol)
Essential tremors	Beta blockers (eg, Propranolol)
Migraine	β-blockers, Calcium channel blockers

DISEASE	ADVERSE EFFECT ON COMORBID CONDITIONS
Depression	β-blockers, Central-acting alpha-2 agonists
Gout	Thiazides and Loop diuretics
Hyperkalemia	ACEI, ARBs, renin inhibitors, aldosterone antagonists
Hyponatremia	Thiazides
SEVERE renal disease	ACEI, ARBs, renin inhibitors

DISEASE	CONTRAINDICATED
Angioedema	ACEI
SEVERE renovascular disease	ACEI, ARBs, renin inhibitors
2nd or 3rd degree heart block	Beta blockers, Non-dihydropyridine CCBs (Verapamil, Diltiazem)

PHARMACOLOGIC MANAGEMENT OF HYPERTENSION

	DRUG/INTERVENTION	COMMENTS
DIURETICS	**DIURETICS** **Hydrochlorothiazide** **Chlorthalidone** Metolazone	Mechanism of action: • Affect blood pressure by reducing blood volume, prevent kidney Na$^+$/water reabsorption at **distal diluting tubule**. Lower urinary calcium excretion. Adverse effects: • **Hyponatremia, hypokalemia,** mild cholesterol elevations, **hyperuricemia, & hyperglycemia** (therefore caution in patients with Diabetes or Gout). **Hypercalcemia.**
	Loop diuretics **Furosemide, Bumetanide**	Mechanism of action: • Inhibit water transport across <u>Loop of Henle</u> ⇨ ↑excretion of water, Cl, Na, K. Strongest class of diuretics. Adverse effects: • Volume depletion, **hypokalemia**/natremia/calcemia, hyperuricemia, hypochloremic metabolic alkalosis, ototoxicity; **hyperlipidemia, hyperglycemia.** • **Contraindicated if sulfa allergy.**
	Potassium sparing diuretics **Spironolactone** **Amiloride** **Eplerenone**	Mechanism of action: • **Inhibit aldosterone-mediated Na/H$_2$O absorption** (spares potassium). Weak diuretic, most useful in combination with Loop diuretics to minimize potassium loss. Adverse effects: • **Hyperkalemia,** metabolic acidosis, **Gynecomastia with Spironolactone.** • <u>Contraindications</u>: renal failure, hyponatremia
VASODILATORS	**ACE INHIBITORS** Captopril Enalapril Ramipril Benazepril	Mechanism of action: • **Cardioprotective, synergistic effect when used with thiazides;** ↓preload/afterload, (↓synthesis of AG II/aldosterone production), potentiate other vasodilators (bradykinin, prostaglandins, nitric oxide); ↑exercise tolerance. Improves insulin's action. Indications: • **Hypertension, especially if history of Diabetes mellitus, nephropathy, proteinuria, Heart failure, post ST elevation Myocardial infarction.** Adverse effects • **1st-dose hypotension, azotemia/renal insufficiency, hyperkalemia** (can be ameliorated with low salt, diuretics), **cough & angioedema (due to ↑bradykinin), hyperuricemia.** • <u>Contraindications</u>: pregnancy.
	ANGIOTENSIN II RECEPTOR BLOCKERS (ARB) Los**artan** Vals**artan** Irbe**sartan** Candes**artan**	Mechanism of action: • Similar actions as ACE inhibitors but binds and blocks the angiotensin II receptor. Does not increase bradykinin production. Indications: • **Consider in patients not able to tolerate Beta-blockers/ACEI or in addition to ACEI.** Adverse effects: • **Hyperkalemia. Contraindicated in pregnancy.**

CALCIUM CHANNEL BLOCKERS
 	
Dihydropyridines
  Nifedipine
  Amlodipine
 	
Non-dihydropyridines
  Verapamil
  Diltiazem
	Mechanism of action:
	• **Dihydropyridines: potent vasodilators (little or no effect on cardiac contractility or conduction)** neutral or increased vascular permeability. Dihydropyridines most commonly used in HTN.
	• **Non-dihydropyridines affect cardiac contractility & conduction** as well as potent vasodilators, reduces vascular permeability.
	Adverse effects
	• Vasodilation: **headache, dizziness, lightheadedness, flushing, peripheral edema. Constipation with Verapamil.**
	Contraindications:
	• CHF (especially nondihydropyridines). **2nd/3rd AV heart block.**

β – BLOCKERS
 	
Cardioselective (β1):
  Atenolol, Metoprolol, Esmolol
 	
Nonselective (β1, β2):
  Propranolol
 	
Both α & β1,2:
  Labetalol, Carvedilol
	Mechanism of action:
	• Catecholamine inhibitor. **Blocks "adrenergic" renin release.**
	• Not usually used as first line therapy in general unless there is a comorbid condition in which beta blockade is helpful.
	Adverse effects:
	• **Fatigue, depression, impotence;** may mask tachycardic symptoms of hypoglycemia in DM **(so use with caution in diabetic patients).**
	• Caution if **hypotensive or pulse <50 bpm.**
	Contraindications:
	• **2nd/3rd heart block, decompensated heart failure.**
	• **Nonselective agents contraindicated in asthma/COPD** and may worsen peripheral vascular disease & Raynaud's phenomenon.

α1 BLOCKERS
  Prazosin
  Terazosin
  Doxazosin
	Mechanism of action:
	• Alpha blockade leads to peripheral arterial dilation.
	• Generally, not used as first-line therapy generally but **may be helpful in patients with Hypertension + Benign prostatic hypertrophy.**
	• Adverse effects: **1st-dose syncope, dizziness, headache,** weakness.

HYPERTENSIVE URGENCY

• **SBP >180 mmHg and/or DBP >120 mmHg without evidence of end-organ damage.**

CLINICAL MANIFESTATIONS
• General: headache (most common), dyspnea, chest pain, focal neurologic deficits, altered mental status, delirium, seizures, nausea, or vomiting.

MANAGEMENT
• **Patients without symptoms or signs of target organ damage have not been shown to benefit from aggressive antihypertensive therapy in the acute setting.**
• When treatment is indicated, treatment goal is blood pressure <160/<100 mmHg but the mean arterial pressure should not be lowered by more than 25–30% over the first 2-4 hours.
• **Gradual reduction of mean arterial pressure by no more than 25% over 24-48 hours with oral medications (eg, Clonidine or Captopril most commonly used agents),** Labetalol, Nicardipine, Furosemide.

ORAL MEDICATIONS USED IN THE MANAGEMENT OF HYPERTENSIVE URGENCIES		
Drug	**Mechanism of Action**	**Adverse Effects**
Clonidine	**Centrally acting α-2 adrenergic agonist (short-term use only)**	Headache, tachycardia, nausea, vomiting, **sedation,** fatigue dry mouth, **rebound hypertension if discontinued abruptly.**
Captopril	ACE Inhibitor	Angioedema, Acute kidney injury, teratogenic.
Furosemide	Loop diuretic	Electrolyte abnormalities, metabolic alkalosis.
Labetalol	α1 β1 β2 blocker	CI in severe asthma/COPD, ADHF (CHF)
Nicardipine	Calcium channel blocker	Reflex tachycardia, headache, nausea

HYPERTENSIVE EMERGENCY

- **SBP >180 mmHg and/or DBP >120 mmHg** with <u>**evidence of end-organ damage**</u>.

CLINICAL MANIFESTATIONS

- <u>General:</u> headache (most common), dyspnea, chest pain, focal neurologic deficits, altered mental status, delirium, seizures, nausea, vomiting.
- <u>Neurologic:</u> encephalopathy, stroke (hemorrhagic or ischemic), seizure.
- <u>Cardiac:</u> Acute coronary syndrome, Aortic dissection, Acute heart failure (pulmonary edema). Workup includes CXR, ECG, cardiac enzymes, BNP.
- <u>Renal:</u> Acute kidney injury, proteinuria, hematuria (glomerulonephritis).
- <u>Retinal:</u> malignant Hypertension, severe (Grade IV) retinopathy.

MANAGEMENT

- <u>**IV blood pressure reduction agents**</u>**. For most hypertensive emergencies, mean arterial pressure should be reduced gradually by about 10-20% in the first hour and by an additional 5-15% over the next 23 hours**.

The 3 main exceptions are as follows:
- [1] <u>Acute phase of an ischemic stroke:</u> blood pressure is usually not lowered unless it is ≥185/110 mmHg in patients who are candidates for reperfusion treatment OR ≥220/120 mmHg in patients who are not candidates for reperfusion.
- [2] <u>Acute aortic dissection:</u> systolic blood pressure is rapidly lowered to a goal of 100-120 mmHg within 20 minutes.
- [3] <u>Intracerebral hypertension:</u> treatment depends on different factors.

INTRAVENOUS MEDICATIONS USED IN THE MANAGEMENT OF HYPERTENSIVE EMERGENCIES		
EMERGENCY	**FIRST LINE**	**NOTES**
NEUROLOGIC **HTN ENCEPHALOPATHY**	**Nicardipine or Clevidipine** **Labetalol,** Fenoldopam Sodium Nitroprusside	Must rule out stroke. **HTN encephalopathy often presents with confusion, headache, nausea & vomiting.** Symptoms improve with lowering of BP. Nitroprusside, Nitroglycerin & Hydralazine may increase intracranial pressure.
HEMORRHAGIC STROKE	Nicardipine or Labetalol	Benefits vs. risks of lowering blood pressure must be weighed in hemorrhagic strokes.
ISCHEMIC STROKE	Nicardipine or Labetalol	*Avoid cerebral hypoperfusion if ischemic.* Reduce blood pressure ONLY if BP is: ≥220/120 (not a thrombolytic candidate). ≥185/110 (if a thrombolytic candidate).
CARDIOVASCULAR **AORTIC DISSECTION**	***β-blocker:* Esmolol, Labetalol** Sodium Nitroprusside may be added to Beta blockers Nicardipine, Clevidipine	Decreases shearing forces. Beta blocker therapeutic target: systolic BP 100-120 mmHg & pulse <60 bpm achieved within 20 minutes.
ACUTE CORONARY SYNDROME	**Nitroglycerin** **Beta-blockers** (eg, Esmolol, Metoprolol) Nitroprusside	Nitroglycerin not used if suspected right ventricular infarction or phosphodiesterase -5 inhibitor use within 24-48h (eg, Sildenafil).
ACUTE HEART FAILURE	**Nitroglycerin, Furosemide,** Sodium nitroprusside	Avoid Hydralazine & Beta blockers in CHF. Only if no evidence of cardiac ischemia.

POSTURAL (ORTHOSTATIC) HYPOTENSION

- **Hypotension within 2-5 minutes of quiet standing** (or after a 5-minute period of supine rest) **defined by ≥20 mmHg fall in systolic pressure and/or ≥10 mmHg fall in diastolic pressure.**

ETIOLOGIES

- Impaired autonomic function and/or decreased intravascular volume. Common in elderly >65 years.
- <u>Medications</u>: includes antihypertensives (eg, Alpha blockers, Nitroglycerin, ACE inhibitors), diuretics, narcotics, antipsychotics, antidepressants, and alcohol consumption.
- <u>Neurologic</u>: include diabetic neuropathy, Parkinson disease, polyneuropathies etc.
- Hypovolemia (eg, Loop diuretics, hemorrhage or vomiting).

CLINICAL MANIFESTATIONS

- Due to cerebral hypoperfusion — dizziness, lightheadedness, palpitations, blurred vision, darkening of visual fields, and/or syncope.

WORKUP

- **Blood pressure measurement for orthostatic changes is the first diagnostic test.**
- <u>Tilt table test</u>: **Tilt table test can help confirm a diagnosis of suspected Orthostatic hypotension when orthostatic vital signs are nondiagnostic.** Blood pressure reduction at a 60° angle.
- <u>Labs</u>: to evaluate for anemia or dehydration — eg, hematocrit, electrolytes, BUN, creatine, glucose.

MANAGEMENT

- <u>**Conservative**</u> initial management of choice — **increasing salt and fluid intake (volume resuscitation), gradual positional changes** (eg, rising slowly from a supine or sitting position), **compression stockings or abdominal binders, exercise, and discontinuation of offending medications if polypharmacy is the cause. Caffeine may be helpful.** Management of any contributing disease (eg, Diabetes mellitus). In the acute phase, place patient in prior position.
- <u>**Medical:**</u> **Both Fludrocortisone & Midodrine are first-line agents to increase vascular tone.**
- <u>**Fludrocortisone acetate**</u> **is the first-line medical management if persistent symptoms despite nonpharmacologic measures.** Fludrocortisone is a synthetic mineralocorticoid (similar to aldosterone) that causes blood volume expansion and increased vascular tone. Adverse effects include Hypokalemia (may require potassium supplementation), edema, CHF, or worsening seated or supine hypertension, which may require dose reduction or discontinuation.
- <u>**Pressor agents:**</u> **Midodrine is an alpha-1 adrenergic agonist and Droxidopa is a norepinephrine precursor that increase vascular tone.** May be used in combination with Fludrocortisone or first-line monotherapy in those unable or unwilling to tolerate Fludrocortisone adverse effects.
- Avoiding the flat position, sleeping with the head of the bed raised 30-45°.

REFLEX-MEDIATED (NEURAL-MEDIATED) SYNCOPE

VASOVAGAL SYNCOPE

- <u>Due to vasovagal hypotension</u>: self-limited systemic hypotension associated with bradycardia and/or peripheral venodilation/vasodilation.
- **Most common cause of syncope**, especially without apparent neurologic or cardiovascular disease.
- <u>Triggers:</u> blood phobia, emotional stress/fear, pain, trauma.
- <u>Manifestations:</u> **prodromal phase** (eg, dizziness, lightheadedness, epigastric pain, palpitations, blurred vision, darkening of visual fields, warmth, pallor, diaphoresis) followed by syncope & postdromal phase.

CAROTID SINUS SYNCOPE

- Syncope with minor stimulation of the carotid sinus (eg, shaving, putting on neckties, wearing a tight collar, head turning, or applying minor pressure to the carotids).

SITUATIONAL SYNCOPE

- Triggers include defecation, micturition, straining, coughing, sneezing, post-prandial, & trigger points.

INFECTIVE ENDOCARDITIS

- Infection of the endothelium/valves 2^{ry} to colonization (eg, during transient/persistent bacteremia).
- **Mitral valve most common valve involved** (M>A>T>P).
   Exception is IV drug use — tricuspid valve most common valve in IV drug users.
- <u>Risk factors</u>: increased age (>60 years of age), rheumatic heart disease, IV drug use, immunosuppression, prosthetic heart valves, congenital heart disease.

Acute bacterial endocarditis:
- Infection of **normal valves** with a virulent organism (eg, *Staphylococcus aureus*).
Subacute bacterial endocarditis:
- Indolent infection of **abnormal valves** with less virulent organism (eg, *Streptococcus viridans*).
IV drug-related endocarditis:
- **Most commonly due to** *Staphylococcal aureus* **(especially MRSA).** *Pseudomonas aeruginosa*, Candida.
Prosthetic valve endocarditis:
- **Early (within 60 days): usually caused by** *S. aureus* **(including MRSA) &** *S. epidermidis*.

MICROBIOLOGY
Staphylococcus aureus:
- **Most common cause of IE, including <u>ACUTE</u> infective endocarditis, prosthetic valve IE, and IVDA infective endocarditis (especially MRSA).** Often affects normal valves.
Streptococcus viridans
- Most common cause of **SUBACUTE** infective endocarditis, often **affecting damaged valves.**
- Because it is part of the oral flora, ***S. viridans* is associated with Endocarditis from transient bacteremia secondary to gingivitis, poor dentition, or dental procedures.**
Staphylococcus epidermidis:
- **Early Prosthetic valve endocarditis (especially within 60 days of the procedure), is usually caused by** *S. aureus* **or** *S. epidermidis* **(coagulase-negative staphylococci).**
Enterococcus spp. (eg, *E. faecalis*):
- Seen especially in men >50 years with a recent history of **gastrointestinal or genitourinary procedure.**
HACEK organisms:
- (<u>H</u>aemophilus aphrophilus, <u>A</u>ctinobacillus, <u>C</u>ardiobacterium hominis, <u>E</u>ikenella corrodens, <u>K</u>ingella kingae) are gram- negative organisms that are hard to culture.
- **Suspect these organisms in patients with endocarditis & negative blood cultures.**
Streptococcus gallolyticus (bovis):
- Commensal bacteria of the gut seen with **increased incidence in patients with Colorectal cancer and Ulcerative colitis** (Colonoscopy should be performed in these patients to rule out both).

CLINICAL MANIFESTATIONS
- <u>Constitutional</u>: **persistent fever most common symptom**, chills, anorexia, weight loss, malaise.
- **New onset or worsening of an existing murmur** (85%) — eg, Mitral or Tricuspid regurgitation.
- <u>Osler nodes</u>: **painful or tender raised violaceous nodules on the pads of the digits and the palms**; may be seen on the thenar or hypothenar eminence.
- <u>Janeway lesions</u>: **painless erythematous macules on the palms & soles.**
- <u>Splinter hemorrhages:</u> linear reddish-brown lesions under the nail bed, petechiae (skin or mucous membranes). **Roth spots: retinal hemorrhages with central clearing.**
- Splenomegaly, septic arterial or pulmonary emboli, glomerulonephritis.
- <u>Right-sided IE:</u> **in addition to fever & constitutional symptoms, especially with tricuspid involvement, pulmonary symptoms are common** (eg, cough, dyspnea, pleuritic chest pain, and hemoptysis) may mimic URI. **~90% of patients with right-sided IE are IV drug users.**

DIAGNOSTIC STUDIES

- **The 2 most important tests for suspected Endocarditis are [1] blood cultures and [2] echocardiography,** as they help to establish the 2 major Duke criteria.
- <u>Blood cultures:</u> (before antibiotic initiation). **3 sets at least 1 hour apart** if the patient is stable.
- <u>ECG:</u> at regular intervals to assess for new conduction abnormalities (prone to arrhythmias).
- **Echocardiogram:** obtain Transthoracic echo first; consider TEE if TTE is nondiagnostic or increased suspicion. **Transesophageal echocardiogram (TEE) much more sensitive than TTE** (>90% v. 50% in NVE) (82% v. 36% in PVE) so may be used in patients with suspected Prosthetic valve endocarditis.
- **Labs:** CBC: leukocytosis, anemia (normochromic, normocytic); ↑ ESR/Rheumatoid Factor.

MODIFIED DUKE CRITERIA	
<u>MAJOR</u>	<u>MINOR</u>

• <u>SUSTAINED BACTEREMIA</u> 2 ⊕ **blood cultures** by organism known to cause endocarditis.
 	
• <u>ENDOCARDIAL INVOLVEMENT</u>: documented by either:
  - ⊕ **echocardiogram**: (vegetation, abscess, valve perforation, prosthetic dehiscence)
 	
  - clearly established <u>**new** valvular **regurgitation**</u> (aortic or mitral regurgitation)
	• <u>Predisposing condition</u>
	  abnormal valves, IVDA, indwelling catheters, etc.
	• **Fever** (>38° C/100.4°F).
	• <u>**Vascular & embolic phenomena:**</u> Janeway lesions, septic arterial or pulmonary emboli, ICH.
	• <u>**Immunologic phenomena:**</u>
	  - Osler's nodes, Roth spots, ⊕ Rheumatoid factor
	  - Acute glomerulonephritis
	• ⊕ Blood culture not meeting major criteria.
	• ⊕ echocardiogram not meeting major criteria (eg, worsening of existing murmur).

Clinical criteria for infective endocarditis: (1) 2 major OR (2) 1 major + 3 minor OR (3) 5 minor have 80% accuracy	

MANAGEMENT OF INFECTIVE ENDOCARDITIS: suggested **Empiric therapy:**

NATIVE VALVE (MRSA) OR UNKNOWN • Methicillin resistant *S. aureus*	• **Empiric treatment includes (1) Vancomycin or (2) Vancomycin plus EITHER Ceftriaxone or Gentamicin**. • Daptomycin is an alternative to Vancomycin in patients unable to tolerate Vancomycin.
NATIVE VALVE (MSSA) • Methicillin sensitive *S. aureus*	• <u>**Anti-staphylococcal Penicillin**</u> eg, Nafcillin, Oxacillin. • Empiric management of suspected MSSA may include Anti-staphylococcal Penicillin plus EITHER Ceftriaxone or Gentamicin. • <u>**Penicillin allergy:**</u> **Cefazolin is an alternative if non-anaphylactoid allergy;** Vancomycin or Daptomycin.
PROSTHETIC VALVE	• **Vancomycin + Gentamicin + Rifampin.** Rifampin is efficient at killing Staphylococci that are adherent to foreign material.
FUNGAL	• <u>**Parenteral antifungal agent:**</u> eg, **Amphotericin-containing product with or without combination therapy (eg, Amphotericin B and Flucytosine).** • Antifungal therapy is usually given for 6 weeks or more. • Patients often need surgical intervention for fungal cases

Penicillin & Vancomycin have great gram-positive coverage.

Gentamicin has great gram-negative coverage.

Ceftriaxone has great gram-positive & gram-negative coverage.

- Refractory CHF; persistent or refractory infection, invasive infection, prosthetic valve, recurrent systemic emboli, fungal infections.
- In acute Endocarditis, antibiotics are started promptly after culture data is obtained.
- In subacute Endocarditis, if the patient is hemodynamically stable, antibiotics may be delayed in order to properly obtain blood culture data, especially if prior treatment with antibiotics.
- Adjust the antibiotic regimen based on organism, culture & sensitivities. Fever may persist up to 1 week after appropriate antibiotic therapy has been initiated.
- **Duration of therapy usually 4-6 weeks** (with aminoglycosides used only for the first 2 weeks).

ENDOCARDITIS PROPHYLAXIS INDICATIONS	
Cardiac conditions	1. **Prosthetic (artificial) heart valves.** 2. **Heart repairs using prosthetic material (not including stents).** 3. **Prior history of endocarditis.** 4. **Congenital heart disease.** 5. Cardiac valvulopathy in a transplanted heart.
Procedures	1. **Dental:** involving manipulation of gums, roots of the teeth, oral mucosa perforation. 2. **Respiratory:** surgery on respiratory mucosa, rigid bronchoscopy. 3. **Procedures involving infected skin/musculoskeletal tissues** (including abscess incision & drainage).
Regimens	- **Amoxicillin 2g 30-60 minutes before** the procedures listed above. - **Penicillin allergy**: **Macrolides, Doxycycline, or Cephalexin** are other options.

Prophylaxis is no longer routinely recommended for gastrointestinal or genitourinary procedures.
Prophylaxis no longer routinely recommended for most types of valvular heart disease (including mitral valve prolapse, bicuspid aortic valve, acquired mitral or aortic valve disease, hypertrophic cardiomyopathy).
Good oral hygiene recommended to reduce temporary episodes of bacteremia.

- In May 2021, the American Heart Association updated its 2007 guidelines on antibiotic prophylaxis for prevention of streptococcal Infective endocarditis among patients with relevant cardiac **risk factors undergoing dental procedures**. In such patients, the preferred oral regimen is Amoxicillin; alternatives for patients with Amoxicillin allergy include Cephalexin, Azithromycin, Clarithromycin, and Doxycycline. Clindamycin is no longer a suggested alternative in patients undergoing dental procedures because it is associated with more frequent and severe adverse effects (particularly *Clostridioides difficile* infection) than the others.

LIBMAN-SACKS ENDOCARDITIS

- **Nonbacterial thrombotic (marantic) endocarditis** is a noninfectious endocarditis due to sterile platelet thrombi deposition on the affected valve, usually affecting the mitral & aortic valves.

ETIOLOGIES

- Can be seen with malignancy, **Systemic lupus erythematosus**, Antiphospholipid antibody syndrome, rheumatic fever, and other inflammatory conditions.

CLINICAL MANIFESTATIONS

- Most patients are asymptomatic and are usually afebrile.
- Symptoms are usually due to emboli to the skin, kidney, extremities, and spleen.

MANAGEMENT

- Manage the SLE. May need anticoagulation.

THE 5 GOLDEN RULES TO CONQUER MURMURS

RULE 1 - QUALITY OF THE MURMUR

- **HARSH/RUMBLE SOUNDS = think STENOSIS or HCM:** AS, MS, PS, TS, or Hypertrophic cardiomyopathy; abnormal forward flow of blood through (stenotic) valve that should be open. Stenotic lesions lead to <u>pressure overload</u>.

- <u>BLOWING sound</u> – **think REGURGITATION:** AR, MR, PR, TR: abnormal backflow of blood (regurgitation) through an incompletely closed valve. Regurgitation lesions lead to <u>volume overload.</u>

RULE 2 VALVE DISEASE GOLDEN RULE:

- Increase in venous return increases the intensity of ALL murmurs <u>EXCEPT</u> hypertrophic cardiomyopathy & the click of mitral valve prolapse (murmur of hypertrophic cardiomyopathy is **d**ecreased & ejection click is **d**elayed/occurs later).

When the **MVP** with **hypertrophied** arms **squatted**, the sound of the crowd **got quiet** in anticipation

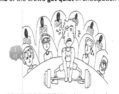

Increase venous return
- Supine position

- Squatting

- Leg elevation

RULE 2 Continued

- **Decrease in venous return decreased the intensity of ALL murmurs EXCEPT hypertrophic cardiomyopathy & the click of mitral valve prolapse** (murmur of hypertrophic cardiomopathy is **i**ntensified (**i**ncreased) & ejection click occurs **e**arlier) [2 vowels].

When the **MVP** with **hypertrophied** arms **stood up**, the sound of the crowd **got louder.**

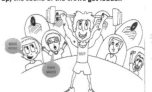

decrease venous return
- Standing

- Valsalva maneuver

PART 3 OF THE VALVE DISEASE GOLDEN RULE:

Since they sound similar, the 2 things that <u>distinguish R-sided from L-sided</u> are

- ❶ inspiration increases the intensity of Right-sided murmurs; inspiration decreas the intensity of left-sided murmurs. Expiration increases intensity of the left murm

- ❷ the location of intensity

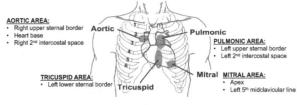

AORTIC AREA:
- Right upper sternal border
- Heart base
- Right 2nd intercostal space

PULMONIC AREA:
- Left upper sternal border
- Left 2nd intercostal space

TRICUSPID AREA:
- Left lower sternal border

MITRAL AREA:
- Apex
- Left 5th midclavicular line

MURMURS ARE BEST HEARD WHERE THE BLOOD FLOWS <u>NOT</u> WHERE THE VALVE IS LOC/

PART 3 OF THE VALVE DISEASE GOLDEN RULE (continued):

The left-sided "cousins" sound like their right-sided "cousins"

- <u>Left sided valves:</u> Mitral and Aortic valves

- <u>Right-sided valves:</u> Tricuspid and Pulmonic valves

MR sounds like TR; MS sounds like TS; AR sounds like PR; AS sounds like PS

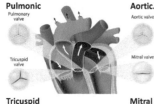

RIGHT		LEFT		
Pulmonic		Aortic.	PR/AR	PS/AS
Tricuspid		Mitral	TR/MR	TS/MS

RULE 4

Radiation of the murmur
- **Axilla – Mitral regurgitation**
- **Carotid – Aortic stenosis, Pulmonic stenosis**

RULE 5

"AR MS' rest: Diastolic ("rest") murmurs
Diastolic murmurs:
- **A**ortic **R**egurgitation; Pulmonic regurgitation.
- **M**itral **S**tenosis; Tricuspid stenosis

Systolic murmurs:
- Aortic stenosis, Pulmonic stenosis
- Mitral regurgitation, Tricuspid regurgitation

MURMUR ACCENTUATION MANEUVERS

POSITION
- **AORTIC:** SITTING UP & LEANING FORWARD ACCENTUATES AORTIC MURMURS (AS, AR).
- **MITRAL:** LYING IN LEFT LATERAL DECUBITUS POSITION ACCENTUATES MITRAL MURMURS (MS, MR).

INCREASED VENOUS RETURN
- ↑venous return INCREASES ALL MURMURS/opening Snap (left & right) - squatting, leg raise, lying down
- Exceptions: ↓murmur of Hypertrophic cardiomyopathy & delayed ejection click (decreased prolapse/shorter murmur duration) of mitral valve prolapse (MVP)

DECREASED VENOUS RETURN
- ↓venous return (Valsalva/standing) DECREASES ALL major MURMURS/Opening Snap (left & right side).
- Exceptions: ↑murmur of Hypertrophic cardiomyopathy & earlier ejection click (increased prolapse & longer murmur duration) of MVP.

INSPIRATION
- Inspiration ↑'es venous return on right side:

   ↑ **ALL murmurs/opening snap on the R side** (↓ejection click R side)
   - **Right-sided murmurs (pulmonic, tricuspid) are best heard with inspiration.**

- Inspiration ↓'es venous return on left side:
   - ↓ ALL murmurs/opening snap on the L side (earlier ejection click on the L side)

EXPIRATION
- Expiration ↑'es venous return on left side:

   ↑ **ALL murmurs/opening snap on the L side** (delayed ejection click on the L side)
   - **Left-sided murmurs (aortic, mitral) are best heard after maximal expiration.**

- Expiration ↓'es venous return on right side:

   ↓ ALL murmurs/opening snap on the R side (earlier ejection click R side).

HANDGRIP
- ↑**'es afterload** (by compressing the arteries of the upper extremity) leading to ↓LV emptying (decreased forward flow & **increased backward flow**).
   - **Outflow murmurs (eg. AS, hypertrophic cardiomyopathy)** and MVP ↓ **with handgrip** (note that *handgrip & amyl nitrate are the only maneuvers that affect Hypertrophic cardiomyopathy & AS in the same direction* – because both maneuvers affect AFTERLOAD & FORWARD FLOW). Because handgrip increases afterload, the increased afterload prevents blood from being ejected from the ventricles, lessening the blood flowing through the stenotic aortic valve and less blood ejected in hypertrophic cardiomyopathy.
   - **Regurgitant murmurs (AR, MR) ↑with handgrip** ↑backward flow; MS ↑'es due to ↑afterload.

AMYL NITRATE
- ↓**'es afterload** (direct arteriolar vasodilator) leading to ↑LV emptying (increases forward flow & decreases backward flow of blood).
   - AS, MVP, hypertrophic cardiomyopathy murmur ↑ with amyl nitrate
   - **Regurgitant murmurs (AR, MR) ↓ with Amyl nitrate**
      This is why afterload reducers like ACEI are used in the management of AR, MR.

- **Aortic stenosis (AS) VS. Hypertrophic obstructive cardiomyopathy (HOCM)**
- Both: angina, syncope, systolic murmur. Both murmurs go in the same direction with afterload maneuvers (eg, both increase with Amyl nitrate & both decrease with handgrip).
- **HOCM:** preload maneuvers that decrease LV volume **(eg, Valsalva, standing) will worsen the murmur of HOCM** whereas these maneuvers will decrease the intensity of most other murmurs (including AS). **Increased LV volume (eg, squatting, leg raise) will decrease the murmur of HOCM** whereas these maneuvers will increase the intensity AS. No carotid radiation.

AORTIC STENOSIS (AS)

- **Pathophysiology:** LV outflow obstruction leads to a fixed cardiac output, increased afterload, Left ventricular hypertrophy (LVH), and eventually LV failure.
- Most common valvular disease. Symptoms usually occur when Aov orifice <1 cm^2 (Normal 3-4 cm^2).

ETIOLOGIES
- **Degenerative:** calcifications, wear and tear, especially >70 years of age.
- **Congenital & Bicuspid valve** more common in patients <70 years of age.
- Rheumatic heart disease: may be isolated or accompanied with Aortic regurgitation.

CLINICAL MANIFESTATIONS
Once symptomatic, lifespan is dramatically reduced.
- **Exertional dyspnea is often the most common presenting symptom in patients with AS. Decreased exercise tolerance.** Increased LV filling pressures with exercise, diastolic dysfunction, & inability of the LV to increase cardiac output during exercise - fixed cardiac output.
- **Angina:** (5 year mean survival if valve not replaced), **syncope** (3 years), and **CHF** (2 years).

PHYSICAL EXAMINATION
- **Harsh, low-pitched, mid-late peaking, systolic, crescendo-decrescendo murmur best heard at the right upper sternal border** (R 2nd intercostal space at base); **radiates to the carotid arteries.**
- **Increased murmur intensity:** sitting while leaning forward (all aortic murmurs), **increased venous return (eg, squatting, supine, and leg raise), expiration** (increased flow to the left side during expiration), and **decreased afterload (inhalation of Amyl nitrate).**
- **Decreased murmur intensity:** decreased venous return (eg, Valsalva, standing), **inspiration** (decreased flow to the left side of the heart), **or increased afterload (eg, handgrip).**
- **Weak, delayed carotid pulse** (slow rising, low volume), **narrow pulse pressure** (↓stroke volume).
- **Single or soft second heart sound (S2):** soft, absent, or paradoxically split S2.
- Fourth heart sound (S4), also known as an atrial gallop, occurs during left ventricular (LV) filling when vigorous left atrial contraction forces blood into a noncompliant (stiff and hypertrophic) LV.

DIAGNOSTIC STUDIES
- **Echocardiogram: test of choice** — small aortic orifice, LVH, thickened or calcified aortic valve.
- **ECG: left ventricular hypertrophy classic.** Left atrial enlargement, Atrial fibrillation.
- Chest radiograph: nonspecific: postaortic dilatation, aortic valve calcification, pulmonary congestion.
- Cardiac catheterization: definitive diagnosis (may be used prior to surgery or if Echo is undiagnostic).

MANAGEMENT
- **Surgical therapy: aortic valve replacement only effective treatment (treatment of choice)**
  Indications: symptomatic AS, severe AS [eg, aortic area < 0.8 cm^2 (normal 3-4cm^2)], or decreased ejection fraction (<50%).
    - Mechanical: prolonged durability but thrombogenic (eg, stroke), bleeding. Must be placed on long-term anticoagulant therapy.
    - Bioprosthetic: less durable but minimally thrombogenic (usually used in patients that that are not candidates for anticoagulant). Heterograft (porcine valve); pericardial.
- Percutaneous aortic valvuloplasty (PAV): results in 50% ↑AoV area, but 50% restenosis at 6-12 months, so used as a bridge to AVR, if not a surgical candidate, or in pediatric patients.
- Intraaortic balloon pump: used for temporary stabilization as a bridge to valve replacement.
- Medical therapy: no medical treatment truly effective. No exercise restrictions in mild AS.
Severe AS prior to surgery:
- Because patients are dependent on preload to maintain cardiac output ⇨ **avoid physical exertion/venodilators** (eg, nitrates)/**negative inotropes** (Ca^{+2} channel blockers, β-blockers).

AORTIC REGURGITATION (AR) or AORTIC INSUFFICIENCY(AI)

- **Incomplete aortic valve closure, leading to regurgitation of blood through the aortic valve into the left ventricle (LV) during diastole.** LV overload leads to LV dilation & hypertrophy.

ETIOLOGIES
- **Chronic AR: usually a slowly progressive disease over decades** before becoming symptomatic. Causes include congenital bicuspid valve, Rheumatic heart disease, Hypertension, autoimmunity, Syphilis, Collagen vascular disease: Ehlers-Danlos syndrome, and Marfan syndrome.
- **Acute AR: acute onset is usually a medical emergency** due to the inability of the left ventricle to rapidly adapt to the abrupt increase in end-diastolic volume caused by the regurgitant flow. **The two most common causes of acute AR of a native aortic valve are [1] Endocarditis & [2] Aortic dissection.** If not surgically corrected, acute severe AR commonly results in cardiogenic shock.

CLINICAL MANIFESTATIONS:
- Chronic AR: Patients may be asymptomatic for decades until severe left ventricular dysfunction has developed — exertional dyspnea, orthopnea, paroxysmal nocturnal dyspnea, decreased exercise tolerance, fatigue, angina, palpitations.
- In acute severe AR, compensatory mechanisms of the LV do not develop rapidly enough to adapt to the regurgitant volume load, increased preload & afterload. LV diastolic pressures rise rapidly leading to acute pulmonary edema (↑pulmonary capillary wedge pressure) and cardiogenic shock.

PHYSICAL EXAMINATION
- **High-pitched, blowing (soft), decrescendo or sustained, diastolic murmur best heard over the left sternal border at Erb's point (third or fourth intercostal space).**
- **Increased murmur intensity: sitting up while leaning forward** (all aortic murmurs), **holding breath in end-expiration** (left-sided murmurs), **increased venous return (eg, squatting, lying supine, and leg raise), increased afterload (eg, handgrip),** and isometric exercise.
- **Decreased murmur intensity: decreased venous return (eg, Valsalva, standing),** inspiration. Decreased afterload (eg, **Amyl nitrate**).
- Austin-Flint murmur: mid-late diastolic rumble at the apex secondary to retrograde regurgitant jet competing with antegrade flow from the left atrium into the left ventricle.
- **Bounding pulses** due to increased stroke volume. Pulsus bisferiens can be seen (especially with combined AS + AR or severe AR). **Wide pulse pressure** (increased SBP and decreased DBP) .

Classic Signs of WIDENED PULSE PRESSURE in AR/AI (seen ONLY with chronic AR/AI)	
SIGN	DESCRIPTION
Water Hammer pulse	**Swift upstroke & rapid fall of radial pulse accentuated with wrist elevation.**
Corrigan's pulse	Similar to water hammer pulse but referring specifically to the carotid artery.
Hill's sign	Popliteal artery systolic pressure > brachial artery by 60mmHg **(most sensitive).**
Duroziez's sign	Gradual pressure over femoral artery ⇨ systolic and diastolic bruits.
Traube's sound (pistol shot)	Double sound heard @ femoral artery with partial compression of femoral artery.
De Musset's sign	**Head-bobbing** (rhythmic jerking) with each heartbeat (low sensitivity).
Müller's sign	**Visible systolic pulsations of the uvula.**
Quincke's pulses	**Visible fingernail bed pulsations** with light compression of the fingernail bed.

DIAGNOSTIC STUDIES
- **Echocardiogram: primary diagnostic test of choice to diagnose AR/AI — regurgitant jet.**
- Cardiac catheterization: definitive diagnosis; may be used prior to surgery.

MANAGEMENT
- Medical therapy: **afterload reduction** improves forward flow (ACEI, ARBs, Nifedipine, Hydralazine).
- Surgical therapy: definitive management. Indicated in symptomatic AR, asymptomatic with LV decompensation (EF < 55% - patients with AR normally have higher than normal ejection fraction). **The management for acute severe AR is emergency aortic valve replacement or repair.**

MITRAL STENOSIS (MS)

- **Narrowing of the mitral valve orifice, leading to obstruction of flow from the left atrium (LA) to the left ventricle (LV) & backflow of blood into the left atrium.**

PATHOPHYSIOLOGY
- Obstruction of flow from LA to LV 2^{ry} to narrowed mitral orifice ⇨ blood backs up into the left atrium.
- **↑L-atrial pressure/volume overload** ⇨ pulmonary congestion ⇨ **pulmonary HTN** ⇨ CHF.

ETIOLOGIES
- **Rheumatic heart disease is almost always the cause.*** Most common in the 3rd/4th decade.
- Congenital, left atrial myxoma, thrombus, valvulitis (SLE, amyloid, carcinoid).

CLINICAL MANIFESTATIONS
- Pulmonary: **exertional dyspnea (most common symptom), exercise intolerance,** fatigue, **hemoptysis,** cough, frequent bronchitis, **pulmonary HTN** (if rheumatic, may occur in 20s – 30s).
- **Atrial fibrillation:** secondary to atrial enlargement ⇨ thromboembolic events (eg, CVA).
- Right-sided heart failure: due to prolonged Pulmonary hypertension.
- **Mitral facies: ruddy (flushed) cheeks with facial pallor** due to chronic hypoxia.
- Signs of left atrial enlargement: dysphagia (esophageal compression), **Ortner's syndrome: hoarseness** due to recurrent laryngeal nerve palsy from compression by the dilated left atrium.

PHYSICAL EXAMINATION
- **Prominent (loud) S1** due to forceful closure of mitral valve. **Opening snap: (OS)** may be heard after the A2 component of the second heart sound (S2) due to forceful opening of the mitral valve when the pressure in the left atrium > than the left ventricle.
- **Loud P2:** The P2 (pulmonic) component of the second heart sound (S2) will be loud if severe Pulmonary hypertension due to Mitral stenosis occurs.
- Mitral facies: chronic severe MS, Pulmonary hypertension, ↓cardiac output, & vasoconstriction may lead to cutaneous vasodilation results in pinkish-purple patches (ruddy appearance) on the cheeks.
- **Low-pitched, mid-diastolic, rumbling murmur best heard at the mitral area/apex (left fifth intercostal space at the mid-clavicular line).** Often heard after the opening snap. Best heard with the bell of the stethoscope at the apex with the patient lying on the left side in held expiration.
- **Increased murmur intensity:** left lateral decubitus position, **expiration,** isometric exercise, **increased venous return (eg, squatting, leg raise, lying supine).**
- **Decreased intensity:** decreased venous return (eg, **Valsalva, standing**), inspiration. Amyl nitrate.
- **Increased severity of MS: [1] shorter A2-OS interval** (as the MS progresses and left atrial pressure is higher, the OS occurs earlier after S2 or A2), and **[2] prolonged murmur duration.**

DIAGNOSIS
- ECG: **left atrial enlargement** (P wave >3 mm, biphasic P wave in V1 and V2), **Atrial fibrillation, Pulmonary hypertension** (RVH, right axis deviation).
- **Echocardiography: most useful noninvasive tool** — mitral valve thickening, decreased valve area.
- Chest radiograph: left atrial enlargement (eg, straightening of the left border, prominent pulmonary arteries, posterior displacement of the esophagus, elevation of left mainstem bronchus).

MANAGEMENT
- **Valve repair: Percutaneous balloon valvuloplasty (commissurotomy): best treatment for symptomatic MS in young patients with noncalcified valves or refractory to medical therapy.**
- Valve replacement: reserved if mitral valvuloplasty is contraindicated or unfavorable valve morphology.
- Medical: diuretics and sodium restriction for edema & volume overload. Rate control of Atrial fibrillation with Beta blockers, Calcium channel blockers, or Digoxin. Anticoagulation if A fib.

MITRAL REGURGITATION (MR)

- Incomplete closure of the mitral valve apparatus, leading to retrograde blood flow from the left ventricle (LV) into the left atrium (LA) during systole.

PATHOPHYSIOLOGY

- Abnormal, retrograde blood flow from the left ventricle into the left atrium, leading to **increased left atrial pressure, subsequent LV volume overload & preload, & increased pulmonary pressure.**
- **With chronic MR, left atrial dilation and left ventricular hypertrophy are compensatory consequences** to better tolerate the regurgitant volume. Later it decompensates.

ETIOLOGIES

- <u>Leaflet abnormalities:</u> **Mitral valve prolapse most common cause in the US** (Rheumatic fever in developing countries). Endocarditis, valvulitis, annulus or **LV dilation,** Marfan syndrome.
- <u>Papillary muscle dysfunction:</u> myocardial ischemia or infarction, cardiomyopathy.
- <u>Ruptured chordae tendineae:</u> collagen vascular disease, dilated cardiomyopathy.

CLINICAL MANIFESTATIONS

- <u>Chronic:</u> Many are asymptomatic. Heart failure symptoms (eg, **exertional dyspnea most common, fatigue**), **Atrial fibrillation**, hemoptysis, Hypertension.
- <u>Acute:</u> **Significant dyspnea at rest, pulmonary edema, hypotension, tachypnea, hypoxemia, cyanosis, decreased cardiac output, and possible cardiogenic shock.** Usually due to either papillary muscle in Acute myocardial infarction or in the setting of Infective endocarditis.

PHYSICAL EXAMINATION

- **High-pitched, blowing, holosystolic murmur best heard at the apex, often with radiation to the left axilla, subscapular region,** or the upper sternal borders.
- **<u>Increased murmur intensity:</u> left lateral decubitus position,** expiration, isometric exercise, **increased venous return (eg, squatting, leg raise, lying supine); increased afterload (eg, handgrip)** due to increased atrial pressure.
- **<u>Decreased murmur intensity:</u> decreased venous return (eg, Valsalva, standing),** inspiration, decreased afterload (eg, **Amyl nitrate**). Widely split S2, laterally displaced PMI, S3. Soft (diminished) S1 if severe.
- With MVP, the murmur may appear in mid-late systole with or without mid-systolic click.

DIAGNOSIS

- **<u>Echocardiogram:</u> primary and most commonly used noninvasive test to diagnose MR** — allows for assessment of MR etiology, morphology, severity, assessment of ventricular size & function, and the need for mitral valve repair. Hyperdynamic LV, regurgitant jet in MR.
- <u>ECG:</u> nonspecific — left atrial enlargement, LVH, or Atrial fibrillation.
- <u>Chest radiograph:</u> nonspecific — left atrial enlargement, LVH, or pulmonary edema.

MANAGEMENT

- **<u>Hypertension + MR:</u> afterload reducers eg, ACE inhibitors (ACEIs), Angiotensin receptor blockers (ARBs),** Hydralazine, Nitrates. ACEI & ARBs have been used to delay MR progression.

Surgical

- **<u>Repair</u> is generally preferred over replacement when possible** (decreased recurrence of MR after repair, lower rate of mortality, & better late outcome). Replacement if extensive tissue destruction.
- <u>Indications:</u> left ventricular dysfunction even in the absence of symptoms (eg, ejection fraction 60% or less or left ventricular end systolic dimension is 40 mm or greater), refractory to medical therapy, moderate to severe symptomatic MR. **Due to abrupt hemodynamic decompensation, acute MR typically requires urgent surgical or percutaneous intervention.**

MITRAL VALVE PROLAPSE (MVP)

- Mitral valve leaflets extend abnormally above the mitral annulus into the left atrium during systole.
- **Most common in young women** (15–35 years of age). Seen in 2-5% of the population.

ETIOLOGIES:
- **Myxomatous degeneration of one or both leaflets of the mitral valve** — weakened and elongated chordae tendineae, mitral annular dilatation, or thickened leaflet tissue.
- Connective tissue diseases eg, Marfan or Ehlers-Danlos syndromes, Osteogenesis imperfecta.

CLINICAL MANIFESTATIONS:
- **Most patients are asymptomatic.** MVP is the most common cause of Mitral regurgitation in the US.
- **MVP syndrome: combination of symptoms & signs with Mitral valve prolapse** — eg, atypical chest pain, palpitations (arrhythmias), exertional dyspnea, exercise intolerance, dizziness, & fatigue. Anxiety, low blood pressure, supraventricular arrhythmias, and syncope suggest autonomic nervous system dysfunction.
- Symptoms associated with Mitral regurgitation progression (not common) — dyspnea, fatigue, CHF.
- In rare cases, it may present with arrhythmias, sudden cardiac death, Infective endocarditis, or stroke.

PHYSICAL EXAMINATION:
- **Mid-late systolic click best heard at the apex** due to tensing of the chordae tendineae & mitral valve apparatus as the leaflets prolapse into the left atrium. **The click may be followed by the high-pitched mid-late systolic murmur of Mitral regurgitation** (the murmur of MR is late systolic early in the disease and becomes holosystolic with severe prolapse).
- **Earlier click: any maneuver that makes the LV smaller or decreases preload (eg, Valsalva, standing) results in an earlier click & longer murmur duration** due to increased prolapse (although the murmur of MR will be fainter).
- **Delayed click: any maneuver that increases preload (eg, squatting, leg raise, supine) results in a delayed click & shorter murmur duration** due to decreased prolapse. **Handgrip.**
- The handgrip maneuver increases the intensity of the Mitral regurgitation associated with MVP and decreases the murmur of Hypertrophic cardiomyopathy.
- Skeletal abnormalities: may have narrow anteroposterior diameter, hypotension, scoliosis, and pectus excavatum deformity. Patients tend to have a lower BMI compared to controls.

DIAGNOSIS
Echocardiography:
- **Diagnostic test of choice (key imaging study) in the diagnosis of MVP** — helps to identify MVP and other associated valvular abnormalities. Two- or three-dimensional echocardiogram allows measurement of leaflet thickness and displacement relative to the annulus.
- Findings of MVP include **displacement of any portion of the mitral leaflets ≥2 mm above the annular plane into the left atrium (systolic billowing)** in a long axis view, posterior bulging leaflets with tissue redundancy.

MANAGEMENT
- **Asymptomatic: MVP patients with no symptoms often require no treatment other than reassurance, conservative management, observation, and monitoring.** Patients with no concomitant mitral regurgitation can be followed every 3-5 years and patients with Mitral regurgitation can be followed annually. **Reassurance is a major component of management of most patients with MVP** — MVP is associated with a good prognosis, has a benign nature, and has a low incidence of serious complications (for most patients, it is of no clinical significance).
- **Autonomic dysfunction: In addition to reassurance and lifestyle changes, Beta-blockers may be used in select patients with autonomic dysfunction.**

PULMONIC REGURGITATION (PR)

ETIOLOGIES
- **Primary PR is almost always congenital.**
- Secondary (functional) PR can occur in the setting of Pulmonary hypertension or pulmonary artery dilatation. Tetralogy of Fallot, endocarditis, and Rheumatic heart disease.

PATHOPHYSIOLOGY
- Retrograde blood flow from pulmonary artery into RV ⇨ R-sided volume overload.

CLINICAL MANIFESTATIONS
- Most clinically insignificant. If symptomatic, **may be associated with right-sided Heart failure symptoms and signs — hepatic congestion (abdominal fullness and bloating), ascites, jugular venous distention, and lower extremity (pedal) edema.**

PHYSICAL EXAMINATION
- **Graham Steell murmur: brief high-pitched decrescendo early diastolic blowing murmur heard maximally at the left upper sternal border (left second or third intercostal space).**
- Increased murmur intensity: inspiration, increased venous return (eg, squatting, leg raise, supine).
- Decreased murmur intensity: decreased venous return (eg, Valsalva, standing), expiration.

MANAGEMENT
- No treatment needed in most (well tolerated). Pulmonic valve replacement (definitive treatment).

TRICUSPID STENOSIS (TS)

- Blood backs up into the right atrium ⇨↑ right atrial enlargement ⇨ right-sided Heart failure.

PHYSICAL EXAMINATION
Mid-diastolic murmur at the left lower sternal border (Xyphoid, 4th intercostal space). Low frequency.
- **↑ intensity**: ↑venous return: eg, squatting, laying down, leg raising, **inspiration.**
- Opening snap (OS): usually occurs later than the opening snap of mitral stenosis.

MANAGEMENT
- Medical: decrease right atrial volume overload with diuretics & Na+ restriction.
- Surgical: commissurotomy or replacement if right heart failure or ↓cardiac output.

TRICUSPID REGURGITATION

Any cause of RV dilation: LV failure, right ventricular/inferior infarction, pulmonary HTN, IV drug use associated Infective endocarditis.
- Clinical manifestations: may present with RV failure (ascites, jugular vein distension, edema).

PHYSICAL EXAMINATION
- **High-pitched holosystolic soft (blowing) murmur at the subxiphoid area, left mid sternal border,** or right mid sternal border with little to no murmur radiation.
- **Increased murmur intensity: inspiration, increased venous return (eg, squatting, leg raise, supine),** hepatic compression, and exercise.
- **Decreased murmur intensity: decreased venous return (eg, standing, Valsalva), expiration.**
- **Carvallo's sign: increased murmur intensity with inspiration** (due to increased right sided blood flow during inspiration). Helps to distinguish TR from MR. ±Pulsatile liver.

MANAGEMENT
- Medical: diuretics (for volume overload & congestion). If LV dysfunction — standard HF therapy.
- Surgical: suggested for patients with severe TR despite medical therapy. Repair >replacement

	AORTIC STENOSIS	MITRAL STENOSIS	AORTIC REGURGITATION	MITRAL REGURGITATION	MITRAL VALVE PROLAPSE
PATHOPHYSIOLOGY	• LV outflow obstruction ⇨ **fixed CO.** • ↑afterload ⇨ LVH	• Obstruction of flow from LA to LV ⇨ ↑left atrial enlargement & pressure ⇨ pulmonary HTN.	• Backflow from aorta to LV ⇨ **LV volume overload & LVH.**	• Backflow from LV into the LA to LV ⇨ **LV volume overload.**	• Myxomatous degeneration of the mitral valve
ETIOLOGIES	• Degeneration: >70 years • Congenital: <70 years • Rheumatic disease	• **Rheumatic heart disease most common** cause by far.	• Rheumatic disease • Endocarditis, Marfan • Syphilis • Ankylosing spondylitis	• **Mitral valve prolapse most common.** • Rheumatic, Ischemia. • Endocarditis	• Most common in young women • Connective tissue disease: Marfan
CLINICAL MANIFESTATIONS	• Dyspnea • Angina • Syncope • Heart failure	• Right-sided heart failure • Pulmonary hypertension • Atrial fibrillation • Mitral facies • Hoarseness	• L-sided heart failure: dyspnea, fatigue	• Acute: dyspnea, pulmonary edema. • Chronic: dyspnea, fatigue, heart failure, atrial fibrillation	• **Most are asymptomatic** • Autonomic symptoms: palpitations, chest pain
MURMUR	• **Harsh systolic ejection crescendo-decrescendo best heard @ RUSB (heart base)** • Late-peaking murmur = ↑severity	• Diastolic rumbling murmur best heard at the apex & in left lateral decubitus position. • May be preceded by opening snap • Shorter S2-OS interval = ↑severity	• **Early diastolic blowing murmur best heard @LUSB.** • Austin flint murmur: apical diastolic rumbling murmur.	• **Blowing holosystolic murmur best at the apex** • ↑ with handgrip • ↓ with Amyl nitrate	**Mid-late systolic ejection click** • ↓venous return results in earlier click • ↑venous return results in delayed click
RADIATION	• Carotids (delayed and diminished)	• No radiation	• Along left sternal border	• Axilla	
HEART SOUNDS	• **S2: soft, absent, paradoxically split** • **S4 gallop** if LVH	• **Opening snap** • **Prominent S1**		• Widely split S2	
PULSE	• **Narrow pulse pressure: weak delayed upstroke**	• Usually reduced intensity	• **Bounding pulses: wide pulse pressure**	• May have brisk upstroke	• Narrow AP diameter • Low body weight • Hypotension • Scoliosis
PHYSICAL EXAM	• LV heave due to LVH	• Left atrial enlargement	Wide pulse pressure: • head bobbing • fingernail pulsations • thrill over femoral arteries		
MANAGEMENT	• **Aortic valve replacement** if symptomatic or if aortic valve area <0.8 cm^2	• **Valve repair preferred over replacement: valvuloplasty (percutaneous mitral balloon commissurotomy)** in young patients.	• Meds: vasodilators • Surgery: acute AR, chronic AR with EF <55%	• Vasodilators (ACE inhibitors) • Surgery: valve repair preferred vs valve replacement	• **Reassurance in most that it is benign** • Autonomic symptoms: Beta blockers

ACUTE PERICARDITIS

- Infection of the endothelium/valves 2ʳʸ to colonization (eg, during transient/persistent bacteremia).

ETIOLOGIES:
- **Idiopathic most common.** Most cases of "idiopathic" Pericarditis are presumed viral in etiology.
- **Viral: 2 most common causes of Pericarditis are idiopathic & viral (especially Coxsackieviruses A and B & Echovirus).** Adenoviruses, Parvovirus B19, HIV, Influenza, EBV, and CMV.
- **Dressler syndrome post MI pericarditis + fever + pleural effusion that may occur after several weeks after the Myocardial infarction** due to delayed autoimmune process post MI.
- Autoimmune, uremia, bacterial, radiation, medications: Procainamide, Isoniazid, Doxorubicin.

CLINICAL MANIFESTATIONS
- **Chest pain:** most common symptom (>95%) — **classically sudden onset of pleuritic (sharp, worse with deep inspiration or coughing) anterior chest pain that is often persistent and positional: worse when supine & improved with the seated position or by leaning forward** (sitting & leaning forward reduces pressure on the parietal pericardium). **The pain may radiate to the shoulder & trapezius ridge** (due to phrenic nerve irritation), back, neck, arm, or epigastrium.
- **Pericardial friction rub:** often best heard at the left parasternal area and the **intensity may be increased during auscultation by having the patient sitting up and leaning forward** or resting the elbows on the knees, applying firm pressure on the stethoscope diaphragm during suspended respiration. Consists of a scratchy or squeaking sound with 3 components (triphasic).

DIAGNOSTIC STUDIES
ECG: diagnostic test of choice — **Precordial leads: widespread diffuse (typically concave up) ST segment elevation in V1-V6 with associated PR depression in those leads** and without reciprocal T-wave inversions or Q waves. **PR segment deviation is highly specific** (less sensitive).
- **Lead aVR: is associated with reciprocal ST depression and PR elevation.**

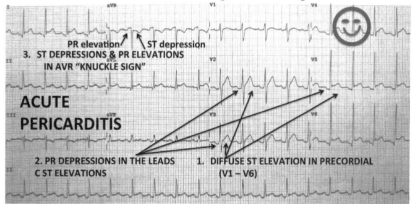

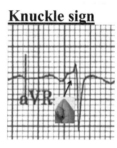

Knuckle sign

Echocardiogram: Useful to evaluate for associated pericardial effusion &/or signs of cardiac tamponade.
Laboratory evaluation: increased ESR &/or CRP. May have slightly elevated cardiac enzymes.

MANAGEMENT
- **High-dose NSAIDs or Aspirin, often with Colchicine, first-line for nearly all patients with acute idiopathic or viral Pericarditis x 7-14 days** (symptoms usually subside in 1-2 days). The addition of Colchicine decreases pain, symptom length, complications, and recurrence rate.
- **Colchicine: second-line or first-line in conjunction with Aspirin or NSAIDs or as monotherapy.**
- **Glucocorticoids: usually reserved for severe or refractory cases, if NSAIDs/ASA or Colchicine is contraindicated,** in connective tissue disease, autoreactivity, uremia, **SLE, or pregnancy.**

Dressler syndrome:
- **Aspirin and/or Colchicine first-line agents; avoid NSAIDs other than Aspirin because they can interfere with myocardial scar formation.**

PERICARDIAL EFFUSION

- Accumulation of fluid in the pericardial space.
- Normally, about 5-15 ml of fluid is located in the pericardial space.

ETIOLOGIES
- Same causes of Acute pericarditis (eg, viral, idiopathic). Immune, Aortic dissection, uremia.
- Malignancy — lung cancer most common malignant cause, breast second most common;

CLINICAL MANIFESTATIONS
- Chest pain (if associated with Acute pericarditis), dyspnea, fatigue.

Physical examination:
- **Decreased (muffled) heart sounds** due to the pericardial fluid interfering with conduction of the cardiac sounds.

DIAGNOSIS
- **Echocardiogram: test of choice — increased fluid in the pericardial space.**

- ECG: The most common ECG findings in patients with a Pericardial effusion are sinus tachycardia, low QRS voltage, & electrical alternans (alternating amplitudes of the QRS complexes in large effusions).

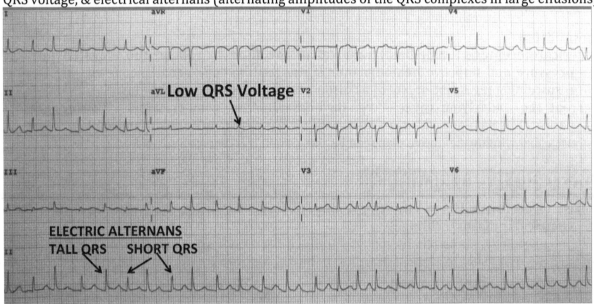

- Chest radiograph: not used in the diagnosis. Findings may include appearance of the heart as a "water bottle" (not sensitive or specific).

MANAGEMENT
- Treat the underlying cause (eg, acute Pericarditis). Serial echocardiography if necessary.
- Large effusions may need pericardiocentesis for symptomatic relief.

CARDIAC (PERICARDIAL) TAMPONADE

- **Pericardial effusion causing significant pressure on the heart, impeding cardiac filling, leading to decreased cardiac output and obstructive shock** (medical emergency).
- **The rate of accumulation of fluid is more critical than the volume.** Rapid accumulation of as little as 150 ml of fluid can cause tamponade, while as much as 1 liter can slowly accumulate if compliant.
- Etiologies: complication of Pericarditis or trauma. Malignancy most common nontraumatic cause.

CLINICAL MANIFESTATIONS

- **Beck's triad:** 3 "Ds" — **D**istant (muffled) heart sounds, **D**istended neck veins (increased JVP), and **D**ecreased blood pressure (systemic hypotension). Classic but uncommon.
- Pulsus paradoxus: exaggerated (>10 mmHg) decrease in systolic blood pressure with inspiration.
- Dyspnea, fatigue, peripheral edema, shock, **reflex tachycardia is common**, cool extremities.

DIAGNOSTIC STUDIES

- **Patients suspected of having Cardiac tamponade should be evaluated with an ECG, chest radiograph, and echocardiography** (echocardiogram may be performed first if unstable).
- **Echocardiogram: pericardial effusion + diastolic collapse of cardiac chambers.**
- ECG: signs of pericardial effusion — low voltage QRS complexes, electrical alternans.
- Chest radiograph: may show an enlarged cardiac silhouette.

MANAGEMENT

- **Pericardiocentesis (immediate) removal of the fluid to relieve the elevated intracardiac pressure and improve hemodynamic status** (can be done percutaneous vs. surgical). Volume resuscitation (eg, saline or blood) or vasopressors if needed.
- **Treat the underlying cause** — eg, High-dose NSAIDs, with or without Colchicine for Acute pericarditis. High-dose Aspirin with or without Colchicine for Dressler syndrome.
- Pericardial window definitive management for drainage if recurrent.

CONSTRICTIVE PERICARDITIS

- **Loss of pericardial elasticity (thickening, fibrosis, & calcification) leading to restriction of ventricular diastolic filling.**
- Pathophysiology: fibrosis limits ventricular filling, decreasing stroke volume and cardiac output.
- Etiologies: any cause of acute Pericarditis. In the US, idiopathic and viral Tuberculosis (worldwide).

CLINICAL MANIFESTATIONS

- Dyspnea most common symptom, fatigue, orthopnea.
- **Right-sided heart failure signs: increased jugular venous distention,** peripheral edema, nausea, vomiting, increased hepatojugular reflex, **Kussmaul's sign (the lack of an inspiratory decline or an increase in jugular vein pressure with inspiration).**
- **Pericardial knock:** high pitched diastolic sound similar to S3 (sudden cessation of ventricular filling).

DIAGNOSTIC STUDIES

- Chest radiograph: pericardial calcification may be seen especially on lateral view, clear lung fields. Normal or slightly increased heart size, Square root sign on cardiac catheterization.
- **Echocardiography: pericardial thickening and/or calcification. "Square root" sign** — early diastolic dip followed by a plateau of diastasis. Also used to rule out Restrictive cardiomyopathy.
- **CT scan or MRI:** more sensitive than echocardiography — **pericardial thickening or calcification.**

MANAGEMENT

- Diuretics for symptom relief & reduction of edema and venous pressure. Pericardiectomy (definitive).

	ACUTE PERICARDITIS	PERICARDIAL EFFUSION	CARDIAC TAMPONADE	CONSTRICTIVE PERICARDITIS
DEFINITION	• Inflammation of the pericardium	• ↑fluid in the pericardial space	• **Pericardial effusion** ⇨ pressure on the heart limits ventricular diastolic filling ⇨↓cardiac output.	• **Fibrotic, calcified limits ventricular diastolic filling.**
ETIOLOGIES	• **The 2 most common causes include idiopathic & viral** (Coxsackievirus, Echovirus) • Neoplastic, Autoimmune • Inflammatory, vascular <u>Dressler syndrome:</u> • post MI pericarditis + pleural effusion	• Same as pericarditis	• Same as pericarditis • May be traumatic	• Same as pericarditis • Chronic inflammation
CLINICAL MANIFESTATIONS	<u>5 Ps of Pericarditis:</u> • **Pleuritic chest pain** (sharp & worse with inspiration) • **Postural:** worse when supine; improved with sitting & leaning forward • **Persistent** pain • **Pyrosis:** fever • **Pericardial friction rub**	• Distant (muffled) heart sounds • May have symptoms of Pericarditis	<u>Beck's triad:</u> • **(1) Distant heart sounds** • **(2) ↑jugular venous distention** • **(3) Systemic hypotension** <u>Pulsus paradoxus:</u> • Drop of systolic BP >10 mmHg with inspiration. <u>Kussmaul sign:</u> • **No fall or ↑JVD with inspiration.**	• Dyspnea most common • **Pericardial knock:** diastolic **sound** (ventricular filling) • Pulsus paradoxus • Kussmaul sign <u>R-sided heart failure:</u> • ↑**jugular venous distention** • **peripheral edema** • **hepatic congestion** • **GI symptoms:** nausea, vomiting
DIAGNOSIS	<u>ECG:</u> • **Diffuse ST elevations:** (concave up) in precordial leads with PR depressions in the same leads • Lead aVR: ST depression; PR elevation <u>Echocardiogram:</u> • Normal; may have pericardial effusions (used to rule out cardiac tamponade)	<u>ECG:</u> • **Low voltage QRS complexes** • **Electrical alternans** <u>Echocardiogram:</u> • ↑pericardial fluid • No hemodynamic compromise	<u>ECG:</u> • **Low voltage QRS complexes** • **Electrical alternans** <u>Echocardiogram:</u> • ↑**pericardial fluid +** • **diastolic ventricular collapse**	<u>Echocardiogram:</u> • ↑**pericardial thickening & calcification**
MANAGEMENT	• **Either Aspirin or NSAID PLUS Colchicine** • Colchicine monotherapy • Glucocorticoids • **Dressler syndrome: Aspirin &/or Colchicine first-line;** avoid steroids & other NSAIDs.	• Treat the underlying cause • Pericardial window if recurrent	• **Pericardiocentesis** (emergent)	• **Pericardiectomy**

AORTIC DISSECTION

- Tear through the innermost layer of the aorta (intima) due to cystic medial necrosis.
- **Ascending most common near the aortic arch or left subclavian (65%),** 20% descending, 10% aortic arch. **Ascending = high mortality.**

RISK FACTORS
- **Hypertension (most important risk factor)**, age >50 years (20-30 years of age in patients with Marfan syndrome), men, vasculitis (rare), trauma, family history of aortic dissection, Turner's syndrome, Collagen disorders: (eg, Marfan syndrome, Ehlers-Danlos), pregnancy.

PATHOPHYSIOLOGY
- **Intimal tear:** constant exposure to high pulsatile pressure and shear stress lead to weakening of the aortic wall in susceptible patients, resulting in an intimal tear, the primary event in Aortic dissection. Degeneration of the aortic media (cystic medial necrosis) is a predisposing factor.
- Site of intimal tear: 95% occur in two places. **The most common site of an intimal tear is the first few centimeters of the ascending aorta (90% occur within 10 cm of the aortic valve).** Second most common is just beyond the ligamentum arteriosum in the descending aorta.

CLINICAL MANIFESTATIONS
- **Chest or back pain**: **most common symptom (90%)** — **sudden onset of severe** (maximal severity at onset) **chest and/or upper back pain with a sharp, ripping, knife-like, or tearing quality that may radiate between the scapulae.** The pain is more often located in the anterior chest in ascending (type A) dissection, back or abdomen in descending (type B) dissection, or may migrate with propagation.
- Accompanied symptoms: **the chest pain may be accompanied with abdominal pain, neurological findings** (eg, limb weakness or paresthesias due to spine ischemia), syncope, Acute coronary syndrome, Heart failure, or Cerebrovascular accident.

PHYSICAL EXAMINATION:
- Blood pressure: **May be hypertensive (common) or hypotensive (ominous sign, indicating rupture). Hypertension more common in descending (type B) dissections** (70%) but seen in only 25-35% of type A. **Hypotension in 25% involving the ascending aorta** but <5% in type B.
- Pulse variation: **variation or discrepancy in blood pressure** — **asymmetric blood pressure (eg, >20 mmHg blood pressure difference between the right & left arms). Asymmetric, decreased, or absent pulses** (eg, carotid, brachial, radial, or femoral). May have wide pulse pressure.
- **Aortic regurgitation of new onset if ascending (blowing diastolic decrescendo murmur).**
- Neurological deficits present in 20% of cases — focal neurologic deficits include stroke, altered consciousness, acute paraplegia (spinal cord ischemia), Horner syndrome (compression of the superior cervical sympathetic ganglion), and hoarseness (vocal cord paralysis due to compression of the left recurrent laryngeal nerve).
- Muffled heart sounds if Cardiac tamponade is present.

Ascending vs. descending:
- Type A: Ascending aorta involvement should be suspected if anterior chest pain more so than the back or abdomen, syncope, hypotension, shock, Acute Aortic valve regurgitation, Acute coronary syndrome, Cardiac tamponade, Hemothorax, focal neurologic deficits related to cerebrovascular ischemia, and upper extremity pulse deficit. Often will have elements of descending dissections.
- Type B: Descending aorta should be suspected if posterior chest/upper back pain that may radiate to the abdomen; Other clinical features include malperfusion syndromes (eg, abdominal pain from visceral ischemia, lower extremity ischemia, focal neurologic deficits related to spinal ischemia, or acute kidney injury).

INITIAL EVALUATION

- <u>ECG</u>: part of the initial evaluation of chest pain to rule out MI. Ischemic changes in 15% & nonspecific ST and T changes in 30%. Extension of type A dissection can cause coronary ischemia.
- **Chest radiograph:** commonly obtained to help rapidly differentiate the various causes of chest pain. **Widening of the mediastinum or widened aortic silhouette (loss of normal aortic knob contour) are common. May be normal in 10% so a normal CXR does <u>not</u> rule out dissection.**

Advanced vascular imaging:

- CT angiogram, Transesophageal echocardiogram, & MR angiogram are all acceptable first-line imaging modalities to confirm and visualize the tear in suspected Aortic dissection and determine the appropriate management.
- **CT angiography: in most EDs, CT angiography with contrast is the most commonly used first vascular imaging technique if the patient is <u>hemodynamically stable</u>** (especially if not strong suspicion of ascending dissection) to determine the type and extent of dissection.
- **Transesophageal echocardiogram performed at the bedside or in the OR is the recommended initial advanced imaging if <u>hemodynamically unstable,</u> impaired renal function (eg, elevated creatinine), contrast allergy, or strong suspicion of an ascending dissection.** Yields diagnosis in minutes, & better compared to CT at seeing a tear, flap, or regurgitation.
- <u>Aortography:</u> may be performed if the diagnosis is uncertain after advanced imaging. CT angiography has largely replaced Aortography.

MANAGEMENT

Surgical management:

- <u>Indications:</u> **used in acute proximal (Stanford A/DeBakey I and II) OR acute distal with complications (Stanford B/Debakey Type III with ischemia, progression, impending rupture,** etc.). Open repair may include excision of the intimal tear, obliteration of entry into the false lumen proximally, reconstitution of the aorta with interposition of a synthetic vascular graft, and repair or replacement of the aortic valve as needed. Endovascular repair an option.
- <u>Preoperative blood pressure control</u> — blood pressure and heart rate may rise during induction for emergency surgery, so lower readings prior to surgery are recommended (eg, Beta blockers).

Medical management:

- <u>Indications:</u> **acute descending dissection** (Stanford B/Debakey III) **<u>without</u> complications.**
- **IV Beta blockers (eg, Esmolol, Labetalol)** — Beta blockers help lower the systolic blood pressure, heart rate, prevent reflex tachycardia, and decrease left ventricular contractility (all of which reduce aortic wall stress). **The vasodilators Sodium nitroprusside or Nicardipine may be added <u>after</u> Beta blockers** to reach target blood pressure goal if additional therapy is needed (they are not used alone or prior to Beta Blockers because they can cause reflex tachycardia).
- **Blood pressure goal: systolic blood pressure is rapidly lowered to a goal of SBP 100-120 mmHg and maintain a heart rate <60 bpm within 20 minutes** to reduce shearing forces, propagation, and rupture.

AORTIC DISSECTION CLASSIFICATION

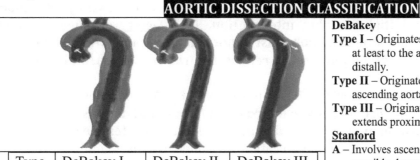

Type	DeBakey I	DeBakey II	DeBakey III
	Stanford A		Stanford B
	Proximal		Distal

DeBakey
Type I – Originates in ascending aorta, propagates at least to the aortic arch and often beyond it distally.
Type II – Originates in and is confined to the ascending aorta.
Type III – Originates in descending aorta, rarely extends proximally but will extend distally.
Stanford
A – Involves ascending aorta and/or aortic arch, & possibly descending aorta.
B – Involves the descending aorta (distal to left subclavian artery origin), without involvement of the ascending aorta or aortic arch.

PERIPHERAL ARTERIAL DISEASE (PAD)

- Atherosclerotic disease of the peripheral arteries, especially involving the lower extremities.

CLINICAL MANIFESTATIONS
- **Classic claudication** most common symptom — intermittent **lower extremity pain or cramping with ambulation, exercise, or movement and relieved with rest.**

VESSEL INVOLVED	AREA OF CLAUDICATION	PERCENTAGE
AORTIC BIFURCATION/COMMON ILIAC	**Buttock, hip, or groin.**	25-30%
	Leriche's syndrome: triad: ❶ claudication (buttock, thigh pain) ❷ erectile dysfunction, & ❸ decreased femoral pulses.	
FEMORAL ARTERY OR BRANCHES	**Thigh, upper 2/3 of the calf**	80 -90%
POPLITEAL ARTERY	**Lower 1/3 of the calf,** ankle, and foot	
TIBIAL AND PERONEAL ARTERIES	Foot	40-50%

- **Atypical extremity pain:** — [1] **leg pain/carry on**: exertional leg pain that does not cause the patient to stop walking & [2] **leg pain on exertion and rest** is exertional leg pain that may occur at rest.
- **Ischemic rest pain:** in advanced disease. Often described as a **constant intractable, burning pain in the forefoot (soles of the feet), most common at night, aggravated by elevation, and relieved with foot dependency** (minor temporary increase in blood flow due to gravity).

PHYSICAL EXAMINATION:
- Pulses: **Decreased, weak, or absent pulses,** bruits, Decreased capillary refill. Usually no edema.
- Skin: **Atrophic skin changes** — muscle atrophy; **skin that is thin, dry, and shiny; hair loss** or slowed hair & nail growth, thickened nails, **cool limbs to the touch,** and areas of necrosis.
- **Nonhealing wound/ulcer:** often starts as a traumatic wound that fails to heal). They are commonly found on the tips of the toes and between the digits. Ischemic ulcers also form at sites of increased focal pressure (eg, **lateral malleolus** and metatarsal heads).
- Color: **Foot & leg pallor on elevation. Dependent rubor** dusky red color of the leg when it is placed in the dependent position (increase in blood flow due to gravity temporarily diminishes the pain).

DIAGNOSIS
- **Ankle-brachial index: most useful screening test** (simple, quick noninvasive). Normal ABI 1-1.3.
  - ⊕ **PAD if ABI <0.90** (0.50 is severe). Rest pain if 0.2-0.4. Tissue loss (ulcer, gangrene): 0-0.4.
  - **>1.3 ⇨ possible noncompressible (calcified) vessels — may lead to a false reading.**
- Duplex ultrasonography: Performed to evaluate the further extent of vascular disease. A classic finding of PAD is low-velocity flow through the affected arteries.
- Arteriography: criterion standard. Usually only performed if revascularization is planned.

MANAGEMENT
- **Supportive: first-line therapy** — risk reduction (eg, **smoking cessation associated with greatest benefit,** hyperlipidemia, DM), **supervised exercise therapy, and possibly pharmacologic therapy, rather than initial vascular intervention.** Risk factor reduction: with lifestyle modifications foot care. **Smoking cessation most important modifiable CAD risk factor.**
- **Platelet inhibitors: Aspirin or Clopidogrel to reduce the risk of Myocardial infarction and Stroke.**
- **Statin therapy:** indicated for all patients with PAD to reduce risk of MI and Stroke.
- **Cilostazol most effective medical therapy to improve symptoms and increase walking distance in patients with claudication with continued pain with exercise & lifestyle changes.** Cilostazol is an ADP inhibitor that prevents platelet aggregation, phosphodiesterase-3 inhibitor that promotes direct arterial vasodilation, increases red blood cell flexibility, and suppresses the proliferation of vascular smooth muscle cells. Naftidrofuryl; Pentoxifylline improves oxygen delivery.
- Revascularization: for rest pain, refractory disease, ulceration — Percutaneous transluminal angioplasty (first-line revascularization procedure), bypass grafts, endarterectomy (last-line).

ACUTE ARTERIAL OCCLUSION

- **Acute limb ischemia** — rapidly developing or abrupt decrease in limb perfusion, usually associated with new or worsening symptoms or signs of limb ischemia.
- **Considered a vascular emergency** — Acute arterial occlusion is time-sensitive and if left untreated, can lead to rapid development of infarction and loss of limb.

ETIOLOGIES
- **[1] Thrombotic occlusion — in situ acute thrombosis of a diseased but previously patent vessel most common etiology** (eg, **preexisting Coronary artery disease or Peripheral arterial disease associated with intermittent claudication,** history of limb revascularization, or atherosclerotic risk factors).
- **[2] Embolic occlusion** from a proximal source lodging into a more distal vessel — the left heart (eg, **atrial thrombus due to Atrial fibrillation**), Infective endocarditis.

CLINICAL MANIFESTATIONS
- **6 Ps — paresthesias (often early), pain, pallor, pulselessness, poikilothermia, paralysis (late finding associated with a worse prognosis).** Symptoms usually distal to the occlusion.
- Physical examination: **classic findings of Acute limb ischemia include decreased capillary refill, decreased or absent pulses, & cool temperature.**

WORKUP
- **Bedside arterial Doppler** A handheld Doppler should be used to confirm the presence of distal pulses (eg, dorsalis pedis, posterior tibial Doppler signals).
- **Vascular imaging: Duplex ultrasound: often the first imaging choice** to assess Acute limb ischemia because it is low cost, widely available, non-invasive, non-irradiant, and can be performed rapidly. In emergent situations, angiography is often performed.
- **Angiography: CT angiography (quicker & more readily available) or catheter-based angiography used in patients with viable or marginally threatened limbs to assess arterial anatomy,** distinguish between thrombus and embolus, and allows for possible catheter-based therapeutic intervention (eg, thrombolysis, angioplasty).
- Catheter-based angiography with digital subtraction provides the most useful information and plays a role in therapeutic strategy (eg, also allows for treatment).
- **An immediately threatened limb may undergo further evaluation & treatment in a surgical suite**.

MANAGEMENT
- Therapeutic management depends on the type of occlusion (thrombus or embolus), location, type of conduit (artery of graft), Rutherford class, duration of ischemia, co-morbidities.
- **Supportive management: In immediately threatened limb, anticoagulation with IV unfractionated Heparin should be initiated following a clinical diagnosis of embolism prior to proceeding with imaging to minimize thrombus propagation and preserve microcirculation** (target aPTT 2.0-2.5 above baseline); **fluid resuscitation, & pain control.**
- **Revascularization for reperfusion is the mainstay of treatment** — surgical procedures include surgical or catheter-based thrombectomy with a balloon catheter (Fogarty), bypass surgery and adjuncts such as endarterectomy, patch angioplasty, and intra-operative thrombolysis depending on the duration of the ischemia and the extent of occlusion. Frequently, a combination of these techniques is required.
- Catheter-directed thrombolysis is often reserved for patients with a salvageable limb.
- Open revascularization: may be indicated as the best option in an immediately threatened or nonviable limb, bypass graft with suspected infection, or if contraindication to thrombolysis.
- Amputation: indicated in irreversible ischemia (eg, profound paralysis and absent pain with inaudible arterial and venous pulses).

ABDOMINAL AORTIC ANEURYSM (AAA)

- Focal aortic dilation > 1.5 normal (>3.0 cm considered aneurysmal). **Infrarenal most common site.**
- Pathophysiology: proteolytic degeneration of aortic wall & connective tissue inflammation.

RISK FACTORS
- **Smoking (main modifiable risk factor), atherosclerosis, age >60 years, Caucasians, males,** hyperlipidemia, connective tissue disorder (eg, Marfan, Ehlers-Danlos), Syphilis, Hypertension.
- Protective factors: female sex, Diabetes mellitus, non-Caucasian race, moderate alcohol consumption.

CLINICAL MANIFESTATIONS
- **Asymptomatic: Most patients are asymptomatic** — may be found to incidentally on imaging or in patients with an abdominal bruit or a palpable abdominal mass.
- **Symptomatic + unruptured: abdominal, flank, or back pain. On examination, an abdominal bruit may be auscultated, and a pulsatile abdominal mass may be palpated.**
- **Symptomatic + ruptured: Classic triad of [1] acute abdominal, flank, or back pain (may be diffuse), [2] abdominal distention or palpable mass, & [3] hemodynamic instability (eg, shock, hypotension, syncope).** Flank ecchymosis or pulsatile mass.
- Aortoenteric fistula: presents as acute GI bleed in patients who underwent prior aortic grafting.

DIAGNOSIS
- **CT scan with IV contrast: best initial test in symptomatic, hemodynamically stable patients** to confirm rupture, exact location, size, extent, and whether endovascular repair is feasible.
- **Focused bedside ultrasound: initial study of choice in hemodynamically unstable patients with suspected AAA prior to abdominal exploration if possible.**
- Patients with known AAA who present with classic symptoms or signs of rupture can be taken to the operating room for surgical repair without preoperative imaging.

Asymptomatic with suspected AAA:
- Abdominal ultrasound: **initial test in asymptomatic patients & to monitor progression.**

MANAGEMENT
- **Symptomatic or ruptured: immediate surgical repair** (endovascular stent graft or open repair). Endovascular repair from a femoral arterial approach is now preferred for most repairs when possible, especially in older and higher-risk patients.
- β-blockers reduces shearing forces, ↓'es expansion & rupture risk.

Asymptomatic:
- The usual threshold for treatment for asymptomatic AAA is 5.5 cm in men & 5.0 cm in women.

AAA SCREENING Society for Vascular Surgery guidelines:
- **One-time screening via abdominal ultrasound in men 65-75 years of age who ever smoked.**

≥5.5 cm in men OR > 0.5 cm expansion in 6 months.	IMMEDIATE SURGICAL REPAIR (even if asymptomatic), symptomatic patients or patients with acute rupture.
5-5.4 cm	Ultrasonography every 3-6 months
4.0-4.9 cm	Ultrasonography every 12 months
3.0-3.9 cm	Ultrasonography every 3 years.

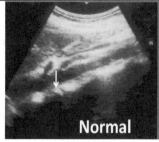
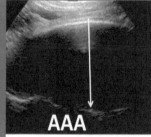

Normal | AAA

THROMBOANGIITIS OBLITERANS [TAO (BUERGER's DISEASE)]

- Nonatherosclerotic inflammatory **small and medium vessel vasculitis,** leading to vaso-occlusive phenomena.
- **Suspect in young smokers/tobacco users with distal extremity ischemia/ischemic ulcers or gangrene of the digits.**

RISK FACTORS
- **Strong association with tobacco use.**
- Most commonly seen in **young men 20-45 years of age** especially in India, Asia, and the Middle East.

CLINICAL MANIFESTATIONS
- Triad: **[1] distal extremity ischemia both upper & lower extremities** (eg, claudication in the lower calf or arch of the foot, ischemic ulcers), **[2] Raynaud's phenomenon,** & **[3] superficial migratory thrombophlebitis** — due to decrease blood flow in the medium and small arteries and veins.

DIAGNOSIS
- Abnormal Allen test: delayed perfusion of the radial and ulnar arteries.
- **Aortography: "corkscrewing" of small collateral arteries** around associated occlusions.
- Biopsy: definitive diagnosis (rarely needed) — segmental vascular inflammation.

MANAGEMENT
- **Strict cessation of smoking/tobacco use is the cornerstone of management of TAO.**
- Wound care — debridement, moist dressings, negative pressure wound therapy.
- Amputation if gangrene occurs or to avoid the spread of infection in severe ischemic cases.
- Intermittent pneumatic compression for patients with ischemic pain, digit ulceration, or gangrene.
- Iloprost: prostaglandin analog that may help with critical limb ischemia while smoking cessation is in progress.
- Raynaud's phenomenon: Calcium channel blockers.

ATRIAL MYXOMA

- Most common primary cardiac tumor. **80% occur in the left atrium** (most found near fossa ovalis).

PATHOPHYSIOLOGY
- **Because many are pedunculated, some can cause a "ball-valve" obstruction of the mitral orifice, mimicking Mitral stenosis.**

CLINICAL MANIFESTATIONS
- Dyspnea, weight loss, and syncope (from mitral valve obstruction). Triad of embolic phenomenon, Mitral stenosis-like symptoms, and constitutional "flu-like" symptoms (fever, weight loss).
- Physical examination: classically also associated **Mitral stenosis-like findings (eg, Prominent S1, low-pitched diastolic murmur).**

DIAGNOSIS
- **Transesophageal echocardiogram — pedunculated mass with "ball-valve" obstruction of the mitral valve orifice.**

MANAGEMENT
- Surgical removal — although a majority of them are benign, prompt surgical resection is recommended due to increased risk of embolization, cardiovascular complications, & sudden death.

GIANT CELL (TEMPORAL) ARTERITIS (GCA)

- Immune-mediated large- & medium-vessel granulomatous vasculitis of the extracranial branches of the carotid artery (eg, temporal, occipital, ophthalmic, & posterior ciliary arteries).

PATHOPHYSIOLOGY
- T-cells and monocytes are mobilized to the vessel wall, resulting in an inflammatory response.
- If not recognized & treated early, ischemic complications may cause permanent vision loss (15–25%).

EPIDEMIOLOGY
- **Same clinical spectrum as Polymyalgia Rheumatica — PMR & GCA frequently overlap**; 20% of patients with PMR will get diagnosed with GCA later; In GCA, PMR features occur in up to 50%.

RISK FACTORS
- **Women, >50 years of age** — peaks 70-79 years (80% of patients are ≥70 years).
- **Northeastern Europeans and Caucasians.** Smoking cigarettes.

CLINICAL MANIFESTATIONS
- **Headache** — **new-onset headaches or change in baseline headaches is the most common systemic symptom** (75%). Headache is usually temporal but can be occipital, periorbital, or non-focal as well. Headaches have an insidious onset and gradually progress over time, although they may spontaneously resolve rarely, even in the absence of treatment. Scalp tenderness while combing or brushing hair is common and can be focal in the temporal areas or diffuse.
- **Jaw claudication exertional ischemia — mandibular pain, discomfort, or fatigue brought on by chewing, talking, or using the jaw, relieved by stopping** (due to ischemia of the masseter muscles supplied by the maxillary artery). **Vision loss due to anterior ischemic optic neuropathy**, central/branch retinal artery occlusion, posterior ischemic neuropathy, or rarely cerebral ischemia.
- **Visual changes: ocular involvement may include eye pain, monocular (rarely binocular) vision loss, diplopia, & Amaurosis fugax (transient monocular vision loss).**
- Abnormal superficial temporal artery: **absent or decreased pulsation, local tenderness to palpation (including scalp tenderness),** localized erythema, beading (nodularity), or thickening. A clinically normal temporal artery does not rule out GCA.
- Constitutional symptoms: fever (usually low-grade), fatigue, weight loss, anorexia, malaise.

DIAGNOSIS
- **Elevated ESR & CRP** hallmark of GCA. Most have a normocytic normochromic anemia.
- **Temporal artery biopsy: Criterion standard** — histopathology reveals inflammatory infiltrate surrounding a fragmented internal elastic lamina within the media of an arterial wall. **The infiltrate consists predominantly of mononuclear cell infiltration or granulomatous inflammation, or multinucleated giant cells.** Biopsy may be normal as there may be skip lesions of normal tissue.
- **Scheduling of temporal artery biopsy should not interfere with or delay initiation of treatment in a patient with a high likelihood of GCA, since delay increase complications (eg, vision loss).** The yield of biopsy is still very high up to 2 weeks after initiation of glucocorticoids.

MANAGEMENT
- **High-dose systemic glucocorticoids: initiated once GCA is suspected to prevent blindness and suppress disease activity (do not delay treatment to biopsy or for biopsy results).**
  IV Methylprednisolone pulses for 3–5 days prior to oral may be used in some with visual changes.
- **Low dose Aspirin** helps to reduce the risk of vision loss, transient ischemic attacks, & Strokes in GCA and can be considered as adjuvant therapy if no contraindications exist.
- **IL-6 inhibitors: Tocilizumab** may be an alternative in patients who are intolerant to corticosteroids. IL-6 levels are significantly elevated in patients with GCA, and IL-6 is thought to play a pathogenic role in GCA by activating the T-cells and promote IFN-gamma release from the T-cells.

SUPERFICIAL THROMBOPHLEBITIS

- **Superficial phlebitis** — **The presence of pain and inflammation involving a superficial vein in the absence of thrombus.** Great saphenous vein (60-80%) small/short saphenous vein (10-20%).
- Superficial thrombophlebitis — Pain and inflammation involving a superficial vein + a thrombus apparent as a thickened cord or more accurately identified on imaging studies (eg, Ultrasound).

RISK FACTORS
- **Varicose veins** — **phlebitis and thrombosis of the lower extremity superficial veins most commonly occur in varicose veins**, especially with a history of lack of physical activity or trauma.
- **Malignancy & hypercoagulable states** — malignancy, hypercoagulable states, and Thromboangiitis obliterans (eg, Buerger disease). **Trousseau sign: migratory thrombophlebitis associated with underlying malignancy** (eg, Carcinoma of the pancreas most common). May be seen with other vasculitic disorders. Pregnancy and estrogen therapy. Vein excision/ablation.
- **Intravenous catheter use** — phlebitis & thrombosis can occur due to a combination of endothelial injury and venous stasis. The upper extremity veins are affected much more commonly.

CLINICAL MANIFESTATIONS
- **Local phlebitis: tenderness, pain, induration, &/or erythema along the course of a superficial vein.** Edema or pruritus may occur.
- **Recurrent or migratory thrombophlebitis** — Phlebitis and thrombosis can be recurrent in the same vein. Migratory thrombophlebitis occurs in distinctly different vein segments over time.
- **Suppurative thrombophlebitis** — High fever, fluctuance, erythema beyond the vein margins, and/or purulent drainage suggest infection within the vein (eg, suppurative or septic thrombophlebitis). May occur in the setting of recent venipuncture or catheterization.

PHYSICAL EXAMINATION
- **A palpable sometimes nodular cord due to thrombus within the affected vein may occur.**
- Tenderness, induration, edema, &/or erythema along the course of a superficial vein.

DIAGNOSIS
- **Venous Duplex ultrasound: performed especially with lower extremity involvement to rule out the presence of coexistent DVT and to determine the exact location & extent of thrombosis** (eg, thrombus within the axial veins) due to the high rate of concurrent deep vein thrombosis (DVT). **Duplex findings include vein wall thickening and perivenous or subcutaneous edema. Noncompressibility of the vein if thrombosis is present**. Perivenous fluid collections or air in the tissues indicated infection (Suppurative thrombophlebitis).

MANAGEMENT
- **Low-risk for VTE: Supportive mainstay** — **NSAIDs for pain and inflammation, extremity elevation (eg, waist level), warm or cool compresses, compression stocking therapy as tolerated if not contraindicated (eg, Peripheral arterial disease).** Low risk = eg, Focal SVT with axial vein involvement ≤5 cm in length, remote from the saphenopopliteal or saphenofemoral junction (eg, SVT involving the below knee), no medical risk factors for VTE.
- **Intermediate risk: Prophylactic anticoagulation** with uncomplicated axial vein thrombosis (eg, SVT) at intermediate risk for thromboembolism. Intermediate risk: eg, SVT in proximity (3-5 cm) to the deep venous system, SVT in the above-knee great saphenous vein, SVT 5 cm or greater, rather than focal involvement, SVT that propagates with conservative management, and the patient has no medical risk factors for VTE.
- **High-risk for thromboembolism: Supportive + therapeutic anticoagulation** (eg, subcutaneous Fondaparinux, Enoxaparin, oral Rivaroxaban). High risk: eg, thrombus ≤5 cm to the deep venous system, especially involving the great saphenous vein above the knee within 10 cm of the saphenofemoral junction, affected vein segment ≥5 cm, positive medical risk factors for VTE.

DEEP VENOUS THROMBOSIS (DVT)

Most important consequence is pulmonary embolism (50%): both are manifestations of a single entity.

RISK FACTORS (Virchow's triad)
- **Intimal damage:** trauma, infection, inflammation Endothelial damage triggers the clotting cascade.
- **Stasis:** eg, Immobilization or prolonged sitting >4 hours, surgery (typically within 12 weeks of surgery or trauma), Stroke with hemiplegia or immobility.
- **Hypercoagulability:** eg, Protein C or S Deficiency, Factor V Leiden mutation, antithrombin III deficiency, oral contraceptive use, malignancy, pregnancy, cigarette smoking.

CLINICAL MANIFESTATIONS
- DVT should be suspected in patients who present with **leg swelling, pain, warmth, and erythema.**

Physical examination:
- **Unilateral calf swelling (edema) ≥3 cm than the other leg, measured 10 cm below the tibial tuberosity most specific sign. Calf pain & tenderness.** May be warm to palpation.
- Homan sign: deep calf pain with foot dorsiflexion while squeezing the calf (not reliable).

DIAGNOSIS
- **Venous Duplex Ultrasound:** usually first-line imaging. **Most DVTs originate in the calf.**
- **Compression ultrasonography** (CUS) with Doppler is the diagnostic test of choice in patients with suspected DVT. Non-compressibility of the affected vein = DVT.
- D-dimer: highly sensitive but not specific. There are 2 main uses of D-dimer: **negative D-dimer with a low-risk for DVT can exclude DVT as the diagnosis.** In a patient with moderate risk, a positive D-dimer and a negative initial ultrasound, serial ultrasounds are recommended. In general, any positive DVT should be followed by ultrasonography.
- Contrast venography: definitive diagnosis (gold standard). It is invasive, difficult to perform, and rarely used. CT venography and MR venography rarely used.

MANAGEMENT
- **Anticoagulation: first-line treatment for most patients with DVT** (eg, popliteal, femoral, iliac veins). Options include [1] Low molecular weight heparin + Warfarin, [2] LMWH + either Dabigatran or Edoxaban or [3] monotherapy with either Rivaroxaban or Apixaban. **A minimum of 3 months of oral therapy has been suggested after a first episode of DVT or PE.**
- **IVC filter:** 3 main reasons for IVC filter placement: **recurrent DVT/PE despite adequate anticoagulation** OR **stable patients in whom anticoagulation is contraindicated** OR right ventricular dysfunction with an enlarged RV on echocardiogram.
- **In general, subcutaneous LMWH (eg, Enoxaparin) is preferred over IV Unfractionated Heparin (UFH) or subcutaneous UFH in most pregnant patients with DVT/PE** because it is easier to use, appears to be more efficacious, and has a better safety profile.
- Thrombolysis or Thrombectomy: generally not performed (reserved for massive DVT or if severe).

RISK FACTORS VENOUS THROMBOEMBOLISM (VTE)	RECOMMENDED DURATION OF THERAPY
1st event with reversible or time-limiting RF for VTE	at least **3 months** (Risk factors: trauma, surgery, OCPs etc).

1st episode of IDIOPATHIC DVT (no malignancy)
  - **Proximal DVT or PE**
  - **Distal DVT**
	Long-term anticoagulation
	3 months if severely symptomatic distal DVT
	  No treatment & surveillance (ultrasound) if asymptomatic distal DVT

Pregnancy	**LMWH preferred as initial & long-term therapy.**
Malignancy	**LMWH** as initial & long-term therapy. Warfarin or direct oral anticoagulants are alternatives to LMWH in these patients.
Antiphospholipid syndrome	**Warfarin** is the preferred agent in nonpregnant individuals.

2016 ACCP guidelines: direct oral anticoagulants (Apixaban, Dabigatran, Edoxaban, Rivaroxaban) are preferred over Warfarin therapy in the management of DVT/PE (if no cancer is present).

WELL'S CRITERIA FOR DVT

Clinical feature	Points	Interpretation:
Active cancer (including treatment within 6 months, or palliation)	1	• Low probability of DVT: -2 to 0 points
Paralysis, paresis, or immobilization of lower extremity	1	• Moderate probability: 1- 2 points
Bedridden for more than 3 days because of surgery (within 4 weeks)	1	• High probability: 3 – 8 points
Localized tenderness along distribution of deep veins	1	
Swelling of entire leg	1	
Unilateral calf swelling of greater than 3 cm (below tibial tuberosity)	1	
Unilateral pitting edema	1	
Collateral superficial veins	1	
Alternative diagnosis as likely or more likely than DVT	-2	
Total points		

PERIPHERAL ARTERIAL DISEASE VS. CHRONIC VENOUS INSUFFICIENCY

PERIPHERAL ARTERIAL DISEASE

Skin
- **Atrophic changes**: hairless, thin, shiny, mottled appearance
- **Cool or cold to touch**
- **Dependent rubor**
- **Cyanosis with elevation**

Pain:
- **Worse** with walking, elevation
- **Better** with leg dependency, rest

Ulcers
- **Lateral malleolar ulcers**
- Clean margins

Pulses
- Diminished, absent

Edema:
- Infrequent

PERIPHERAL VENOUS DISEASE

Skin
- **Stasis dermatitis**: thick skin, eczematous, **brown hyperpigmentation**
- Warm to the touch
- May be cyanotic with dependency

Pain:
- **Worse** leg dependency, prolonged sitting or standing
- **Better** walking, leg elevation

Ulcers
- **Medial malleolar ulcers**
- Uneven ulcer margins

Pulses
- Usually present and normal

Edema:
- **Hallmark symptom & finding**

CHRONIC VENOUS INSUFFICIENCY

- **Changes due to venous hypertension of the lower extremities as a result of venous valvular incompetency.**
- Most commonly occurs after superficial thrombophlebitis, after DVT, or trauma to the affected leg.

CLINICAL MANIFESTATIONS
- **Leg pain worsened with prolonged standing,** prolonged sitting with the feet dependent.
- **Leg pain improved with ambulation and leg elevation.**
- Pain classically described as a burning, aching, throbbing, cramping or "heavy leg".

PHYSICAL EXAM FINDINGS
- **Stasis Dermatitis: itchy eczematous rash** (inflammatory papules, crusts, or scales), excoriations, weeping erosions & **brownish or dark purple hyperpigmentation of the skin** (hemosiderin deposition).
- **Venous stasis ulcers, especially at the medial malleolus,** may be seen.
- **Dependent pitting leg edema,** increased leg circumference, varicosities, & erythema with normal pulse and temperature.
- Atrophie blanche: atrophic, hypopigmented areas with telangiectasias, & punctate red dots.

MANAGEMENT
- **Nonoperative:** initial management of choice for most includes compression stockings **(cornerstone of treatment), leg elevation, skin care, exercise** (improves the calf muscle pump), **weight management,** and avoidance of prolonged sitting or standing. Treat the underlying cause.
- Stasis dermatitis: wet compresses & topical corticosteroids for acute erythema, vesicles, oozing, and pruritus.
- Ulcer management: compression bandaging systems (eg, zinc impregnated gauze/Unna boots), wound debridement if needed, Aspirin (accelerates ulcer healing).
- Surgical intervention usually reserved for patients not responsive to conservative therapy.

VARICOSE VEINS

- **Dilation of superficial veins due to failure of the venous valves in the saphenous veins,** leading to retrograde flow, venous stasis, and pooling of blood.

RISK FACTORS
- Family history, female gender, increased age, standing for long periods, obesity, increased estrogen (eg, OCP use, pregnancy), or chronic venous insufficiency.

CLINICAL MANIFESTATIONS
- **Most are asymptomatic but may present due to cosmetic issues.**
- Dull ache or pressure sensation. Pain is worse with prolonged standing or sitting with the leg dependent and is relieved with elevation.
- Physical examination: **visibly dilated tortuous veins,** telangiectasias, swelling, discoloration, Venous stasis ulcers: severe varicosities resulting in skin ulcerations. ± Mild ankle edema.

MANAGEMENT
- **Conservative: graduated compression stockings, leg elevation, pain control, exercise.**
- Ablation: catheter-based endovenous thermal ablation (laser or radiofrequency).
- Ligation and stripping, compression sclerotherapy.

NORMAL FETAL CIRCULATION

FETAL CARDIAC PHYSIOLOGY

- **FETAL CIRCULATION USES RIGHT TO LEFT SHUNTS.** The **fetus receives its nutrients & oxygen from the placenta** (not the fetal lungs). The oxygenated & nutrient-rich blood goes from the placenta to the right atrium. There are 2 right to left shunts that bypass the nonfunctioning fetal lungs:

  1. **FORAMEN OVALE: which shunts** about 2/3 of the blood **from the right atrium directly into the left atrium.** The remaining 1/3 passes into the right ventricle. Most of the remaining 1/3 goes through the right ventricle and gets pumped into the pulmonary artery.

  2. **DUCTUS ARTERIOSUS: shunts blood from the pulmonary artery directly into the aorta** (systemic circulation), bypassing the fetal lungs.

Note: as a baby takes its first breath, left side pressure becomes > right side pressure, promoting closure of these openings.

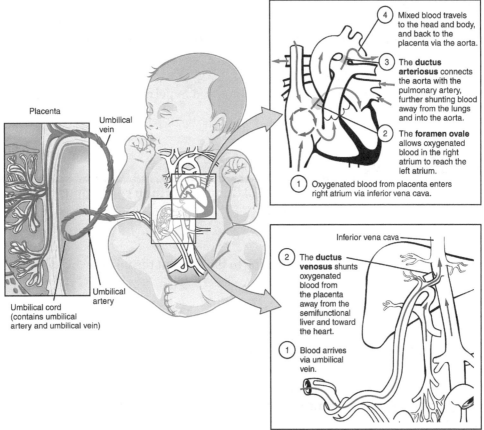

By OpenStax College [CC BY 3.0 (http://creativecommons.org/licenses/by/3.0)], via Wikimedia Commons

CLINICAL CORRELATION
Prostaglandins keep the ductus arteriosus patent (prostaglandins are vasodilators).
1. To **close a patent ductus arteriosus**, a **prostaglandin inhibitor** is given (eg, **IV indomethacin** or Ibuprofen).   Most commonly used in preterm infants or within the 1st 10-14 days of life.

2. To **keep the ductus arteriosus open, administer prostaglandins.** In severe cyanotic diseases (eg, severe coarctation of the aorta, tetralogy of Fallot or transposition of the great vessels), a patent ductus arteriosus allows for mixing of the blood to improve cyanosis. **Prostaglandin E1 analogs** (eg, Alprostadil) maintains the ductus arteriosus open, reducing the cyanosis and improving circulation until surgical correction can be performed.

PEDIATRIC FUNCTIONAL MURMURS

Innocent (functional, physiologic) murmurs: non-pathologic, "functioning" murmurs caused by blood moving through the chambers.

Innocent murmurs tend to be soft, not associated with symptoms, position-dependent, often occurs during systole & seen in up to 40% of children at some point in their lives.

Systolic murmurs may be innocent or pathologic. Diastolic murmurs are almost always pathological.

STILL MURMUR

- **Most common innocent (physiologic) murmur of childhood.**
- Usually heard from 2 months of age until preadolescence. Usually resolves by early adolescence.
- Pathophysiology: thought to be due to the vibration of the valve leaflets.

PHYSICAL EXAMINATION
- **Musical, vibratory, noisy, twanging, low-pitched early to mid-systolic ejection murmur that is best heard in the inferior aspect of the left lower sternal border & apex.**
- Minimal to no radiation (may radiate to the carotids).
- Diminishes with sitting up, standing, or Valsalva.
- Accentuated in the supine position than when sitting, and hyperdynamic states (eg, fever, anxiety).

CERVICAL VENOUS HUM

- 2nd most common innocent murmur (after Still's) & **most common <u>continuous</u> benign murmur.**
- Most commonly seen between 2-8 years of life.

PATHOPHYSIOLOGY
- Due to turbulent blood flow from blood returning to the heart at the junction between the jugular vein and the superior vena cava.

PHYSICAL EXAMINATION
- Soft, whirling, low-pitched **continuous murmur, best heard in the left or right sternal borders or right infraclavicular or supraclavicular areas in the upright position.** The murmur does not radiate.
- Increased intensity: sitting or upright position with the head extended.
- **Decreased murmur intensity: supine, light jugular compression, & rotation or flexion of the head,** Valsalva.

PULMONARY EJECTION MURMUR

- Usually heard in older children and adolescents.
- It is best heard in mid systole and in the left second intercostal space (or superior aspect of the left lower sternal border).
- Due to blood flowing across the pulmonary valve into the pulmonary artery. Commonly heard in older children & adolescents. Best heard in *mid-systole* in the **second left intercostal space** (or superior aspect of the left lower sternal border). Harsh in quality.

PATENT FORAMEN OVALE (PFO)

- Covered but not sealed open communication between the right and left atria; however, a PFO is not considered an ASD because no septal tissue is missing (it is due to failed septal fusion).

CLINICAL MANIFESTATIONS
- Most are asymptomatic
- **Strokes from paradoxical embolism, <u>cryptogenic stroke</u>*** (stroke with no other underlying cause), decompression sickness, migraine, and acute limb ischemia secondary to emboli.

DIAGNOSIS
- **<u>Echocardiogram:</u> best test to make the diagnosis.** Transthoracic echocardiogram is usually performed first but Transesophageal echocardiogram is more sensitive.

MANAGEMENT
- Percutaneous device closure, surgical PFO closure. <u>Cryptogenic stroke:</u> antiplatelet or anticoagulants.

ATRIAL SEPTAL DEFECT (ASD)

- Abnormal opening in the atrial septum between the right and left atrium.
- <u>Pathophysiology:</u> allows for a left to right shunt (noncyanotic).
- <u>Types:</u> **<u>Ostium secundum</u> most common type (75-80%). <u>Ostium primum:</u> (15-20%) & are nearly always associated with anomalies of the atrioventricular (AV) valves (especially mitral valve abnormalities).** Sinus venosus: (5-10%); Coronary sinus: (<1%).

CLINICAL MANIFESTATIONS
- Most patients are asymptomatic or minimally symptomatic in childhood.
- Symptoms often initially occur in the third decade of life or later.
- <u>Infants & young children:</u> recurrent respiratory infection, failure to thrive, exertional dyspnea.
- <u>Adolescents & young adults:</u> exertional dyspnea, easy fatigability, palpitations, atrial arrhythmias, syncope, heart failure.
- **May develop paradoxical emboli** (stroke from venous clots) or dysrhythmias later in life.

PHYSICAL EXAMINATION
- **Soft systolic ejection crescendo-decrescendo flow murmur over the <u>pulmonic area</u> (left upper sternal border second intercostal space).**
- **<u>Wide, fixed split S2 that does not vary with respirations</u>**, loud S1, & hyperdynamic right ventricle.
- <u>Eisenmenger syndrome</u> development may lead to cyanosis and clubbing.

DIAGNOSIS
- **<u>Transthoracic echocardiography</u> with Doppler — initial test for diagnosis & evaluation of ASDs.**
- <u>ECG:</u> incomplete RBBB. **<u>Crochetage sign</u>** notching of the peak of the R wave in the inferior leads.
- <u>CXR:</u> cardiomegaly & increased cardiovascular markings.
- <u>Cardiac catheterization:</u> definitive but rarely needed.

MANAGEMENT
- **Small ASD <5 mm may be observed** (most small ASD spontaneously close in the first year if life).

- <u>Surgical correction:</u> if >1 cm or symptomatic (usually between 2-4 years of age).
  Percutaneous transcatheter closure vs. surgical intervention.

PATENT DUCTUS ARTERIOSUS (PDA)

- Persistent aortic-pulmonary artery shunt (communication between the descending thoracic aorta and main pulmonary artery) via the ductus arteriosus that fails to completely close soon after birth.
- Risk factor: **Preterm — infants born <1,000 grams at greatest risk for PDA, Female** (2 times more common), Fetal hypoxia, In utero alcohol exposure, Congenital rubella.

PATHOPHYSIOLOGY:
- Normally, after the first breath, pulmonary vascular resistance decreases and stimulates bradykinin release from the infant's lungs in addition to high oxygen, which causes the ductus to begin to close.
- **In PDA, continued prostaglandin E2 production & low arterial oxygen content promote patency of the ductus arteriosus.**
- A large PDA can lead to left-to-right shunting of blood in the heart (noncyanotic), leading to increased pulmonary blood flow & alterations in the pulmonary vasculature. The cardiac output increases in order to overcome the left to right flow at the ductus arteriosus and to compensate for the "steal" from the aorta via the PDA during diastole.

CLINICAL MANIFESTATIONS
- **Most are asymptomatic.** Infants may develop poor feeding and poor weight gain, weight loss, frequent lower respiratory tract infections, pulmonary congestion, easy fatigability, or endocarditis.
- **Eisenmenger syndrome: Pulmonary hypertension & cyanotic heart disease occurring when a left-to-right shunt switches & becomes a right-to-left shunt (cyanotic).** Cyanosis and clubbing.

PHYSICAL EXAMINATION
- **Continuous "machine-like" or "to and fro" murmur loudest at the pulmonic area (left infraclavicular region along the left upper sternal border).** May radiate to the back.
- **Wide pulse pressure (>30 mmHg), bounding peripheral pulses,** & prominent precordial impulse due to increased cardiac output & lower diastolic blood pressure from the run-off.
- Loud S2. Respiratory distress may present as tachypnea, tachycardia, grunting, & flaring.

DIAGNOSIS
- Electrocardiogram: LVH, left atrial enlargement. ECG indicated to assess for arrhythmias.
- Chest radiograph: Normal or cardiomegaly.
- **Echocardiogram: Best initial test to make the diagnosis of PDA** — evidence of a patent ductus arteriosus, left to right flow is classically seen. A hemodynamically significant PDA manifests on echo with increased left atrial and left ventricular enlargement.

MANAGEMENT
- Asymptomatic infant >1,000 g: Conservative: includes watchful waiting for spontaneous closure, fluid restriction (eg, 110-113 ml/kg/d while monitoring urine output), observing for signs of heart failure or pulmonary edema, is appropriate for a small, asymptomatic patent ductus arteriosus in an infant > 1,000 grams who is gestationally more mature.
- Infants born >1,000 g are likely to close the ductus arteriosus prior to hospital discharge spontaneously. Asymptomatic PDA does not require immediate pharmacologic treatment.
- **NSAIDs Indications: First-line medical therapy for symptomatic preterm infants & infants who do not need the PDA (eg, IV Indomethacin or Ibuprofen).** Acetaminophen is an alternative. NSAIDs are cyclooxygenase 2 inhibitors that interfere with prostaglandin synthesis, promoting PDA closure (vasodilatory prostaglandins are responsible for maintaining ductus arteriosus patency).
- Surgical correction: Percutaneous catheter occlusion or surgical ligation. Indications: rarely necessary and is reserved for hemodynamically significant PDA despite 1 or 2 courses of pharmacologic therapy and results in increased respiratory support, renal impairment, or if there are contraindications to use of pharmacologic therapy. Best if done before 1-3 years of age.

COARCTATION OF THE AORTA

- **Congenital narrowing of the aortic lumen at the distal arch or descending aorta, causing Hypertension in the upper extremities relative to the lower extremities.**
- Usually located at the insertion of the ductus arteriosus (ligamentum arteriosum after regression) just distal to the left subclavian artery.

EPIDEMIOLOGY:
- Males more common. 4–6% of all congenital heart defects. Most cases are sporadic.

ASSOCIATIONS:
- **Bicuspid aortic valve seen in 70%;** Mitral valve defects, Patent ductus arteriosus
- **Turner syndrome:** 5–15% of girls with CoA have Turner syndrome. Karyotype screening is recommended for females diagnosed with coarctation.

PATHOPHYSIOLOGY
- Narrowing of the aorta most commonly at the insertion of the ductus arteriosus distal to the origin of the left subclavian vein results in hypertension in the arteries proximal to the lesion (eg, primary arteries supplying the upper extremities) with relative hypotension in the lower extremities.
- Compensates occurs with development of collateral around the coarctation (eg, intercostal arteries).

TYPES
- Post-ductal (adult type) — narrowing occurs distal to the ductus arteriosum.
- Pre-ductal (infantile type) — narrowing occurs proximal to ductus arteriosum.

CLINICAL MANIFESTATIONS
- Most patients are asymptomatic. **Hypertension** — eg, headache, epistaxis due to elevated pressures. Hypertension is the most common presentation in adults. Intracranial aneurysms.
- **Bilateral claudication.** Dyspnea on exertion, exercise intolerance, fatigue, syncope.
- Neonatal presentation: failure to thrive in infants, poor feeding 1-2 weeks after birth.

PHYSICAL EXAMINATION
- **Upper extremity systolic hypertension with lower extremity hypotension with relative lower extremity hypotension** (eg, SBP >10 mmHg or higher in the right arm compared to the right leg)
- **Diminished or delayed lower extremity pulses:** eg, femoral & dorsalis pedis pulses.
- Systolic murmur: **harsh systolic murmur along the left sternal border radiating to the back, left infrascapular region, or chest** (best heard on the back between the scapulae near the aortic isthmus where coarctation usually occurs).

DIAGNOSIS
- **Echocardiography: confirmatory test** — narrowing of the aorta.
- **CXR: posterior rib notching (due to increased intercostal artery collateral flow), figure 3 sign (narrowed indented aorta looks like the notch of the 3).** Barium swallow: "reverse 3" or "E" sign.
- ECG: left ventricular hypertrophy.
- Angiography: criterion standard.

MANAGEMENT
- **Repair: Corrective surgery or transcatheter-based intervention** (eg, balloon angioplasty with or without stent placement), preferably in early childhood.
- **Prostaglandin E1 (eg, Alprostadil) preoperatively in neonates to stabilize the condition** — maintains a patent ductus arteriosus, reduces symptoms & improves lower extremity blood flow by relaxing the tissue of the coarctation segment.

TETRALOGY OF FALLOT (TOF)

- Constellation of [1] RV outflow obstruction, [2] Right ventricular hypertrophy (RVH), [3] large unrestrictive VSD, and [4] overriding aorta.
- **Most common cyanotic congenital heart disease (associated with a right-to-left shunt).**

CLINICAL MANIFESTATIONS
- Infancy: **cyanosis most common presentation** (blue baby syndrome), poor feeding, hemoptysis.
- Older children: exertional dyspnea, cyanosis that worsens with age. **Tet spells — paroxysms of cyanosis relieved with squatting** (decreases right-to-left shunting, improving oxygenation).

PHYSICAL EXAMINATION
- **Harsh systolic murmur at left mid to upper sternal border** (VSD), **right ventricular heave** (RVH).
- Digital clubbing, cyanosis.
- **Loud single S2** because the pulmonic component is rarely audible.
- Systolic thrill may be palpable along the left sternal border. **Right ventricular heave** (RVH)

DIAGNOSIS
- **Echocardiogram: Test of choice to establish the diagnosis** — features include a VSD and overriding aorta. Many infants with TOF are diagnosed prenatally.
- Chest radiograph: **"Boot-shaped" heart — upturned apex and a concave main pulmonary artery segment.** The heart size is often normal, pulmonary flow normal or decreased.
- Electrocardiogram: RVH, right atrial enlargement, and right axis deviation.

MANAGEMENT
- Neonates with severe RVOT obstruction may require intravenous prostaglandin therapy (eg, Alprostadil) to maintain ductus arteriosus patency, ductal stenting, or palliative shunt placement to maintain adequate pulmonary blood flow prior to surgical repair.
- **Surgical repair definitive management.** Usually performed in the first 12 months of life (ideally 3-6 months of age). Surgical repair includes patch closure of the ventricular septal defect and enlargement of the RVOT to relieve the pulmonary outflow obstruction.
- **Prostaglandin infusion prior to surgery to maintain a patent ductus arteriosus** — improves circulation and provides adequate lower extremity perfusion.
- Beta blockers used in some prior to surgical repair to decreases the risk of Tet spells. IV beta-blocker therapy improves relaxation of the RV outflow obstruction & improved pulmonary blood flow.

Hypercyanotic spells:
- **The stepwise management approach of patients who experience hypercyanotic ("Tet") spells includes knee-chest positioning in infants or squatting in older children** (increases preload and systemic vascular resistance), supplemental oxygen, intravenous (IV) Morphine, IV fluid bolus.
- If these measures fail, IV Beta blockers (eg, Propranolol, Esmolol) can be given and if symptoms persist, IV Phenylephrine is the next step. Palliative surgical procedure if medical therapy fails.

PULMONIC STENOSIS (PS)

- Right ventricular outflow obstruction of blood across the pulmonic valve.
- **Almost always congenital & a disease of the young** (eg, Congenital rubella syndrome).

PHYSICAL EXAMINATION
- Harsh mid-systolic ejection crescendo-decrescendo murmur (maximal at the left upper sternal border) radiates to the neck.
  - **Murmur increases with inspiration.** The longer the murmur duration = ↑stenosis.
  - Systolic ejection click (often "buried" in S1), Wide split S_2 (delayed P_2), ± S_4

MANAGEMENT
- Balloon valvuloplasty is the preferred treatment.

TRANSPOSITION OF THE GREAT ARTERIES (TOGA)

- Discordance between the aorta and pulmonary trunk (the aorta arises from the right ventricle and the pulmonary trunk arises from the left ventricle).
- Most common cyanotic heart disease presenting in the neonatal period (dextro).

TYPES
- **Dextro-TGA: most common. The aorta arises from the right ventricle & the pulmonary artery from the left ventricle,** leading to **two parallel circuits.** The systemic circuit sends systemic deoxygenated blood back to the systemic circulation. The pulmonary circuit sends oxygenated pulmonary venous blood back to the lungs. **Prior to surgical correction, survival is dependent upon the presence of shunts between the right and left circulations** (eg, patent ductus arteriosus, ASD, VSD).
- **Levo-TGA: is usually acyanotic.** The right atrium (RA) sends blood to the morphologic left ventricle (LV), which is on the right side physically. This morphologic LV sends blood to pulmonary system. The left atrium (LA) sends blood to morphologic right ventricle (RV) located on the left side; The morphologic right ventricle sends blood to the systemic circulation.

CLINICAL MANIFESTATIONS
- **Severe cyanosis & tachypnea within the first 30 days of life** not affected by exertion or oxygen use.
- **Neonatal cyanosis: severe cyanosis within the first 30 days of life not affected by exertion or the use of oxygen.** The degree of cyanosis is dependent on the amount of mixing between the two parallel circuits. Factors affecting intracardiac mixing include the size & presence of an ASD or VSD.
- **Tachypnea**: Patients usually have a respiratory rate >60 breaths per minute but they often appear comfortable without retractions, grunting, or flaring.
- **Diaphoresis and poor feeding.**
- Patients with L-TGA are typically unaffected until later in life when the right ventricle can no longer compensate for the increased afterload of the systemic circulation. These patients present with signs and symptoms of Heart failure.

PHYSICAL EXAMINATION
- **Central cyanosis. Loud and single second heart sound (S2).**
- **Murmurs**: Murmurs are not typically present unless a small VSD or pulmonic stenosis exists.

DIAGNOSIS
- **Echocardiogram: primary means of diagnosis.**
- **Electrocardiography**: may be normal or show right axis deviation or right ventricular hypertrophy.
- **Chest radiography**: **"egg on a string" appearance — cardiomegaly + narrowed mediastinum**: the heart appears as an egg on its side with the narrowed, atrophic thymus of the superior mediastinum appearing as the string. Mildly increased pulmonary vascular congestion, & mild cardiomegaly.
- **Cardiac catheterization**: criterion standard but rarely used to make the diagnosis but may be used in therapeutic treatment (eg, balloon atrial septostomy).

MANAGEMENT
- **Initial management of patients with D-TGA is to ensure adequate oxygenation (eg, Prostaglandin E1 administration [eg, Alprostadil] & Balloon atrial septostomy) & corrective surgery (eg, Arterial switch operation) once the patient is hemodynamically stable.**
- Prostaglandin E1 analog to maintain a patent ductus arteriosus & balloon atrial septostomy may be needed for temporary intercirculatory mixing prior to definitive surgical repair.
- Without treatment, 90% die by 1 year. 5-year survival rate after surgery >80%.

VENTRICULAR SEPTAL DEFECT (VSD)

- Hole in the ventricular septum. Usually associated with a left to right shunt.
- **Most common type of congenital heart disease in childhood.**
- Small to moderate associated with a left to right shunt.
- Large (unrestricted) defects may eventually develop a right to left shunt (Eisenmenger syndrome).

TYPES

- **Membranous: most common type (80%). Hole in the LV outflow tract** just beneath the aortic valve & behind the septal leaflet of the tricuspid valve. **Involvement of muscular septum.**
- Muscular: usually multiple holes in a **"swiss cheese"** pattern.
- AV canal (inlet, posterior): located posterior to the septal leaflet of the tricuspid valve just inferior to the inlet valves (tricuspid and mitral) within the inlet part of the right ventricular septum.
- **Supracristal (outlet) (subpulmonic, infundibular)** — located below the semilunar valves (aortic and pulmonic valves) in the outlet septum of the right ventricle above the crista supraventricularis. They commonly are associated with prolapse of the right coronary cusp of the aortic valve **with or without Aortic insufficiency**. Outlet defects rarely close spontaneously.

CLINICAL MANIFESTATIONS

- **Small (restrictive): asymptomatic or mild symptoms and are often incidentally found on examination. Normal pressure differences between the ventricles maintained.**
- Moderate: excessive sweating or fatigue, especially during feeds, poor feeding (may appear hungry but tires easily; sweats with feeds), lack of adequate growth, frequent respiratory infections, tachypnea, tachycardia, hepatomegaly, pallor, and mild congestive heart failure (eg, pulmonary rales, grunting, retractions) due to moderate LV volume overload and absent to mild PAH.
- **Large (unrestricted):** severe symptoms. **No pressure differences between the ventricles.** Larger VSDs with significant left-to-right shunting may cause failure to thrive in infancy or signs of heart failure by 3-4 weeks of age due to severe LV volume overload and severe PAH.
- Eisenmenger syndrome: right to left shunt occurring with large (unrestricted) VSDs. **Eisenmenger syndrome manifests in cyanosis, dyspnea, syncope, desaturation, secondary erythrocytosis, and clubbing.** The typical murmur of VSD may be absent and accentuated pulmonic component of the second heart sound (P2) may be heard.

PHYSICAL EXAMINATION

- **High-pitched harsh holosystolic murmur best heard at the third or fourth intercostal spaces along the left lower sternal border.**
- Smaller VSDs are usually louder and associated with more palpable thrills than larger ones.
- May be associated with a thrill or diastolic rumble at the mitral area.
- **Handgrip maneuver: increases the intensity of the murmur of VSD** due to increase flow of blood from the left to right ventricles as a result of increased systemic vascular resistance and afterload.

DIAGNOSIS

- **Echocardiogram:** determines the size and location of VSD. **Echocardiogram usually preferred over catheterization.**
- ECG: LVH in mild to moderate disease. Combines RVH + LVH (Katz-Wachtel phenomenon).
- Chest radiograph: may be normal, show left atrial enlargement or right ventricular hypertrophy.

MANAGEMENT

- Observation: in small, asymptomatic VSDs (most close within 12 months).
- Patch closure: symptomatic infants or uncontrolled CHF, growth delay, recurrent respiratory infections. Large shunts repaired by 2 years of age to prevent pulmonary hypertension.

	ATRIAL SEPTAL DEFECT	PATENT DUCTUS ARTERIOSUS	COARCTATION OF AORTA	TETRALOGY OF FALLOT
DEFINITION	Hole in atrial septum (opening between right & left atrium).	Communication between descending thoracic aorta & pulmonary artery	Congenital narrowing of descending thoracic aorta. Male:female 2:1	MC cyanotic congenital heart disease
SHUNT	Left to Right (Noncyanotic)	Left to Right (Noncyanotic)	Noncyanotic usually	Right to Left (Cyanotic)*
ETIOLOGIES PATHOPHYSIOLOGY	• Ostium secundum MC* (80%) • Ostium primum – associated with mitral regurgitation • Sinus venosus, coronary sinus • ASD 2nd MC cause of CHD (VSD MC)	Prematurity, perinatal distress & hypoxia delays closure, Rubella infection in the 1st trimester. Continued Prostaglandin E_2 production promotes patency	↑LV afterload with SNS activity & RAAS activation ⇨ HTN, LVH, CHF. 70% ALSO HAVE BICUSPID AORTIC VALVE*	❶ RV outflow obstruction – pulmonary artery stenosis ❷ RV Hypertrophy ❸ VSD (large unrestrictive) ❹ overriding aorta – between ventricles
CLINICAL MANIFESTATIONS	• Most patients asymptomatic or minimal in childhood until >30y. • Infants/young children: recurrent respiratory infections, failure to thrive, exertional dyspnea. • Adolescents/Adults: exertional dyspnea, easy fatigability, palpitations, atrial arrhythmias, syncope, heart failure. • Stroke (paroxysmal embolus)	• Most asymptomatic • Poor feeding, weight loss, frequent lower respiratory tract infections, pulmonary congestion • Eisenmenger's syndrome: left to right shunt switches & becomes right to left shunt (cyanotic) pulmonary HTN ⇨ left to right shunt switches & becomes right to left shunt (cyanotic)	• Secondary HTN* • bilateral claudication, dyspnea on exertion, syncope. • Infants: failure to thrive, poor feeding, shock. Types • Infantile: preductal • Adult: postductal	• Blue Baby syndrome (cyanosis) •Older: exertional dyspnea, cyanosis worsens with age. • "Tet-spells"*: paroxysms of cyanosis – older children relieve spells by squatting*. • Eisenmenger's syndrome: seen with PDA, VSD, TOF (±ASD)
PHYSICAL EXAM FINDINGS	• Systolic ejection crescendo-decrescendo flow murmur @ pulmonic area* (left upper sternal border). Sounds like PS (functional flow murmur). • WIDELY SPLIT FIXED S_2:* DOES NOT VARY WITH RESPIRATIONS.* • Loud S_1, hyperdynamic RV*	• CONTINUOUS MACHINERY MURMUR* loudest @ pulmonic area. • Wide pulse pressure: BOUNDING PERIPHERAL PULSES* LOUD S2 • Eisenmenger: normal hands (upper extremities) with cyanotic lower extremities (clubbed, blue toes)	• Systolic murmur that radiates to the back/scapula/chest* • ↑BP upper > lower extremities*. • Delayed/weak femoral pulses* ↓flow distal to obstruction in the lower extremities.	• Harsh holosystolic murmur @ left upper sternal border (sounds like PS). • Right ventricular heave. • Digital clubbing
DIAGNOSIS	• CXR: - cardiomegaly • ECG: - Incomplete RBB (rsR' in V_1 RAD) - Crochetage sign: notching of the peak of the R wave in inferior leads. • Echocardiogram: gold standard	• CXR: Normal or cardiomegaly • ECG: LVH, left atrial enlargement • Echocardiogram: gold standard	• CXR: - Rib notching*: ↑collateral circulation via intercostal arteries. - "3 sign".* Narrowed aorta looks like the notch of the number 3 • ECG: LVH • Angiogram: gold standard.* CT scan	• CXR: - Boot-shaped heart* Prominent right ventricle • ECG: Right ventricular hypertrophy* Right atrial enlargement (RAE) • Echocardiogram: gold standard
MANAGEMENT	• Spontaneous closure likely in 1st year so may observe if small. • Surgical correction if symptomatic (usually between 2-4y)	• IV indomethacin 1st line tx* (closes the PDA) • Surgical correction if indomethacin fails. Best if done before 1-3y of age.	• Surgical Correction • Balloon angioplasty ± stent • Prostaglandin E_1 (PGE$_1$) preoperatively (reduces symptoms, improves lower extremity blood flow)	Surgical repair performed in the first 4 – 12 months of life. PGE1 infusion: prevents ductal closure if patient in cyanotic patients prior to surgery.

ATRIAL SEPTAL DEFECT

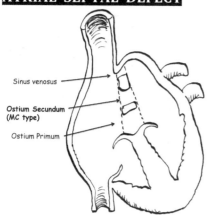

HALLMARKS

- Usually asymptomatic until >30y

- **Systolic ejection murmur** best heard at the pulmonic area.
- May develop stroke due to paradoxical emboli.
- <u>**Widely fixed, split** S2 **(doesn't vary with respirations).**</u>

PATENT DUCTUS ARTERIOSUS

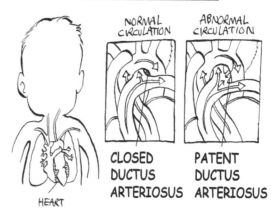

HALLMARKS

- **Continuous machinery murmur** loudest at the pulmonic area

- Wide pulse pressure - **bounding pulses**

- **IV Indomethacin 1st line to close a PDA in infants** (prostaglandin inhibition).

TETRALOGY OF FALLOT

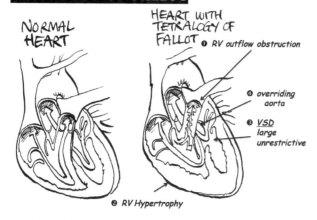

HALLMARKS

- MC cyanotic heart disease overall.

- Cyanosis in infants, <u>**Tet spells**</u> in older children **(periodic episodes of cyanosis relived with squatting** or putting an infant's knees to its chest).

- <u>CXR:</u> **boot-shaped heart**

- <u>Management:</u> surgical correction. Prostaglandin E1 prior to surgery to maintain patency of the ductus arteriosus.

COARCTATION OF THE AORTA

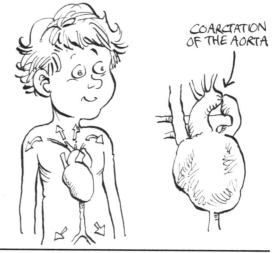

HALLMARKS

- 70% have a bicuspid aortic valve.
- Suspect in a child with 2ry **hypertension,** bilateral lower extremity claudication.
- Systolic murmur that radiates to the back, scapula or chest.
- **Systolic blood pressure in upper extremities > lower extremities.**
- Delayed or weak femoral pulses.
- <u>CXR:</u> **rib notching** (due to dilation of the intercostal arteries), **"3" sign** (shape of the coarctation).

CONGENITAL CYANOTIC HEART DISEASES

5 Ts:

1. **T**RUNCUS ARTERIOSUS **1 vessel** instead of 2 normal vessels (aorta & pulmonary artery)

2. **T**RANSPOSITION OF GREAT ARTERIES **2 vessels switched** (aorta & pulmonary artery).

3. **T**RICUSPID ATRESIA (**3= tri**) absence of the **tri**cuspid valve leads to a hypoplastic right ventricle. An ASD & VSD must be present for blood to flow out of the right atrium.

4. **T**ETRALOGY OF FALLOT (**4- tetra**): 4 problems: ❶ right ventricular outflow obstruction ex. pulmonary stenosis ❷ right ventricular hypertrophy ❸ overriding aorta & ❹ ventricular septal defect (large, unrestrictive).

5. **T**OTAL ANOMALOUS PULMONARY VENOUS RETURN (**5 vessels involved**): all 4 pulmonary veins connect to 1 vessel (superior vena cava) instead of the left atrium.

Hypoplastic left heart syndrome is often associated with mitral valve &/or aortic valve atresia.

PULMONARY ATRESIA

- Pulmonary atresia with intact intraventricular septum (PA/IVS) is characterized by **complete obstruction to right ventricular outflow** with varying degrees of right ventricular & tricuspid valve hypoplasia — **blood is unable to flow from the right ventricle into the pulmonary artery & the lungs.**

TYPES
- Valvular (membranous): atretic pulmonary valve, small valve annulus with fused valve leaflets leading to a thin, intact membrane that causes right ventricular outflow tract obstruction.
- Muscular: obliteration of the muscular infundibulum. It is associated with severe right ventricular hypoplasia and increased coronary artery abnormalities.

CLINICAL MANIFESTATIONS
- Cyanosis due to right-to-left shunting at the atrial level. Improved survival if there is a patent ductus arteriosus.
- Single heart sound (due to a single semilunar valve – the aortic valve).
- Systolic murmur of tricuspid regurgitation

MANAGEMENT
- Maintain the patency of the ductus arteriosus (eg, prostaglandin E1 analog Alprostadil) to stabilize initially. Balloon atrial septostomy to improve the right to left atrial shunting.
- Surgical repair: definitive. If untreated, approximately 50% of these children die within 2 weeks of birth & 85% by six months.

TRICUSPID ATRESIA

- 2% of all congenital heart disease. Absence of the tricuspid valve leads to a hypoplastic right ventricle. A PDA or VSD is necessary for pulmonary blood flow and survival.

CLINICAL MANIFESTATIONS
- **Cyanosis due to right-to-left shunting.** Improved survival if there is a patent ductus arteriosus.
- Single heart sound (S_2).

DIAGNOSIS
- ECG: left ventricular hypertrophy.
- CXR: normal or enlarged cardiac silhouette with *decreased* pulmonary flow.

MANAGEMENT
- Maintain the patency of the ductus arteriosus (eg, prostaglandin E1 analog Alprostadil) to stabilize initially. Presence of VSD improves oxygenation of blood.
- Surgical repair: definitive. Subclavian artery to pulmonary shunt followed by a 2-staged surgical correction to direct systemic venous return directly to the pulmonary arteries.

HYPOPLASTIC LEFT HEART SYNDROME

- Failure of the development of the mitral valve, aortic valve, or the aortic arch ⇨ small ventricle unable to supply the normal systemic circulation requirements. 1% of all congenital heart disease.

CLINICAL MANIFESTATIONS
- Symptoms begin when the ductus arteriosus constricts, leading to cyanosis and heart failure.

DIAGNOSIS
- ECG: right ventricular hypertrophy.
- CXR: cardiomegaly.

MANAGEMENT
- Prostaglandin E1 to open the ductus arteriosus followed by surgical repair.

CIRCULATORY SHOCK

- **<u>Inadequate organ perfusion & tissue oxygenation</u>** to meet the body's oxygenation requirements.
  Often associated with hypotension (but not always). Shock is determined by <u>EITHER</u>:
  - **(1) <u>Low cardiac output (CO)</u> &/OR**
  - **(2) <u>Low systemic vascular resistance</u>** (SVR). SVR = the resistance to blood flow through the circulatory system (determined by peripheral blood vessels). Peripheral vasoconstriction increases SVR. Vasodilation decreases SVR.
  Remember Blood pressure = Cardiac output (CO) x Systemic vascular resistance (SVR)

4 MAIN TYPES OF SHOCK	
1. **HYPOVOLEMIC**	**loss of blood or fluid volume** (eg, hemorrhage).
2. **CARDIOGENIC**	**primary myocardial dysfunction** ⇨ reduced cardiac output (eg, MI).
3. **OBSTRUCTIVE**	**extrinsic or intrinsic obstruction to circulation** (eg, pericardial tamponade).
4. **DISTRIBUTIVE**	**maldistribution of blood flow** from essential organs to nonessential organs due to loss of autonomic control of the vasculature (eg, **septic, endocrine, neurogenic shock**).

PATHOPHYSIOLOGY OF SHOCK
1. **<u>Inadequate tissue perfusion:</u>** inability to meet the body's metabolic oxygen requirements ⇨ metabolic acidosis & organ dysfunction.
2. **<u>Autonomic nervous system activation:</u>** in an attempt to improve systemic O_2 delivery.
   - <u>Sympathetic nervous system activation:</u> causes vasoconstriction (↑SVR) & ↑contractility (to ↑CO). ↑Norepinephrine, dopamine, & cortisol release. The ↑SVR helps to maintain cerebral & cardiac perfusion by causing vasoconstriction of splanchnic, musculoskeletal, & renal blood flow.
   - <u>RAAS activation:</u> water & sodium retention (↓urine output to minimize renal water & salt loss). Also causes vasoconstriction to help maintain cardiac output.
3. **<u>Systemic effects of shock:</u>**
   - ATP depletion ⇨ ion pump dysfunction leading to cellular dysfunction, cell swelling, & death.
   - **<u>Metabolic acidosis</u>:** due to lack of oxygen ⇨ cells resort to anaerobic metabolism, producing **lactic acid** as a byproduct. **Order lactate levels as part of workup.**
   - <u>Multiorgan Dysfunction Syndrome (MODS):</u> physiologic consequences of shock on organ systems. Includes lung, kidney, heart, & brain dysfunction as well as DIC (disseminated intravascular coagulation).
   - <u>Multisystemic Organ Failure (MSOF):</u> organ failure if the conditions persist.

CLINICAL MANIFESTATIONS OF SHOCK
1. Often acutely ill, altered mental status, decreased peripheral pulses, tachycardia, skin usually cool and mottled (may be warm and flushed in distributive shock), systolic blood pressure <110 mmHg (some patients in shock may be normotensive initially). **Oliguria or anuria.**
2. <u>Laboratory tests:</u> include CBC, BMP (Chem-7), **lactic acidosis**, coagulation studies, cultures (to look for potential infectious sources), ABG and other studies depending on the likely etiology.

GENERAL MANAGEMENT OF SHOCK ABCDE's
1. <u>Airway:</u> may need intubation.
2. <u>Breathing:</u> mechanical ventilation & sedation decreases the work of breathing (reducing the oxygen demand associated with tachypnea).
3. <u>Circulation:</u> isotonic crystalloids (Normal Saline, Lactated Ringer's). Often given multiple liters & titrated to central venous pressure (CVP) of 8-12mmHg OR urine output of 0.5ml/kg/hr (30ml/hr) OR an improved heart rate.
4. <u>Delivery of Oxygen:</u> monitor lactate levels.
5. <u>Endpoint of Resuscitation:</u> urine output (UOP): 0.5ml/kg/hr, CVP 8-12mmHg, mean arterial pressure (MAP) 65-90mmHg, central venous oxygen concentration >70%.

HYPOVOLEMIC SHOCK

- Shock secondary to reduced intravascular volume (eg, reduced preload), primarily due to loss of blood (hemorrhagic) or nonhemorrhagic fluid losses (eg, diarrhea).

ETIOLOGIES
- **Hemorrhagic — blunt or penetrating trauma (includes multiple fractures without vessel injury) is the most common cause of Hypovolemic shock by far**. GI bleed, AAA rupture, massive hemoptysis, trauma, ectopic pregnancy, postpartum hemorrhage.
- **Non-blood fluid loss:** GI: vomiting, bowel obstruction, pancreatitis; severe burns, diabetic ketoacidosis (causes osmotic diuresis in response to hyperglycemia).

PATHOPHYSIOLOGY
Loss of blood or fluid volume ⇨ ↑heart rate, vasoconstriction [↑systemic vascular resistance (SVR)], hypotension, ↓cardiac output, and pulmonary capillary wedge pressure.
Body's response to hypovolemia:
  - rapid: peripheral vasoconstriction, ↑cardiac activity.
  - sustained: arterial vasoconstriction, Na$^+$/water retention, ↑cortisol.

CLINICAL MANIFESTATIONS
Loss of volume ⇨ ↑heart rate (tachycardia), hypotension, ↓CO (oliguria or anuria), vasoconstriction (↑SVR) ⇨ **pale cool dry skin/extremities, slow capillary refill >2 seconds, ↓skin turgor, dry mucous membranes, altered mental status.**
Usually does not cause profound respiratory distress.

PHYSICAL EXAMINATION
- Skin examination: pale, cool, clammy skin (most common initial finding); mottling, **prolonged capillary refill, decreased skin turgor, dry mucous membranes,** nondistended jugular veins.
- **Tachycardia most common initial vital sign change. Hypotension.**

CLASSES OF HEMORRHAGIC SHOCK		
I	< 15% blood loss	Pulse usually normal, systolic blood pressure (SBP) usually normal.
II	15–30% blood loss	**Tachycardia** (pulse >100 BPM). SBP usually >100 mmHg.
III	30–40% blood loss	Tachycardia, **decreased systolic blood pressure** (<100 mmHg), confusion, decreased urine output.
IV	>40% blood loss	Tachycardia, decreased SBP, **lethargy, no urine output.**

DIAGNOSIS
- **Vasoconstriction (↑SVR), hypotension, ↓CO, & decreased pulmonary capillary pressure.**
- Decreased CVP (central venous pressure)/PCWP (pulmonary capillary wedge pressure).
- CBC: ↑Hgb/Hct = dehydration (hemoconcentration). ↓Hgb/Hct is late sign in hemorrhagic shock.

MANAGEMENT:
- ABCDE's, Insert 2 large bore IV lines or a central line.
- **When etiology of Hypovolemic shock is established, replacement of blood or fluid loss should be done as soon as possible to minimize tissue ischemia.** Factors to consider when replacing fluid loss include the rate of fluid replacement and type of fluid to be used.
- **Volume resuscitation — crystalloid fluids (eg, Normal saline or Lactated ringers).** Blood products superior if hemorrhagic. Fluid repletion can be monitored by measuring blood pressure, urine output, mental status, and peripheral edema. Adverse effect of the solution used include (eg, hyponatremia [Lactated Ringer] & hyperchloremic acidosis [normal saline]).
- Control the source of hemorrhage to prevent further sequelae. ±Packed RBC blood transfusion if severe hemorrhage: (O-negative or cross-matched).
- Surgical exploration may be necessary for non-responders, so the bleeding source may be identified.
- In hypovolemic shock, vasopressors generally not be used because they can worsen tissue perfusion.

CARDIOGENIC SHOCK

- **PRIMARY CARDIAC/MYOCARDIAL DYSFUNCTION** ⇨ inadequate tissue perfusion ⇨ ↓CO (cardiac output) with ↑systemic vascular resistance (SVR). Often systolic in nature.
- Cardiogenic often produces increased respiratory effort/distress whereas hypovolemic does not.

ETIOLOGIES

Cardiac disease: myocardial infarction, myocarditis, valve dysfunction, congenital heart disease, cardiomyopathy, arrhythmias (bradycardia or tachycardia).

PATHOPHYSIOLOGY

↓CO & evidence of tissue hypoxia in the presence of adequate intravascular volume. Sustained hypotension in the presence of **↑pulmonary capillary wedge pressure** (>15 mmHg).
Vasoconstriction (↑SVR), hypotension, ↓CO, & ↑pulmonary capillary wedge pressure.

MANAGEMENT

- Treat the underlying cause: Reperfusion: early and definitive restoration of coronary blood flow if due to myocardial ischemia — PCI, CABG, or Fibrinolytic therapy. Avoid Beta blockers.
- **Avoid aggressive IV fluid resuscitation — Cardiogenic shock is the only type of shock in which large amounts of IV fluids aren't given** to prevent pulmonary edema.
- **Norepinephrine is a potent vasopressor with some positive inotropic properties that is often the initial vasopressor of choice in cardiogenic, septic, and hypovolemic shock** [preferred over Dopamine in patients with severe hypotension (SBP <70 mm Hg)].
- **Dobutamine initial agent of choice in cardiogenic shock with low cardiac output and maintained blood pressure (fewer sick patients with borderline low BP without severe hypotension).** Inotrope (nonadrenergic, PDE3 inhibitor): Milrinone: if refractory.

OBSTRUCTIVE SHOCK

- **Obstruction of blood flow due to physical or vascular obstruction of the heart or great vessels.**
- Intrinsic or extrinsic (↑ external pressure on the heart decreases the heart's ability to pump blood).
- Similar to Hypovolemic shock but the **combination of poor perfusion associated with distended neck veins (↑ JVD) is seen with Obstructive & Cardiogenic shock.** Hypotension, cold & clammy skin, & tachycardia.
- ↓PCWP <15 mmHg in most cases (↑ PCWP in cardiac tamponade), normal or ↓CO, ↑ SVR.

ETIOLOGIES:

1. **Massive pulmonary embolism**: obstruction to pulmonary artery blood flow. Cyanosis, tachycardia, hypotension, VQ mismatch, hemoptysis. ECG: $S_1Q_3T_3$, sinus tachycardia. ABG: PaO_2 <80 mmHg, ↑A-a gradient. Low CO, ↑peripheral resistance, ↑CVP.
2. **Pericardial Tamponade:** blood in the pericardial space prevents venous return to the heart, causing obstruction. **Beck's triad**: muffled heart sounds, systemic hypotension, & ↑JVP.
3. **Tension pneumothorax**: positive air pressure causes external pressure on the heart. **Hyperresonance to percussion & decreased breath sounds on the affected side. Mediastinal & tracheal shift to the contralateral side**, SQ emphysema, and ↑JVP.
4. **Aortic dissection:** proximal dissections. May also cause hypovolemic shock.

MANAGEMENT

Oxygen, isotonic fluids, inotropic support: dobutamine, epinephrine, intra-aortic balloon pump.
Because this shock is mechanical or vascular obstruction, treat the underlying cause:
Pulmonary Embolism: heparin, thrombolytics. ± Embolectomy.
Pericardial tamponade ⇨ pericardiocentesis.
Tension pneumothorax ⇨ needle decompression.
Proximal dissections usually require surgical intervention.

DISTRIBUTIVE SHOCK

- **EXCESS VASODILATION & ALTERED DISTRIBUTION OF BLOOD FLOW** (increased venous capacity) with shunting of blood flow from vital organs (ex. heart, kidney) to non-vital tissues (eg, skin, skeletal muscle). **Hallmark: ↓CO, ↓SVR, ↓PCWP.**
- An **important EXCEPTION IS EARLY SEPTIC SHOCK - ASSOCIATED WITH ↑CO & ↓SVR so warm extremities often noted in these patients.** Septic shock is the most common type of distributive shock.
- **Systemic inflammatory response syndrome (SIRS):** defined by the presence of any 2 of the following criteria: (1) body temperature over 38 or under 36 degrees Celsius, (2) heart rate > 90/min, (3) a respiratory rate >20 breaths/min or partial pressure of CO2 <32 mmHg, (4) a leukocyte count >12,000 or <4,000 cells/microliters, or >10% immature forms or bands.
- Sepsis: life-threatening organ dysfunction caused by host systemic inflammation due to infection.

CLINICAL MANIFESTATIONS
- **Septic shock consists of [1] low cardiac filling pressures, or [2] low central venous pressures (CVP) and capillary wedge pressure, and [3] decreased systemic vascular resistance (SVR).**
- **In early Septic shock due to the Frank-Starling mechanism, cardiac output is often increased to maintain blood pressure in the presence of systemic vasodilatation.** With low preload & afterload, cardiac output (CO) must increase to compensate with **increased heart rate.**
- Early in Septic shock, the rise in cardiac output is often limited by hypovolemia and a fall in preload because of low cardiac filling pressures. When intravascular volume is augmented, the cardiac output usually is elevated (hyperdynamic or warm shock).

MANAGEMENT
- 3-hour bundle obtain appropriate cultures before administration of antibiotics if possible, obtain plasma lactate level, broad-spectrum antibiotics [eg, Vancomycin PLUS 1 of the following Third- or fourth-generation Cephalosporin: eg, Ceftriaxone, Cefotaxime; or Cefepime, Beta-lactam/beta-lactamase inhibitor: eg, Piperacillin-Tazobactam or Carbapenem: eg, Imipenem or Meropenem], and administer of crystalloid (eg, Normal saline or Lactated ringers) at 30 ml/kg for hypotension or lactate level ≥4 mmol/L, within the first 3 hours.
- If hypotensive despite adequate fluid resuscitation (eg, 3L in first 3 hours), vasopressor therapy (eg, Norepinephrine) to maintain mean arterial pressure >65 mmHg.

1. **ANAPHYLACTIC SHOCK:** **IgE-mediated severe systemic hypersensitivity reaction.** History of insect bite/stings, food or drug allergy, recent IV contrast. Symptoms usually begin within 60 minutes of exposure.
    PHYSICAL EXAM: pruritus, hives, angioedema ⇨ respiratory distress, stridor, sensation of "lump in throat", and hoarseness (life threatening laryngeal edema).
    MANAGEMENT: **IM Epinephrine 1st line** (0.3 mg IM of 1:1000 repeat q 5-10 min as needed). If cardiovascular collapse, give Epinephrine 1 mg IV (1:10,000). **Airway management, antihistamines** (Diphenhydramine 25-50 mg IV blocks H_1, Famotidine blocks H_2), IV fluids. **Observe patient for 4-6 hours** because up to 20% of patients have a biphasic phenomenon (return of symptoms 3-4 hours after the initial reaction).

2. **NEUROGENIC SHOCK:** due to **acute spinal cord injury**, regional anesthesia.
    PATHOPHYSIOLOGY: autonomic sympathetic blockade ⇨ unopposed ↑vagal tone ⇨ **bradycardia & hypotension.** Loss of sympathetic tone ⇨ warm, dry skin.
    CLINICAL: warm skin, normal or ↓HR, ↓SVR, hypovolemia, **WIDE pulse pressure.**
    Management: fluids, pressors, ± corticosteroids.

3. **ENDOCRINE SHOCK:** eg, **Adrenal insufficiency (Addisonian crisis).**
    Management: **Hydrocortisone 100mg IV** (often unresponsive to fluids & pressors).

	PATHOPHYSIOLOGY	ETIOLOGIES	CO	PCWP	SVR	CLINICAL MANIFESTATIONS
HYPOVOLEMIC	*LOSS OF BLOOD OR FLUID VOLUME* ⟹ ↑PVR & ↑HR to maintain CO.	**Hemorrhage:** GI bleed, AAA rupture etc. **Fluid loss:** GI: vomiting, diarrhea, pancreatitis, severe burns etc.	Decreased	*Decreased*	Increased	•*Pale, cool, mottled skin* •*Prolonged capillary refill* •*Decreased skin turgor, dry mucous membranes* •Usually no severe respiratory distress
CARDIOGENIC	*PRIMARY MYOCARDIAL ABNORMALITY* ⟹ heart unable to maintain CO	•Myocardial Infarction •Myocarditis •Valvular disease •Cardiomyopathies •Arrhythmias	Decreased	*Increased*	Increased	•*Severe respiratory distress* •*Cool clammy skin*
OBSTRUCTIVE	*EXTRINSIC OR INTRINSIC OBSTRUCTION of heart or great vessels*	•Pericardial tamponade •Massive Pulmonary Embolism •Tension Pneumothorax •Aortic dissection	Decreased	*Increased*	Increased	•*Severe respiratory distress* •*Cool clammy skin*
DISTRIBUTIVE 4 types (below)	*MALDISTRIBUTION OF BLOOD & VASODILATION with shunting of blood away from vital to non vital organs*				*Decreased*	
1. SEPTIC	Severe host immune response	Bacteria				
Early (warm)	Vasodilation		*Increased**	↑ or ↓	*Decreased*	•*↑CO*: WARM, FLUSHED EXTREMITIES & skin, brisk capillary refill, bounding pulses, WIDE pulse pressure* •*ONLY SHOCK ASSOC WITH ↑CO**
Late (cool)			Decreased	Decreased	Increased	Cool clammy skin
2. NEUROGENIC	Sympathetic blockade ⟹ unopposed vagal tone on vessels ⟹ vasodilation	Acute spine injury	Decreased	Decreased	Decreased	•*Hypotension without tachycardia** •± *Bradycardia**
3. ANAPHYLACTIC	*IgE mediated* systemic HSN reaction with histamine release ⟹ vasodilation leading to ↑capillary permeability	•Insect bites/stings •Food allergies •Drug allergies •Recent IV contrast	Decreased	Decreased	Decreased	•*Pruritus, hives, ± angioedema* ± throat fullness, hoarseness, wheezing •Recent h/o of insect bite/sting, food, drug or IV contrast
4. HYPOADRENAL	Decreased corticosteroid & mineralocorticoid activity	Adrenal insufficiency (Addisonian crisis)	Decreased	Decreased	Decreased	•*Low serum glucose.* •*Hypotension refractory to fluids & pressors*

SVR = Systemic Vascular Resistance   CO = Cardiac Output   PCWP = Pulmonary Capillary Wedge Pressure

CARDIOLOGY PHOTO CREDITS

CHAPTER 2 – PULMONARY SYSTEM

NEONATAL RESPIRATORY DISTRESS SYNDROME

- **Diffuse atelectasis, alveolar collapse, & pulmonary perfusion without ventilation due to insufficient surfactant production by an immature lung**. Primarily a disease of **preterm infants**.
- Surfactant production begins 24–28 weeks & enough is produced by 35 weeks. Surfactant reduces alveolar surface tension, decreases the pressure needed to keep the alveoli inflated and maintains alveolar stability.
- In ARDS, the infant is not be able to generate the increased inspiratory pressure needed to inflate alveolar units without surfactant, resulting in the development of progressive & diffuse atelectasis.

RISK FACTORS
- **Caucasians, males, multiple births, maternal Diabetes**, C-section delivery, perinatal infections.

CLINICAL MANIFESTATIONS
- **Usually presents at birth or shortly after birth with respiratory distress** (eg, tachypnea > 60/min, tachycardia, labored breathing, chest wall retractions, expiratory grunting, nasal flaring, cyanosis).

DIAGNOSIS
- CXR: **bilateral diffuse reticular (ground-glass) opacities + air bronchograms, bilateral atelectasis,** poor lung expansion, and domed diaphragms.
- ABG: hypoxia (often unresponsive to oxygen supplementation). Normal or slightly increased PCO_2.
- Postmortem histopathology: waxy-appearing layers lining the collapsed alveoli. Airway distention.

MANAGEMENT
- **Strong respiratory drive noninvasive support — either nasal continuous positive airway pressure or nasal intermittent positive pressure ventilation** rather than high-flow nasal cannula.
- **Apneic or poor respiratory effort** — with a heart rate <100 beats per minute require **resuscitation with bag mask ventilation (BMV)**. Infants who do not respond to BMV require intubation and initiation of invasive mechanical ventilation with Continuous positive airway pressure (CPAP).
- For neonates with an inadequate response to noninvasive respiratory support, Surfactant is given.
- Clinical course is 2-3 days with or without treatment. 90% survival rate with treatment and normal return of lung function within 1 month. Most common single cause of death in the first month of life.
- **Prevention: Pregnant women <34 weeks' gestation at high risk for preterm delivery should receive antenatal corticosteroids to enhance fetal lung maturity.**

MECONIUM ASPIRATION

- Entrance of meconium-containing amniotic fluid into the respiratory tract ⇨ respiratory distress, hypoxia & acidosis. Increased incidence in **POSTterm infants &/or infants small for gestational age.**

CLINICAL MANIFESTATIONS
- **Signs of respiratory distress usually after birth** — cyanosis, severe tachypnea, use of accessory muscles, intercostal retractions, grunting, nasal flaring. May occur with fetal distress & hypoxia.

DIAGNOSIS
- **Evidence of meconium-stained amniotic fluid**. May be seen in the trachea, vernix, or umbilical cord.
- Chest radiograph: **coarse, irregular infiltrates with lung hyperinflation/hyperexpansion** (flattened diaphragms, increased AP diameter). May show pneumothorax.

MANAGEMENT
- Mild to moderate disease, supplemental oxygen & ventilation via an oxygen hood or nasal cannula. Continuous positive airway pressure CPAP to reduce the need for invasive mechanical ventilation.
- Severe disease often requires intubation and mechanical ventilation. Empiric antibiotic therapy.
- **Prevention is the most effective therapy — prevention of postterm delivery (>41 weeks) via labor induction & prevention of fetal hypoxia.**

LUNG VOLUMES

- **Tidal volume (TV):** the volume of air moved into or out of the lungs during quiet breathing.

- **Residual Volume (RV):** the volume of air remaining in the lungs after maximal expiration. This residual volume functions to maintain alveolar patency, especially during end expiration.

- **Expiratory reserve volume (ERV):** the volume of air that can be further exhaled at the end of normal expiration.

- **Inspiratory reserve volume (IRV):** the volume of air that can be further inhaled at the end of normal inspiration.

- **Vital Capacity (VC):** maximum volume of air that can be exhaled following maximum inspiration (IRV + TV + ERV).

- **Total Lung Capacity (TLC):** the volume in the lungs at maximum inspiration (VC + RV).

- **Functional residual capacity (FRC):** volume of gas in the lungs at normal tidal volume end expiration (ERV + RV). This is the air in which gas exchange takes place.
    - ↑FRC seen in disorders with hyperinflation (due to loss of elastic recoil, PEEP).
    - ↓FRC seen in restrictive lung diseases.

- **FEV₁ Forced Expiratory Volume in 1 second**: the volume of air that has been exhaled at the end of the first second of forced expiration.

- **Forced Vital Capacity (FVC):** measurement of the volume of air that can be expelled from a maximally inflated lung, with the patient breathing as hard & fast as possible.

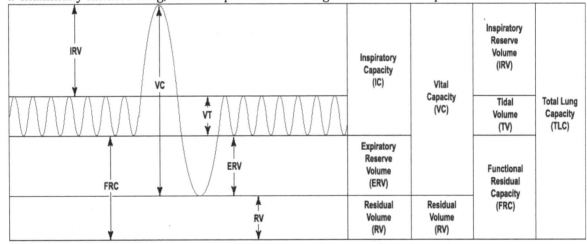

4 MAIN ATYPICAL SOUNDS

1. **WHEEZING:** high-pitched, **whistling, continuous,** musical sound (**usually louder during expiration** compared to inspiration) **produced by narrowed/obstructed airways.** Seen with obstructive lung diseases (Asthma, COPD), Bronchiectasis, Bronchiolitis, Lung cancer, Sleep apnea, CHF, GERD, anaphylaxis, foreign body etc.
2. **RHONCHI:** continuous, rumbling (rattling), coarse, **low-pitched sounds** (sounds like snoring) that **may clear with cough** or suctioning. Rhonchi are caused by increased secretions or obstruction in the bronchial airways.
3. **CRACKLES (RALES):** discontinuous high-pitched sounds **heard during inspiration** (usually not cleared by cough). Due to the "popping" open of collapsed alveoli & small airways (from fluid, exudates or lack of aeration). Seen with pneumonia, atelectasis, bronchitis, bronchiectasis, pulmonary edema & pulmonary fibrosis.
4. **STRIDOR:** monophonic sound usually loudest over the anterior neck due to **narrowing of the larynx or anywhere over the trachea.** Can be heard during inspiration, expiration or throughout the respiratory cycle.

OBSTRUCTIVE VS. RESTRICTIVE DISEASES

	OBSTRUCTIVE DISORDERS	RESTRICTIVE DISORDERS
PULMONARY FUNCTION TESTS (PFT)	**INCREASED lung volumes** **Hyperinflation:** ↑TLC, RV, RV/TLC, FRC **Obstruction:** ↓FEV1, ↓FVC; ↓FEV1/FVC FEV1 decreases more than the FVC	**DECREASED lung volumes** ↓TLC, RV, RV/TLC, FRC, FVC **Normal or ↑FEV₁/FVC**, ↓FEV1 FVC decreases more than FEV1
COMPLIANCE	↑ compliance with Emphysema	↓ compliance
EXAMPLES	• Asthma • COPD (Chronic bronchitis, Emphysema) • Bronchiectasis • Cystic Fibrosis • **Coal Workers Pneumoconiosis often presents with an obstructive pattern**	• Sarcoidosis • Pneumoconiosis • Idiopathic Pulmonary Fibrosis • ↓Muscular effort: Myasthenia Gravis, Polio • Scoliosis, Mesothelioma

CHRONIC OBSTRUCTIVE PULMONARY DISEASE (COPD)

- **COPD:** progressive, **largely irreversible airflow obstruction** due to ❶ **loss of elastic recoil** & ❷ **increased airway resistance.**
- COPD includes: ❶ EMPHYSEMA & ❷ CHRONIC BRONCHITIS.
- **Common >55y.** Chronic bronchitis usually episodic; Emphysema usually has a steady decline.
- Both usually coexist with one being more dominant.

RISK FACTORS
- **Cigarette smoking/exposure most important risk** (90%). Only 15% of smokers develop COPD.
- **Alpha-1 antitrypsin deficiency: only genetic disease linked to COPD in younger patients (<40y).**
- Occupational or environmental exposures, recurrent airway infections.

	EMPHYSEMA	CHRONIC BRONCHITIS
CLINICAL MANIFESTATIONS	• **Dyspnea most common symptom.** • Accessory muscle use, tachypnea, prolonged expiration. Mild cough. • Thin body habitus ("pink puffers")	• **Productive cough hallmark** symptom, prolonged expiration. • Cyanotic & obese "blue bloaters"
PHYSICAL EXAMINATION	**Hyperinflation:** • **Hyperresonance** to percussion • **↓/absent breath sounds, ↓fremitus** • **Barrel chest (↑AP diameter),** quiet chest. • Pursed-lip breathing.	• **"noisy lungs": rales (crackles), rhonchi, wheezing** ± change in location with cough. • ±Signs of cor pulmonale **(peripheral edema & cyanosis)**
LABS	Hemoglobin often normal initially.	• **↑Hematocrit/hemoglobin:** hypoxia stimulates erythropoiesis.
V/Q MISMATCH	**Matched V/Q defects:** Mild to moderate hypoxemia • **PaO2 normal to slightly reduced:** 65–75 mm Hg but SaO2 normal at rest. • **PaCO2 normal to slightly reduced:** 35–40 mmHg Can develop respiratory acidosis if severe	**Severe V/Q mismatch:** • **Severe hypoxemia:** PaO2 reduced: 45–60 mmHg • **Hypercapnia: Respiratory acidosis:** PaCO2 **slightly to markedly elevated** (50–60 mmHg).
APPEARANCE	**Pink puffers:** cachectic, pursed lip breathing- noncyanotic	**Blue bloaters:** obese & cyanotic

COPD RADIOLOGIC FINDINGS

NORMAL PA CXR

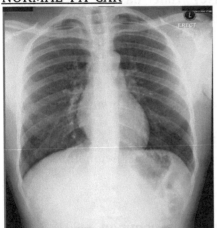

Note roundness of
the diaphragms.

EMPHYSEMA

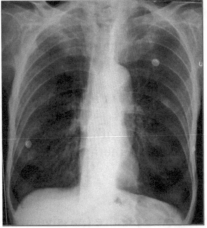

1. **Enlarged lung fields, flattened diaphragms.**
2. **Trapped air** (darker lung areas).
3. **Decreased vascular markings.**
4. **Bullae** seen (right side).

CHRONIC BRONCHITIS

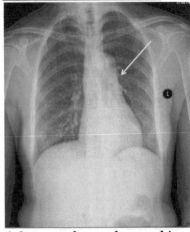

1. **Increased vascular markings, normal diaphragms.**
2. Prominent pulmonary artery & pulmonary hypertension (arrow), horizontal heart.
3. Right heart enlargement.

NORMAL LATERAL CXR

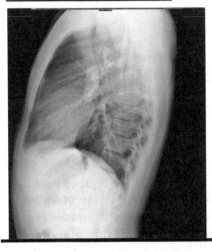

EMPHYSEMA

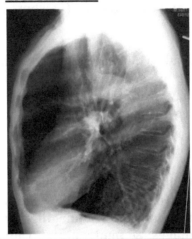

EMPHYSEMA LATERAL CXR:
1. **barrel chest**
2. **increased AP diameter**

NORMAL CT SCAN

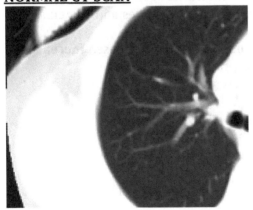

EMPHYSEMA

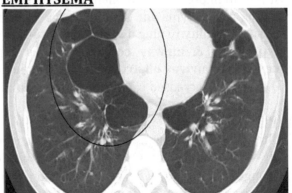

Emphysema: bullae (circular areas of darkness), which signifies airspace loss.

135

EMPHYSEMA

- **A type of COPD (Chronic obstructive pulmonary disease) that has a pathologic definition — <u>abnormal permanent enlargement of the terminal airspaces</u> distal to the terminal bronchioles, including the alveolar septae, with no obvious fibrosis.**
- Pulmonary Emphysema is often a progressive lung disease.

TYPES
- **<u>Centrilobar</u> (proximal acinar) involvement is most commonly associated with smoking.** May also be seen in Coal workers' pneumoconiosis.
- **<u>Panacinar</u> (panlobar, diffuse) is associated with Alpha-1 antitrypsin deficiency.**
- <u>Paraseptal</u> (distal acinar) can be seen with the above 2 or with spontaneous Pneumothorax (if isolated).

ETIOLOGIES
- **<u>Cigarette smoking</u> and tobacco use or exposure (passive or active) most common** — 80%-90% of patients with COPD are cigarette smokers, with 10%-15% smokers developing COPD, especially after at least 20 packs per year of tobacco exposure.
- <u>Occupational exposure:</u> — eg, hazardous occupational dust or chemicals, industrial pollutants, indoor or outdoor air pollution (eg, biomass fuels).
- Cystic fibrosis
- **<u>Alpha-1 antitrypsin (AAT) deficiency</u> — suspect Alpha-1 antitrypsin deficiency in nonsmokers or minimal smokers who develop young onset Emphysema (<45 years), especially bibasilar panacinar (diffuse) Emphysema and liver disease (Cirrhosis).** 1-2% of all cases of COPD.

EPIDEMIOLOGY
- COPD is the fourth-ranked cause of death in the United States, killing > 120,000 individuals each year.
- COPD includes patients with Chronic bronchitis and Emphysema. Although identified as separate entities, most patients with COPD have features of both.
- It is slowly increasing in incidence primarily due to the increase in cigarette smoking and environmental pollution.

PATHOPHYSIOLOGY
- Long-term exposure to noxious stimuli (eg, smoke) recruits inflammatory cells (eg, macrophages, neutrophils, and T lymphocytes), leading to **chronic inflammation, decreased protective enzymes (eg, alpha1-antitrypsin), & increased damaging enzymes known as proteinases (eg, elastase release from macrophages & neutrophils) cause destruction of the alveolar-capillary membrane (<u>destruction of the capillaries + alveolar wall destruction and dilation</u>).**
- Because elastin is an important component of the extracellular framework required to maintain the integrity of lung parenchyma and small airways, elastin destruction by elastases and proteinases increase the susceptibility to lung destruction, resulting in airspace enlargement.
- **<u>Loss of elastic recoil</u> & airway collapse makes expiration an active process. Increased compliance leads to airway obstruction (increased air trapping).**
- Matched V/Q defects & decreased capillary surface area cause decreased gas exchange.

CLINICAL MANIFESTATIONS
- **<u>Dyspnea</u> hallmark of Emphysema.** Progressively worsens as the disease advances.
- <u>Chronic cough</u> — often mild, with or without sputum production.
- May have prolonged expiration, hyperventilation, and generalized malaise.
- <u>Weight loss</u> due to systemic inflammation and increased energy spent on the work of breathing.

PHYSICAL EXAMINATION
- **Hyperinflation: decreased (distant) breath sounds, increased anteroposterior diameter (barrel chest), hyperresonance to percussion.**
- Obstruction: end-expiratory wheezing and/or prolonged expiration. Accessory muscle use.
- **Cachectic and non-cyanotic = "pink puffers".**
- Severe disease = **pursed-lip expiration** increases airway pressure & prevents airway collapse; semi-tripod positioning (sitting forward) to improve breathing, and use of accessory muscles.
- AAT deficiency may also be associated with hepatomegaly and/or signs of Cirrhosis.

DIAGNOSIS:
Chest radiograph:
- **Hyperinflation: — flattened diaphragms, increased anteroposterior (AP) diameter, decreased vascular markings; parenchymal bullae and/or subpleural blebs.**
- Computed tomography (CT): Although not needed for the routine diagnosis of COPD, CT has a greater sensitivity and specificity than Chest radiograph and can differentiate whether the Emphysema is centriacinar (centrilobular), panacinar, or paraseptal.

Pulmonary function test:
- **Criterion standard** — Pulmonary function tests (PFTs), especially spirometry, are the **cornerstone of the diagnostic evaluation of patients with suspected COPD.**
- Obstructive pattern that is not fully reversible and, in many cases, is progressive:
- **Airway obstruction: normal or decreased FVC (Forced vital capacity), post bronchodilator decreased FEV1/FVC <70% predicted (incompletely reversible); decreased FEV1** (Forced expiratory volume in 1 second) used to categorize severity based on Global initiative for chronic Obstructive Lung Disease (GOLD) — Mild: >80%, moderate: 50-79%, severe: 30-49%, very severe: <30%.
- **Hyperinflation: increased volumes — eg, RV, TLC, RV/TLC, FRC.** RV = Residual volume; TLC = Total lung capacity; FRC = Functional residual capacity.
- **Decreased DLCO in Emphysema** due to the emphysematous destruction of the alveolar-capillary pulmonary membrane (vs. the roughly normal DLCO in Chronic bronchitis.). DLCO = diffusing capacity of the lungs for carbon monoxide.

Arterial blood gas (ABG):
- **Hypoxemia mild to moderate decrease in PO2.** Normal or decreased PCO2.
- **May develop respiratory acidosis in acute disease.**
- ABG may be obtained for O2 saturation <92%, altered mental status, or acute exacerbation.

MANAGEMENT:
- **Smoking cessation: and avoidance of all contact with cigarette smoke has the greatest impact on mortality & is the single most important step in the management of COPD.** Smoking cessation reduces the rate of FEV1 decline and mortality in patients with COPD. Pharmacologic therapy for smoking cessation may include Nicotine replacement, Bupropion, &/or Varenicline.
- Vaccinations: Influenza, Pneumococcal, & SARS-CoV-2 vaccines help to reduce mortality.
- **Bronchodilators: Bronchodilators do not reduce mortality but improve symptoms,** exercise tolerance, & FEV_1,. **Anticholinergic inhalers (eg, Tiotropium or Ipratropium) are superior to β-adrenergic agonists in achieving bronchodilation in patients with COPD.**
- **Home oxygen: indicated if severe resting hypoxia (PaO2 ≤55 mmHg or oxygen saturation ≤88% or Cor pulmonale).** Oxygen can lead to a reduction of right atrial pressure. **Long-term use of oxygen reduces mortality** and improves the quality of life in patients with severe COPD.
- Pulmonary rehabilitation — education, lifestyle modification, regular physical activity, and avoidance of exposure to known pollutants either at work or living environment.
- Lung resection or transplantation: may be beneficial in severe cases refractory to medical management.

CHRONIC BRONCHITIS

- **A type of COPD (Chronic obstructive pulmonary disease) defined clinically as chronic productive cough for at least 3 months a year for 2 consecutive years.**
- **Airway disease**: COPD is a common respiratory condition characterized by airflow limitation.

ETIOLOGIES:
- **Smoking and tobacco use or exposure (passive or active) most common** — 80% of patients with Chronic bronchitis in the US have a smoking history.
- Occupational exposure: — eg, hazardous occupational dust or chemicals, industrial pollutants, and indoor or outdoor air pollution (eg, biomass fuels).
- Cystic fibrosis, Alpha-1 antitrypsin deficiency.

EPIDEMIOLOGY:
- Chronic bronchitis affects >5% of the population and is associated with high morbidity and mortality.
- It is the fourth-ranked cause of death in the United States, killing >120,000 individuals each year.
- Most common in adults >35 years with significant smoking history.

PATHOPHYSIOLOGY
- **Airway disease: Chronic inflammation (eg, due to cigarette smoke) leads to mucous gland hyperplasia, goblet cell mucus production, mucus hypersecretion, dysfunctional and damaged cilia, & infiltration of neutrophils and CD8+ T cells.**
- These changes increase susceptibility to infections (eg, *S. pneumoniae, H. influenzae, Staphylococcus,* and *Mycoplasma pneumoniae)* as well as viruses (eg, Influenza A & B, Rhinovirus, SARS-CoV-2).

CLINICAL MANIFESTATIONS
- 3 cardinal symptoms: **[1] chronic cough most common and earliest symptom, [2] sputum production** 50% (but may be nonproductive), and **[3] dyspnea, especially on exertion.**
- May have prolonged expiration and generalized malaise.

PHYSICAL EXAMINATION
- **Noisy lungs: crackles (rales), coarse rhonchi, and wheezing.**
- Signs of cor pulmonale include enlarged tender liver, jugular venous distention, and peripheral edema.
- **"Blue bloaters": cyanosis, peripheral edema, and obesity.**

DIAGNOSIS
Pulmonary function test:
- **Criterion standard** — **Pulmonary function tests (PFTs), especially spirometry, are the cornerstone of the diagnostic evaluation of patients with suspected COPD.**
- Obstructive pattern that is not fully reversible:
- **Airway obstruction: decreased FEV1, normal or decreased FVC, postbronchodilator decreased FEV1/FVC <70%** predicted. Mild: > 80%, moderate: 50-79%, severe: 30-49%, very severe: < 30%.
- **Hyperinflation: increased volumes — eg, RV, TLC, RV/TLC, FRC.** RV = Residual volume; TLC = Total lung capacity; FRC = Functional residual capacity.
- **Roughly normal DLCO in Chronic bronchitis** (vs. decreased DLCO in emphysema). DLCO = diffusing capacity of the lungs for carbon monoxide.

Chest radiograph:
- Pulmonary hypertension: — eg, enlarged right heart border, increased AP diameter, and increased vascular markings.
- Electrocardiogram: **Cor pulmonale — eg, RVH, right atrial enlargement, & right axis deviation.**
- May see Multifocal atrial tachycardia.

Laboratory:
- CBC: **increased hemoglobin and hematocrit** to compensate for chronic hypoxia.
- ABG: **respiratory acidosis (severe hypoxemia and hypercapnia).**

MANAGEMENT
- **Smoking cessation: and avoidance of all contact with cigarette smoke has the greatest impact on mortality & is the single most important step in the management of COPD.** Smoking cessation reduces the rate of FEV1 decline and mortality in patients with COPD. Pharmacologic therapy for smoking cessation may include Nicotine replacement, Bupropion, &/or Varenicline.
- Vaccinations: Influenza, Pneumococcal, & SARS-CoV-2 vaccines help to reduce mortality.
- **Bronchodilators: Bronchodilators do not reduce mortality but improve symptoms,** exercise tolerance, & FEV$_1$. **Anticholinergic inhalers (eg, Tiotropium or Ipratropium) are superior to β-adrenergic agonists in achieving bronchodilation in patients with COPD** with longer duration.
- **Home oxygen: indicated if severe resting hypoxia (PaO2 ≤55 mmHg or oxygen saturation ≤88% or Cor pulmonale).** Oxygen can lead to a reduction of right atrial pressure. **Long-term use of oxygen reduces mortality** and improves the quality of life in patients with severe COPD.
- Pulmonary rehabilitation: is an important part of treatment for Chronic bronchitis — rehabilitation consists of education, lifestyle modification, regular physical activity, and avoidance of exposure to known pollutants either at work or living environment.
- The GOLD criteria looks at FEV1 and FEV1/FVC ratio. The revised GOLD criteria also looks at additional factors such as risk of exacerbations.
- Lung resection or transplantation: may be beneficial in severe cases refractory to medical management.

OXYGEN THERAPY IN COPD
Rationale:
- Patients develop Pulmonary hypertension and subsequent right-sided Heart failure (cor pulmonale) as a result of hypoxic vasoconstriction, which increases right-sided pulmonary arterial pressure.
- Oxygen can lead to a reduction of right atrial pressure, reversing hypoxic vasoconstriction, and reducing pulmonary arterial pressure.
- **Long-term use of oxygen reduces mortality & improves quality of life in severe COPD.**

Indications for home oxygen (O$_2$) therapy:
- **Cor pulmonale**
- **O2 saturation ≤88%**
- **PaO2 ≤55 mmHg.**

- For those with paO2 ≤55 mmHg or saturation ≤88%; mortality benefit is directly proportional to the number of hours that oxygen is used.

MANAGEMENT OF COPD

FACTORS THAT REDUCE MORTALITY

- **[1] Smoking cessation most important step in the management of COPD** (immediate effects).
- **[2] Oxygen therapy only medication that reduces mortality in COPD** if paO2 ≤55 mmHg or saturation ≤88%; mortality benefit directly proportional to the number of hours that oxygen is used.
- **[3] Vaccinations**: eg, Pneumococcal, annual Influenza, and SARS-CoV-2 vaccinations.

SYMPTOM CONTROL

Rescue bronchodilator therapy in all patients:

- **Short-acting bronchodilator: For all patients with COPD, a short-acting bronchodilator (eg, SAMA &/or SABA) is used as needed for relief of episodic dyspnea and early treatment of exacerbations**. Options include a beta agonist [SABA (eg, Albuterol, Levalbuterol)] or anticholinergic agent [SAMA (eg, Ipratropium)] as needed if infrequent intermittent dyspnea.
- SABA-SAMA therapy preferred — achieves a greater bronchodilator response with more bronchodilator effectiveness than either short-acting agent alone. SAMA more effective vs. SABA.

Group A: Minimally symptomatic, low risk of exacerbation (0-1 exacerbations/year):

- The Global Initiative for Chronic Obstructive Lung Disease (GOLD) 2023 report identifies key changes for patients with COPD, specifically more aggressive initial bronchodilator therapy: **Single-agent long-acting bronchodilator therapy for less severe symptoms (Group A).**
- **Long-acting bronchodilator agent — In addition to short-acting bronchodilator rescue therapy, Group A patients often receive a long-acting bronchodilator**. Long-acting bronchodilators have been shown to be effective even in patients with mild symptoms.
- **If needed, LAMA [eg, Tiotropium, Aclidinium, Umeclidinium, Glycopyrrolate] is often preferred rather than a long-acting beta-agonist (LABA). Once daily LABA [eg, Salmeterol, Formoterol, Indacaterol, Vilanterol, (Arformoterol available in nebulized form)] is an appropriate alternative to LAMA. Both LAMAs and LABAs reduce exacerbations, but LAMAs have a greater effect.**
- Patient preference: Individual patients may prefer one bronchodilator over the other.

Group B: More symptomatic, low risk of exacerbation (0-1 exacerbations/year):

- **LAMA + LABA: Dual long-acting bronchodilator therapy (LAMA-LABA) for more severe symptoms and low exacerbation risk (Group B).** Dual bronchodilator (LAMA-LABA) therapy as a fixed-dose LAMA-LABA combinations, rather than two separate inhalers, may be preferred due to a potential for improved adherence, which may lead to improved outcomes (eg, improved breathlessness) and lung function compared with short-acting therapy alone.
- **When a single agent is used (eg, patients unable to take combination LAMA-LABA), LAMA (long-acting antimuscarinic/anticholinergic agent) [eg, Tiotropium] is often preferred single agent because it may be slightly more efficacious than a LABA (eg, Salmeterol)**; both LAMAs and LABAs reduce exacerbations, but LAMAs have a greater effect. LAMAs include Tiotropium, Aclidinium, Umeclidinium, and Glycopyrrolate.
- In COPD, LABAs are effective bronchodilators that may be used alone or in combination with anticholinergics or ICSs. LABAs include Salmeterol, Formoterol, Indacaterol, and Vilanterol.

Group E (Higher symptom burden) ≥2 exacerbations/yr; ≥1 exacerbation leading to hospitalization:

- **LAMA + LABA: Dual long-acting bronchodilator therapy LAMA + LABA (preferred rather than either alone) for high exacerbation risk, regardless of symptoms (Group E, replacing previous Groups C and D categories).**
- LABA + inhaled glucocorticoid an alternative. The preference for using LAMA-LABA therapy over a LABA-ICS combination is largely based on evidence of improved lung function, better control of mild exacerbations, and fewer episodes of pneumonia.
- If persistent, triple inhaler therapy is recommended [LAMA + LABA + ICS]. Triple therapy is also used for patients with hospitalization due to exacerbation or highly elevated blood eosinophils (≥300 cells/microL).

BRONCHODILATORS	Improve symptoms but do not decrease progression or reduce mortality.
LAMAs **Tiotropium** (inhaled powder) Aclidinium, Umeclidinium Glycopyrrolate	Mechanism of action • **LAMA: Long-acting anticholinergics (antimuscarinics) that lead to bronchodilation** (M1 and M3 selectivity) **and decreased secretions.** Benefits: • Improve lung function, decrease hyperinflation, & improve quality of life. • As long-term monotherapy, **LAMAs slightly more efficacious than LABAs.** Adverse effects • **Anticholinergic:** dry mouth, thirst, blurred vision, urinary retention, difficulty swallowing. May exacerbate Acute angle-closure glaucoma.
SAMA **Ipratropium**	Mechanism of action • SAMA: Short-acting anticholinergic (antimuscarinic) that leads to bronchodilation via the M1, M2, and M3 receptors. Indications: • As-needed relief of intermittent increases in dyspnea; may be combined with a short-acting beta agonist (SABA). Adverse effects • **Anticholinergic:** dry mouth, thirst, blurred vision, urinary retention, difficulty swallowing. May exacerbate Acute angle-closure glaucoma.
LABA: **Salmeterol** **Formoterol** Indacaterol Vilanterol Arformoterol (nebulized form)	Mechanism of action • LABA: Long-acting beta-2 agonists. **Formoterol has both a rapid onset & long duration of action** (up to 12 hours of bronchodilation). Indications: • Decrease exacerbation rates; improve quality of life and lung function. Adverse effects of LABAs and SABAs: • **Muscle tremors, restlessness, tachycardia, Hypokalemia.** • Metabolic effects: ↑FFA (free fatty acids), glucose, lactate, pyruvate, insulin.
SABA: **Albuterol** **Levalbuterol**	Mechanism of action • Short-acting beta-2 agonist. Indications: • As-needed relief of intermittent increases in dyspnea; may combined with a short-acting antimuscarinic agent. Adverse reactions • Beta-1 cross reactivity: tachycardia, palpitations, tremors, CNS stimulation.
INHALED GLUCOCORTICOIDS **Fluticasone** **Budesonide**	Indications: • Can be added to a LABA and/or LAMA for severe or persistent disease. • Fluticasone furoate is a different molecule than Fluticasone propionate and 2x duration of action, 2 times as potent (dosed once daily unlike other ICS). Adverse reactions • Oral candidiasis (reduced by using spacer or washing out mouth after use).

THEOPHYLLINE
• Fourth line agent: Oral Theophylline is reserved for add-on treatment in refractory disease.
• Its use is limited due to a narrow therapeutic index, adverse effects, & drug interactions with the cytochrome P450 system, but mainly because of more effective therapy with β_2 agonists and ICSs.
• Mechanism: Theophylline is a bronchodilator (cousin of caffeine) with anti-inflammatory effects.

Surgery:
• Lung reduction surgery: improves dyspnea by removing damaged lung, which allows the remaining lung to expand & function more efficiently.
• Lung transplantation. Replacement of α-1 antitrypsin in some patients.

ACUTE COPD EXACERBATIONS

An event characterized by
- [1] dyspnea &/or cough and sputum that worsens over ≤14 days, may be accompanied by
- [2] tachypnea and/or tachycardia, and is often associated with
- [3] **increased local and systemic inflammation caused by airway infection (eg, viral or bacterial) most common**, pollution, or other insult to the airways.

CLINICAL FEATURES
- Diffuse wheezing, distant breath sounds, barrel-shaped chest, tachypnea, tachycardia, change in quality or amount of sputum production, acute worsening of usual symptoms.
- Features of severe respiratory insufficiency: use of accessory muscles; brief, fragmented speech; inability to lie supine; profound diaphoresis; agitation.

EXACERBATION WORKUP
- Pulse oximetry: to assess oxygen saturation; ABG if severe.
- Chest radiograph: to assess for signs of pneumonia, acute heart failure, pneumothorax. When evidence of acute infection is absent & chest radiograph is unrevealing, CT pulmonary angiogram for PE.
- Laboratory evaluation: CBC, electrolytes, BUN, creatinine; troponin, BNP, or NT-proBNP.
- ECG: to assess for ischemia, arrhythmia, cor pulmonale. Test for Influenza during Influenza season.

MANAGEMENT
Management of COPD exacerbations include [1] short course of systemic corticosteroids & aggressive short-acting bronchodilator therapy [SAMA &/or SABA] to reverse airflow limitation, [2] antibacterial or antiviral agents if indicated, [3] oxygen supplementation, & [4] ventilatory support.

[1] Short-acting bronchodilators:
- **For all patients with COPD exacerbation, short-acting beta-agonist (SABA; eg, Albuterol) or combined SABA + short-acting muscarinic antagonist (SAMA; eg, Ipratropium) are used.**
- **SABA-SAMA combination therapy is often preferred rather than either alone.** The combination is well tolerated and might achieve better bronchodilation. Magnesium sulfate added if severe.

[2] Systemic (oral, IV) glucocorticoids:
- **Systemic glucocorticoids added to bronchodilators improve lung function, reduce airway inflammation, reverse airflow, limitation, promote shorter hospital stay, & reduce relapse.**

[3] Antibiotics and/or antiviral agents if indicated:
- No *Pseudomonas* risk factor(s): **Ceftriaxone, or Cefotaxime, Levofloxacin or Moxifloxacin.**
- **For outpatients who do not have risk factors for poor outcomes or *Pseudomonas* infection — Macrolide (eg, Azithromycin, Clarithromycin) or a second- or third-generation cephalosporin** (eg, Cefuroxime, Cefpodoxime, Cefdinir). **Trimethoprim-sulfamethoxazole. Amoxicillin-clavulanate; respiratory Fluoroquinolone (eg, Levofloxacin or Moxifloxacin).**
- *Pseudomonas* risk factor(s): Piperacillin-tazobactam or Cefepime or Ceftazidime.
- Antiviral therapy (Influenza suspected): Oseltamivir 75 mg orally every 12 hours or Peramivir 600 mg IV once (for patients unable to take oral medication) or others as needed for respiratory viruses.

[4] Titrating supplemental oxygen:
- **Patients with hypoxemia due to an exacerbation of COPD should receive supplemental oxygen, often titrated to a target SpO2 of 88-92% or an arterial oxygen tension (PaO2) of ~60-70 mmHg, to minimize the risk of worsening hypercapnia with excess supplemental oxygen.** This is because they have chronic hypercapnia and are more dependent on their hypoxic respiratory drive sensed by peripheral carotid bodies.

[5] Ventilatory support:
- Ventilatory support is necessary for patients who develop respiratory fatigue despite supportive therapy with medications and oxygen.
- Noninvasive ventilation (NIV) preferred method in most patients. Mechanical ventilation if severe.

CYSTIC FIBROSIS (CF)

- Autosomal recessive exocrinopathy. **Most common in Caucasians & Northern Europeans.**

PATHOPHYSIOLOGY
- **Mutation in the Cystic fibrosis transmembrane conductance receptor (CFTR) gene leads to abnormal chloride and water transport** across exocrine glands throughout the body, leading to **thick, viscous secretions of the lungs,** pancreas, sinuses, intestines, liver, and genitourinary tract.

CLINICAL MANIFESTATIONS
- Infancy: **meconium ileus** — delayed passage of meconium leading to obstruction of the bowel by meconium in a newborn infant (20%). **Failure to thrive**, prolonged neonatal jaundice, diarrhea (malabsorption), rectal prolapse. The lungs are usually normal in utero & at birth.
- **Bronchiectasis: CF is the most common cause of Bronchiectasis in the US (persistent cough with thick purulent sputum production and recurrent infections).** Bacterial colonization with pathogens such as *Pseudomonas aeruginosa,* **the most common colonizer of the respiratory tract -** mucoid *Pseudomonas aeruginosa* more common in adults; nonmucoid *P.* common in children.
- **Recurrent pulmonary infections:** *S. aureus* & *Pseudomonal spp.* are more common in older children & adults. Respiratory symptoms are more prominent in adulthood. **Chronis sinusitis**, nasal polyps.
- **GI:** malabsorption especially of fat-soluble vitamins A, D, E, & K, steatorrhea, diarrhea, recurrent pancreatitis (may lead to pancreatic insufficiency), distal intestinal obstruction, biliary cirrhosis.
- Genitourinary: **Infertility in men** due to azoospermia — 95% of males with Cystic fibrosis will **also have congenital absence of the vas deferens, which causes infertility later in life.**

DIAGNOSIS
- **Elevated sweat chloride: test of choice (most accurate).** Chloride levels ≥60 mmol/L on 2 occasions after Pilocarpine administration (Pilocarpine is a cholinergic drug that induces sweating).
- Chest radiographs: Bronchiectasis common, hyperinflation of the lungs.
- Pulmonary function test: obstructive pattern classic (usually irreversible).
- CFTR gene sequencing (DNA analysis) — performed if positive or intermediate sweat test (sweat chloride 30-59 mmol/L). Genotyping is not as accurate as sweat chloride testing because there are more types of mutations than those tested with genotyping.
- **Abnormal nasal potential difference if inconclusive sweat chloride &/or DNA testing.**

MANAGEMENT
- **Airway clearance treatment — eg, bronchodilators, mucolytics, antibiotics, and decongestants.** Inhaled dornase alfa or inhaled hypertonic saline are prescribed to promote airway secretion clearance in conjunction with chest physiotherapy. Glucocorticoids.
- **Diet: high-fat diet with supplemental fat-soluble vitamins (A, D, E, and K)** to compensate for malabsorption. Additionally, patients living with CF are encouraged to consume a high-calorie diet to maintain a healthy weight and decrease chronic inflammation (women should consume 2,500 to 3000 calories a day; men should consume 3,000 – 3,700 calories a day).
- **Pancreatic enzyme replacement often needed.** Lung & pancreatic transplantation in selected cases.
- Vaccinations — Influenza and Pneumococcal to prevent pulmonary infections
- CFTR modulators: Ivacaftor, Lumacaftor, Tezacaftor, and Elexacaftor.

Pulmonary infections:
- Because pulmonary disease is the most common cause of mortality in Cystic fibrosis, diagnosis and intervention in pulmonary illness exacerbations is paramount.
- **Antibiotics are often needed** — Macrolides (eg, Azithromycin, Clarithromycin); Cephalosporins (eg, Cefuroxime, Cefixime), Amoxicillin-clavulanate, Fluoroquinolones. Inhaled Aminoglycosides.
- *S. aureus* (treat with Vancomycin). *Pseudomonal spp.* (treat with Amikacin, Ceftazidime, or Ciprofloxacin).

BRONCHIECTASIS

- **Chronic lung disease characterized by permanent and irreversible dilatation of the bronchial airways,** with dysfunction of the mucociliary transport mechanism.

ETIOLOGIES

- **Cystic fibrosis is the most common cause in US** (50%). **Recurrent lung infections:**
  Pseudomonas aeruginosa **most common colonizer if due to Cystic fibrosis.**
  Haemophilus influenzae **most common colonized bacteria if not due to Cystic Fibrosis.**
- Airway foreign body, tumors, Alpha-1 antitrypsin deficiency, collagen vascular disease (eg, Rheumatoid arthritis, Aspergillosis, panhypogammaglobulinemia, & immune deficiency.

PATHOPHYSIOLOGY

- Airway inflammation (eg, neutrophils), dilatation of the bronchi, & impairment of the mucociliary escalator due to damage to the muscular & elastic components of the bronchial wall due to chronic lung disease lead to mucus pooling in the bronchial tree & **the 3 main components — [1] recurrent infections, [2] airway obstruction, and [3] peribronchial fibrosis.**
- Increased risk for _Pseudomonas aeruginosa, Mycobacterium avium_ complex, and Aspergillus.

CLINICAL MANIFESTATIONS

- **Daily production of <u>thick tenacious/dark brown</u> & mucopurulent sputum**, dyspnea, pleuritic chest pain.
- **<u>Hemoptysis</u>** due to bronchial artery erosion. <u>Nonspecific:</u> fatigue, weight loss, recurrent infections.
- <u>Physical examination:</u> nonspecific — **crackles most common** (often bibasilar), wheezing, & rhonchi.

DIAGNOSIS

- <u>Chest radiographs:</u> usually abnormal but nonspecific. Findings include linear atelectasis, tram-track appearance, opacities, and increased bronchial markings.
- **<u>High-resolution CT scan:</u> preferred imaging of choice.** <u>Findings</u> include **thickened bronchial walls, airway dilatation & lack of tapering of the airway (parallel or tram-track appearance).** <u>Signet ring sign</u> increased airway diameter > adjacent vessel diameter.
- **<u>Pulmonary function test:</u> criterion standard. <u>Obstructive pattern</u>** that is not fully reversible:
  <u>Airway obstruction:</u> decreased FEV1, decreased FEV1/FVC <70% predicted, decreased FVC.
  <u>Hyperinflation</u>: increased lung volumes (eg, RV, TLC, RV/TLC, FRC). Also, test for Cystic fibrosis.

MANAGEMENT

- **<u>Conservative:</u> <u>Mucus clearance:</u> chest physiotherapy, mucolytics (eg, nebulized hypertonic saline solution, Acetylcysteine), postural drainage.** Inhaled bronchodilators and corticosteroids.
- **<u>Vaccination</u> against influenza and pneumococcal disease recommended.**
- <u>Massive hemoptysis:</u> Bronchial artery embolization and/or surgery is first-line therapy.

Antibiotics:

- <u>Oral:</u> <u>Sputum culture data not available</u> — Fluoroquinolone (eg, Moxifloxacin, Levofloxacin).
- <u>Sputum growing sensitive organisms</u> — if sputum cultures do not show beta-lactamase-positive _H. influenzae_ or _Pseudomonas_, options may include Amoxicillin or Macrolides.
- <u>Beta-lactamase-positive organism</u> — in the presence of _M. catarrhalis_ or beta-lactamase producing _H. influenzae_: Amoxicillin/clavulanate, Macrolides (eg, Clarithromycin, Azithromycin), second- or third generation Cephalosporins, Doxycycline, or Fluoroquinolones.
- <u>Sputum growing sensitive Pseudomonas</u> — Ciprofloxacin is often the initial treatment if choice. Quinolone resistance often requires administration of intravenous antibiotics.
- <u>Intravenous:</u> Aminoglycosides (eg, Gentamicin, Tobramycin), Ceftriaxone, Fluoroquinolones. Antibiotic cycling may be needed.
- <u>Surgery:</u> Resection or transplantation is adjunct to therapy in some patients with severe or refractor disease, young patients with unilateral Bronchiectasis, confined to a single lobe or segment on CT).

BRONCHIECTASIS

NORMAL CXR

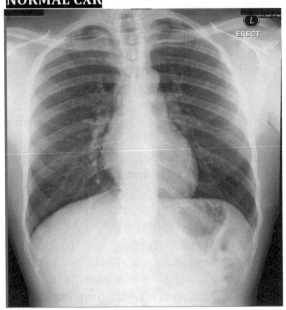

BRONCHIECTASIS

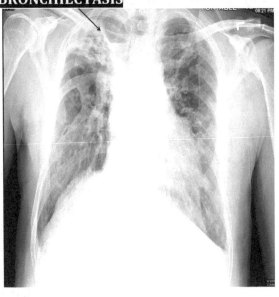

Bronchiectasis: irregular opacities, crowded bronchial markings, "tram track" markings.

NORMAL CT SCAN

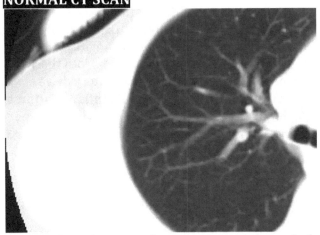

Signet ring sign: pulmonary artery coupled with a dilated bronchus (white arrow).

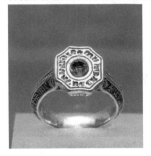

BRONCHIECTASIS

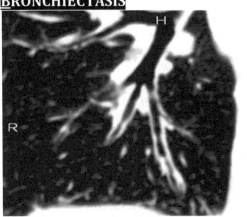

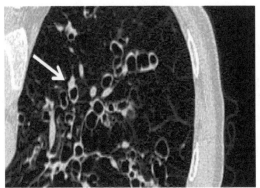

- Proximal airway dilation with thick walls, lack of airway tapering giving a "tram-track" appearance (above photo).
- Signet ring sign (arrow).

ASTHMA

- **Reversible, often intermittent, obstructive disease of the small airways.**

EPIDEMIOLOGY:
- **Asthma may develop at any age, but initial occurrence most commonly in childhood.**
- Hospitalization rates are highest among Blacks & children; death rates highest in Blacks 15–24 years.

PATHOPHYSIOLOGY:
3 components — **[1] airway inflammation, [2] airway hyperreactivity (hyperresponsiveness), and [3] bronchoconstriction.**
- **[1] Airway inflammation: The earliest event in asthmatic airway responses is the activation of local inflammatory cells, principally mast cells and eosinophils.** Inflammatory cell activation can occur directly by specific IgE-dependent mechanisms or indirectly via other processes (eg, chemical irritant exposure). Increased IgE binds to mast cells, initiating an inflammatory response, including increased leukotrienes, eosinophils, neutrophils, & lymphocytes (especially T cells).
- **[2] Hyperreactivity: Type I hypersensitivity reaction** to certain triggers lead to release of mediators that alter airway smooth muscle tone & responsiveness, induce mucus hypersecretion, & damage airway epithelium. Atopy of IgE antibodies attack specific antigens, allergens, or pollutants.
- **[3] Bronchoconstriction:** Airway wall thickening & airway narrowing can result from inflammation or from bronchial smooth muscle contraction, leading to wheezing and increased work of breathing.

PHENOTYPES
- **Allergic Asthma: most common phenotype, usually begins in childhood and is associated with other allergic diseases such as Eczema, Allergic rhinitis, or food allergy.** Exposure of sensitive patients to inhaled allergens may cause symptoms immediately (immediate asthmatic response) or 4–6 hours after allergen exposure (late asthmatic response). Allergic asthma falls into the T2-high endotype, as do late-onset T2-high asthma and aspirin/NSAID-associated respiratory disease.
- **Nonallergic Asthma: tends to occur in adults & associated with neutrophilic inflammation and variable response to standard therapies.** Nonallergic Asthma is a T2-low Asthma phenotype.
- Asthma with obesity refers to prominent respiratory symptoms in obese patients with little airway inflammation.

RISK FACTORS
- **Atopy strongest risk factor,** family history, pollution, obesity, environmental tobacco smoke, male.

TRIGGERS
Extrinsic (allergic):
- **Associated with increased IgE — animal dander, seasonal pollen, mold, dust mites** (often found in pillows, mattresses, upholstered furniture, carpets, and drapes), **cockroaches, mice.**
Intrinsic (non-allergic):
- Physiologic & pharmacologic: **Histamine, Methacholine, Adenosine** triphosphate.
- **Exercise, physical activity, hyperventilation with cold, dry air.** Exercise-induced bronchoconstriction begins during exercise or within 3 minutes after its end, peaks within 10–15 minutes, and then resolves by 60 minutes. It is thought to be a result of the airways warming and humidifying an increased volume of expired air during exercise. Temperature and weather.
- Inhaled respiratory irritants — air pollutants (eg, sulfur dioxide, nitrogen dioxide, diesel fuel), **tobacco and cannabis smoke.**
- **Respiratory infections eg, viruses (eg, influenza A),** bacteria. Emotional factors: eg, anxiety, stress.
- **Medications: Aspirin, NSAIDs, Beta blockers.**
- Comorbidities: Rhinitis, rhinovirus infection, postnasal drip gastroesophageal reflux, obesity, obstructive sleep apnea, depression, and anxiety can trigger asthma symptoms as well.

CLINICAL MANIFESTATIONS
- **Classic triad**: episodic dyspnea, wheezing, and cough (especially at night), provoked by typical triggers. **May have chest tightness or fatigue.**
- Symptoms vary over time and in intensity and are often worse at night or in the early morning. Asthma symptoms may occur spontaneously or be precipitated or exacerbated by many different triggers.
- Clues to severity include previous intubations, hospital admissions, or ICU admission.

PHYSICAL EXAMINATION
- Chest examination may be normal between exacerbations in patients with mild Asthma.
- **Wheezing and/or prolonged expiratory phase during normal breathing due to the presence of airflow obstruction, hyperresonance to percussion, decreased breath sounds, tachycardia, tachypnea, use of accessory muscles** (due to increased work of breathing) are suggestive but are not specific.
- Asthmatic wheezing is typically composed of multiple high-pitched sounds audible most prominently during expiration.
- Allergic Asthma: nasal mucosal swelling, increased secretions, and nasal polyps are often seen in patients with allergic Asthma. Atopic dermatitis (Eczema) or other allergic skin disorders may also be present.
- **Severe Asthma & Status asthmaticus: inability to speak in full sentences, "tripod" positioning, silent chest** (no air movement due to limited airflow), **altered mental status** (ominous), **pulsus paradoxus** (inspiratory blood pressure drop >10 mmHg), PEFR <40% predicted.

DIAGNOSIS OF ACUTE ASTHMA EXACERBATION
Peak expiratory flow rate:
- **Best & most objective way to assess acute Asthma exacerbation severity & patient response to treatment.**
- **PEFR >15% from initial attempt = response to treatment**. Comparison with reference values is less helpful than comparison with the patient's own baseline.
- PEFR values <200 L/min indicate severe airflow obstruction.

Pulse oximetry:
- SaO2 <90% is indicative of respiratory distress.

Arterial blood gas (ABG):
- **ABG: not usually ordered in most exacerbations; may be normal during a mild Asthma exacerbation, but respiratory alkalosis (from tachypnea) is expected** and an increase in the alveolar arterial oxygen difference is common.
- During severe exacerbations, hypoxemia develops and the PaCO2 returns to normal (pseudonormalization).
- **Pseudonormalization of the PaCO2 or the combination of an increased PaCO2 and respiratory acidosis may indicate impending respiratory failure and the need for mechanical ventilation.**

Chest radiographs:
- Not helpful in the diagnosis of Asthma but may be used to rule out other causes of symptoms.
- Routine chest radiographs in patients with Asthma are usually normal or show only hyperinflation.

DIAGNOSIS OF CHRONIC ASTHMA IN THE OFFICE

Pulmonary function tests:

- **Spirometry pre- and post-bronchodilator to identify <u>reversible</u> airflow obstruction is the criterion standard and most helpful in making the diagnosis of Asthma.**
- **<u>Airflow obstruction</u>** — Expiratory airflow obstruction with a reversible reduction in the forced expiratory volume in one second (decreased FEV1), decreased FEV1/FVC (<70%); Increased lung volumes due to hyperinflation: increased Residual volume (RV), Total lung capacity (TLC), and RV/TLC.
- **<u>Significant reversibility of airflow obstruction</u> is defined by an increase of ≥12% and 200 mL in FEV1 or FVC after inhaling a short-acting bronchodilator,** especially if post-bronchodilator spirometry is normal, strongly supports the diagnosis of Asthma.
- <u>Bronchial provocation:</u> **Bronchial provocation testing with Methacholine or Histamine challenge (a decrease in the FEV1 ≥20% after exposure to Methacholine). Bronchoprovocation may be reserved for use when Asthma is suspected but baseline spirometry is normal or nondiagnostic.** After provocation, reversible obstruction is defined by an increase of FEV1 ≥12% after short-acting bronchodilator challenge.
- Exercise challenge testing may be useful in patients with symptoms of exercise-induced bronchospasm.

MANAGEMENT

Asthma medications can be divided into 3 main categories:

- (1) long-term controller medications used long-term to reduce airway inflammation, symptoms, and risk of future exacerbations
- (2) reliever medications used on an as-needed basis to relieve breakthrough symptoms, and
- (3) add-on therapies for severe Asthma.
- <u>Reliever medications</u> include Beta-2 adrenergic agonists (eg, Albuterol, Levalbuterol), Anticholinergics (eg, Ipratropium), Systemic corticosteroids.
- <u>Long-term controller medications:</u> include Inhaled corticosteroids, systemic corticosteroids, inhaled long-acting beta-adrenergic agonists (LABAs), Mast cell modifiers, Leukotriene modifiers, 5-lipoxygenase inhibitor.

Acute exacerbation

- **<u>Inhaled short-acting Beta-2 agonist</u>** — **for all patients with symptoms of an Asthma exacerbation, prompt administration of an inhaled short-acting beta-agonist (SABA; eg, Albuterol, Levalbuterol) is the mainstay of bronchodilator treatment.**
- **<u>Inhaled muscarinic antagonists</u>** — addition of inhaled short-acting antimuscarinic (SAMA; also called anticholinergic agents) eg, Ipratropium. **Ipratropium often added to SABA in patients with moderate to severe exacerbation of Asthma.**
- **<u>Systemic glucocorticoids</u>: with the exception of a mild exacerbation, Acute exacerbation of Asthma often requires an initial, brief course of systemic glucocorticoids** (eg, Prednisone 40-60 mg daily, Methylprednisolone, Prednisolone).
- **<u>IV Magnesium sulfate</u>** — Intravenous administration of a single dose of IV Magnesium sulfate for bronchodilation (2 g infused over 20 min) may be needed for patients who present with a life-threatening exacerbation or have a severe exacerbation that is not responding to initial therapy.
- <u>Respiratory support:</u> **Mechanical ventilation (intubation) and noninvasive positive pressure ventilation may be needed in some severe Asthma exacerbations** (eg, unresponsive to above therapies, worsening hypercapnia and associated respiratory acidosis, or inability to maintain an oxygen saturation >92% despite face mask supplemental oxygen). A short trial of Noninvasive ventilation (NIV) may be attempted in select patients not responding to medical therapy who do not require immediate intubation and if they are cooperative.

QUICK RELIEF FOR ACUTE EXACERBATION (RESCUE DRUGS)

SHORT-ACTING β₂ AGONISTS (SABAs)

Albuterol, Levalbuterol. Terbutaline, Epinephrine

- Indications: **first-line treatment for acute exacerbation — most effective & fastest meds** (2-5 minutes).
- MOA: **bronchodilators** (especially **peripherally**), decrease bronchospasm, inhibit the release of bronchospastic mediators, increase ciliary movement, airway edema & resistance.
- Administration: MDI, nebulizer. **Nebulizers most common used in ED** (MDI ± slightly more efficacious). Generally given every 20 minutes x 3 doses (or continuous) + reevaluation after 3 doses (at least q 1-2 hours).
- S/E: **β₋₁ cross reaction: tachycardia/arrhythmias; muscle tremors, CNS stimulation, hypokalemia.**

ANTICHOLINERGICS (ANTIMUSCARINIC) Ipratropium

- MOA: **central bronchodilator** (inhibits vagal-mediated bronchoconstriction) & inhibits nasal mucosal secretions. ⊕ synergy between β₂ agonists & anticholinergics. Most useful in the first hour.
- S/E: **thirst, blurred vision (pupil dilation), dry mouth, urinary retention, dysphagia, glaucoma, BPH.**

CORTICOSTEROIDS

Prednisone, Methylprednisolone, Prednisolone

- MOA: **anti-inflammatory. All but the mildest exacerbations should be discharged on a short course of oral corticosteroids** (eg, 3-5 days) unless contraindicated. **Steroids decrease relapse** & reverse the late pathophysiology. Short courses don't need tapering (unless on chronic steroids, or recent treatment with repeated short courses in a short period). Onset of action 4-8 hours for both oral & IV.
- S/E: **immunosuppression, catabolic, hyperglycemia, fluid retention, osteoporosis, growth delays.**

LONG-TERM (CHRONIC, CONTROL) MAINTENANCE

INHALED CORTICOSTEROIDS (ICS)

Beclomethasone, Flunisolide, Triamcinolone, Budesonide

- Indications: **first-line long term, persistent (chronic maintenance).** Effective long-term control with very low incidence of systemic adverse effects. MOA: cytokine & inflammation inhibition.
- S/E: **oral candidiasis** (using spacer & rinsing mouth after inhaler use decreases risk), dysphonia.

LONG ACTING β₂ AGONISTS (LABAs)

Salmeterol, ICS/LABA: Budesonide/**Formoterol,** Fluticasone/Salmeterol

- Mechanism: bronchodilator that prevents symptoms (especially nocturnal asthma).
- **Formoterol has both a rapid onset & long duration of action** (up to 12 hours of bronchodilation).
- Indications: **Long acting β₂ agonists added to steroids** (or other long term asthma medications) **ONLY if persistent Asthma not controlled with ICS alone.**
- CI: **NOT used as [1] a rescue drug in acute exacerbations or [2] as monotherapy for long-term Asthma.**

MAST CELL MODIFIERS

Cromolyn, Nedocromil

- MOA: inhibits mast cell & leukotriene-mediated degranulation. Used as prophylaxis only.
- Indications: improved lung function, ↓airway reactivity **(inhibits acute response to cold air, exercise, sulfites).** Effective prophylaxis may take several weeks. **Minimal adverse effects** (throat irritation).
- **Adverse effects: Relatively good adverse effect profile** (minimal because they are not absorbed from the site of administration). Localized effects may include cough and throat irritation.

LEUKOTRIENE MODIFIERS/RECEPTOR ANTAGONISTS (LTRA)

Montelukast, Zafirlukast, Zileuton

- MOA: blocks leukotriene-mediated neutrophil migration, capillary permeability, smooth muscle contraction via leukotriene receptor inhibition. Zileuton does so via 5-lipoxygenase inhibition.
- Indications: **prophylaxis only — allergic rhinitis/aspirin-induced Asthma, exercise-induced bronchospasm,** and antigen-induced bronchospasm.
- Adverse effects: minimal side effects (increased LFTs, headache, GI, myalgias). Zafirlukast has been associated with Churg-Strauss syndrome.

LONG-TERM ASTHMA MANAGEMENT

Intermittent (Step 1)

- <u>Definition</u>: daytime symptoms up to 2 days/week, nocturnal awakenings up 2 times a month, Normal FEV1, Exacerbations ≤1 time/year.
- **NAEPP guidelines: Short Acting Beta Agonist (SABA) as needed** (eg, Albuterol).
- **GINA guidelines: as needed combination inhaler of low-dose combination inhaled corticosteroid (ICS) + fast-acting long-acting beta-agonist Formoterol (eg, Budesonide-Formoterol) as needed for symptom relief.** Formoterol has both a rapid onset and long duration of action (up to 12 hours of bronchodilation).

Mild persistent (Step 2)

- <u>Definition</u>: daytime symptoms >2 but <7 days/week; Nocturnal awakenings 3-4 nights/month; minor interference with activities; FEV1 within the normal range, Exacerbations ≥2/year.
- **Inhaled Corticosteroids (ICS) first-line long-term treatment for persistent Asthma.** Regular use of ICS reduce symptom frequency, improve quality of life, & decrease risk of serious exacerbations.
- **NAEPP guidelines: Low-dose ICS daily and SABA as needed.**
  <u>Alternative option(s)</u>: Daily LTRA **and** SABA as needed.
- **GINA guidelines: Low-dose ICS-Formoterol as needed (preferred).** Alternative: Low-dose ICS daily **and** SABA as needed

Moderate persistent (Step 3)

- Daily symptoms; nocturnal awakenings >1/week; daily need for SABA; some activity limitation, FEV1 60 - 80% predicted; Exacerbations 2/year or greater.
- **NAEPP guidelines: Low-dose ICS-Formoterol as maintenance and reliever therapy (preferred).**
  <u>Alternative option(s)</u>: **Medium-dose ICS daily** and **SABA as needed.**
- Addition of an inhaled long-acting muscarinic antagonist (LAMA; Tiotropium) to an inhaled glucocorticoid is equally effective compared to the combination of an inhaled glucocorticoid and LABA. However, it requires two separate inhaler devices with distinct inhaler techniques.
- **GINA guidelines: Low-dose ICS-Formoterol as maintenance and reliever (preferred).** Low-dose ICS-LABA combination daily **and** SABA as needed

Severe persistent (Step 4):

- Symptoms all day; nocturnal awakenings nightly; need for SABA several times/day; extreme limitation in activity, FEV1 <60% predicted; exacerbations 2/year or greater.
- **NAEPP guidelines: Medium-dose ICS-Formoterol as maintenance + reliever (preferred).**
  <u>Alternative</u>: medium-dose ICS-LABA daily or medium-dose ICS **plus** LAMA daily or Medium-dose ICS daily **plus** anti-leukotriene **plus** SABA as needed.
- **GINA guidelines: Medium-dose ICS-Formoterol as maintenance + reliever (preferred)**

Step 5:

- **High-dose ICS + LABA. Additional agent either LAMA or anti-IgE medication.**
- **Triple: high ICS + LABA + LAMA (Fluticasone + Umeclidinium-Vilanterol).**

Step 6:

- High-dose ICS-LABA daily; consider LAMA as substitute for LABA or as add-on therapy if not done previously; Oral glucocorticoids, titrated to optimize asthma control and minimize adverse effects; Possible addition of asthma biologics [eg, Omalizumab (Anti-IgE), Dupilumab].
- Additional therapy with a Leukotriene modifier, Tiotropium, or biologic agent may be needed, guided by the treatment response.

Step down therapy: "step down" (remove) from the last thing placed on "step up" therapy **after 3 months** of improved symptoms.

National Asthma Education & prevention program (NAEPP): Expert panel working group		Global initiative for Asthma (GINA)	
Symptoms/lung function	Therapy	Asthma symptoms	Therapy
STEP 1		**STEP 1**	
All of the following: • Daytime symptoms ≤2 days/week • Nocturnal awakenings ≤2/month • Normal FEV$_1$ • Exacerbations ≤1/year.	• **SABA, as needed**	• Infrequent asthma symptoms (eg, <2 times/week) • No risk factors for exacerbations	• **Low-dose ICS-Formoterol as needed (preferred)** • Low-dose ICS whenever SABA used or as-needed low-dose ICS-SABA.
STEP 2		**STEP 2**	
Any of the following: • Daytime symptoms >2 but <7 days/week • Nocturnal awakenings up to 3 to 4 nights/month • Minor interference with activities • Exacerbations ≥2/year	• **Low-dose ICS daily and SABA as needed** • Low-dose ICS-SABA or ICS **plus** SABA, concomitantly administered, as needed Alternative option(s) • Daily LTRA **and** SABA as needed	• Asthma symptoms or need for reliever inhaler ≥2 times/week, but without troublesome daily symptoms	• **Low-dose ICS-Formoterol as needed (preferred)** • Low-dose ICS daily **and** SABA as needed Other options • Low-dose ICS-SABA or ICS **plus** SABA, concomitantly administered, prn • LTRA daily + prn SABA
STEP 3		**STEP 3**	
Any of the following: • Daily symptoms • Nocturnal awakenings >1/week • Daily need for reliever • Some activity limitation • FEV$_1$ 60-80% predicted • Exacerbations ≥2/year	• **Low-dose ICS-Formoterol as maintenance and reliever (preferred)** Alternative option(s) • **Medium-dose ICS daily <u>and</u> SABA as needed** • Low-dose ICS-LABA combination daily or low-dose ICS **plus** LAMA daily or low-dose ICS **plus** anti-leukotriene daily & SABA as needed	• Troublesome asthma symptoms most days, nocturnal awakening due to asthma ≥1 time/month, multiple risk factors for exacerbations.	• **Low-dose ICS-Formoterol as maintenance and reliever (preferred)** • Low-dose ICS-LABA combination daily **and** SABA as needed Other options • Medium-dose ICS daily **and** SABA or ICS-SABA as needed. • Low-dose ICS plus LTRA daily **and** SABA or ICS-SABA as needed.
STEP 4		**STEP 4**	
Any of the following: • Symptoms all day • Nocturnal awakenings nightly • Need for SABA several times/day • Extreme limitation in activity • FEV$_1$ <60% predicted • Exacerbations ≥2/year • An acute exacerbation	• **Medium-dose ICS-formoterol as maintenance + reliever (preferred)** Alternative option(s) • Medium-dose ICS-LABA daily or medium-dose ICS **plus** LAMA daily or Medium-dose ICS daily **plus** anti-leukotriene **and** SABA as needed.	Severely uncontrolled asthma with ≥3 of the following: • Daytime asthma symptoms >2 times/week • Nocturnal awakening due to asthma • Reliever for symptoms >2 times/week • Activity limitation due to asthma	• **Medium-dose ICS-formoterol as maintenance + reliever (preferred)** • Medium dose ICS-LABA daily **and** SABA or ICS-SABA as needed Other options • Possible add-on LAMA or switch to ICS-LAMA-LABA • Possible add-on LTRA

EXERCISE INDUCED BRONCHOSPASM

[1] Pre-exercise treatments for Exercise-induced bronchospasm:
- **Albuterol** 2 puffs 5-20 minutes prior to exercise first-line.
- **Budesonide-Formoterol** combination is an alternative 5-20 minutes prior to exercise.

[2] Daily therapy for EIB:
- **Leukotriene modifiers (LTRAs) for patients who require daily therapy for EIB** due to prolonged or recurrent exercise.
- Regular use of an LTRA or an inhaled corticosteroid in addition to a short-acting beta-agonist preferred, rather than regular daily use of a beta-agonist alone.

CLASSIFICATION OF ASTHMA SEVERITY				
	INTERMITTENT	**PERSISTENT**		
		MILD	**MODERATE**	**SEVERE**
Symptoms	≤2 x /day ≤2/ week	>2days/week (but not daily)	Daily	Throughout the day
SABA use for symptoms	≤2x/day ≤2x/week	>2days/week (but not >1x/day)	Daily	Several times a day
Nighttime awakenings	≤2x/month	3-4 x/month	>1x/week (but not nightly)	Often Usually nightly
Interference with normal activity	None	Minor limitation	Some limitation	Extremely limited
Lung Function	• Normal FEV1 between exacerbations • FEV1 >80% predicted • FEV1/FVC normal	• FEV1 ≥80% predicted • FEV1/FVC normal	• **FEV1 60 – 80% predicted** • FEV1/FVC reduced by 5%	• **FEV1 <60% predicted** FEV1/FVC reduced >5%
Recommended Management	• Inhaled SABA as needed	• Inhaled SABA as needed + **Low-dose ICS**	• **Low ICS + LABA** OR • **Increase ICS dose (medium)** or • Add LTRA	• High dose ICS + LABA • **± Omalizumab** (Anti-IgE drug)
Exacerbations requiring PO steroids	0-1/year	≥2/year		

ICS=Inhaled Corticosteroid; LABA=Long Acting β2 Agonist; SA = short, LTRA + Leukotriene Receptor Antagonists

NORMAL

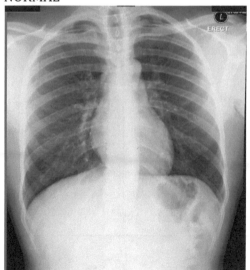

SARCOIDOSIS
Bilateral hilar lymphadenopathy (Stage I)

SARCOIDOSIS

- Idiopathic chronic multisystemic inflammatory non-caseating granulomatous disease.

RISK FACTORS
- **Females, Black Americans, Northern Europeans,** 20-40 years of age (but can affect any age).

PATHOPHYSIOLOGY
- Exaggerated T cell response to a variety of antigens or self-antigens, leading to central immune system activation, granuloma formation, and peripheral immune depression.

CLINICAL MANIFESTATIONS
- **50% are asymptomatic** — incidentally found on imaging.
- Constitutional symptoms: fever, anorexia, weight loss, malaise, myalgias.
- **Pulmonary: (>90%)** — **dry (nonproductive) cough, dyspnea,** chest pain, & **rales** on examination.
- **Lymphadenopathy:** intrathoracic (hilar nodes, paratracheal). Hepatosplenomegaly.
- **Skin: erythema nodosum (classic), lupus pernio (most specific),** maculopapular rash (most common). Parotid gland enlargement. Cutaneous anergy.
- **Eyes: Anterior uveitis most common ocular finding.** Dry eyes and visual loss.
- Cardiac: Restrictive cardiomyopathy, Dilated cardiomyopathy, arrhythmias, heart blocks.
- Rheumatologic: arthralgias, arthritis, bone lesions.
- Neurologic **cranial nerve palsies (especially facial nerve — CN VII [7]),** Diabetes insipidus.
- Löfgren syndrome: triad of erythema nodosum + bilateral hilar LAD + polyarthralgia with fever.

DIAGNOSIS
- Based on compatible clinical/radiologic findings, noncaseating granulomas, & excluding other causes.
- **Chest radiographs: best initial test — bilateral hilar lymphadenopathy (BHL) classic.**
  Interstitial lung disease: reticular opacities, ground glass appearance. Eggshell calcifications, fibrosis.

Stage I: BHL only	**Stage III:** interstitial lung disease (ILD) only.
Stage II: BHL + interstitial lung disease (ILD).	**Stage IV:** fibrosis (restrictive disease).

- Pulmonary function tests: **restrictive pattern is classic**:
  - Normal or increased FEV_1/FVC; normal or decreased FVC, decreased FEV1.
  - Decreased lung volumes (eg, RV, TLC, VC, FRC). Decreased DLCO.
  - PFTs primarily used to monitor response to treatment.

- **Tissue Biopsy: most accurate — noncaseating granulomas** classic nonspecific histological finding.
- Labs: **increased ACE levels, hypercalciuria, hypercalcemia,** increased vitamin D. Cutaneous anergy.

MANAGEMENT
- **Asymptomatic: observation** — spontaneous remission within 2 years in most without treatment.
- **Symptomatic: oral corticosteroids first-line management of choice when treatment is needed.**
  Indications: worsening or bothersome symptoms (eg, cough, dyspnea, chest pain, hemoptysis), deteriorating lung function, progressive radiologic decline, cardiac and/or eye involvement.
- Cytotoxic agents (eg, Methotrexate, Leflunomide, Azathioprine), and biologic anti-TNF agents (eg, Infliximab) may be used as a corticosteroid alternative or corticosteroid-refractory disease.

PROGNOSIS
- Prognosis good overall. 40% spontaneously resolve; 40% improve with treatment; 20% progress to irreversible lung injury.
- Good prognosis: Stage I, erythema nodosum.
- Interstitial lung disease & lupus pernio associated with poorer prognosis.

IDIOPATHIC FIBROSING INTERSTITIAL PNEUMONIA (PULMONARY FIBROSIS)

- Progressive extensive remodeling and scarring of the lungs due to an unknown cause.

RISK FACTORS
- **Men >50 years of age; <u>Cigarette smoking</u> is most strongly associated with IPF.**

CLINICAL MANIFESTATIONS
- Gradual onset of progressive dyspnea, nonproductive cough, and constitutional symptoms (eg, fatigue, weight loss, anorexia, malaise).
- **Most common symptoms are dyspnea on exertion & cough, followed by fatigue** (gradual onset).

PHYSICAL EXAMINATION
- **Diffuse, fine, dry, bibasilar end-inspiratory "Velcro" crackles** (rales). Clubbing of the fingers.

DIAGNOSIS
Chest radiographs:
- **<u>Patchy reticular opacities</u> (<u>honeycombing</u>, ground glass opacities), most marked at lung bases.**
High-resolution Chest CT:
- **<u>High-resolution Chest CT</u> preferred imaging modality: <u>Usual interstitial pneumonia</u> (UIP) — <u>peripheral, basilar predominant opacities</u> associated with <u>reticular honeycombing</u> (focal ground-grass opacification) and traction bronchiectasis;** Bronchiolectasis.

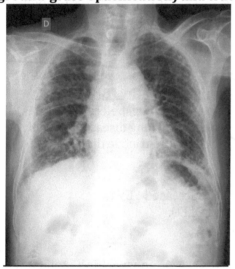
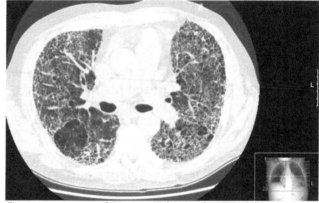

Case courtesy of Bruno Di Muzio rID:28155
Radiopaedia

Pulmonary function test:
- **<u>Restrictive pattern</u> — normal or increased FEV1/FVC**, normal or decreased FVC.
  Decreased lung volumes (eg, RV, TLC, FRC, VC), decreased DLCO.
Histopathology:
- **<u>Usual interstitial pneumonia</u> (UIP) —** abnormal proliferation of mesenchymal cells; **Patchy, temporally and nonuniform distribution of fibrosis. Subpleural cystic airspaces (3-10 mm) honeycomb cysts** (large cystic airspaces from cystic fibrotic alveolitis).

MANAGEMENT
- **<u>No effective medical management</u>.** Most do not respond to treatment and experience gradual respiratory decline. Mean survival 3-7 years after diagnosis.
- **<u>Lung transplant</u> only possible cure** (poor prognosis without transplant). Strategies include smoking cessation and oxygen.
- **<u>Pirfenidone and Nintedanib</u>** are antifibrotic agents that may slow progression but do not significantly benefit mortality.

PNEUMOCONIOSES/ENVIRONMENTAL LUNG DISEASES

PNEUMOCONIOSIS: chronic fibrotic lung disease secondary to **inhalation of mineral dust.**

SILICOSIS

- Occupational pulmonary disease caused by inhalation of silicon dioxide.
- **Silicosis greatly increases the risk for Tuberculosis** and non-TB mycobacterium infections.
- Pathophysiology: silica deposits activate alveolar macrophages, stimulating fibrogenesis.

RISK FACTORS
- **Silica dust inhalation: coal mining, quarry work with granite, slate, quartz, stone cutting, pottery makers, sandblasting, glass & cement manufacturing, masonry, hydraulic fracturing.**

CLINICAL MANIFESTATIONS
- Chronic: often asymptomatic, dyspnea on exertion, nonproductive cough, crackles (rales).
- Acute: dyspnea, cough, weight loss, fatigue. Increased incidence of Tuberculosis.

DIAGNOSIS
- Chest radiographs:
  - Multiple small (<10 mm) round nodular opacities (miliary pattern) **primarily in the upper lobes.**
  - **Eggshell calcifications of hilar & mediastinal nodes classic** (but only seen in 5-20%).
  - Bilateral nodular densities progress from periphery to the hilum.

- High resolution CT: "crazy paving" — multiple small nodules consistent with Silicosis but also diffuse ground glass densities with thickened intralobular and interlobular septa with polygonal shapes.
- PFTs: mixed picture of obstructive & restrictive ventilatory impairment with **decreased compliance,** decreased FEV1 and FEV1FVC ratio, and **decreased DLCO.**
- Lung Biopsy: dust-laden macrophages and loose reticulin fibers in the lung.
- All patients with Silicosis should have a tuberculin skin test and a CXR to rule out Tuberculosis.

MANAGEMENT
- **Complete avoidance or minimization of further exposure to silica mainstay of treatment.** Proper use of respirators or protective equipment.
- Nonspecific supportive management — smoking cessation, bronchodilators, oxygen, rehabilitation.

COAL WORKER'S PNEUMOCONIOSIS (black lung disease)

- Lung disease from inhalation and deposition of coal dust particles.

CLINICAL MANIFESTATIONS
- Usually asymptomatic. Dyspnea, cough; fine crackles (rales) often heard.
- **Caplan syndrome: Coal worker pneumoconiosis + Rheumatoid Arthritis (serology-positive).**

DIAGNOSIS
- Chest radiograph: **small nodules predominantly in the upper lung** with hyperinflation of lower lobes in an obstructive pattern (resembles Emphysema).
- Pulmonary function test: **obstructive pattern** increased lung volumes — RV, TLC, RV/TLC.
- Lung biopsy: shows dark "black" lungs — interstitial pigment deposition and an anthracitic macrophage (black pigment-ladened macrophages). Not needed for diagnosis.

MANAGEMENT
- **Supportive** —Pulmonary rehabilitation programs: breathing re-training, low to high-intensity exercise training, endurance training, & strength training.
- Proper use of respirators or protective equipment.

BERYLLIOSIS

- **Granulomatous pulmonary disease similar to Sarcoidosis, caused by beryllium exposure.**

RISK FACTORS
- Beryllium is often alloyed with nickel, aluminum, and copper so people working in those industries are at increased exposure.
- **High-risk occupations: Aerospace, high technology electronics, ceramics, tool & dye manufacturing, alloy manufacturing (eg, jewelry making), fluorescent light bulbs etc.**

CLINICAL MANIFESTATIONS
- **Dyspnea and dry cough are the most common symptoms.**
- Joint pain, fever, night sweats, fatigue, weight loss are less common

DIAGNOSIS
- Chest radiograph: normal 50%, hilar lymphadenopathy & increased interstitial lung markings similar to Sarcoidosis.
- **The blood Beryllium lymphocyte proliferation test (BeLPT) is the most appropriate initial diagnostic test for patients suspected of having Berylliosis (clinical or radiographic evidence of Berylliosis)** for identifying beryllium-sensitization. Beryllium lymphocyte proliferation test assesses lymphocyte uptake of thymidine.
- Pulmonary function test: As with Sarcoidosis, Pulmonary function test results may show restrictive and/or obstructive ventilatory deficits.
- Biopsy: noncaseating granulomas.

MANAGEMENT
- **Supportive therapy** — influenza and pneumococcal vaccination and smoking cessation counselling, are provided to all patients. Supplemental oxygen and pulmonary rehabilitation as needed.
Asymptomatic or mild disease:
- Patients with mild Berylliosis who are asymptomatic or have mild exertional dyspnea can be observed for stabilization or improvement with beryllium avoidance.
- **In early disease, treatment with Inhaled corticosteroids (ICS) has been shown to improve symptoms of cough and dyspnea especially in patients with obstruction and air trapping.**
Symptomatic with respiratory impairment:
- **Systemic glucocorticoid therapy (eg, Prednisone) is the standard treatment for symptomatic Berylliosis (bothersome dyspnea or cough) with evidence of respiratory impairment on pulmonary function tests** [>10% decline in lung volumes or gas exchange compared with baseline; lung volumes or diffusing lung capacity for carbon monoxide (DLCO) >70% of predicted].

COMPLICATIONS
- Associated with increased risk of lung, stomach, and colon cancer.

BYSSINOSIS

- Lung disease due to **cotton exposure** in those employed in the **textile industry** (may be caused by flax or hemp dust exposure).

CLINICAL MANIFESTATIONS:
- Dyspnea, wheezing, cough, chest tightness.

- The symptoms tend to get worse at the beginning of the work week then improve later in the week or on the weekend "Monday fever'. May be progressive in some patients.

ASBESTOSIS

- Slow, progressive diffuse pulmonary fibrosis as a result of inhalation of asbestos fibers.
- Seen 15-20 years after lengthy exposure to asbestos.

RISK FACTORS
- Asbestos was commonly used due to its fire-resistant, thermal, & electrical insulation properties.
- **High-risk occupations: destruction, repair or renovation of old buildings, insulators, pipefitting, boiler makers, shipbuilding and shipyard workers, fire-resistant products.**

CLINICAL MANIFESTATIONS
- Slowly progressive dyspnea on exertion, cough.
- Physical examination: Bibasilar end-inspiratory crackles may be heard. Clubbing or cyanosis.

DIAGNOSIS
- **Chest radiographs:**
  - **Pleural plaques** — bilateral mid-lung zone parietal pleural thickening or calcification, especially along the lower lung fields and diaphragmatic pleura are hallmark of prior asbestos exposure. Diffuse pleural thickening.
  - Interstitial fibrosis (honeycomb lung) — irregular linear opacities especially in the lower lobes.
  - **"Shaggy heart" sign** — indistinct heart border, "ground glass" appearance of the lung fields.
- **Pulmonary function tests: restrictive lung pattern — normal or increased FEV1/FVC**, normal or decreased FVC, **decreased lung volumes** (RV, FRC, TLC, VC). Decreased DLCO & lung compliance.
- Biopsy: **may show linear asbestos bodies in the lung tissue (ferruginous bodies).**

MANAGEMENT
- No specific therapy. Management includes: bronchodilators, O_2, corticosteroids, ± lung transplant.

COMPLICATIONS
- **The major health effects from exposure to asbestos are [1] pleural and pulmonary fibrosis, [2] cancers of the respiratory tract (eg, Bronchogenic carcinoma) most common, and [3] Mesothelioma (eg, pleural and peritoneal)** rare in incidence but most specific to Asbestosis.

ALPHA-1 ANTITRYPSIN DEFICIENCY

- **Genetic disorder leading to panacinar Emphysema, Bronchiectasis, hepatomegaly, & Cirrhosis.**

CLINICAL MANIFESTATIONS
- **Lung: dyspnea due to Emphysema** most common symptom, **Bronchiectasis**, cough, wheezing, recurrent infections. **Young onset (<45 years) of basilar-dominant pattern Emphysema.**
- **Liver:** Hepatomegaly, chronic hepatitis, cirrhosis, or Hepatocellular carcinoma.
- **Panniculitis:** painful, hot, red nodules or plaques most commonly occurring on the thigh or buttocks.

DIAGNOSIS
- **The diagnosis of AATD is confirmed by demonstrating a serum alpha-1 antitrypsin level <11 micromol/L** (~57 mg/dL by nephelometry) **+ deficient phenotype, generally via genotype or isoelectric focusing.**
- Chest radiographs: **bullous pattern of Emphysema more prominent at the lung bases.**
- CT scan: bibasilar panacinar (diffuse) Emphysema (dilation of terminal airways)
- PFTs: obstructive pattern. Liver biopsy: PAS-positive globules in hepatocytes.

MANAGEMENT
- Medical: IV pooled alpha-1 antitrypsin. Surgical: lung transplantation

HYPERSENSITIVITY PNEUMONITIS (EXTRINSIC ALLERGIC ALVEOLITIS)

- Immunologic reaction occurring within the pulmonary parenchyma caused by **hypersensitivity to an organic agent (eg, microbial, avian, and animal antigens and, less commonly, other organic compounds.** Less commonly due to an inorganic agent.

TRIGGERS
- Farming, vegetable and dairy cattle workers; Exposure to ventilation systems and water reservoirs.
- Bird and poultry handlers; Animal handlers, Grain and flour processing; Lumber milling, construction, bark stripping, Plastics, paint/epoxy, electronics industries.

DISEASE	ANTIGEN	SOURCE
Farmer's lung Cattle worker's lung	Thermophilic actinomycetes, such as *Saccharopolyspora rectivirgula* (*Micropolyspora faeni* or *Faenia rectivirgula*)	Moldy hay, grain, silage
Humidifier lung	*Thermoactinomyces spp* (*T vulgaris, T sacchari, T candidus*)	Contaminated water or heating
Bird breeder lung	Avian proteins	Bird feces, feathers, and proteins
Sequoiosis	Graphium, Trichoderma spp, fungi	Moldy redwood sawdust
Mushroom lung	Actinomycetes	Moldy spores in compost

CLINICAL MANIFESTATIONS

[1] Acute HP:
- **Rapid onset of low-grade fever, chills, dyspnea, productive cough, chest tightness, malaise, or nausea** occurring 4-8 hours after prolonged exposure to the antigen.

[2] Subacute HP:
- **Gradual development of dyspnea, productive cough, anorexia, weight loss, pleuritis** (similar to acute but slower onset, longer duration, and less severe).

[3] Chronic HP:
- Slow onset of progressive dyspnea, weight loss, clubbing, tachypnea.

PHYSICAL EXAMINATION
- Crackles, mid-inspiratory squeaks, and rarely wheezes, may be heard on examination.
- Clubbing may be noted.

DIAGNOSIS

[1] Chest radiograph:
- **Acute**: **diffuse micronodular interstitial pattern**. Subacute & chronic more predominant the lower lung fields.

[2] High resolution Computed tomography (HRCT)
- **Nonfibrotic HP:** **mid-to-upper lung zone predominance of centrilobular ground-glass or nodular opacities with a mosaic attenuation** pattern and signs of air-trapping.
- **Fibrotic HP:** irregular linear opacities/coarse reticulation with lung distortion in a random or mid-lung zone predominant location.

[3] Pulmonary function testing:
- **Restrictive pattern often seen on Spirometry.** An obstructive or a mixed pattern can be seen.
- **Decreased DLCO: Marked impairment in diffusion capacity (DLCO)** is also noted.

MANAGEMENT
- **Acute HP: Identification of the offending agent with removal or avoidance of ongoing exposure to the provocative antigen(s), particularly patients with progressive disease.** Some patients, such as those with farmers' lung who have prompt resolution of initial symptoms, may not progress despite continued low-level exposure.
- **Symptomatic acute, subacute, or chronic HP: Oral glucocorticoids** with gradual taper once symptoms & lung function improve.
- Supportive care: eg, smoking cessation, seasonal Influenza and Pneumococcal vaccinations, pulmonary rehabilitation, and supplemental oxygen.

SILO FILLER DISEASE

- **Organic dust toxic syndrome from** Nitrogen dioxide (NO$_2$) gas exposure released from plant matter (eg, grain) stored in silos as they ferment, especially at the chute & base of the silo.
- Also seen with combustion exposure (eg, fires, diesel fume). Smoking increases the risk.
- Pathophysiology: The gas is converted to nitric acid in the lungs when inhaled.

CLINICAL MANIFESTATIONS
- Cough, dyspnea, fatigue, cardiopulmonary edema. May develop Bronchiolitis obliterans.

MANAGEMENT
- **Occupational reduction of exposure — not entering recently filled silos for 2 weeks;** If entrance is imperative during the filling process, a blower should be run for 30 minutes prior to entering the silo and kept running while anyone is inside; **and use of respiratory N95 masks.**

DIFFERENTIAL DIAGNOSIS
- Farmer's lung (allergic alveolitis/pneumonitis specifically due to moldy hay exposure).

PARROT FEVER (PSITTACOSIS)

- ***Chlamydophila psittaci* infection due to exposure to infected birds** (eg, parrots, ducks, etc.).

TRANSMISSION
- Inhalation of organism in dried feces (eg, cleaning cages, mouth to beak contact, bird exposure).
- 5-14 day incubation period. *C. psittaci* is a Gram-negative, obligate intracellular organism.

CLINICAL MANIFESTATIONS
- **Systemic (Influenza-like) manifestations: abrupt onset of fever, chills, myalgias, profound headache,** photophobia, nausea, vomiting, diarrhea.
- **Atypical pneumonia: dry cough,** dyspnea, chest pain, hemoptysis **in the setting of bird exposure.**

PHYSICAL EXAMINATION
- Rales most common. May have pleural friction rub.
- **Splenomegaly and hepatomegaly occur in ~10%.**

DIAGNOSIS
- Chest radiograph: **atypical pneumonia, multilobar changes, ground-glass opacities.** ± Normal.
- High-resolution CT scan: may show nodular pulmonary infiltrates surrounded by ground-glass opacities.
- **Serologic testing: microimmunofluorescent antibody testing preferred, but complement fixation assay may be used as an alternative.**
- Culture not usually performed as it can be hazardous to lab personnel (*C. psittaci* is highly infectious).
- Suspect Psittacosis if bird exposure and Pneumonia, especially if not responsive to beta lactams.

MANAGEMENT
- **Tetracyclines first-line therapy for Psittacosis (eg, Doxycycline** 100 mg twice daily for 7-10 days). Tetracycline in severe disease.
- **Macrolides (eg, Erythromycin, Azithromycin) are second-line therapy when Tetracyclines are contraindicated.**

COMPLICATIONS
- Rare — hepatitis, respiratory failure, encephalitis, and endocarditis. Infection in pregnancy may be life-threatening.

INFLUENZA

- **Influenza viruses are part of the Orthomyxoviridae RNA virus family**, leads to a highly contagious disease transmitted by the respiratory route in humans.
- It occurs in outbreaks and epidemics worldwide, primarily during the winter season.

TRANSMISSION

- **Primarily via airborne respiratory secretions and droplet nuclei (eg, sneezing, coughing, talking, breathing).**
- Less commonly via fomites and contaminated objects.
- In otherwise healthy adults with influenza infection, viral shedding can be detected 24-48 hours before illness onset but is generally at much lower titers than during the symptomatic period.

ETIOLOGIES

- Type A viruses are further divided into subtypes based on the hemagglutinin (H) and the neuraminidase (N) expressed on their surface.
- **Influenza A associated with more severe outbreaks compared to Influenza B.**

EPIDEMIOLOGY

- Annual epidemics usually appear in the fall or winter in temperate climates, although sporadic cases occur as summer outbreaks in northern areas such as Alaska or the southern hemisphere.
- **Children are important vectors for the disease; the highest rates of infection are seen among children but individuals ≥65 years are at the highest risk for complications.**
- Influenza epidemics affect 10–20% of the global population on average each year and are typically the result of minor antigenic variations of the virus, or antigenic drift, which occur often in influenza A virus.
- Pandemics, associated with higher mortality, appear at longer and varying intervals (decades) as a consequence of major genetic reassortment of the virus (antigenic shift) or adaptation of an avian or swine virus to humans (as with the pandemic H1N1 virus).

INCREASED RISK

Higher risk for complications:

- **Age ≥65 years, pregnancy, immunocompromised.**
- Residents of nursing homes and long-term care facilities.
- **Underlying medical conditions**: eg, Asthma, morbid obesity, and persons with underlying medical conditions (pulmonary, renal, cardiovascular, hepatic, hematologic, neurologic, and neurodevelopmental conditions; and immune-deficient conditions, such as HIV, Diabetes, and Cirrhosis), long-term Aspirin therapy in patients younger than 19 years.

CLINICAL MANIFESTATIONS

The incubation period is 1–4 days.

- **In unvaccinated individuals, uncomplicated Influenza often begins abruptly.**
- **Systemic symptoms** — eg, abrupt onset of fever, chills, headache, malaise, myalgias (most commonly involving the legs and lumbosacral areas). Fever lasts 1–7 days (usually 3–5). Frontal or retro-orbital headache is common and may occur with ocular symptoms (eg, photophobia, pain).
- **Respiratory symptoms often accompany systemic symptoms** — eg, rhinorrhea, congestion, nasal discharge, pharyngitis, hoarseness, nonproductive cough, and substernal soreness.
- Gastrointestinal symptoms (eg, vomiting and diarrhea), rare in adults but can be seen in 10-20% of young children, especially with Influenza B virus infections.
- Elderly patients especially may present with lassitude and confusion, often without fever or respiratory symptoms.

PHYSICAL EXAMINATION
- Signs include mild pharyngeal injection, flushed face, and conjunctival redness. Findings are few.
- Cervical lymphadenopathy and tracheal tenderness may be observed, especially in younger children.
- The presence of fever (>38.2°C) and cough during Influenza season is highly predictive of Influenza infection in those older than 4 years.

COMPLICATIONS
- **Pneumonia is the most common complication of Influenza, especially in high-risk individuals.**
- **Primary Influenza pneumonia** — occurs when Influenza virus infection directly involves the lung, typically producing a severe pneumonia. Primary influenza pneumonia should be suspected when the symptoms persist & increase instead of resolving in a patient with acute Influenza & high fever.
- **Bacterial pneumonia: Pneumococcal pneumonia is the most common secondary infection, and** *Staphylococcal aureus* **pneumonia is the most serious.** *Haemophilus* spp. infections also occur. If the fever recurs or persists for >4 days with productive cough and white cell count >10,000/mcL, secondary bacterial infection should be suspected.

DIAGNOSIS
- **Routine Influenza testing is not necessary unless the patient is ill enough to require admission.**
- Rapid Influenza testing: **Rapid molecular assays [eg, Nucleic acid amplification tests (NAAT)] are preferred over rapid Influenza diagnostic tests in outpatients.** Because of low sensitivity leading to high false-negative results, the CDC recommends empirically treating patients in whom Influenza is suspected.
- Viral cultures: Viral culture may also be used.

MANAGEMENT
Mild disease & healthy:
- **Supportive management is the mainstay of treatment in healthy patients** (eg, Acetaminophen, Salicylates may be used in adults, rest).
- **The CDC suggests that antiviral treatment (eg, Oseltamivir) can be considered for any previously healthy, symptomatic outpatient not at high risk for Influenza complications, who is diagnosed with confirmed or suspected Influenza, based on clinical judgement, if treatment can be initiated within 48 hours of illness onset.**
- Oseltamivir can reduce the duration of uncomplicated influenza A and B illness by ~1 day when administered within 48 hours of illness onset
- For outpatients with acute uncomplicated Influenza, the CDC recommends oral Oseltamivir, inhaled Zanamivir, intravenous Peramivir, or oral Baloxavir for treatment.
- **Patients with uncomplicated Influenza that are not at high risk who have had more than 48 hours of Influenza signs and symptoms are usually not treated with antivirals.**

High-risk for complications:
- **Antivirals (eg, Oseltamivir) are recommended in patients that are hospitalized or have high risk of complications: ≥65 years of age,** cardiovascular disease (except isolated hypertension), pulmonary disease, immunosuppression (eg, malignancy, Diabetes mellitus, HIV infection, post-transplant), chronic liver disease, and hemoglobinopathies (eg, Sickle cell disease).
- **Oral Oseltamivir (75 mg twice daily for 5 days) is the drug of choice for patients of any age, pregnant women, and patients who are hospitalized or have complicated infection. Oseltamivir best if initiated within 48 hours of symptom onset.** Works against both A and B. Adverse reactions: skin reactions, nausea, vomiting, and transient neuropsychiatric events.
- Inhaled Zanamivir (10 mg, 2 inhalations twice daily for 5 days) is indicated for uncomplicated acute Influenza in patients 7 years and older. Relatively contraindicated among persons with Asthma because of the risk of bronchospasm.
- Baloxavir marboxil is a novel agent that inhibits the initiation of Influenza mRNA synthesis. Not used for treatment in pregnant women, breastfeeding mothers, or severely immunosuppressed.

CHEMOPROPHYLAXIS
- **Oseltamivir can be used for individuals one year or older in cases of outbreaks & exposure in high-risk groups.**
- Chemoprophylaxis against influenza A and B is accomplished with daily administration of the neuraminidase inhibitors Oseltamivir (75 mg/day, oral) or Zanamivir (10 mg/day, inhaled) to continue through 7 days after last known exposure.
- For outbreak control in long-term care facilities and hospitals, a minimum of 2 weeks is recommended, including in vaccinated persons if the seasonal vaccine is not well matched to the circulating strain, to continue until 1 week after identification of the last known case.

PROGNOSIS
- **The duration of the uncomplicated illness is 1–7 days, and the prognosis is excellent in healthy adults and children.**
- Hospitalization typically occurs in those with underlying medical disease, at the extremes of age, and in pregnant women.
- **Most fatalities are due to bacterial pneumonia, although exacerbations of other disease processes (eg, cardiac diseases) may cause fatality.**
- Pneumonia resulting from Influenza has a high mortality rate among pregnant women and persons with a history of rheumatic heart disease.
- **An estimated 80-90% of seasonal flu-related deaths and 50-70% of hospitalizations occur among people ≥65 years of age**, who comprise only 15% of the population.

PREVENTION:
- **Annual administration of Influenza vaccine is the most effective measure for preventing influenza and its complications.** Seasonal Influenza vaccines can reduce Influenza hospitalizations by ~60%.
- **Annual influenza vaccination is recommended for all persons over 6 months of age (including pregnancy) with no contraindications.** Vaccination is emphasized for high-risk groups and their contacts and caregivers.
- Vaccination of health care workers is associated with decreased mortality among hospitalized patients and those in long-term care facilities.
- Vaccination prevents Influenza illness among pregnant women and their infants during the first months of life.

INFLUENZA VACCINE
QUADRIVALENT VACCINES:
Inactivated influenza vaccines (IIV4s).
- For the IIV4s produced from cell culture, the approved age indication has been expanded from 4 years or older to 6 months of age or older as per the updated ACIP guidance on Influenza vaccination in the United States (September 2021).
- **Egg based:** (1) **Standard dose, parenterally administered** — (Fluarix, FluLaval, and Fluzone). They are approved by the US Food and Drug Administration (FDA) for intramuscular injection in all adults. These vaccines are produced in embryonated chicken eggs. (2) **Standard dose, "needle free"** — inactivated IIV (Afluria) is administered intramuscularly using a jet injector device approved for adults 18 to 64 years of age; (3) **Standard dose, adjuvanted** — An adjuvanted IIV (Fluad Quadrivalent) is approved for use in individuals 65 years of age or older; **(4) High dose** — An intramuscular high-dose quadrivalent IIV (Fluzone High-Dose) is approved for individuals 65 years of age or older.
- **Cell culture based, standard dose** — A non-egg-based IIV produced in cultured mammalian cells (Flucelvax) is approved for individuals 6 months of age or older.

1 recombinant influenza vaccine (RIV4)

- A recombinant HA influenza vaccine (Flublok), produced using recombinant DNA technology.
- FDA approved and available for individuals 18 years of age or older.
- Unlike the other formulations, which contain both HA and neuraminidase antigens, the recombinant vaccine contains only HA antigens.

1 Live attenuated Influenza vaccine (LAIV4).

- The intranasally administered LAIV (FluMist) is approved for healthy nonpregnant individuals between 2-49 years of age. The vaccine is produced in embryonated chicken eggs.

INDICATIONS:

Inactivated vaccine:

- Advisory Committee on Immunization Practices (ACIP) recommends **annual Influenza vaccination for all individuals 6 months of age or older (including pregnancy, and immunocompromised individuals,** such as HIV, malignancy, post-transplant, etc.) **who do not have contraindications.**
- **Ideally before the onset of Influenza activity in the community (by the end of October in the northern hemisphere** and by April in the southern hemisphere).
- Influenza vaccination may be co-administered with COVID-19 vaccination, at different anatomic sites.

Live attenuated (intranasal):

- Can be used for annual vaccination in ages 2-49 years of age if there are no contraindications.

CHOICE OF VACCINE FORMULATION:

- **For healthy nonpregnant adults up to 49 years of age**, any of the inactivated influenza vaccines (IIVs) or LAIV may be given.
- **For individuals between 50 and 64 years of age and for individuals 49 years of age or younger who have a contraindication to receiving LAIV** (eg, immunocompromise; chronic cardiovascular, pulmonary, or metabolic disease; pregnancy), any of the IIVs may be given.
- **For individuals 65 years of age or older, high-dose IIV (Fluzone High-Dose) is preferred, rather than a standard-dose IIV, particularly in those taking a statin,** when available.
- Individuals who are needle phobic may prefer to receive the single-dose LAIV administered intranasal sprayer or needle-free intramuscular administration for individuals 18 and 64 years of age.
- Live attenuated (intranasal): can be an alternative for annual vaccination in ages 2 to 49 years of age.

ADVERSE REACTIONS:

- **Soreness at the injection site most common** (64%). Injection site reaction, fever, myalgia, irritability. Nasal spray may cause upper or lower respiratory tract symptoms. Anaphylaxis rare.
- Needle-free intramuscular administration — jet injector device is associated with a higher frequency of local injection site reactions than the use of needle and syringe (eg, pain, tenderness, itching, redness, swelling, and bruising).
- Live attenuated vaccine — rhinorrhea, nasal congestion, headache, and sore throat.

CONTRAINDICATIONS & PRECAUTIONS:

- Anaphylaxis to the influenza vaccine. **Guillain-Barré syndrome** within 6 weeks after a previous dose.
- **High fever** with an acute respiratory illness. Most patients with an active infection should delay vaccination until they are better. **Infants <6 months of age.**
- **Although allergy to protein egg used to be a contraindication, individuals with egg allergy of any severity (including anaphylaxis) can safely receive the egg-based inactivated Influenza vaccine in a medical setting supervised by a health care provider or use the non-egg option.**

Live attenuated vaccine only:

- **Immunocompromised patients** (including HIV), **pregnancy, adults age 50 years or older**.
- Chronic cardiovascular, pulmonary, or metabolic disease
- Individuals who have taken an Influenza antiviral medication within the last 48 hours, close contacts and caregivers of severely immunocompromised persons who require a protected environment.

ACUTE BRONCHITIS

- Self-limited lower respiratory tract infection causing inflammation of the large airways.

ETIOLOGIES:
- **Respiratory viruses most common** — The most common viral isolates are Influenza A and B viruses, parainfluenza virus, respiratory syncytial virus, coronavirus, adenovirus, and rhinovirus.
- Bacterial — *S. pneumoniae, H. influenzae, M. catarrhalis, Mycoplasma pneumoniae, Chlamydia pneumoniae,* and *Bordetella pertussis.*

EPIDEMIOLOGY: Acute bronchitis occurs most commonly during the winter months.

PATHOPHYSIOLOGY:
- Epithelial infection of the bronchi leads to inflammation and thickening of the bronchial and tracheal mucosa. The inflammation results in airflow obstruction and bronchial hyperresponsiveness [eg, reversible decrease in forced expiratory volume in 1 second (FEV1)].

CLINICAL MANIFESTATIONS
- **Cough is hallmark (cardinal) symptom of Acute bronchitis.** The cough is acute & often persistent (1-3 weeks). Initially, the cough is nonproductive, but later, a productive cough with mucoid sputum may develop. The presence of purulent sputum is a nonspecific finding and is not predictive of bacterial infection or antibiotic response.
- URI symptoms may precede or occur with the cough — runny nose, sore throat, low-grade fever, headache, malaise, myalgias. With involvement of the lower tract, the cough becomes the predominant symptom. **Fever is rare in Acute bronchitis.**
- **Wheezing or mild dyspnea may accompany the cough.**
- **Hemoptysis** — The most common causes of non-life-threatening hemoptysis in developed countries are Acute bronchitis, Bronchial neoplasms (primary or secondary), and Bronchiectasis.
- Physical examination: **Often normal but both wheezing and rhonchi may be auscultated on physical examination; rhonchi that usually clear with coughing.**

DIAGNOSIS:
- **Clinical diagnosis:** Acute bronchitis is usually a clinical diagnosis without the need for imaging — acute onset of persistent cough (often lasting 1-3 weeks) + no findings suggestive of pneumonia (eg, fever, tachypnea, rales, hypoxia, or signs of parenchymal consolidation, such as dullness to percussion, decreased or bronchial breath sounds, rales, egophony).
- No further workup is needed if vital signs are normal and there are no exam findings suggestive of pneumonia.
- Chest radiographs: **Chest radiographs not usually needed as they are usually normal or nonspecific.** Indications: **chest radiographs are indicated when Acute bronchitis cannot be clinically distinguished from Pneumonia** — (1) chest examination findings of consolidation (eg, rales, egophony, or increased tactile fremitus), (2) abnormal vital signs, such as heart rate is >100/min, respiratory rate > 24 breaths/min, oral body temperature is >38°C [100.4°F] or (3) mental status or behavioral changes in patients >75 years old.

MANAGEMENT:
- **Supportive management:** Acute bronchitis is self-limited (often lasts 1-3 weeks); patient education & symptom control are the cornerstones of management — eg, fluids, antitussives, antipyretics, analgesics, expectorants, & mucolytics.
- Cough relief (nonpharmacologic) — throat lozenges, hot tea, and smoking cessation.
- Cough relief (pharmacologic) — Dextromethorphan, Guaifenesin if >2 years of age.
- **Avoid antibiotic overuse — don't treat with empiric antibiotic therapy in most cases of Acute bronchitis in otherwise healthy adults.** Antibiotics do not provide significant benefit.

ACUTE EPIGLOTTITIS (SUPRAGLOTTITIS)

- **Inflammation of the epiglottis and adjacent supraglottic structures (Supraglottitis).**
- The median age of children with Epiglottitis has increased from 3 years of age to ~6-12 years of age.

ETIOLOGIES
- **_Haemophilus influenzae B_ historically was the most common cause** (reduced in the US due to Hib vaccination). **Hib Epiglottitis still occurs in _unvaccinated children or foreign immigrants._**
- **In an individual with a history of vaccinations, suspect <u>Streptococcus species</u>** [eg, _Streptococcus pyogenes_ (Group A Streptococcus), _S. pneumoniae_] or other _H. influenzae._

PATHOPHYSIOLOGY
- <u>Swelling of the epiglottitis:</u> serious & rapidly progressive infection and swelling of the epiglottis and contiguous structures (eg, aryepiglottic folds, aretynoids, and vallecula).
- <u>Airway obstruction:</u> swelling of the epiglottis (edema & accumulation of inflammatory cells) reduces the lumen of the airway, leading to rapid deterioration, airflow obstruction, & respiratory distress.

CLINICAL MANIFESTATIONS
- **<u>Rapid onset of "3 Ds":</u> <u>D</u>ysphagia, <u>D</u>rooling, & <u>D</u>istress (respiratory) — high fever** (>38.8-40.0°C), **dysphagia, odynophagia, drooling, inspiratory stridor, muffled "hot potato" voice, anxiety, and respiratory distress** (eg, dyspnea, respiratory retraction, choking sensation).
- **<u>Tripoding:</u> may prefer the "tripod" or "sniffing" position** — trunk leaning forward with the neck hyperextended and chin thrusted forward in a "sniffing" posture; reluctant to lie supine.
- The patient often has an ill, uncomfortable, anxious, or restless appearance, and may appear toxic.
- Older children, adolescents, and adults may complain of severe sore throat (most common major complaint) with a relatively benign oropharyngeal examination.

PHYSICAL EXAMINATION
- **In young children, avoid attempting to visualize the throat using a tongue depressor (may result in the loss of the airway).**

DIAGNOSIS
- **Primarily a clinical diagnosis.** Laboratory studies should **<u>not</u>** be done in young children in whom Epiglottitis is suspected until the airway is secured (agitation may worsen respiratory distress).
- **<u>Laryngoscopy:</u> definitive diagnosis** — visualization of an edematous, erythematous (cherry-red) epiglottis performed when securing the airway during direct laryngoscopy or nasolaryngoscopy.
- <u>Cervical radiographs:</u> **soft-tissue lateral neck radiographs — enlarged epiglottis "thumb or thumbprint sign"**, loss of the vallecular air space, thickened aryepiglottic folds, a distended hypopharynx, and straightening of the cervical spine. **May be obtained in patients without airway obstruction but not necessary for diagnosis** (may be performed only if stable & comfortable).

MANAGEMENT
- **<u>Airway maintenance:</u> the single, most important, aspect of treatment is securing &/or maintenance the airway (if needed).** In patients with signs of total or near-total airway obstruction, airway control necessarily precedes diagnostic evaluation.
- **<u>Supportive:</u> every attempt should be made to keep the child as calm and comfortable as possible until an airway is secured** as symptoms can be exacerbated by patient discomfort.
- **<u>Antibiotics:</u> second- or third-generation Cephalosporin (eg, Ceftriaxone, Cefotaxime, Cefuroxime), often with anti-staphylococcal coverage added (eg, Vancomycin).** Penicillin or Ampicillin; Dexamethasone for swelling in some.

PREVENTION
- Rifampin given to close contacts. Routine use of Hib vaccine.

LARYNGOTRACHEITIS (CROUP)

- **Respiratory illness characterized by inflammation of the larynx, trachea, and subglottic airway, resulting in <u>barking cough</u>, inspiratory stridor, and <u>hoarseness</u>.**

ETIOLOGIES
- **<u>Parainfluenza virus type 1</u> most common cause.** Parainfluenza type 2 sometimes causes croup outbreaks but usually with milder disease than type 1.
- <u>Other viruses:</u> Adenovirus, Respiratory syncytial virus (RSV), Rhinovirus, Influenza A and B, Measles.

PATHOPHYSIOLOGY
- The viruses that cause Croup typically infect the nasal and pharyngeal mucosal epithelia prior to local spread along the respiratory epithelium, leading to swelling of the larynx, trachea, and large bronchi.
- **<u>Subglottic narrowing</u>: Swelling results in partial airway obstruction** which, when significant, results in significantly increased work of breathing, and stridor due to turbulent, noisy airflow.

EPIDEMIOLOGY
- **Most common <6 years of age (peaks 6 months–3 years of age). Most cases of Croup occur in the fall or early winter**, coinciding with the major incidence peaks of Parainfluenza type 1 activity.

CLINICAL MANIFESTATIONS
- **<u>Upper airway & larynx involvement</u>: harsh, "<u>seal-like barking" cough</u> — hallmark of the disease in infants & young children, inspiratory stridor, hoarseness** (especially in older children and adults), dyspnea, low-grade fever. **Symptoms often worse at night.**
- URI symptoms (eg, **coryza**) prior, during, or after the acute presentation.
- Significant upper airway obstruction, respiratory distress, and rarely death.

DIAGNOSIS
- **<u>Clinical diagnosis</u>** once Epiglottitis & foreign body aspiration are excluded. Neither radiographs nor laboratory tests are necessary to make the diagnosis.
- **<u>Frontal cervical radiograph</u>: steeple sign (subglottic narrowing of the airway) — 50%. A frontal radiograph of the neck may be considered but is not routinely performed.** Radiographic evaluation of the chest and/or upper trachea is indicated if the child has severe symptoms, is unresponsive to therapeutic interventions, or another diagnosis is suspected.
- **<u>Westley Croup score (WCS)</u>:** used to classify the severity of Croup.

MANAGEMENT
- **<u>Glucocorticoids</u> should be administered in <u>all</u> stages of Croup — they are the best initial therapy and primary treatment for Croup [eg, <u>Dexamethasone</u> (oral, IV, or IM) or oral Prednisolone]. Glucocorticoids result in faster resolution of symptoms, decreased length of stay**, & decreased relapse (provides significant relief as early as 6 hours after single dose oral or IM).
- **<u>Supportive management</u> includes cool humidified air mist, antipyretics, and encouragement of oral fluid intake** (Croup may be associated with decreased oral intake and increased insensible losses from fever and tachypnea, leading to dehydration). **Supplemental oxygen in patients with SaO2 <92%** by "blow-by" administration causes less agitation than mask or nasal cannula.
- **<u>Nebulized Epinephrine</u>** (Racemic or L-Epinephrine) **is reserved as add-on therapy in those with moderate to severe Croup. <u>Epinephrine provides rapid relief</u> within 1 hour.**

<u>**Mild** [no stridor at rest (may be present with agitation), no respiratory distress] WCS 1-2:</u>
- **Symptomatically with glucocorticoids and supportive management** (eg, humidity, fever reduction, and oral fluids). Supplemental oxygen in patients with SaO2 <92%. **Patients can be discharged home.** >85% of children present with mild disease.

Moderate (stridor at rest with mild to moderate retractions) WCS 3-7:
- **All** of the following: **corticosteroids (eg, Dexamethasone), nebulized Epinephrine, & supportive care** (including antipyretics, humidified air or oxygen, & encouragement of fluid intake).
- Disposition: **patients are observed for 3-4 hours after initial treatment.** The majority of children with moderate Croup + symptomatic improvement after treatment can be discharged home.

Severe (significant stridor at rest with marked retractions, anxious, pale, or fatigued child) ≥WCS 8:
- Stridor at rest, marked retractions (suprasternal, subcostal, intercostal), and the child may appear anxious, agitated, fatigued, or pale.
- **Immediate pharmacologic treatment — eg, nebulized Epinephrine (provides relief within 1 hour), systemic or nebulized corticosteroids (eg, Dexamethasone), supportive management, & hospitalization.**

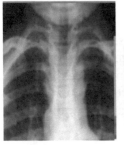
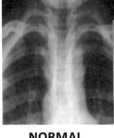
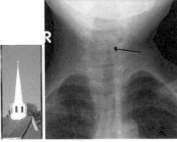
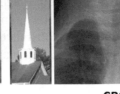

NORMAL　　　　　**CROUP**

Croup:
- **Steeple sign**: narrowing of the trachea seen on frontal radiographs.

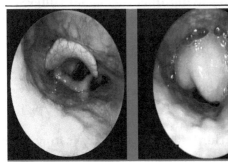
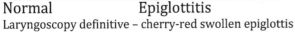

Normal　　　　Epiglottitis
Laryngoscopy definitive – cherry-red swollen epiglottis

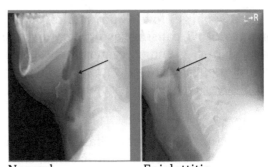

Normal　　　　Epiglottitis
Lateral views: Thumb or thumbprinting sign

BACTERIAL TRACHEITIS (BACTERIAL CROUP)

- Rare invasive exudative inflammation and bacterial infection of the soft tissues of the trachea.
- *Staphylococcus aureus* is the most common cause of Bacterial tracheitis.
- **Bacterial tracheitis may occur as a primary infection or as a complication of viral Croup.**

CLINICAL MANIFESTATIONS
- Most common in children 3-5 years. **Children will appear similar to Croup but appear toxic.**
- With secondary infection, patients present with symptoms of **viral Croup & then have marked worsening with high fevers, toxic appearance, cough, stridor, & severe respiratory distress.**

DIAGNOSIS
- The lateral radiograph in children with Bacterial tracheitis may demonstrate only nonspecific edema or intraluminal membranes and irregularities of the tracheal wall.

MANAGEMENT
- Racemic nebulized Epinephrine. May become an airway emergency.
- Antibiotics: empiric Vancomycin **plus** either a third-generation Cephalosporin (eg, Ceftriaxone, Cefotaxime) or Ampicillin-sulbactam.

ACUTE BRONCHIOLITIS

- Infection and inflammation of the small airways (bronchioles).

'ETIOLOGIES:
- **Respiratory syncytial virus (RSV) most common cause,** followed by Rhinovirus.
- Adenovirus, Influenza virus, Parainfluenza virus, etc.

RISK FACTORS:
- **Infants 2 months to children 2 years most commonly affected**, especially during the fall & winter.
- <6 months in age, exposure to cigarette smoke, lack of breastfeeding, preterm (<37 weeks' gestation), & crowded conditions (eg, day care).

PATHOPHYSIOLOGY
- Inflammation: Viruses infect the upper tract initially and within a few days, travel to the lower respiratory tract (terminal bronchiolar epithelial cells), causing direct damage and inflammation.
- Lower airway obstruction: Direct damage and inflammation results in edema, excessive mucus, epithelial cell necrosis and sloughing, and bronchospasm leading to obstruction of small airways, atelectasis, air trapping, & lower airway hyperinflation, ultimately causing respiratory distress.

CLINICAL MANIFESTATIONS
- **[1] Viral URI prodrome: low-grade fever, upper respiratory symptoms (eg, nasal congestion &/or discharge) for 1-3 days followed by [2] lower respiratory infection with inflammation on days 2 to 3, causing respiratory distress** — eg, bilateral wheezing, crackles (rales), tachypnea, nasal flaring, grunting, cyanosis, chest retractions, use of accessory muscles, rales, prolonged expiratory phase. Lower tract signs and symptoms peak on days 3 to 5 and then gradually resolve.
- Signs of severity: hypoxemia, apnea (especially if age <6 weeks), poor feeding, respiratory failure.

DIAGNOSIS:
- **Mainly a clinical diagnosis (based on history and examination).** Routine ancillary testing (chest radiograph, blood tests, viral/bacterial cultures) is not recommended and should be used only in the context of clinical suspicion of severe bacterial infections.
- **Pulse oximetry single best predictor of disease in children.**
- Chest radiograph: Not routinely performed but may be used to rule out other causes. Nonspecific findings — hyperinflation, peribronchial cuffing or thickening, atelectasis etc.

MANAGEMENT:
- **Supportive care mainstay of treatment — adequate hydration (oral or IV fluids), relief of nasal congestion/obstruction (eg, nasal suctioning), supplemental oxygen and respiratory support (if needed), antipyretics (eg, Acetaminophen), and monitoring of disease progression.**
- Respiratory support: Supplemental oxygen should be provided by nasal cannula, face mask, or head box to maintain SpO_2 >90-92%. Mechanical ventilation may be indicated if severe.
- Heated humidified high-flow nasal cannula (warm humidified oxygen) therapy and/or continuous positive airway pressure (CPAP) are used to reduce the work of breathing, improve gas exchange, and avoid endotracheal intubation in children at risk for progression to respiratory failure.
- **Medications play a limited role:** nebulized hypertonic saline, inhaled bronchodilators (eg, Beta-agonists, nebulized racemic Epinephrine), & antibiotics are **not** routinely used. Corticosteroids are **not** indicated in the **first** episode, unless there is a history of underlying reactive airway disease.

PREVENTION IN HIGH-RISK
- **Immunoprophylaxis with Palivizumab,** a human monoclonal antibody against RSV F glycoprotein, may be given during the first year of life for preterm infants <29 weeks, symptomatic chronic lung disease of prematurity, congenital heart disease, neuromuscular difficulties, immunodeficiency.
- **Handwashing is preventative and limits the spread of disease. RSV vaccination.**

BORDETELLA PERTUSSIS INFECTION (WHOOPING COUGH)

- Highly contagious infection due to *Bordetella pertussis*, a gram-negative aerobic coccobacillus.

EPIDEMIOLOGY
- 38% of cases occur in infants <6 months and 71% of cases occurring in children <5 years of age.
- Risk factors: Pregnancy, exposure; Lack of immunization, incomplete vaccination, or lapse in vaccination.
- Transmission: Respiratory droplets during coughing fits. 7–10-day incubation period.
- Bacteria colonize the mucosal surface and ciliated respiratory epithelial cells. Released toxins (pertussis toxin, dermonecrotic toxin, adenylate cyclase toxin, and tracheal cytotoxin) act locally and systemically.

CLINICAL MANIFESTATIONS
- **[1] Catarrhal phase**: **URI symptoms** — eg, rhinorrhea, sneezing, coryza, anorexia, conjunctival injection, fever, **hacking cough at night that becomes diurnal and increases**, lasting 1-2 weeks.
- **[2] Paroxysmal phase: Severe paroxysmal coughing fits with inspiratory high-pitched inspiratory whooping sound after cough fits*** due to strong rapid inspiration against a closed glottis. Episodes often worse at night. Often lasts 2-4 weeks. **Posttussive vomiting: May have post coughing emesis, syncope, or apnea.** Prolonged cough in adults (nicknamed cough of "100 days")
- **[3] Convalescent phase**: Begins about 4 weeks after symptom onset and associated with resolution of the cough (coughing stage may last for up to 6 weeks).
- Complications: Pneumonia (*B. pertussis* pneumonia in infants, secondary bacterial Pneumonia in adults). Young infants: failure to thrive; Death and apnea may occur.

DIAGNOSIS
- When available, order both throat culture & PCR; **However, confirmatory tests are not necessary for a clear case of Pertussis clinically, which can be treated without further testing.**
- CBC: **absolute lymphocytosis common, especially in younger children, and is often striking** — WBC count usually 15,000–20,000/mcL (60–80% are lymphocytes).
- Nasopharyngeal culture and Polymerase chain reaction (PCR) may yield laboratory confirmation, but the slow-growing *Bordetella* organisms require specialized media (eg, Bordet-Gengou agar or Regan-Lowe) and cultures are typically not positive for 3 to 7 days.

MANAGEMENT
- **Supportive management as needed + antibiotics** in suspected cases of Pertussis within 3 weeks of symptom onset (up to 6 weeks in patients with Asthma, COPD, immunocompromising conditions, 65 years or older, and in pregnant women, especially near term).
- **Supportive management:** oxygenation, suctioning, hydration, avoidance of respiratory irritants as needed. Use of β-adrenergic agonists &/or glucocorticoids are used by some but not proven to be effective. Cough suppressants are not effective in Pertussis, but Dextromethorphan used in some.
- Young infants have the highest rates of complication and death from Pertussis, so most infants (and older children with severe disease) should be hospitalized. **Droplet precautions if admitted.**

Antibiotics:
- Indications: **Antibiotics given to patients AND close contacts**. Treatment shortens the duration of carriage, decreases contagiousness of the affected patient, and may diminish the severity of coughing paroxysms. **Often initiated empirically once there is sufficient clinical suspicion of Pertussis without awaiting diagnostic testing results.**
- **Macrolides drug of choice** — eg, Azithromycin (preferred if young or pregnant), **Clarithromycin.**
- **Trimethoprim-sulfamethoxazole second-line or if allergic to Macrolides.**

PREVENTION
- **DTaP vaccine** Diphtheria, Tetanus, and acellular Pertussis vaccine — **5 doses** (2 months, 4 months, 6 months, 15-18 months, and 4-6 years of age). Tdap vaccine booster dose administered 11-18 years of age and should also be given to pregnant mothers and those around them.

PNEUMONIA

ETIOLOGIES
- <u>Typical</u>: **Streptococcus pneumoniae (most common)**, *Haemophilus influenzae, Klebsiella pneumoniae, Staphylococcus aureus.*
- <u>Atypical</u>: *Mycoplasma pneumoniae, Chlamydophila pneumoniae, Legionella pneumophila,* viruses.

CLINICAL MANIFESTATIONS
- <u>Typical</u>: fever, productive cough, pleuritic chest pain, dyspnea. Rigors (severe chills with violent shaking) is classically associated with *Streptococcus pneumoniae.*
- <u>Atypical</u>: low-grade fever, dry nonproductive cough, <u>extrapulmonary symptoms</u> — eg, myalgias, malaise, pharyngitis, nausea, vomiting, diarrhea.

PHYSICAL EXAMINATION
- **<u>Typical</u>:** tachypnea, tachycardia, **<u>signs of consolidation</u>: bronchial breath sounds, dullness to percussion, increased tactile fremitus, egophony, whispered pectoriloquy,** inspiratory rales (crackles).
- **<u>Atypical</u>: pulmonary exam often normal** (signs of consolidation usually absent).
  May have crackles (rales).
- Elderly, diabetic, and immunocompromised patients may have minimal exam findings even with typical pneumonia.

	PERCUSSION	FREMITUS	BREATH SOUNDS
PNEUMONIA	Dullness	**INCREASED**	**Bronchial, EGOPHONY**
PLEURAL EFFUSION	Dullness	Decreased	Decreased
PNEUMOTHORAX or OBSTRUCTIVE LUNG DISEASE	**HYPERRESONANCE**	Decreased	Decreased

MICROBIOLOGY
Streptococcus pneumoniae
- **Most common cause of Community-acquired pneumonia (65%).**
- <u>Classic presentation</u>: **sudden onset of one-time chills & rigors (violent shivering),** fever, productive cough with **blood-tinged (rusty) sputum.**
- <u>Gram stain</u>: **gram-positive diplococci (cocci in pairs).**

Haemophilus influenzae
- **Second most common cause of Community-acquired pneumonia (CAP).**
- <u>Increased risk</u>: **extremes of age** (<6y, elderly), **immunocompromised** (eg, Diabetes mellitus, HIV, chemotherapy), **underlying pulmonary disease** (eg, Asthma, **COPD, Bronchiectasis, Cystic fibrosis**), alcoholism.
- Gram-negative rod that is often a colonizer of the respiratory tract.

Klebsiella pneumoniae
- *K. pneumoniae* **as a cause of community-acquired pneumonia (CAP) most often occurs in individuals with <u>impaired host defenses</u> (alcoholics, Diabetes mellitus, or severe COPD).**
- *K. pneumoniae* pneumonia is also associated with marked inflammation and necrosis that can lead to **thick, mucoid with blood-tinged ("<u>currant jelly</u>") sputum.**
- <u>Chest radiograph</u>: **cavitary lesions** (necrosis) are hallmark but nonspecific; lobar consolidations.
- <u>Sputum gram stain</u>: gram-negative rods.

Staphylococcus aureus
- **Commonly associated as a <u>superimposed infection after a viral infection</u>** (eg, post Influenza bacterial pneumonia), **hospital-acquired pneumonia (eg, MRSA).**
- <u>Chest radiograph:</u> classically associated with **bilateral, multilobar infiltrates or abscesses (cavitary lesions).** Sputum gram stain: **gram-positive cocci in clusters.**

MYCOPLASMA PNEUMONIAE
- **Most common cause of Atypical (walking) Pneumonia.**
- <u>Risk factors:</u> **<u>Young & healthy</u> — eg, school-aged children, age 5–40 years, college students, military recruits.** Outbreaks often occur in the late summer & early fall.

CLINICAL MANIFESTATIONS
- <u>Extrapulmonary symptoms:</u> commonly presents with **pharyngitis & URI prodrome** (rhinorrhea, headache, malaise, fever) followed by persistent **cough most prominent respiratory complaint** [dry (nonproductive) or productive]. Physical examination often normal. Maculopapular rash.
- Bullous myringitis (fluid-filled blisters on the tympanic membrane) is a rare, nonspecific finding.
- <u>Complications:</u> Stevens-Johnson syndrome/TEN, Erythema multiforme, **Cold agglutinin disease (Autoimmune hemolytic anemia) that is direct antiglobulin (Coombs) test positive.**

DIAGNOSTIC TESTS
- <u>Chest radiograph:</u> **<u>Atypical pattern</u> — reticulonodular pattern most common, diffuse, patchy or interstitial infiltrates;** can be unilateral or bilateral and are more prominent in the lower lobes.
- **<u>Cold agglutinin titers</u> elevated in >50% of patients;** However, not specific to Mycoplasma infection.
- PCR, special culture media; because Mycoplasma have no cell wall, gram-stain is not useful.

MANAGEMENT
- **Macrolides (eg, Azithromycin, Clarithromycin) or Doxycycline are first line agents.**
- Levofloxacin or Moxifloxacin. Because *M. pneumoniae* lacks a cell wall, beta lactams are ineffective.

LEGIONELLA PNEUMOPHILA
- Aerobic, pleomorphic intracellular Gram-negative bacterium.
- <u>Transmission:</u> **Outbreaks related to contaminated water sources, especially in summer & early fall (eg, air conditioners, potable water, cooling towers, ventilation systems, hot tubs, etc.)** in large facilities (eg, hospitals, hotels, or apartment buildings). No person to person transmission.
- <u>Risk factors:</u> immunosuppressed patients, smokers, elderly, chronic lung disease.

CLINICAL MANIFESTATIONS
- **Predominant symptoms include fever, chills, cough, dyspnea,** chest pain, malaise, anorexia. Fever and fatigue often precede the onset of cough. Although "atypical", patients can be very ill.
- <u>Extrapulmonary symptoms:</u> **GI symptoms prominent: diarrhea (watery and non-bloody), nausea, vomiting. <u>Neurologic symptoms:</u> headache, confusion, altered mental status.**
- <u>Physical examination:</u> Rales and/or other signs of consolidation can be present. Relative bradycardia also may be present, which is low or low-normal heart rate despite the presence of a fever.

DIAGNOSIS
- Radiographic findings nonspecific — Patchy unilobar infiltrates that may progress to consolidations.
- Nucleic acid detection — **PCR preferred test; urine antigen (if PCR not available);** culture.
- <u>Labs:</u> **Hyponatremia (due to SIADH). Elevated transaminases (ALT & AST).**

MANAGEMENT
- **Macrolides** (eg, **Azithromycin,** Clarithromycin) **or respiratory Fluoroquinolones** (eg, **Levofloxacin,** Moxifloxacin, and Gemifloxacin) **are the preferred agents.**

ASPIRATION PNEUMONIA
- **Most commonly caused by anaerobes** (eg, *Peptostreptococcus, Bacteroides, Fusobacterium*, etc.). Increased incidence: periodontal disease.
- In chronically ill, gram-negative rods and Staphylococcus aureus may also be a cause.

PATHOPHYSIOLOGY
- Inhalation of oropharyngeal & gastric microbes.

RISK FACTORS
- Reduced consciousness, protracted vomiting, etc.
- **Most common in the right lower lobe** due to vertical angle of the right mainstem bronchus.
- Associated with **foul-smelling sputum ("rotten egg" smell)**, pulmonary abscesses, & Empyema.

2019 guideline update:
- **The 2019 ATS/IDSA new guidelines recommend against routinely adding coverage against anaerobes in suspected aspiration pneumonia unless empyema or lung abscess is present.**
- Several more recent studies did not find a major role for anaerobes in etiology; therefore, adding anaerobic coverage might cause harm without added benefit.

ANTIBIOTICS
- <u>First-line:</u> **Ampicillin-Sulbactam first line (parenteral) or Amoxicillin-clavulanate (oral).**
- <u>Alternative:</u> Metronidazole plus either Amoxicillin or Penicillin G.
- <u>Hospital-acquired aspiration:</u> Imipenem, Meropenem, Piperacillin-tazobactam.

COMMUNITY ACQUIRED PNEUMONIA: ❶ acquired OUTSIDE of the hospital setting & patient is not a resident of a long-term care facility (eg, nursing home) OR ❷ patient that was ambulatory prior to admission who develops pneumonia **within 48 hours of initial hospital admission.**

HOSPITAL ACQUIRED (NOSOCOMIAL) PNEUMONIA: pneumonia occurring **>48 hours after hospital admission.** Often caused by **Pseudomonas, MRSA,** & other organisms found in the hospital.

	TYPICAL PNEUMONIA	ATYPICAL PNEUMONIA
ORGANISMS	*S. pneumoniae* *H. influenzae* *Klebsiella pneumoniae* *S. Aureus*	*Mycoplasma pneumoniae* *Chlamydophila pneumoniae* *Legionella pneumophila* Viruses
CHEST X RAY	Lobar pneumonia	Diffuse, patchy interstitial or reticulonodular infiltrates.
CLINICAL MANIFESTATIONS	• Sudden onset of fever • Productive cough + purulent sputum • Pleuritic chest pain • **Rigors (especially *S. pneumoniae*)** • Tachycardia, tachypnea	• Low grade fever • Dry, nonproductive cough • **Extrapulmonary symptoms:** myalgias, malaise, sore throat, headache, N/V/D.
PHYSICAL EXAMINATION	<u>Signs of consolidation:</u> • **bronchial breath sounds** • **dullness on percussion** • **↑TACTILE FREMITUS, EGOPHONY** • Inspiratory rales (crackles)	**Often normal.** ± crackles, rhonchi. Signs of consolidation usually absent.

CURB65 admission if at least 2 (1 point each)
<u>C</u>onfusion, <u>U</u>remia (>30 mg/dL), <u>R</u>espiratory rate ≥30, <u>B</u>P low (SBP <90 or DBP < 60), Age >**65**

MANAGEMENT

- As per ATS/IDSA 2019 guidelines, for healthy outpatient adults aged <65 years without comorbidities, recent antibiotic use, or risk factors for antibiotic resistant pathogens, options include:

Community-acquired treated as outpatient (otherwise healthy):

- **Amoxicillin** 1 g three times daily **OR**
- **Macrolide** (eg, **Azithromycin** 500 mg on first day then 250 mg daily or **Clarithromycin** 500 mg twice daily or Clarithromycin extended release 1,000 mg daily) only in areas with pneumococcal resistance to Macrolides <25%. **OR**
- **Doxycycline** 100 mg twice daily.
- Beta-lactams which primarily targets *S. pneumoniae* (eg, high-dose Amoxicillin) are preferred because they remain active against most strains of *S. pneumoniae* & *H. influenzae*, despite rising resistance rates among Macrolides, Tetracyclines, and other antibiotic classes. Amoxicillin-clavulanate rather than Amoxicillin may be used in older patients, smokers, and those with comorbidities because of its extended spectrum.
- High-dose Amoxicillin (eg, 1g orally three times daily) plus atypical pathogen coverage with either a Macrolide (eg, Azithromycin or Clarithromycin) or Doxycycline) can be used in some healthy patients < 65 years of age with no recent antibiotic use. **If *M. pneumoniae* is suspected, a Macrolide or Doxycycline is often used or added because beta-lactams and cell wall synthesis inhibitors (eg, Amoxicillin) are ineffective against *M. pneumoniae*.** Macrolides are generally preferred over Doxycycline, unless there are contraindications.
- For mild non-(Ig)E-mediated reactions to penicillin (eg maculopapular rash) or known tolerance to Cephalosporins, a third-generation cephalosporin (eg, Cefpodoxime) is an alternative to Amoxicillin.

Community-acquired treated as outpatient (with comorbidities):

- **Combination therapy: Amoxicillin clavulanate OR a Cephalosporin (eg, Cefpodoxime or Cefuroxime) PLUS a Macrolide (eg, Azithromycin or Clarithromycin).**
- **Monotherapy: respiratory Fluoroquinolones** (eg, Levofloxacin, Moxifloxacin, Gemifloxacin). Fluoroquinolone use is discouraged in ambulatory patients with CAP without comorbid conditions or recent antimicrobial use unless use of other regimens is not feasible.

Community-acquired treated as inpatient (nonsevere):

- Combination therapy: **Beta lactam** (eg, **Ceftriaxone, Ceftaroline) plus a Macrolide.**
- Monotherapy: **respiratory Fluoroquinolone** (eg, Levofloxacin, Moxifloxacin).

Community-acquired treated as inpatient (severe without risk factors for MRSA or *P. aeruginosa*):

- Beta lactam plus a Macrolide OR Beta lactam plus a Respiratory fluoroquinolone.

Extended spectrum antibiotic therapy for MRSA or *P. aeruginosa*:

- **MRSA: Vancomycin OR Linezolid**
- ***P. aeruginosa*: antipseudomonal beta-lactam (Piperacillin/tazobactam, Cefepime,** Aztreonam, Imipenem, Meropenem).

PEDIATRIC MANAGEMENT

6 months–5 years of age:

- Outpatient: **Amoxicillin is usually considered the drug of choice** — eg, high-dose Amoxicillin (90 - 100 mg/kg per day divided into two or three doses; maximum dose 4 g/day). **Alternatives include a second- or third-generation Cephalosporin (eg, Cefdinir), Macrolide**, or Clindamycin.

Children 5 years or older:

- **Amoxicillin is usually considered the drug of choice.**
- **Macrolide antibiotics for initial empiric therapy for suspected atypical CAP treated as an outpatient.** Macrolide antibiotics cover atypical pathogens & provide some *S. pneumoniae* coverage.

PNEUMOCOCCAL VACCINES

VACCINE TYPES

Pneumococcal conjugate vaccine (PCV):

- Pneumococcal protein-conjugate vaccine (PCV13, PCV15, PCV20) that includes capsular polysaccharide antigens covalently linked to a nontoxic protein nearly identical to diphtheria toxin.

Pneumococcal Polysaccharide vaccine (PPSV23)

- PPSV23 includes 23 purified capsular polysaccharide antigens.

Initial vaccination in children:

- Four doses of a pneumococcal vaccine (PCV15 or PCV20) are recommended as a **4-dose immunization series (eg, given at 2 months, 4 months, 6 months, and 12-15 months of age).**
- May also be indicated in older high-risk patients.

PNEUMOCOCCAL VACCINATION IN ADULTS

Adult Pneumococcal Vaccines

- **Indicated in adults ≥65 years or <65 years with risk factors.**

(1) Never received a pneumococcal conjugate vaccine:
For adults ≥65 years with no medical conditions:

- **(1) Administer 1 dose of PCV20 OR**
- **(2) Sequential PCV15 ⇨ PPSV23: 1 dose of PCV15 followed by one dose of PPSV23 at least 1 year later.**
- For those who previously received PCV13 but not PPSV23, administer PPSV at least 1 year after PCV13

For adults ≥65 years PLUS medical conditions:

- **(1) Administer one dose of PCV20 OR**
- **(2) Sequential PCV15 ⇨ PPSV23: 1 dose of PCV15 followed by one dose of PPSV23 at least 1 year later**
- No additional doses are indicated at this age if PCV15 or PCV20 was administered at a younger age.
- For those who previously received PCV13 but not PPSV23, administer PPSV at least 1 year after PCV13

Ages 19-64 with underlying medical condition:

- **Administer one dose of PCV20**

OR

- **One dose of PCV15 followed by one dose of PPSV23 at least 1 year later**

The minimum interval (8 weeks) can be considered in adults with an immunocompromising condition*, cochlear implant, or cerebrospinal fluid leak.

Ages 19-64 no underlying medical condition:

- **None**

(2) For those who have not previously received PCV (or vaccine status unknown):

- **Administer one dose of PCV20**

OR

- **One dose of PCV15 followed by one dose of PPSV23 at least 1 year later** (except in patients with certain risk factors where an interval ≥ 8 weeks can be considered)
- For those who previously received PCV13 but not PPSV23: Administer PPSV23 at least 1 year after PCV13.

HISTOPLASMOSIS
- *Histoplasma capsulatum* — **dimorphic oval yeast that is <u>not</u> encapsulated** (despite its name).

TRANSMISSION:
- **The mycelial form of *H. capsulatum* is found in the soil, especially in areas contaminated with <u>bird/bat droppings</u>**, altering the soil characteristics. Associated with activities involving disruption of the soil (eg, farming, demolition, construction projects, excavation, **spelunking in caves**)].
- **Especially seen in the Midwestern states in the <u>Mississippi & Ohio river valleys</u>, SE US.**

RISK FACTORS
- <u>Immunocompromised states</u> — **AIDS-defining illness, especially CD4+ counts ≤150 cells/microL.**
- <u>Infants and children</u> are affected more frequently than adults because cellular immunity derived from prior exposure decreases the incidence and severity of symptomatic infections.

CLINICAL MANIFESTATIONS
[1] Acute Pulmonary Histoplasmosis
- **<u>Asymptomatic pulmonary Histoplasmosis</u> is the most common syndrome following infection especially in immunocompetent individuals** (90%). May show evidence of granulomatous disease on chest imaging (solitary pulmonary nodule most common abnormality).
- **<u>Atypical pneumonia</u>**: Fever, nonproductive cough, chest pain, myalgias. **Can mimic Tuberculosis.** Occasionally it presents with hemoptysis due to erosion of the nodes into the bronchus.
- **<u>Flu-like symptoms</u>:** fever, chills, headache, cough, myalgias, malaise, anorexia, weight loss chest pain.
[2] Disseminated Histoplasmosis:
- **Rare and occurs primarily in immunocompromised individuals (eg, HIV, especially if CD4+ count ≤150 cells/microL)** — fever (most common symptom), headache, anorexia, weight loss, malaise. Hepatosplenomegaly, lymphadenopathy, mucocutaneous lesions (including ulcerations).
[3] Extrapulmonary manifestations:
- Extrapulmonary manifestations of Histoplasmosis are often caused by a hyperinflammatory response to *H. capsulatum* rather than the infection. Adrenal insufficiency due to adrenal gland involvement.
- <u>Rheumatologic manifestations</u>: **arthralgias or arthritis often accompanied by Erythema nodosum or Erythema multiforme** in a small number of patients (6%), mostly women.

DIAGNOSIS
- **<u>PCR Antigen testing</u> via sputum or urine highly specific.**
- <u>Antibody testing</u> either immunodiffusion assay, enzyme immunoassay, or complement fixation.
- **<u>Cultures</u>: <u>Most specific test</u>** — Culture (eg, sputum, blood) remains the criterion standard for diagnosis but requires a lengthy incubation period (may not be positive for as long as 6 weeks). Blood culture positivity if disseminated/HIV.
- <u>Histopathology & cytology</u>: biopsy findings of lung or mediastinal tissues with special staining include granulomas (in a majority of cases), Yeast-phase organisms of *H. capsulatum* at 37°C appear as **<u>narrow-based, ovoid, budding yeast cells</u>, measuring 2-5 micrometers in diameter.**
Chest radiographs:
- **<u>Acute pulmonary Histoplasmosis</u>: focal or patchy pulmonary infiltrates, often with hilar or mediastinal lymphadenopathy but may be normal.**

MANAGEMENT
- **<u>Asymptomatic</u>: no treatment required (eg, patients with pulmonary symptoms <4 weeks).**
- **<u>Mild-moderate disease</u>: <u>Itraconazole</u> first-line treatment.** Posoconazole or Voriconazole.
- **<u>Severe disease</u>: Amphotericin B.** Also used if Itraconazole therapy is ineffective. Because of its potential toxicity (eg, nephrotoxicity, hypokalemia), Amphotericin B is often reserved for the initial treatment of moderately severe or severe infection. Lipid preparations of Amphotericin B (eg, liposomal Amphotericin B) are preferred because lipid formulations are less nephrotoxic.

PNEUMOCYSTIS (PCP) PNEUMONIA

- **_Pneumocystis jirovecii_** (formerly *carinii*) is a yeast-like fungus (doesn't respond to antifungals).

RISK FACTORS
- Immunocompromised states — eg, HIV, malignancy, chemotherapy, transplant recipients.
- **Most common opportunistic infection in HIV, especially if CD4+ ≤200 cells/microL.**

CLINICAL MANIFESTATIONS
- Classic triad: **progressive dyspnea on exertion (most common), fever, & nonproductive cough.**
- Fatigue with usual activities. Other symptoms may include chills, weight loss, or chest pain.
- Physical examination: **Nearly all patients with PCP will have either hypoxemia at rest or with exertion (eg, oxygen desaturation with ambulation is highly suggestive of PCP).**

DIAGNOSIS
- **Almost all patients with PCP have ≥2 of the following: fever, cough, dyspnea, lactate dehydrogenase (LDH) >460 U/L or arterial partial pressure of oxygen (PaO2) <75 mmHg.**
- **Induced sputum sample** usually the initial procedure for the diagnosis of PCP. If PCP is not identified by induction, bronchoscopy with bronchoalveolar lavage should be performed.
- **Chest radiographs: Diffuse bilateral interstitial, perihilar, or alveolar (ground-glass) infiltrates are classic, and lower lung predominant opacities but can be normal in at least one third of cases,** so a normal chest radiograph does not exclude the diagnosis.
- **Increased LDH (lactate dehydrogenase) >200 U/L used as a clinical indicator if HIV-positive.**
- Increased 1-3-beta-D-glucan levels >80 pg/mL, especially if markedly elevated, suggests PCP.
- Bronchoalveolar lavage specimen or induced sputum: Direct fluorescent antibody staining of the sample to see both trophic & cyst forms most common technique used.
  - Trophic forms: Wright-Giemsa stain. Cysts: methenamine silver & toluidine blue stains. If induced sputum is negative, bronchoscopy should be performed.

MANAGEMENT
- **Trimethoprim-sulfamethoxazole drug of choice for 21 days (oral for mild to moderate disease and IV for severe disease).** Trimethoprim-sulfamethoxazole is the drug of choice for both treatment and prophylaxis.
- **Adjunctive corticosteroid therapy in HIV+ patients if hypoxic (eg, PaO$_2$ <70 mmHg, A-a gradient ≥35 mmHg, or hypoxia on pulse oximetry) to decrease the incidence of mortality and respiratory failure associated with PCP.** Without glucocorticoids, patients with PCP may worsen clinically after 2-3 days of therapy, due to increased inflammatory response.
- **Sulfa allergies: Trimethoprim-Dapsone, Clindamycin-Primaquine, Atovaquone** usually limited to patients with mild disease, or to complete a course of therapy in patients improving on TMP-SMX who develop an adverse reaction and need to discontinue it. Desensitization to TMP-SMX an option.
- **Severe disease: Clindamycin-Primaquine** for patients with severe disease who cannot take TMP-SMX. Because Primaquine must be administered orally, **IV Pentamidine must be used for patients with severe PCP who have a life-threatening sulfonamide allergy and cannot take oral medications.** IV Pentamidine should be switched to a less toxic regimen as soon oral therapy is tolerated. Adverse reactions occur in up to 70% of patients on IV Pentamidine and include nausea, taste disturbance, hypotension, cardiac arrhythmias, nephrotoxicity, pancreatitis, electrolyte disorders (eg, hypo- or hyperglycemia, hypo- or hyperkalemia, hypocalcemia).

G6PD deficiency:
- **Avoid Dapsone or Primaquine when possible due to increased risk of hemolytic anemia.**
- **Mild disease: Atovaquone in sulfa-intolerant patients with G6PDD.**
- Moderate disease: in sulfa-intolerant patients — Atovaquone, desensitize to TMP-SMX or switch to IV Pentamidine are options.

TUBERCULOSIS

- **Infection of the respiratory system and possibly other organs by *Mycobacterium tuberculosis,* an acid-fast bacillus.**

EPIDEMIOLOGY
- Tuberculosis is the leading cause of death from an infectious agent worldwide.
- A third of the world's population is said to be infected with *Mycobacterium tuberculosis,* with estimates of 10,000,000 new infections globally each year.

TRANSMISSION
- **Inhalation of infected aerosolized microdroplets.**
- Prolonged exposure is the main factor in increasing the risk of transmission.

RISK FACTORS
- Close contact with someone infected with TB, immigrants from highly endemic regions, crowded conditions eg, prisons, homeless shelters, Health care workers in hospitals and nursing homes. Medical or microbiology department personnel. Immunosuppression eg, **HIV**, Diabetes mellitus, immunosuppressive medications (eg, TNF-inhibitors).

PATHOPHYSIOLOGY
- After inhalation Mtb goes to the alveoli, gets incorporated into macrophages, and can disseminate from there via macrophages.
- Inhalation of *Mycobacterium tuberculosis* and deposition in the lungs lead to one of four possible outcomes: [1] immediate clearance of the organism (rare), [2] **primary disease** rapid progression to active disease, [3] **latent infection** infected with TB but not infectious, or [4] **reactivation (secondary) disease** onset of active disease many years following a period of latent infection.
- The body's ability to effectively limit or eliminate Mtb is determined by the immune status of the individual, genetic factors, and whether it is a primary or secondary exposure to the organism.
- **Caseating granulomas: The major pathology in Tuberculosis is granulomatous inflammation with caseation (central necrosis),** with the lungs being the primary site of involvement. Tuberculosis infection induces a cell-mediated delayed type IV hypersensitivity reaction, leading to granuloma formation.

Primary infection:
- Primary TB is usually localized to the middle portion of the lungs, and this is known as the Ghon focus of primary TB.
- 90% of individuals with an intact immunity control further replication of Mtb, and may experience clearance of the organism or enter a "latent" phase (infected but not infectious). ~2-3 billion people in the world are latently infected with *M. tuberculosis.* **Patients with latent TB are infected [evidenced by a positive screening test (eg, PPD or interferon gamma test) but are not infectious (no symptoms and no evidence of active infection on chest imaging)].**
- **10% of primary infections develop primary progressive TB Pneumonia,** especially if immunocompromised, HIV infection, chronic kidney disease, poorly controlled Diabetes mellitus, young children (<5 years of age), and older adults.

Secondary (reactivation):
- **5-15% of patients with latent TB may "reactivate", progressing to symptomatic disease in their lifetime.**
- Secondary Tuberculosis usually occurs because of reactivation of latent Tuberculosis infection after a long period of latency (usually several years after initial primary infection). The lesions of secondary Tuberculosis are in the lung apices (due to higher oxygen content). A smaller proportion of people who develop secondary Tuberculosis do so after getting infected a second time (re-infection).

CLINICAL MANIFESTATIONS:

Pulmonary:
- **Prolonged fever** (often with a diurnal pattern) is the most commonly reported symptom of primary TB; only one-third of patients with pulmonary involvement develop respiratory symptoms.
- **Cough, often mild & nonproductive, but may become productive** (often present >2 weeks), **chest pain (pleuritic), dyspnea, hemoptysis, fatigue, fever, chills, drenching night sweats.**
- Nonpulmonary symptoms include lymphadenopathy, fatigue, and pharyngitis.
- Advanced disease: **Anorexia, wasting (consumption),** and malaise are common.

Extrapulmonary:
- <u>**Can affect any organ**</u> — cervical lymph nodes **(Scrofula),** meningitis, **Pott disease (vertebrae),** Miliary TB, pericarditis, adrenal gland involvement, genitourinary.

Physical examination:
- <u>Pulmonary findings</u>: Usually normal in mild disease or shows none specific lung findings (eg, crackles or signs of consolidation). Absent breath sounds are noted over consolidation areas.
- <u>Extrapulmonary findings</u> include clubbing and other signs of distant organ involvement.

DIAGNOSIS:
- **Isolation of *M. tuberculosis* from a body secretion or fluid** (eg, culture of sputum, bronchoalveolar lavage, or pleural fluid) **or tissue** (eg, pleural biopsy or lung biopsy).
- **During evaluation, patients are placed on respiratory isolation:** negative pressure room, HEPA filter.

<u>Chest radiograph:</u>
- **Often the initial diagnostic imaging in evaluation of suspected Tuberculosis.**
- **If chest imaging is suggestive of infection, 3 sputum samples should be collected and sent for acid-fast bacilli (AFB) staining and culture, with one sample tested with nucleic acid amplification (NAAT).** If AFB staining and/or NAAT are positive, TB is likely, and treatment should be initiated.
- <u>**Primary TB**</u>**: middle/lower lobe consolidation classic.**
- <u>**Reactivation pulmonary TB**</u> **"classically" presents with focal infiltration (patchy or lobar consolidation) of the upper lobe(s), especially at the lung apices** due to higher oxygen content. In secondary disease, the tissue reaction and hypersensitivity is more severe, resulting in formation of **cavities in the upper portion of the lungs.** Fibrosis with enlargement of hilar and mediastinal lymph nodes may be seen. Pleural effusions.
- <u>**Miliary TB:**</u> **small fibronodular lesions resembling millet seeds due to pulmonary or systemic dissemination of the tubercles.**
- Chest computed tomography (CT) is more sensitive than plain chest radiography for identifying early or subtle parenchymal and nodal processes but usually reserved if chest radiograph is insufficient.

MILIARY TUBERCULOSIS	**CLASSIC PRIMARY TB**	**CLASSIC REACTIVATION TB**

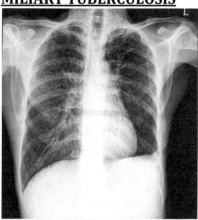 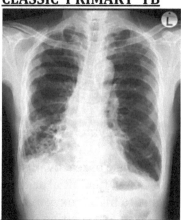 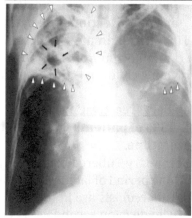

Sputum acid-fast staining:
- **In patients with imaging suspicious of TB, 3 sputum specimens should be submitted for acid-fast bacilli (AFB) smear, mycobacterial culture, and NAA testing** (obtained via cough or induction at least 8 hours apart and including at least one early-morning specimen).
- **The detection of acid-fast bacilli (AFB) on microscopic examination of stained sputum smears is the most rapid and inexpensive TB diagnostic tool.** Diminished sensitivity in HIV positivity.

Sputum cultures:
- At least 3 samples on 3 consecutive days, preferably early morning specimens.
- Culture may take weeks for the results to return.

Nucleic acid amplification testing (NAAT):
- **More sensitive than sputum smears for AFB.** NAA testing should be used for rapid diagnosis (24 to 48 hours) of organisms belonging to the *M. tuberculosis* complex in patients with suspected TB.
- **A positive NAA test (with or without AFB smear positivity) is sufficient to diagnose TB.**
- A negative NAA result is <u>not</u> sufficient to exclude the presence of active TB or drug resistance.

Histology:
- <u>Caseating granulomas</u> **(caseous necrosis) are hallmark of Tuberculosis**, though they may be present in other diseases. The central area undergoes degradation by lysosomal enzymes and appears as cheesy material on gross examination and multinucleated giant cells are present.

Supportive tests:
- In addition, Tuberculin skin test (TST) or Interferon-gamma release assay (IGRA) should be performed to support diagnosis as positive tests signify exposure to TB and support (but cannot be used to establish) a diagnosis of active TB disease. Negative results do not exclude active TB disease.

MANAGEMENT (ACTIVE TB):
Initiate TB treatment AFTER confirmation via AFB smear or NAAT testing:
- <u>Initiate 4-drugs:</u> **RIPE (Rifampin, Isoniazid + Pyridoxine/Vitamin B6, Pyrazinamide, Ethambutol) for the first 2 months followed by a 4-month continuation phase with Rifampin and Isoniazid, pending sensitivity (6-month minimum total treatment duration).** When drug sensitivity is available, and the bacterium is susceptible to both INH and RIF, EMB could be stopped.
- Streptomycin can be used instead of Ethambutol (RIPE or RIPS) if not pregnant.
- <u>Active TB in Pregnancy:</u> **INH + RIF + ETH for 2 months, followed by INH + RIF x 7 months (total of 9 months duration).** Streptomycin and Pyrazinamide are not used in pregnancy.
- Sputum for AFB smear and culture at monthly intervals until 2 consecutive cultures are negative.
- If there is a concern about compliance or difficulty achieving DOT, the dosing for the continuous phase could be modified to 3 times weekly.

DRUG	ADVERSE EFFECTS	CONSIDERATIONS
RIFAMPIN (RIF)	**Thrombocytopenia,** flu-like symptoms. **Orange colored secretions** (eg, tears, urine). GI upset, hypersensitivity, fever, hepatitis.	<u>MOA:</u> inhibits RNA synthesis <u>CI:</u> in patients taking protease inhibitors, NNRTIs
ISONIAZID (INH)	**Hepatitis (especially if ≥35 years of age). Peripheral neuropathy.** Drug-induced lupus, rash. Abdominal pain, high anion gap acidosis. Cytochrome P450 inhibition.	<u>MOA:</u> inhibits mycolic acid synthesis **Peripheral neuropathy prevented by pyridoxine (vitamin B6).** Baseline LFTs recommended.
PYRAZINAMIDE (PZA)	**Hepatitis & hyperuricemia.** GI symptoms, arthritis. **Photosensitive dermatologic rash.**	Pyrazinamide not usually recommended in pregnancy. **Caution in gout & liver disease.**
ETHAMBUTOL (EMB)	<u>Optic neuritis</u> ⇨ scotoma, color perception problems (red-green), visual changes. **Peripheral neuropathy,** GI symptoms, rash.	
STREPTOMYCIN (STM)	**Ototoxicity (CN 8), nephrotoxicity.**	Streptomycin is an aminoglycoside.

TUBERCULOSIS SCREENING

There are 2 major tests for screening & identification of TB infection:
- **[1] Tuberculin skin (TST)/Purified protein derivative (PPD)**
- **[2] Interferon-gamma release assay (IGRA) blood test.**

- **Chest imaging** (eg, radiograph) is the most appropriate next step in **any patient with a positive screening test (eg, TST or IGRA)** to rule out active infection.

[1] Tuberculin skin (TST)/Purified protein derivative (PPD):
- **Determines if the patient is infected (does not determine if infectious).** Read after 48-72 hours.
- **Any positive TST/PPD should be followed by chest imaging to rule out active disease.**
- **Considered positive if transverse induration** is:

REACTION SIZE	PERSONS CONSIDERED TO HAVE ⊕ TEST
≥5 mm	- **HIV⊕ or immunosuppressed** (eg, chemotherapy, post organ transplantation, glucocorticoid therapy >15 mg/day for at least 1 month, TNF-alpha inhibitor). - **Close contacts of patients with active TB.** - **CXR consistent with old/healed TB (eg, calcified granuloma).**
≥10 mm	- **All other high-risk populations/high prevalence populations.** - Recent conversion = ↑induration by >10 mm in the past 2 years.
≥15 mm	Everyone else with no known risk factors for TB.
False negative	**Anergy** (HIV, Sarcoidosis*)*, **Faulty application** (if given SQ instead of TD), acute TB (normally takes 2-10 weeks to convert), acute non-TB infections, malignancy.
False ⊕	**Improper reading, cross reaction with an atypical** (eg, Mycobacterium avium complex), **within 2-10 years of BCG vaccination** (although usually <10 mm).
Booster effect	Infected person's immune system "forgets" about TB until years later when testing "reminds" the immune system. Next PPD will be ⊕ because of initial infection (years ago) NOT because recently converted. Confirmed by 2-step PPD testing.

History of a previous BCG vaccine has no impact or effect on recommendations for the screening and treatment of Latent tuberculosis infection in adults.

[2] Interferon Gamma release assay (IGRA):
- **Blood test with improved specificity, no reader bias, no booster phenomenon, and not affected by prior BCG vaccination compared to TST/PPD.**
- QuantiFERON gold assay is an example.
- <u>Indications</u>: IGRAs are recommended for patients who may not return for the TST reading (history of drug abuse, homelessness), those who were previously vaccinated with the BCG, or individuals > 5 years who are likely to be infected with *Mycobacterium tuberculosis*, have a low or intermediate risk of disease progression, and in whom it has been decided that testing for latent Tuberculosis is warranted.
- Disadvantages of IGRA include high cost, the need for technical expertise to perform the test, and high rates of false-positive and false negatives.

Chest radiographs:
- **Chest imaging** (eg, radiograph) is the most appropriate next step in any patient with a positive screening test (eg, TST or IGRA) to rule out active infection.
- Patients with evidence of an active infection on imaging should undergo further workup (eg, isolation, NAA testing, Acid fast smear) and treated for active infection if NAAT or AFB is positive.
- **Patients who are [1] TST or IGRA positive, [2] asymptomatic, with [3] negative chest imaging (no signs of active disease) are considered to have Latent TB infection.**
- Chest radiographs also used for yearly screening in patients with positive PPD or IGRA who require yearly screening (eg, health care workers).

LATENT TUBERCULOSIS INFECTION (LTBI)

- **Infected with Tuberculosis but without active infection** [individuals with LTBI are not infectious (contagious) to other people]. Evidence of infection via screening test [eg, Tuberculin skin test (usually positive 2-4 weeks after initial infection) or Interferon gamma release assay].
- The main risk is that ~10% of these people (5% in the first 2 years after infection and 0.1% per year thereafter) will go on to develop active Tuberculosis.

PATHOPHYSIOLOGY
- **~90% of people infected with Tuberculosis control the initial primary infection via caseating granuloma formation (latent infection).** These granulomas may become caseating (central necrosis & acidic with low oxygen, making it hostile for Mtb to grow).

DIAGNOSIS
Need ALL 3 to show the patient is infected with TB but NOT infectious (no evidence of active infection).
- **[1] positive screening test (eg, TST/PPD or IFGRA)** identifies infection with TB
PLUS no evidence of active infection:
- **[2] no symptoms of active infection, &**
- **[3] chest imaging shows no findings suggestive of active infection.**

Rationale for management of LTBI:
- The management of LTBI may be offered to reduce the risk of secondary (reactive) TB in the future.
- The lifetime incidence of reactivation is 5-10%; LTBI treatment reduces this by 75%.
- The treatment is NOT mandatory, and patients may decide against management.

MANAGEMENT OF LATENT TB INFECTION:
[1] Rifamycin-based regimens: (preferred)
- **Rifampin (RIF) daily for 4 months** (4R)
- **Isoniazid (INH) and Rifampin daily for 3 months** (3HR)
- Isoniazid (INH) and Rifapentine weekly for 3 months (3HP)
- The guidelines for treatment of LTBI issued by the United States Centers for Disease Control and Prevention (CDC) and National Tuberculosis Controllers Association (NTCA) in 2020, now favor a Rifamycin-based regimen over Isoniazid therapy. Rifamycin-based regimens are preferred given their efficacy, favorable treatment completion rates, relatively low hepatotoxicity rates.

[2] Older regimen:
- **Isoniazid monotherapy [with Pyridoxine (Vitamin B6) for 6-9 months.**

(1) ACTIVE INFECTION	(2) SCREENING FOR TB	(3) LATENT INFECTION
Primary progressive or Secondary (reactive) TB	• PPD (TST) or Interferon gamma release assay	All 3 present?:
• **Symptoms of pneumonia + consumption (eg, weight loss, cachexia) + risk factors** (eg, immigrant, crowded condition).	• **5mm:** immunocompromised, granuloma on CXR, recent contact with + TB.	• **(1) positive screening test [TST/PPD or IGRA] PLUS**
		• **(2) Negative CXR**
	• **10mm:** all other risk factors	• **(3) No symptoms**
⬇		
Testing for active infection:	**Positive screening test:**	**Treatment of LTBI (Optional)**
• **NAA testing or**	• **Chest imaging to rule out active infection**	• **Rifampin x 4 months**
• **Acid fast smear positivity**		• **INH + Rifampin x 3 mos**
⬇		• INH + Rifapentine x 3 mos
		• **Isoniazid monotherapy for 6-9 months.**
Management of active infection:	**Negative screening test**	
• RIPE or RIPS	• **No management; follow-up**	

SOLITARY PULMONARY NODULE

- Single, small (≤30 mm), usually well-circumscribed lesion that is surrounded entirely by pulmonary parenchyma. Lesions measuring >30 mm are considered masses & have higher malignant potential.

ETIOLOGIES
- **Infectious granulomas most common solitary pulmonary nodule** (>75% of all benign nodules), especially Mycobacteria (eg, Tuberculosis) and fungi (eg, Histoplasmosis, Coccidioidomycosis).
- May be benign or malignant tumors (eg, lung cancer, metastasis, carcinoid tumors).
- Thymoma most common mediastinal tumor.

RISK OF MALIGNANCY
- **Increased risk: spiculated** nodule, large (>2 cm), irregular borders, asymmetric calcification, upper lobe location, **>40 years of age, smoker,** female gender, enlarging lesions, Emphysema, asbestos exposure, abnormal PET scan.
- **Decreased risk**: well circumscribed smooth borders, small (<1 cm), **dense diffuse calcification, <30 years of age**, nonsmoker, no change in size, normal CT scan.

DIAGNOSTIC WORKUP
- **Chest radiograph: usually the initial test** that often revealed the presence of a pulmonary nodule.
- **CT of the chest without contrast preferred initial imaging modality to determine the likelihood of malignancy of a nodule found incidentally on chest radiographs**.
- PET scan may be used to determine to determine metabolic functioning of the nodule.

MANAGEMENT
- Low probability: active surveillance with monitoring for changes.
- Intermediate probability: bronchoscopy with biopsy if central lesion. Transthoracic needle aspiration for peripheral lesions.
- High probability: resection with biopsy.

BRONCHIAL CARCINOID TUMORS

- Rare neuroendocrine (enterochromaffin cell) tumors characterized by slow growth, low metastasis, and are usually well-differentiated.
- GI tract is the most common site of carcinoid tumors. Lung is the second most common.
- May secrete serotonin, ACTH, ADH, or melanocyte stimulating hormone. Most common <60 years.

CLINICAL MANIFESTATIONS
- Most patients have a centrally located tumor and are symptomatic from the tumor mass.
- Focal wheezing, cough, hemoptysis, wheezing. SIADH, Cushing's syndrome, obstruction.
- **Carcinoid syndrome: (rare but classic)** — episodes of diarrhea (serotonin release), flushing, tachycardia, bronchoconstriction/wheezing (histamine release), and hemodynamic instability (eg, hypotension). Tryptophan is converted from Niacin (B3) to serotonin by the tumor.

DIAGNOSIS
- **CT of the chest most useful imaging**, with the diagnosis generally confirmed by either by bronchoscopic biopsy (for central lesions) or by transthoracic needle biopsy (peripheral lesions).
- **Bronchoscopy: pink to purple well-vascularized centrally located tumor.**
- Tumor localization: CT scan & Octreotide scintigraphy.

MANAGEMENT
- **Surgical excision definitive management**. Tumors are often resistant to radiation & chemotherapy.
- Octreotide may be used to reduce symptoms (decreases secretion of the active hormones).

BRONCHOGENIC CARCINOMA

- Second most common cancer diagnosed in the US (after prostate in men & breast in women).
- **Most common cause of cancer-related deaths in the US.**
- Greatest tendency to METS to the brain, bone, liver, lymph nodes, & adrenals.

RISK FACTORS
- **Cigarette smoking most common cause** (including second-hand). Smoking associated with 85-90% of cases (exception is lepidic pattern). Asbestosis is the second most common cause.
- **Asbestosis & smoking are synergistic.**
- Radon exposure (eg, uranium miners). Idiopathic Pulmonary Fibrosis, Tuberculosis, & COPD associated with increased lung cancer incidence. Genetic susceptibility is also a factor.

DIVIDED INTO 2 MAIN TYPES
- **[1] Non-small cell cancer:** includes Adenocarcinoma, Large cell, Squamous cell, Lepidic pattern. **Usually treated with surgical resection.**
- **[2] Small cell cancer:** because it is aggressive & usually metastatic at the time of presentation, **chemotherapy is the initial management of choice for most** (with or without radiation).

LUNG CANCER SCREENING
The US Preventative Services Task Force recommends **annual low-dose CT screening** for those **50–80 years old who are at high risk of lung cancer:**
- **at least a 20 pack-year smoking history** and are
- **either current smokers or former smokers having quit within the past 15 years.**
- Screening should be discontinued once a person has not smoked for 15 years or develops a health condition substantially limiting life expectancy or ability or willingness to undergo curative surgery.

ADENOCARCINOMA OF THE LUNG

- **Most common primary lung cancer** in smokers, women, men, & nonsmokers (50% of cases).

RISK FACTORS
- **Cigarette smoking strongest risk factor**. Exposure to silica, asbestos, radon, heavy metals.

CHARACTERISTICS
- **Arises from bronchial mucosal glands. It is a type of non-small cell lung cancer.**
- Common gene mutations include *KRAS, EGFR, ALK*.
- With the new classification, bronchioloalveolar carcinoma and mixed subtypes Adenocarcinoma are eliminated. "Lepidic" has been used to describe non-invasive growth along intact alveolar septae (formerly bronchioloalveolar).
- Lepidic pattern: a rare low-grade subtype characterized by noninvasive growth of tumor cells along intact alveolar septae (has the best prognosis). Classically presents with voluminous sputum & an interstitial lung pattern on chest radiographs.

CLINICAL MANIFESTATIONS
- Asymptomatic in early disease. Cough, dyspnea, hemoptysis, weight loss.

DIAGNOSIS
- Chest radiograph: **Typically peripherally located.**
- CT-guided biopsy: Histology: **gland formation (glandular appearance) with mucin production.**

MANAGEMENT
- **Surgical resection in most cases.**

SQUAMOUS CELL LUNG CARCINOMA

- 60-80% arise from proximal portions of the tracheobronchial epithelium. Most are bronchial in origin.
- Classified as a type of non-small cell lung carcinoma. Often presents as an intraluminal mass.
- **Second most common cause of lung carcinoma (after Adenocarcinoma)** — 23% of cases.

RISK FACTORS
- **Cigarette smoking is strongly associated with Squamous cell carcinoma.**

CHARACTERISTICS
- **"CCCP": typically centrally located** and may be associated with a widened mediastinum. Associated with **cavitary lesions** (central necrosis with cavitation), **hypercalcemia**, & **Pancoast syndrome.**

DIAGNOSIS
- **Sputum cytology:** May be detected in the sputum since it is commonly central. Sputum cytology is highly specific but insensitive; the yield is highest when there are lesions in the central airways.
- **Fiberoptic bronchoscopy:** useful to evaluate lesions & obtain cytology for centrally located lesions.
- Biopsy: **keratinization by tumor cells and/or intracellular desmosomes** ("intercellular bridges").

SMALL CELL (OAT CELL) CARCINOMA (SCLC)

- **Aggressive type of lung cancer associated with early metastasis.**
- Comprises about 15% of all lung cancers. Associated with *MYC* gene mutation.

RISK FACTORS
- **Cigarette smoking** has the strongest association with Small cell lung cancer (SCLC) and Squamous cell carcinoma. SCLC is extremely rare in persons who have never smoked. Male gender.

CLINICAL MANIFESTATIONS
- Cough, chest pain, dyspnea, hemoptysis, wheezing, weight loss.
- **Paraneoplastic syndromes: SVC syndrome, SIADH (hyponatremia), Cushing syndrome (ectopic ACTH production), & Lambert-Eaton syndrome. SCLC is the most common solid tumor to present with paraneoplastic syndromes.**

DIAGNOSIS
- **Chest radiograph: mass often centrally located.** CT scan gives more information.
- Biopsy: usually CT-guided (if peripherally located), or via bronchoscopy (if centrally located).
- Histology: **sheets of small dark blue cells with rosette formation (about 2 times the size of resting lymphocytes)** that lack nucleoli but have a high nuclear: cytoplasm ratio. The size of the cells primarily distinguish small cell from NSCLC.

MANAGEMENT
- **Chemotherapy is the treatment for most (with or without radiation) because they are often metastatic at the time of presentation.**

LARGE CELL CARCINOMA (LCC)

- Large cell carcinoma (LCC) is a malignant epithelial neoplasm lacking glandular, squamous, or neuroendocrine differentiation by light microscopy and immunohistochemistry (diagnosis of exclusion).
- **Highly associated with smoking.**
- **LCC classically presents as a large peripheral mass with prominent necrosis.**
- Histology: **pleomorphic giant cells** — sheets of round to polygonal cells with prominent nucleoli and abundant pale staining cytoplasm without differentiating features.
- Associated with a **poor prognosis.**

PARANEOPLASTIC MANIFESTATIONS OF LUNG CANCER

- Set of systemic symptoms and/or signs due to tumor release of hormones & cytokines or by an immune response against the tumor.
- Examples: SVC syndrome, SIADH (hyponatremia), Cushing syndrome, & Lambert-Eaton syndrome.
- Small cell lung carcinoma is the most common solid tumor to present with paraneoplastic syndromes.

SUPERIOR VENA CAVA (SVC) SYNDROME

- Signs and symptoms due to partial or complete extrinsic obstruction of blood flow through the SVC.

ETIOLOGIES
- **Small cell bronchogenic carcinoma most common**, non-Hodgkin lymphoma, SVC stenosis.

CLINICAL MANIFESTATIONS
- Facial, neck, or upper extremity edema, facial plethora, chest pain, respiratory symptoms, or neurologic manifestations. Dyspnea is the most common presenting symptom.
- Physical examination: **dilated & prominent neck & chest veins**.

DIAGNOSIS
- Chest radiograph: may show right hilar mass or widening of the mediastinum.
- Contrast-enhanced CT scan provides better imaging and can assess the degree of obstruction.

MANAGEMENT
- Histologic diagnosis is required prior to initiating specific antitumor therapy.
- For patients **with life-threatening symptoms** (eg, stridor due to central airway obstruction, respiratory compromise, severe laryngeal edema, or depressed CNS function), **initial stabilization (secure airway, support breathing and circulation), expedient confirmation of the diagnosis, & immediate endovenous intervention (eg, thrombus removal/stent placement).**

LAMBERT-EATON MYASTHENIC SYNDROME

- **Antibodies against presynaptic voltage-gated calcium channels** prevent acetylcholine release in the neuromuscular junction, leading to muscle weakness.
- **Most commonly associated with Small cell lung cancer** & other malignancies.

CLINICAL MANIFESTATIONS
- **Proximal muscle weakness that <u>improves with repeated muscle use</u>** (unlike Myasthenia gravis). The weakness may cause difficulty arising from a chair, gait alteration, or managing stairs. The pattern of progression is often proximal to distal, and caudal to cranial.
- **<u>Autonomic symptoms</u>: dry mouth most common,** postural hypotension, & erectile dysfunction.
Physical examination:
- **Hyporeflexia** & sluggish pupillary response. No significant muscle atrophy.

DIAGNOSIS
- **<u>Voltage-gated calcium channel antibody assay</u>** positive in 85-95% of LEMS.
- **<u>Electrophysiology</u>: <u>Repetitive nerve stimulation (RNS) testing</u> — low CMAP (compound muscle action potential) amplitude at rest, reproducible post-exercise increase in CMAP,** a decremental response at low rates of RNS, and an incremental response at high-rate stimulation.
- CT or MRI of the chest to assess for underlying malignancy.

MANAGEMENT
- **Treat the underlying malignancy.**
- Initial symptomatic management: Amifampridine (3,4-diaminopyridine). Pyridostigmine.
- Second-line: Plasmapheresis, IVIG, oral immunosuppressants.

SUPERIOR SULCUS (PANCOAST) TUMORS

- **Tumors located in the superior sulcus (near the apex)** characterized by a distinct pattern of signs and symptoms.
- The diagnosis of Pancoast tumor is determined by the location of the tumor, not the histology.

ETIOLOGIES
- **Non-small cell lung carcinoma >95% of all cases (eg, Squamous cell lung carcinoma).**

PATHOPHYSIOLOGY
- Tumor compression of the lower brachial plexus, ulnar nerve, and/or cervical sympathetic nerve chain.

CLINICAL MANIFESTATIONS
- **Shoulder & arm pain most common initial symptom** in the distribution of the C8, T1, and T2 dermatomes. Pain can progress and radiate up to the head and neck.
- **Horner syndrome: the triad of ipsilateral ptosis, miosis, and anhidrosis** due to involvement of the paravertebral sympathetic chain. May be preceded by ipsilateral flushing & facial diaphoresis.
- **Weakness and/or atrophy of the muscles of the hand and/or arm.**
- **Ulnar neuropathy** may occur.
- Because the tumors are usually peripheral, pulmonary symptoms (eg, cough, dyspnea, hemoptysis) are uncommon until the disease is advances.

DIAGNOSIS
- **Chest radiograph often initial test ordered** but MRI is better to assess the extent of infiltration of adjacent tissues.
- Core needle biopsy is generally preferred to provide tissue for histology and molecular markers.

MANAGEMENT
- For patients with resectable disease, concurrent chemoradiotherapy is the recommended initial step in management. This is followed by surgical resection if there is no evidence of distant metastases or local progression and postoperative chemotherapy.
- Adjuvant Atezolizumab is now used for patients with stage II to IIIA non-small cell lung cancer (NSCLC) with programmed cell death ligand 1 (PD-L1) expression of ≥1%.

Pancoast tumor labeled as P, non-small cell lung carcinoma, right lung.

Horner's syndrome: miosis, ptosis, anhidrosis (due to cervical cranial nerve sympathetic compression).

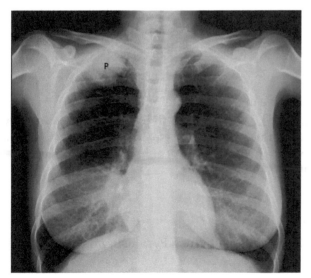

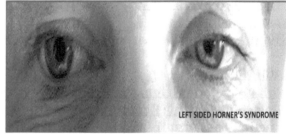

LEFT SIDED HORNER'S SYNDROME

MESOTHELIOMA

- **Rare tumor originating from the mesothelial surface of the pleura (80%), peritoneum** (second most common), tunica vaginalis, or pericardium. ¾ are malignant (poor prognosis if malignant).
- **Chronic asbestos exposure in 80%** (the risk of Mesothelioma is much less than that of Lung cancer). Smoking is <u>not</u> a risk factor for Mesothelioma, compared to other lung cancers.

CLINICAL MANIFESTATIONS
- <u>Pleural mesothelioma:</u> pleuritic chest pain, dyspnea, fever, night sweats, weight loss, hemoptysis.

DIAGNOSIS
- <u>Chest radiograph:</u> **unilateral pleural thickening and bloody pleural effusions are common.**
- <u>Pleural biopsy:</u> closed via video-assisted thoracoscopy (VATS), or open thoracotomy definitive.

MANAGEMENT
- <u>Surgical candidates:</u> Combined approach may include chemotherapy (eg, a platinum agent plus Pemetrexed), macroscopic complete resection with either pleurectomy/decortication or radical extrapleural pneumonectomy, and radiation therapy.
- <u>Not a surgical candidate:</u> systemic chemotherapy and/or palliative radiation therapy.

FOREIGN BODY ASPIRATION

- Aerodigestive foreign body causing varying amounts of obstruction to the airway.
- Common items include food, coins, toys food and balloons. **Peanuts are the most common foreign body aspirated in children.**
- **Mean age is 2 years** (incisors are used to bite the food but absence of molars make it difficult to grind food).
- The main cause of death is due to hypoxic-ischemic brain injury and less commonly, pulmonary hemorrhage.
- Complications include bronchiectasis, pneumonia, lung abscess, and atelectasis.
- **Most common on the right side**, due to wider, more vertical, & shorter right main bronchus.
- <u>Position may influence location:</u>
  <u>Supine:</u> most common in superior segment of the right lower lobe.
  <u>Sitting/standing:</u> most common in posterobasal segment of the right lower lobe.
  <u>Lying on right side:</u> most common in right middle lobe or posterior segment of the right upper lobe.

CLINICAL MANIFESTATIONS
- **Asymptomatic or sudden onset of choking, cough, and dyspnea**.
- <u>Physical examination:</u> **wheezing or asymmetric breath sounds.** May be normal.

DIAGNOSIS
- **Chest radiographs: air trapping most common finding in children,** atelectasis, pneumothorax. A normal chest radiograph does not rule out FB aspiration. May order additional neck films.
- <u>CT chest:</u> may be indicated in symptomatic patients with negative radiographs.
- **Rigid bronchoscopy definitive diagnostic test (also therapeutic** because object can be removed). Flexible rather than rigid bronchoscopy may be used for diagnostic purposes in cases when the diagnosis is not clear or if the FBA is known but the location is unclear.

MANAGEMENT
- **Removal of foreign object via rigid bronchoscopy.** Thoracotomy if refractory to bronchoscopy.
- In acute choking, the Heimlich maneuver should be performed. Emergency tracheostomy performed if Heimlich maneuver is not successful.

PLEURAL EFFUSION

- Abnormal accumulation of fluid in the pleural space; not a disease itself but a sign of a disease.

TYPES
- **Parapneumonic effusions uninfected pleural fluid** associated with bacterial pneumonia, lung abscess, or bronchiectasis. Most common cause of exudative Pleural effusion in the US.
- **Empyema** refers to a grossly purulent (infected) Pleural effusion.
- **Hydrothorax:** fluid in the cavity, including CHF; In Cirrhosis, the effusion is usually right-sided and frequently large enough to produce severe dyspnea.
- Chylothorax: accumulation of lymphatic fluid, often from disruption of the thoracic duct. Associated with persistent turbidity after centrifuge (if not ⇨ empyemic).
- Hemothorax gross blood in the pleural space, usually after chest trauma or instrumentation.

[1] Transudate effusions:
- **Transudative effusions occur when systemic factors lead to either (1) increased hydrostatic pressure or (2) decreased oncotic pressure.** Both are associated with normal capillary integrity.
- **Etiologies: Congestive heart failure (CHF) most common cause (>90%), Nephrotic syndrome, Cirrhosis,** Atelectasis, Hypoalbuminemia, Peritoneal dialysis, Pulmonary embolism.

[2] Exudate effusions:
- **Increased capillary permeability: Any condition associated with (1) infection and/or (2) inflammation** [eg, Pneumonia, Tuberculosis, malignancies (eg, lung cancer, breast cancer, lymphoma), Inflammatory disorders], leading to increased capillary permeability, often via local factors. **Pulmonary embolism can be exudative or rarely transudative.**
- As a result of increased mesothelial and capillary permeability due to the infectious or inflammatory process, exudative effusions contains plasma, proteins, WBCs, platelets, & RBCs.

PRESENTATION
- Clinical manifestations: asymptomatic or may complain of dyspnea, pleuritic chest pain, or cough.
- **Physical examination: dullness to percussion, decreased fremitus, decreased breath sounds.** May have a pleural friction rub (due to pleuritis). Asymmetric chest expansion if large.

DIAGNOSIS
- **Chest radiographs: initial test of choice — blunting of the costophrenic angles (meniscus sign).** Lateral decubitus also helpful to differentiate loculations from empyema and detect smaller effusions. In extreme cases, it may cause lung collapse or mediastinal shift to the contralateral side.
  - PA/lateral: >175 cc can obscure the lateral costophrenic sulcus (500 cc for the diaphragm). **Blunting of costophrenic angles (⊕ menisci sign)** ± loculations (due to Pleural adhesions).
  - **Lateral decubitus films: best** — detects smaller effusions & differentiates loculations & empyema from new effusions or scarring.
- **Thoracentesis: diagnostic criterion standard — determining the cause of a Pleural effusion is greatly facilitated by analysis of the pleural fluid (helps to distinguish between transudate and exudate).** Can be diagnostic and therapeutic. Not usually performed if the cause is clear.
  Light's criteria: an exudate is present if **any** of these 3 are present
      [1] pleural fluid protein: serum protein >0.5 OR
      [2] Pleural fluid LDH: serum LDH >0.6 OR
      [3] Pleural fluid LDH >2/3 the upper limit of normal LDH
  Indications: diagnostic Thoracentesis should be performed if there is a new large Pleural effusion and no obvious clinically apparent cause (obvious causes include CHF, Pneumonia), an atypical presentation, or failure of an effusion to resolve. Observation is appropriate in some situations (symmetric bilateral pleural effusions in the setting of Decompensated heart failure).

- **CT scan or US: more accurate** than Lateral decubitus film to assess loculated effusions or Empyema.

MANAGEMENT

- **Treat the underlying disease** mainstay of treatment (Pleural effusion is a sign of an underlying disease).
- Thoracentesis: diagnostic and therapeutic. Not always needed. Don't remove >1.5 liters during any one procedure.
- **Chest tube fluid drainage:** if empyema (eg, pleural fluid pH <7.2, glucose <40 mg/dL, or positive gram stain of pleural fluid),** along with antibiotics. Instillation of intrapleural fibrinolytics (eg, Streptokinase) and DNAse may improve or facilitate drainage.
- Pleurodesis: if malignant or chronic effusions to remove the fluid and stop accumulation. Talc is most commonly used, Doxycycline, Minocycline. Bleomycin rarely used due toxicity.

PLEURAL EFFUSION

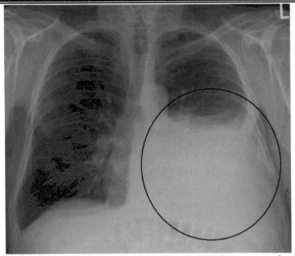

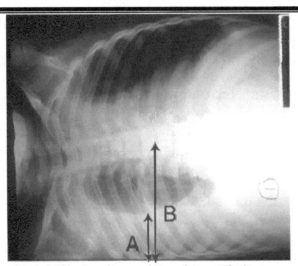

Pleural Effusion PA Film: clear costophrenic angle on the right side with **blunting of the costophrenic angle (meniscus sign)** on the left side.

Pleural Effusion (Lateral Decubitus Film): layering of the fluid.

PNEUMOTHORAX

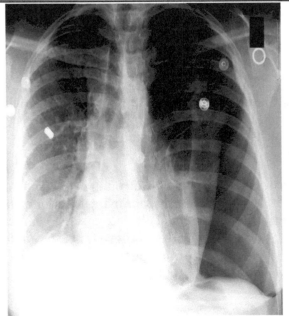

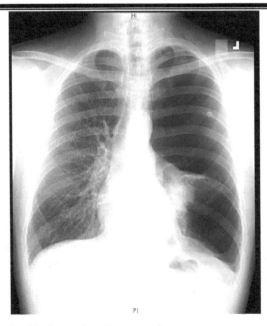

Linear shadow of visceral pleura with **decreased peripheral lung markings on the left side**

L-sided tension Pneumothorax: **mediastinal shift** to the right side.

PNEUMOTHORAX

- Air in the pleural space, leading to collapse of the lung from the positive intrapleural air pressure.

TYPES
- **Primary spontaneous (PSP): atraumatic and idiopathic with no underlying lung disease.** Due to bleb rupture. Mainly affects **tall, thin men 20-40 years of age, smokers,** family history of PTX.
- **Secondary spontaneous (SSP): underlying lung disease** (eg, COPD, Asthma).
- Traumatic: iatrogenic (eg, during CPR, thoracentesis, PEEP ventilation, subclavian line). Car accidents.
- **Tension: any type of Pneumothorax in which positive air pressure pushes the trachea, great vessels, &/or heart to the contralateral side.**
- Catamenial: occurs during menstruation due to ectopic endometrial tissue in the pleural space.

CLINICAL MANIFESTATIONS
- **Sudden onset of dyspnea & chest pain — usually pleuritic, ipsilateral, unilateral,** non-exertional.

Physical examination:
- **Air: Hyperresonance to percussion, decreased fremitus, & decreased breath sounds** over the affected area. Unequal (unilateral) chest expansion, decreased movement of the chest.
- **Tension: increased jugular venous distention (JVP), systemic hypotension, pulsus paradoxus.**

DIAGNOSIS
- **Chest radiograph: initial test of choice (expiratory upright view preferred).**
  - **Decreased peripheral markings extending into the periphery** (collapsed lung tissue).
  - **Companion lines: visceral pleural line running parallel with the ribs.**
  - **Deep sulcus sign** on supine film — an abnormally radiolucent & deeper costophrenic sulcus.

MANAGEMENT
Small PSP: <3 cm from chest wall at the apex or <15-20% the diameter of the hemithorax:
- **Small & first episode: observation for 4-6 hours with or without supplemental oxygen if the patient is reliable.** May be discharged if stable & repeat films after 6 hours excludes progression. Chest tube thoracostomy may be performed if worse on repeat films.

Large PSP (>3 cm from chest the wall at the apex):
- **Needle or small-bore catheter aspiration (either preferred) or if the aspiration fails, chest tube or catheter thoracostomy.** Placement of a small-bore chest tube attached to a one-way Heimlich valve provides protection against the development of Tension pneumothorax.
- Symptomatically treatment and monitoring with serial chest radiographs every 24 hours.

Stable, secondary spontaneous Pneumothorax (SSP):
- **Nearly all patients with secondary spontaneous Pneumothorax should be treated with chest tube placement (tube thoracostomy) and hospitalization.** Most should also be treated with thoracoscopy or thoracotomy with the stapling of blebs and pleural abrasion.

Tension Pneumothorax:
- **Needle aspiration followed by chest tube thoracostomy.** Needle aspiration often performed in the 2nd or 3rd intercostal space (midclavicular line) or 4th or 5th intercostal space in the anterior axillary line above the rib margin. Thoracostomy may be performed without needle decompression in some.
- Other: **Video-assisted thoracoscopic surgery (VATS) may be indicated if there is persistent leak after chest tube placement or no regression with chest tube, persistent or recurrent pneumothoracies.** Thoracotomy is a more invasive option.

PATIENT EDUCATION
- Avoid pressure changes for a minimum of 2 weeks (eg, high altitudes, smoking, unpressurized aircrafts, scuba diving, etc.).

HEMOTHORAX

- A type of Pleural effusion characterized by **blood in the pleural space**.

MECHANISMS OF INJURY
- **Bleeding from direct lung injury** is the most common cause of Hemothorax (lung parenchyma and intercostal or mammary blood vessels). In the setting of trauma (eg, MVA), hypovolemic shock is attributed to hemorrhage until proven otherwise.

DIAGNOSTIC IMAGING
- **Upright chest radiograph:** collections >200-300 mL are visualized on upright or decubitus CXR.
- Ultrasound: allows for more accurate diagnosis but is operator dependent.
- **CT scan of chest: has the highest sensitivity and specificity for detecting Hemothorax.**

MANAGEMENT
- **Tube thoracostomy**: Hemothorax >300-500 mL (eg, tube 28 French or larger). Large hemothoraces that remain undrained can result in infection and pulmonary fibrosis. **IV fluid resuscitation.**
- **Surgical thoracotomy: Immediate bloody drainage of ≥20 mL/kg, massive Hemothorax (≥1,500 mL), shock,** and persistent, substantial bleeding (generally 200-300 mL/hour).
- Small Hemothorax: small (<300 mL) and stable collections in patients not on positive-pressure ventilation may be managed with observation or needle aspiration and drainage.

TENSION PNEUMOTHORAX	SIGNIFICANT HEMOTHORAX
Examination:	**Examination:**
• **Obtructive shock: hypotension, tachycardia, distended neck veins.***	• **Hypovolemic shock: hypotension, tachycardia, and flat neck veins.***
• **Air: Absent breath sounds and hyperresonance to percussion.*** • Contralateral tracheal deviation.	• **Fluid: Decreased breath sounds and dullness to percussion.*** • Contralateral tracheal deviation.
Management • **Needle decompression followed by chest tube thoracostomy.**	**Management** • **Tube thoracostomy** should be performed; with immediate bloody drainage of >20 mL/kg (~1,500 mL) being an indication for emergent surgical thoracotomy.

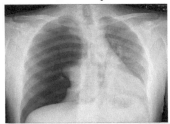
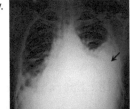

PULMONARY CONTUSION

- Direct injury to the lung resulting in both hemorrhage and edema in the absence of a pulmonary laceration. Damage results in ventilation-perfusion inequalities and decreased lung compliance.
- Pulmonary contusion is a common consequence of blunt chest trauma (compression-decompression injury to the chest), most often occurring from high-speed motor vehicle collisions (MVCs).

DIAGNOSTIC IMAGING
- **Chest radiograph: Irregular, non-lobar patchy ground-glass opacification of pulmonary parenchyma** is classic. ~One-third of the time, the contusion is not evident on initial radiographs.
- Chest CT provides better resolution but rarely alters management.

MANAGEMENT
- **Pain control and pulmonary toilet are the mainstays of treatment**. Prophylactic endotracheal intubation is not usually needed, but patients with hypoxia or difficulty ventilating require airway management. Fluid resuscitation with crystalloid to achieve euvolemia.
- Common complications include Pneumonia and Acute respiratory distress syndrome (ARDS).
- Pulmonary contusions generally develop over the first 24 hours and resolve in ~7-10 days

COSTOCHONDRITIS & TIETZE SYNDROME

COSTOCHONDRITIS

- Acute inflammation of the upper costal cartilages at the costochondral or costosternal junctions.

ETIOLOGIES
- Often idiopathic but can occur postviral or posttraumatic (eg, physical strain, excessive coughing).

CLINICAL MANIFESTATIONS
- **Pleuritic chest pain that may be worse with inspiration, coughing, or certain body movements.**

PHYSICAL EXAMINATION
- **Reproducible point chest wall tenderness** with palpation, most commonly involving the third, fourth, & fifth sternocostal joints. The diagnosis is based solely upon the ability to reproduce pain by palpation of tender areas.
- **The absence of palpable edema helps to distinguish Costochondritis from the less common Tietze syndrome.**

DIAGNOSIS
- Usually a diagnosis of exclusion. Labs, ECG, and radiographs are usually within normal limits.

MANAGEMENT
- **Supportive management — musculoskeletal chest pain from Costochondritis may be reduced with analgesia (eg, NSAIDS), ice or heat,** stretching exercises, and temporary activity restriction.

TIETZE SYNDROME

- Acute benign, painful, nonsuppurative localized swelling (inflammation) of the costal cartilages or the costosternal, sternoclavicular, or costochondral joints, **most often involving the area of the second and third ribs.**
- Most commonly seen in young adults & one area is usually involved.

ETIOLOGIES
- Often idiopathic but can occur postviral or posttraumatic (eg, physical strain, excessive coughing).

CLINICAL MANIFESTATIONS
- **Pleuritic chest pain** that may be worse with inspiration, coughing, or certain body movements.

PHYSICAL EXAMINATION
- **[1] Reproducible point chest wall tenderness with [2] palpable edema.**
  Most commonly involves the second and third costochondral junctions.
- **The presence of palpable edema distinguishes Tietze syndrome from Costochondritis.**

DIAGNOSIS
- Usually a diagnosis of exclusion. Labs, ECG, and radiographs are usually within normal limits.

MANAGEMENT
- **Supportive management — analgesia (eg, NSAIDS), ice or heat,** and temporary activity restriction.

PULMONARY HYPERTENSION

- **Elevated mean pulmonary arterial pressure ≥20 mmHg or ≥25 mmHg on resting cardiac catheterization** and a pulmonary vascular resistance ≥3 Wood units.

PATHOPHYSIOLOGY
- Increased pulmonary vascular resistance leads to right ventricular hypertrophy, increased RV pressure and eventually right-sided Heart failure.
- Primary: **Idiopathic. Most common in middle-aged or young women** (mean age of diagnosis 50 years) due to BMPR2 gene defect. The BMPR2 gene normally inhibits pulmonary vessel smooth muscle growth and vasoconstriction.
- Secondary: pulmonary HTN due to pulmonary disease, sleep apnea, Pulmonary embolism, cardiac, metabolic, or systemic disease (eg, connective tissue diseases).

CLASSIFICATION (GROUPS)

1	**Idiopathic pulmonary arterial hypertension (Primary).** Diagnosis of exclusion.
2	**Pulmonary HTN due to left heart disease** — eg, Left heart failure, mitral valve dysfunction.
3	**Pulmonary HTN due to hypoxemic or chronic lung disease** — eg, COPD, pulmonary fibrosis, interstitial lung disease, obstructive sleep apnea, Bronchiectasis.
4	**Pulmonary HTN due to chronic thromboembolic disease** — eg, Pulmonary embolism.
5	Pulmonary HTN multifactorial or other: eg, Sarcoidosis, Sickle cell disease, Schistosomiasis

CLINICAL MANIFESTATIONS
- **Dyspnea on exertion** (at rest if advanced), **lethargy, and/or fatigue most common.** Chest pain.

Physical examination:
- **Accentuated S2: due to prominent P2.** May have a **fixed or paradoxically split P2.***
- **Signs of right-sided Heart failure:** increased JVP, peripheral leg edema, ascites, hepatomegaly.
- **Tricuspid regurgitation (holosystolic murmur),** right ventricular heave, systolic ejection click.

DIAGNOSIS
- Chest radiograph: enlarged pulmonary arteries, interstitial/alveolar edema, right-sided heart failure.
- ECG: **cor pulmonale** — eg, RVH, right axis deviation, right atrial enlargement, right BBB. LVH.
- **Echocardiography with bubble study is the most important noninvasive screening test for suspected PH to [1] estimate the pulmonary artery pressure (presumptive diagnosis if ≥25 mmHg) and [2] assess ventricular function.** Findings of PH: **elevated right ventricular systolic pressure, hypertrophied and dilated right ventricle, and/or right ventricular dysfunction.**
- **Right heart catheterization: definitive diagnosis (criterion standard)** — [1] recommended as the confirmatory test for Pulmonary hypertension (directly measures pressures) and [2] can also be useful for assessment of the reversibility of PAH with vasodilatory therapy.
- CBC: **polycythemia with increased hematocrit.**

MANAGEMENT
- **Group 1: Oral Calcium channel blockers with extended release (eg, Nifedipine, Diltiazem, and Amlodipine) are useful in patients with a positive vasoreactivity test and significant vasodilator response during cardiac catheterization.** WHO functional class I (monotherapy). Functional class II & III (combination oral therapy) — **endothelin receptor antagonist (ERA)** and an agent that targets the nitric oxide-cyclic guanosine monophosphate (cGMP) pathway, typically a **phosphodiesterase 5 inhibitor** (PDE5I) [eg, **Ambrisentan + Tadalafil**]. Alternatives include PDE5I + Riociguat; or two agents from a different class eg, Macitentan + Sildenafil; Tadalafil + Bosentan; Riociguat + Bosentan; Selexipag plus ERA and/or PDE5I.
- **Group 2: treating Left heart failure and volume overload, primarily with loop diuretics.**
- **Group 3: supplemental oxygen if hypoxemia at rest or with physical activity.**
- **Group 4: long-term anticoagulation is recommended.** The most effective step in effectively reducing the resistance of pulmonary vessels is surgical pulmonary thromboendarterectomy.

PULMONARY EMBOLISM (PE)

- Mechanical obstruction of the pulmonary blood flow secondary to a blood clot — usually a thromboembolism from Deep venous thrombosis (DVT).
- PE and DVT are 2 manifestations of the same disease, known as Venous thromboembolic disease (VTE). Third most common cause of cardiovascular death in hospitalized patients.

ETIOLOGIES
- **DVT: 70% arise from deep veins in the leg/proximal thigh** (iliac, femoral, or popliteal veins). About 50-60% of patients with DVT will have a PE (many are asymptomatic). Rarely, PEs originate from pelvic, renal, or upper extremity veins or from the right heart chambers.
- Septic embolism from right-heart Endocarditis. Fat embolism from a long-bone fracture (eg, femur).

RISK FACTORS
Virchow's triad:
- **[1] Intimal damage:** eg, trauma, infection, inflammation.
- **[2] Venous stasis:** eg, prolonged immobilization, surgery, prolonged sitting >4 hours, stroke, bed rest (especially postoperative).
- **[3] Hypercoagulability:** eg, Factor V Leiden mutation, Protein C or S Deficiency, Antithrombin III deficiency, Oral contraceptives and estrogen replacement, malignancy (high risk of recurrent VTE), pregnancy, smoking, hemolytic anemias, Heparin-induced thrombocytopenia.

PATHOPHYSIOLOGY
- **Pulmonary vasculature occlusion is a mechanical obstruction of the vascular bed, resulting in hypoxemia (impaired gas exchange) and subsequent pulmonary vasoconstriction.**
- Most Pulmonary emboli are multiple, with the lower lobes involved more commonly involved than the upper lobes, and bilateral lung involvement being more common.

CLINICAL MANIFESTATIONS
- **Dyspnea (at rest or with exertion) is the most common presenting symptom (>70%), followed by chest pain (classically pleuritic but may be dull), and cough.** Dyspnea may be milder in peripheral PEs.
- **Classic triad [1] sudden onset of dyspnea (most common symptom), [2] pleuritic chest pain, & [3] hemoptysis (classic but rare — 13%).**
- May have mild or nonspecific symptoms or may be asymptomatic. Syncope if massive PE.

PHYSICAL EXAMINATION
- **Tachypnea most common sign** — respiratory rate >16/min (54%).
- **Hypoxia. Lung exam is usually normal.** Rales may be heard.
- Lower extremities: (47%) — DVT (eg, calf or thigh pain, erythema, tenderness, and/or swelling); signs of thrombophlebitis (eg, tenderness, palpable cords). Positive Homan sign (lacks sensitivity and specificity).
- **Tachycardia** (24%).
- Low-grade fever — temperature >100°F [37.8°C].
- **Loud P2** (accentuated pulmonic component of the second heart sound) in 15%.
- Diaphoresis.
- Phlegmasia curulea dolens: enlarged, blue, and tender leg (very rare finding).
- Massive PE: may present with dyspnea, presyncope or syncope, hypotension (obstructive shock), cyanosis, right ventricular failure, circulatory collapse, cariogenic shock, cardiac arrest, Pulseless electrical activity (PEA). Massive PE = usually due to central PE (saddle embolus) or extensive PE.

ANCILLARY TESTS IN PE:
- Chest radiographs, ECG, D-dimer, and possibly ABG are initial tests that may be ordered, but they don't directly look for PE.

Chest radiographs:
- **The chest radiograph is most often normal** but performed to exclude other common lung conditions (it does not establish the diagnosis of PE by itself). **A normal chest radiograph in the setting of hypoxia is highly suspicious for PE.**
- Abnormal findings: **atelectasis is the most common abnormal finding,** pleural effusion, or other nonspecific abnormalities.
- **Classic but rare findings** include **[1] Westermark's sign: sharp cut-off of pulmonary vessels with avascular markings in a segmental distribution distal to the PE, & [2] Hampton's hump: wedge-shaped, pleural-based opacification in the periphery of the lung,** most commonly due to Pulmonary embolism, pulmonary hemorrhaging, and lung infarction.

Electrocardiogram (ECG):
- **Nonspecific ST/T changes & sinus tachycardia are the most common ECG findings in PE** (70%) — Anterior ST-segment changes and T-wave inversion (V1-V4).
- **S1Q3T3 pattern: uncommon but most specific for PE** — wide deep S in lead I; both an isolated Q as well as T wave inversion in lead III but seen in <10%; right ventricular strain, right bundle branch block, or inferior Q waves. S1Q3T3 pattern may be seen due to right heart dysfunction.

D-dimer:
- **D-dimer testing has a high sensitivity but poor specificity and a high negative predictive value; hence, a normal D-dimer level makes acute PE or DVT unlikely with <u>low</u> pre-test probability for PE.** Normal D dimer is <500 ng/mL (fibrinogen equivalent units).
- **For most patients in whom the risk of PE is thought to be intermediate, a normal D-dimer (<500 ng/mL) also effectively excludes PE, and typically, no further testing is required.**
- **A positive D-dimer must be followed by a confirmatory study (eg, CTA chest).** Since the positive predictive value of elevated D-dimer levels is low, D-dimer is not useful for confirmation of PE.

Arterial blood gas (ABG):
- **Hypoxemia, hypocapnia, acute respiratory alkalosis (due to hyperventilation), and elevated alveolar-arterial gradient for oxygen are common findings — unexplained hypoxemia in the setting of a normal chest radiograph should increase the clinical suspicion for PE.**
- Hypercapnia, respiratory, and/or lactic acidosis are uncommon but can be seen in patients with massive PE associated with obstructive shock and respiratory arrest.

Pretest probability: Wells' criteria: used to determine the clinical probability of PE:
- 3 points for each — clinical signs and symptoms of DVT; PE is #1 diagnosis OR equally likely.
- 1.5 points for each — heart rate >100 bpm, immobilization at least 3 days OR surgery in the previous 4 weeks, or previous objectively diagnosed DVT or PE.
- 1 point for each — hemoptysis or malignancy (even if treated within 6 months).

- **Low probability: <2 points — may consider D-dimer or use PERC rule.**
- **Intermediate probability: 2-6 points — High-sensitivity D-dimer.** If D-dimer is negative [<500 ng/mL (fibrinogen equivalent units)], PE likely excluded and no further testing is generally required. If D-dimer is ≥500 ng/mL, then CTPA is performed. If CTPA is inconclusive or contraindicated, V/Q scan should be performed. **Some experts proceed directly to CTPA in patients on the higher end of the intermediate risk spectrum (eg, Wells score 4-6).**
- **High probability: >6 points — Emergent CTPA should be performed.** If CTPA is inconclusive or not feasible, perform a V/Q scan. In patients with a high clinical suspicion for PE, anticoagulation is started even before diagnostic imaging is obtained.

Low-risk patients: either (1) apply PERC rule OR (2) D-dimer testing may be used if low risk.

- **(1) PERC rule:** used to identify outpatients with a **low** clinical probability of PE in whom the risk of unnecessary testing outweighs the risk of PE. **In patients with a low probability of PE who fulfill all 8 PERC criteria, the likelihood of PE is sufficiently low that further testing is not indicated** (age <50 years, heart rate <100 beats/minute, O2 sat ≥95%, no hemoptysis, no estrogen use, no prior DVT or PE, no unilateral leg swelling, no surgery/trauma requiring hospitalization within the prior 4 weeks).
- **(2) D-dimer:** **testing is indicated in low-risk patients where PERC cannot be applied (eg, inpatients, critically ill patients) or if all 8 PERC criteria are not fulfilled.** If D-dimer is negative [<500 ng/mL (fibrinogen equivalent units)], no further testing is required. If the D-dimer is ≥500 ng/mL, diagnostic imaging should be performed (eg, CT pulmonary angiography).

IMAGING FOR PE:

[1] CT pulmonary angiography (CTPA):

- **CT pulmonary angiography (CTPA, Chest CT angiogram with contrast) is the first-choice diagnostic imaging modality (criterion standard) for PE** because it is >90% sensitive and specific for the diagnosis of PE in most patients, has a high negative predictive value, and excellent ability to identify other conditions that cause dyspnea and chest pain (eg, Pneumonia, Aortic dissection). The risk of PE after a negative CT scan in patients with a low or intermediate clinical probability of PE is <2%.
- Although CTPA requires administration of intravenous radiocontrast dye, it is otherwise noninvasive.
- **Patients with intermediate or high pretest probability of PE (or PE likely) or those with an elevated D-dimer should undergo a CTPA.**
- Results: **A positive CTPA for PE demonstrates a filling defect** in any branch of the pulmonary artery (main, lobar, segmental, subsegmental) by contrast enhancement. A negative CTPA indicates that the likelihood of PE is low (usually, no further testing is required, unless inadequate imaging is suspected). An inconclusive CTPA result may necessitate alternate imaging, such as V/Q scanning.

[2] Ventilation/perfusion (V/Q) scan:

- **V/Q scan used in patients in whom CT scan cannot be performed — eg, [A] pregnancy (due to radiation risk with CT) or [B] increased creatinine (risk of kidney injury due to contrast,** kidney dysfunction), contrast cannot be given (eg, contrast induced anaphylaxis), or if CT is unavailable. VQ scan may also be helpful if CTPA is inconclusive.
- A normal chest radiograph is usually required prior to V/Q scanning.
- **V/Q scanning is often the test of choice for the diagnosis of PE in pregnancy.**
- Results: In patients with normal V/Q scan & any clinical probability, no further testing is necessary. In patients with a low-probability V/Q scan and low clinical probability (eg, Wells score <2), no further testing is necessary. In patients with a high-probability V/Q scan and high clinical probability (eg, Wells score >6), immediate treatment is indicated. All other combinations of V/Q scan results and clinical pretest probabilities are indeterminate (inconclusive), and further testing is required (eg, lower extremity compression ultrasonography with Doppler to evaluate for coexisting DVT).

Venous duplex ultrasound (US)

- Lower extremity compression Doppler US is not usually an initial test in evaluation of suspected PE.
- Indications: Because of the low sensitivity of Doppler ultrasonography in this setting, it is reserved for patients suspected of having a PE but in whom definitive imaging (eg, CTPA, V/Q scanning) is contraindicated or indeterminate. 70% of patients with PE will have DVT on evaluation.
- Results after definitive imaging: If lower-extremity Doppler ultrasonography is positive, patients can be treated (usually anticoagulation). If Doppler ultrasonography is negative and the clinical suspicion for PE is low or intermediate, it is generally considered safe to withhold anticoagulation and monitor for DVT with serial ultrasonography (eg, twice a week for 2 weeks) until chest imaging can be performed (eg, after treatment of contrast allergy).

Catheter-based Pulmonary angiography:
- Invasive catheter-based Pulmonary angiography was the historical criterion standard. With the widespread use of CTPA, Catheter-based angiography is not usually performed.
- Reserved for rare circumstances for patients with a high clinical probability of PE, in whom CTPA or V/Q scanning is nondiagnostic. The primary use for Pulmonary angiography is for catheter-directed therapy (thrombolytics or for mechanical thrombectomy) in the treatment of massive unstable PE.

MANAGEMENT OF PE:

Anticoagulation: mainstay first-line therapy for most patients with stable VTE. 3 major options:
- **[1] parenteral therapy switched after 5 days to a novel oral anticoagulant (eg, Direct thrombin inhibitor or anti-Xa agent).**
- **[2] oral anticoagulant monotherapy with the anti-Xa agents Rivaroxaban or Apixaban** with a 3-week or 1-week loading dose, respectively, followed by a maintenance dose <u>without</u> parenteral anticoagulation. **Direct oral anticoagulants are alternatives and often preferred to Warfarin for prophylaxis and treatment of PE — Factor Xa inhibitors (eg, Apixaban or Rivaroxaban) or Direct thrombin inhibitors (eg, Dabigatran).** Direct acting oral anticoagulants (DOACs) offer predictable pharmacokinetics and pharmacodynamics, few drug interactions, & no lab monitoring.
- **[3]** the classical but waning strategy of **parenteral anticoagulation [eg, subcutaneous LMW Heparin or Fondaparinux, or less commonly unfractionated Heparin (UFH)] "bridged" to Warfarin. In general, the use of LMWH or Fondaparinux is recommended over IV or SC Unfractionated heparin (UFH)** because LMWHs are as effective but have faster therapeutic activity in the treatment of VTE and have a less incidence of inducing major bleeding and Heparin-induced thrombocytopenia. **Warfarin, a vitamin K antagonist should be started on the same day as anticoagulant therapy in patients with acute PE.** Parenteral anticoagulation and Warfarin should be continued together for a minimum of at least 5 days and until the INR is 2-3. **LMWH monotherapy preferred in stable pregnant females and in patients with malignancy.**

Hemodynamically stable:
- **[1] Anticoagulation: is the mainstay first-line therapy for most VTE.** Anticoagulation impedes additional thrombus formation, allowing endogenous fibrinolytic mechanisms to lyse the existing clot, decreasing mortality and recurrence of PE. **In patients with a high clinical suspicion for PE, anticoagulation is started even before diagnostic imaging is obtained.**
- **[2] Inferior vena cava (IVC) filter: The 2 principal indications for insertion of an IVC filter are (1) stable patients in whom anticoagulation is unsuccessful (eg, PE despite adequate anticoagulation) or (2) stable PE in whom anticoagulation is contraindicated** [eg, bleeding disorder or a recent history (past 3 months) of active bleed, CVA, or recent intracranial bleed]. **(3) Right ventricular dysfunction is seen on echocardiogram** (with RV dysfunction, the next PE, even if small, can be fatal). IVC filters block the path of travel of emboli and prevent them from entering the pulmonary circulation. Retrievable filters are preferred, so that once the contraindication has resolved, the filter can be removed, and patients can be anticoagulated.

Hemodynamically unstable:
- **[1] Thrombolysis: to restore reperfusion [eg, Recombinant tissue plasminogen activator (Alteplase),** Streptokinase, Urokinase] **is the first-line management of hemodynamically unstable patients with PE (eg, systolic blood pressure <90 mmHg) or severe PE (eg, right-sided Heart failure,** right ventricular dilation, right ventricular hypokinesis) **if there are no contraindications to systemic thrombolysis.** Thrombolytics increase plasmin levels, directly lysing intravascular thrombi, resulting in rapid restoration of perfusion, resolution of emboli, and hemodynamic stabilization. Thrombolytics are contraindicated if bleeding disorder or a recent history (past 3 months) of active bleed, CVA, or recent intracranial bleed. Relative contraindications: uncontrolled hypertension & surgery or trauma within 6 weeks.
- **[2] Embolectomy:** (mechanical or surgical) **indicated in hemodynamically unstable or massive PE in whom thrombolytic therapy is contraindicated or in those who fail thrombolysis.**

Duration of anticoagulation therapy:
- **First thromboembolic event occurring in the setting of reversible risk factors, such as immobilization, surgery, or trauma, should receive anticoagulation therapy for <u>at least 3 months</u>.**
- All patients with unprovoked PE receive 3 months of treatment with anticoagulation over a shorter duration of treatment and have an assessment of the risk-benefit ratio of extended therapy at the end of 3 months.

<u>SPECIAL POPULATIONS</u>
<u>Pregnant females</u>:
- **<u>LMWH</u>: Adjusted-dose subcutaneous (SC) Low molecular weight heparin (LMWH) first-line anticoagulant therapy for stable pregnant patients**, rather than adjusted dose intravenous (IV) or subcutaneous unfractionated Heparin, because **LMWH does not cross the placenta,** is not associated with fetal or neonatal complications, and LMWH improves the live-birth rate in high-risk pregnancies (eg, Antiphospholipid syndrome, thrombophilia, recurrent fetal loss).
- <u>Avoid</u>: Vitamin K antagonists (eg, Warfarin), oral direct thrombin inhibitors (eg, Dabigatran), or anti-Xa inhibitors (eg, Apixaban, Rivaroxaban) are generally avoided; Warfarin is teratogenic.

<u>Malignancy</u>
- **<u>LMWH</u>: Low molecular weight (LMW) heparin (eg, Enoxaparin, Dalteparin) monotherapy is first-line anticoagulant therapy for most patients with VTE and malignancy**, rather than unfractionated Heparin (UFH), who do not have severe renal insufficiency (eg, creatinine clearance <30 mL/minute) or a contraindication to anticoagulation. LMWH is preferred because compared with patients who do not have malignancy, anticoagulation in patients with malignancy is complicated due to higher than usual rates of recurrent VTE and bleeding while on anticoagulation, in addition to the impact of comorbidities, procedures, and medications.
- <u>Apixaban</u>, a direct oral anticoagulant (DOAC), is an alternative as a monotherapeutic option in patients who do not want to perform injections with LMWH.

<u>Renal dysfunction</u>:
- **<u>Unfractionated Heparin</u> is preferred** (eg, creatinine clearance <30 mL/minute) or those in whom a need to discontinue or reverse anticoagulation is anticipated in the near future. Monitor UFH effectiveness via PTT levels & monitor serum creatinine levels. Renally-dosed LMW Heparin.

<u>Antiphospholipid antibody syndrome</u>:
- <u>Long-term</u>: **Indefinite treatment with a vitamin K antagonist (Warfarin)** may be recommended for prevention of PE in **nonpregnant patients with Antiphospholipid antibody syndrome.**

<u>PROPHYLAXIS</u>
- **Prevention is the single most important step in regard to PE.**
- Patients at highest risk include those with critical illness, cancer, stroke, myocardial infarction, old age (>75 years), prolonged immobility, obesity, kidney disease, previous VTE, and hypercoagulable states.
- Hospitalized patients with one or more of these risk factors and an acute medical illness should receive pharmacologic thromboprophylaxis.

[1] <u>Low risk</u>:
- **Early ambulation for low-risk, minor procedures in patients <40 years of age.**

[2] <u>Moderate risk</u>:
- **<u>Nonpharmacologic</u>:** consider early ambulation in addition to intermittent pneumatic compression devices, venodyne boots, and elastic stockings.

[3] <u>High risk</u>:
- **<u>Combination therapy</u>: of medical & pharmacological measures may be needed. Low molecular weight Heparin in patients undergoing orthopedic or neurosurgical procedures, trauma.**

CLASSIC WORKUP OF PULMONARY EMBOLISM (PE)

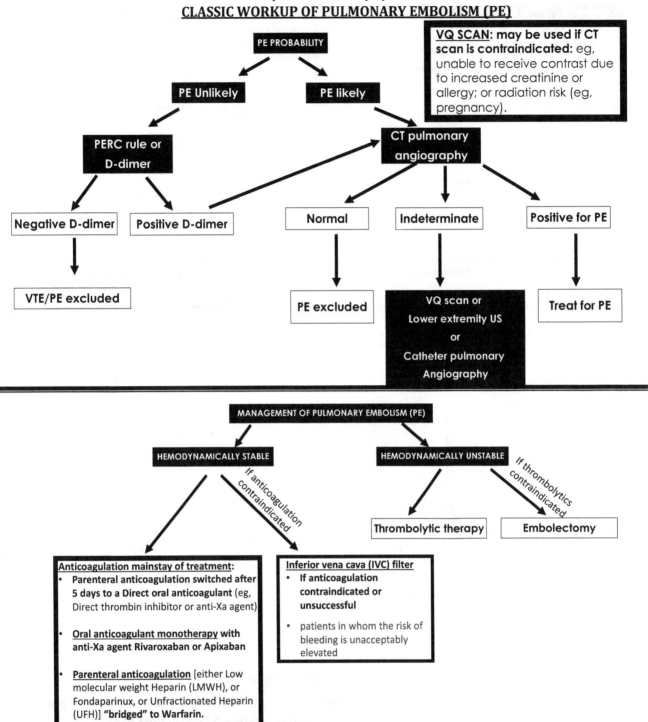

The Pulmonary Embolism Rule Out Criteria (PERC) is used in patients with a **low clinical probability of PE**.
The following 8 are part of the PERC rule:

1. Age <50 years
2. Heart rate <100 beats/minute
3. Oxyhemoglobin saturation ≥95%
4. No hemoptysis
5. No estrogen use
6. No prior DVT or PE
7. No unilateral leg swelling
8. No surgery/trauma requiring hospitalization within the prior four weeks.

- **In patients with low risk who meet all 8 criteria, no further testing for PE is needed.**
- **In patients with low risk but do not fulfill all 8 criteria, D-dimer testing is indicated.**

LOW MOLECULAR WEIGHT HEPARIN (LMWH)	UNFRACTIONATED HEPARIN (UFH)
• **MOA:** potentiates antithrombin III - works more on factor Xa than thrombin (Factor IIa).	• **MOA:** potentiates antithrombin III, inhibits thrombin & other coagulation factors.
• **SQ injection. Compliant, low-risk patients can be discharged home during bridging therapy.**	• Continuous IV drip – requires hospitalization for bridging therapy.
• **Duration of action ~12 hours.**	• **Duration of Action: 1 hour after IV drip is discontinued.**
• **No need to monitor PTT** (weight based – more predictable dosing).	• **Must monitor PTT 1.5-2.5x normal value.**
• **Protamine Sulfate is the antidote** (not as effective as it is for UFH).	• **Protamine Sulfate is the antidote.**
• **Lower risk of HIT:** higher anti Xa-IIa ratio means less potential binding with platelets.	**Heparin Induced Thrombocytopenia:** • Heparin acts as a hapten (stimulates the immune response when attached to platelet factor 4). This complex activates platelets, causing simultaneous thrombocytopenia & thrombosis.
• **Contraindications: Renal failure** (Cr >2.0) because LMWH excreted by kidneys, **Thrombocytopenia.**	• **Management:** Factor Xa inhibitors or Direct thrombin inhibitors (eg, Argatroban or Bivalirudin, Apixaban). DO NOT use Warfarin (may develop necrosis).

CXR FINDINGS IN PULMONARY EMBOLISM

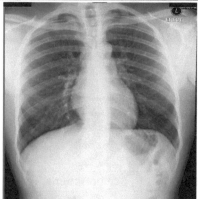

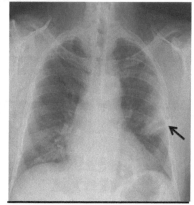

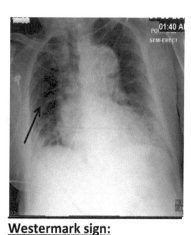

Normal CXR:
Most common finding in PE

Atelectasis most common abnormal finding on CXR

Hampton's Hump:
Wedge-shaped infiltrate or infarction (arrow).
Classic (not common)

Westermark sign:
Avascular markings distal to the area of the embolus (arrow).
Classic (not common)

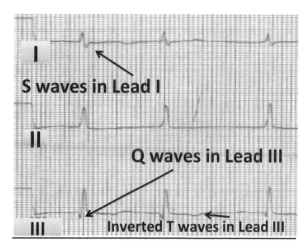

ECG FINDINGS IN PE:
❶ Nonspecific ST/T changes and Sinus tachycardia are the most common ECG findings in PE.

❷ **S1Q3T3:** more specific:
- Deep S in lead I
- Pathological Q wave & T wave inversion in lead III.

S1Q3T3 due to the presence of <u>cor pulmonale</u> with a large Pulmonary embolus.
Classic (not most common).

ACUTE RESPIRATORY DISTRESS SYNDROME (ARDS)

- Acute, diffuse inflammatory form of lung injury characterized by **[1] rapid onset of severe dyspnea, [2] refractory hypoxemia, & [3] diffuse pulmonary infiltrates, leading to respiratory failure** due to a variety of causes not fully explained by Heart failure or volume overload.

PATHOPHYSIOLOGY
- **ARDS is a consequence of an alveolar injury producing <u>diffuse alveolar damage</u> (capillary endothelium and alveolar epithelium damage)** via an inflammatory response.

RISK FACTORS
- **Most commonly develops in critically ill patients — Pneumonia and Sepsis (~40–60%).** Sepsis most common cause. Severe trauma, Pancreatitis, aspiration of gastric contents, near drowning.

CLINICAL MANIFESTATIONS
- <u>Physical examination</u>: labored breathing, tachypnea, intercostal retractions, and crackles.

ARDS should be suspected in patients with:
- **[1] <u>dyspnea</u>: acute onset of progressive symptoms of profound dyspnea** (respiratory distress)
- **[2] <u>hypoxemia</u>** with an increasing requirement for oxygen often progressing to respiratory failure,
- **[3] <u>alveolar infiltrates</u> on chest imaging within 6-72 hours of an inciting event (up to 7 days).**

- **<u>Severe hypoxemia</u> refractory to supplemental oxygen.** PaO/FiO ratio of < 300 mmHg.

HYPOXEMIA	PaO$_2$/FIO$_2$ ratio (mmHg)	VENTILATION
Mild:	201 – 300 mmHg	PEEP or CPAP ≥5cm H$_2$0 (formerly Acute Lung Injury).
Moderate:	101 – 200 mmHg	PEEP ≥5 cm H$_2$0
Severe:	≤100 mmHg	PEEP ≥5 cm H$_2$0

- **<u>Chest radiographs:</u> bilateral diffuse pulmonary infiltrates similar to CHF but ARDS classically spares the costophrenic angles.**

ADULT RESPIRATORY DISTRESS SYNDROME
Pulmonary Capillary Wedge Pressure:
- CXR of ARDS & cardiogenic pulmonary edema looks the same
- PCWP <18mmHg→ ARDS*
- PCWP >18mmHg→ Cardio Pul. Edema

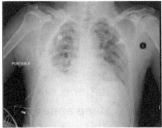
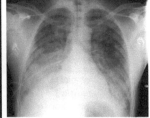

Cardiogenic Pulmonary Edema   **ARDS**

MANAGEMENT
- **Noninvasive or mechanical ventilation + treat the underlying cause that led to ARDS:**
  - **<u>Positive end-expiration pressure</u> (PEEP) improves hypoxemia** by preventing alveolar collapse, improves the VQ mismatch & increases functional residual capacity.
  - **<u>Low tidal volume</u> ventilation** — a tidal volume of ~6 mL/kg of predicted body weight (PBW) or less (4-8 mL/kg) should be used as a first approach in many patients with ARDS prevents "volutrauma". LTVV is typically performed using a volume-limited assist control mode, targets a plateau pressure (Pplat) 30 ≤cm H$_2$0, and applies PEEP, and respiratory rate <35 breaths per minute. LTVV has been shown to decrease non-pulmonary organ failure and weaning.
  - **<u>Positive pressure (PEEP):</u> prevents "atelectrauma" from recurrent alveolar collapse by preventing alveolar collapse at end expiration.**
  - **<u>Supplemental oxygen</u>** PaO2 >55 mmHg or SaO2 88-95%, or FiO2 at ≤0.6 should be used.
  - <u>Prone positioning</u> may improve oxygenation by helping recruit atelectatic alveoli in severe ARDS.

SLEEP APNEA

- Involuntary cessation of breathing during sleep.
- **Complications include Pulmonary hypertension & arrhythmias.**

RISK FACTORS
- **Increased neck circumference**: in men, increased neck circumference has demonstrated the strongest correlation with OSA [>43.2 cm (17 inches)].
- **Obesity**: strong risk factor for OSA (eg, BMI >30 kg/m²).
- Male gender: OSA is 2-3 times more common in men than women.
- Age: most common in the sixth and seventh decades.

TYPES
- **Central sleep apnea**: reduced CNS respiratory drive leads to decreased respiratory effort.
- **Obstructive sleep apnea**: physical airway obstruction (may be due to external airway compression, decreased pharyngeal muscle tone, increased tonsil size, or deviated septum).

CLINICAL MANIFESTATIONS
- Snoring, unrestful sleep (which may lead to chronic daytime sleepiness). Nocturnal choking.
- Physical examination: large neck circumference, crowded oropharynx, micrognathia.

DIAGNOSIS
- **In-laboratory polysomnography**: **first line diagnostic test.** Positive if ≥15 events/hour: obstructive or mixed apneas, hypopneas, respiratory effort arousals etc.
- Labs: **polycythemia (increased hemoglobin & hematocrit) due to chronic hypoxemia.**
- Epworth sleepiness scale: used to quantify patient's perception of fatigue and sleep.

STOP-BANG SURVEY FOR OBSTRUCTIVE SLEEP APNEA	
1 point for each characteristic	• **S**noring • **T**iredness (excessive daytime) • **O**bserved apneas of choking/gasping • **P**ressure elevation: hypertension • **B**MI > 35 kg/m² • **A**ge >50 years • **N**eck size: men >17 in (43.2 cm); women >16 in (40.6) • **G**ender: Male
Low risk: 0-2 points **Intermediate risk**: 3-4 points **High risk**: 5 points or greater	**Patients with a score <3 are unlikely to have sleep apnea and do not need further diagnostic testing.**
Not included in the scoring but **absence of either morning headaches or poor concentration makes OSA less likely.**	

MANAGEMENT
- **Behavioral changes include weight loss, alcohol abstinence, & changes in sleep positioning.**
- **Continuous positive airway pressure (CPAP) is the mainstay of treatment of OSA.**
- Oral appliances can be tried if CPAP is unsuccessful or as an alternative (not as effective as CPAP).
- Surgical correction: Tracheostomy is considered the definitive treatment for Obstructive sleep apnea. Other interventions include nasal septoplasty & uvulopalatopharyngoplasty.

OBESITY HYPOVENTILATION SYNDROME (OHS)/PICKWICKIAN SYNDROME

- **The presence of awake alveolar hypoventilation in an obese individual which cannot be attributed to other conditions associated with hypoventilation** (eg, neuromuscular disease).
- Hypoventilation due to a combination of blunted ventilatory drive and increased mechanical load imposed upon the chest by obesity.
- **90% of patients with OHS have coexistent Obstructive sleep apnea (OSA).**

CLINICAL MANIFESTATIONS
- **Manifestations of obesity & sleep disordered breathing:** eg, dyspnea, fatigue, hypersomnolence, snoring, witnessed apneas, sleep-related desaturation, daytime hypoxemia, and sluggishness.

DIAGNOSIS
- **OHS is a diagnosis of exclusion. Diagnostic criteria include [1] obesity — BMI ≥30 kg/m², [2] hypoventilation — a partial arterial pressure of carbon dioxide (PaCO₂) ≥45 mmHg, [3] sleep disordered breathing (often OSA), & [4] exclusion of other causes of alveolar hypoventilation.**
- Once diagnosed, all patients with OHS should be assessed for common complications, (eg, Pulmonary hypertension and Cardiovascular conditions).

Workup based on suspicion:
- **High suspicion: Arterial blood gas (ABG) obtained to assess for evidence of alveolar hypoventilation (eg, PaCO₂ ≥45 mmHg)** for those in whom OHS is strongly suspected [eg, morbidly obese patients with suspected or known Obstructive sleep apnea (OSA)].
- **Low to moderate suspicion: serum bicarbonate** often ordered in patients when the suspicion is low to moderate (eg, <20%); **an elevated bicarbonate level >27 mEq/L, increases the likelihood of OHS and should prompt an ABG;** a bicarbonate level ≤27 mEq/L suggests that OHS is unlikely, and an ABG is not usually indicated.
- Abnormal ABG findings: For those in whom a chronic respiratory acidosis (PaCO₂ ≥45 mmHg) with compensatory metabolic alkalosis is found, additional testing is necessary to exclude other diseases that can cause or contribute to chronic alveolar hypoventilation or hypercapnia.

Identification of coexistent breathing disorders:
- In-laboratory polysomnography to assess for Obstructive sleep apneas (OSA) if not already diagnosed.

MANAGEMENT
- **Multipronged approach, including [1] immediate initiation of Noninvasive positive airway pressure ventilation (NPPV) and [2] lifestyle modifications for weight loss,** which improves hypoxemia and hypercapnia as well as ventilation response to both; patients with OHS should be followed clinically for their response to noninvasive PAP and/or weight loss (eg, every six months).
- **If present, concomitant severe Obstructive sleep apnea must be treated aggressively (eg, nasal CPAP)** to improve daytime hypercapnia & hypoxemia in >50% of patients with OHS + severe OSA.
- Treatment of comorbid conditions: identify and treat comorbid conditions that may contribute to hypoventilation (eg, COPD) or can complicate OHS (eg, Pulmonary hypertension).
- Avoidance of contributors to hypoventilation including alcohol and sedatives (eg, Opiates, Barbiturates, Benzodiazepines, muscle relaxants).

Second-line:
- For patients with OHS who fail or do not tolerate first-line therapies in whom aggressive attempts have been made to optimize NPPV therapy, options include tracheostomy for the treatment of sleep-disordered breathing and bariatric surgery or rarely medication for weight loss. In general, these therapies are suboptimal and associated with higher risk of adverse events.
- For patients with OHS in whom supplemental oxygen is indicated, oxygen should be administered in conjunction with NPPV; supplemental oxygen alone may worsen hypercapnia.
- Untreated OHS is associated with a high morbidity & mortality, with most deaths due to cardiovascular complications including Pulmonary hypertension, right heart failure, & higher risk of complications in the perioperative period, including respiratory failure, intubation, and Heart failure.

ABNORMAL BREATHING

1. **CHEYNE-STOKES: cyclic breathing in response to hypercapnia.** Smooth increases in respirations & then gradual decrease in respirations with a period of apnea 15-60 seconds.
   Due to **decreased brain blood flow** slowing the impulses to the respiratory center.
2. **BIOT'S BREATHING: irregular respirations (quick shallow breaths of equal depth)* with irregular periods of apnea** (usually of equal depth in comparison to Cheyne-Stokes breathing).
   Can be seen with damage to the medulla oblongata or opioid use.
3. **KUSSMAUL'S RESPIRATION:** (hyperpnea): **deep, rapid, continuous respirations** as a result of **metabolic acidosis** - deep breaths with large tidal volumes (body's attempt to compensate by blowing off excess CO_2). No expiratory pause (no stopping between inhalation & exhalation).

PULMONARY PHOTO CREDITS

CHAPTER 3 – GASTROINTESTINAL/NUTRITION

EOSINOPHILIC ESOPHAGITIS

- Allergic, inflammatory eosinophilic infiltration of the esophageal epithelium after other causes are ruled out.
- **Allergic response to food or environmental antigens trigger esophageal inflammation.**

RISK FACTORS
- Most commonly seen in **children & associated with atopic disease** (eg, Asthma, Eczema, Hay fever).
- **White males between 30-40 years of age.**

CLINICAL MANIFESTATIONS
- <u>Adults and teenagers</u> frequently present with <u>esophageal dysfunction</u> — eg, **dysphagia to solids (most common symptom) and esophageal food impactions.**
- <u>Younger children</u>, symptoms may include feeding difficulties, food refusal, gastroesophageal reflux symptoms, and abdominal pain.

DIAGNOSIS
- **Endoscopy:** normal or multiple corrugated (stacked) circular esophageal rings, strictures (especially proximal), **punctate whitish exudates and white papules** (representing eosinophil microabscesses), loss of vascular markings (edema), and linear, longitudinal furrows.
- **Biopsy:** ≥15 eosinophils/hpf (squamous epithelial eosinophil predominant inflammation).

MANAGEMENT
Dietary therapy:
- **Dietary therapy in addition to avoidance of known allergens is first-line management of Eosinophilic esophagitis in children and adults.** Diets are determined by an allergist and/or dietician highly effective. Empiric elimination of common food allergies (eg, milk, wheat, egg, soy, nuts, and seafood) followed by systematic reintroduction can be used.

Pharmacological therapy:
- <u>Proton pump inhibitors</u> **(PPIs) are among first line treatment options, together with dietary modification and topical glucocorticoids.** PPI responsive esophageal eosinophilia, characterized by elimination of mucosal eosinophilia, occurs in 30–50% of cases of suspected EoE.
- **Topical glucocorticoids**: Patients with persistent symptoms and eosinophilic inflammation following PPI therapy can try elimination diets or swallowed topical glucocorticoids (eg, **inhaled topical corticosteroids, such as Budesonide, <u>without</u> using spacer for local effect**).

<u>Esophageal dilation:</u>
- Esophageal dilation is very effective at relieving dysphagia in patients with fibrostenosis but is associated with increased risk of perforation.

PILL-INDUCED ESOPHAGITIS

- Esophagitis due to prolonged pill contact with the esophagus.
- <u>Medications:</u> **NSAIDS and Aspirin, Bisphosphonates,** Beta blockers, Calcium channel blockers, potassium chloride tablets, iron pills, Tetracyclines, vitamin C, Zidovudine.

CLINICAL MANIFESTATIONS
- Odynophagia, dysphagia, retrosternal chest pain.

DIAGNOSIS
- <u>Endoscopy:</u> small, well-defined discrete ulcers of varying depths.

MANAGEMENT
- Take pills with at least 4 ounces of water.
- Avoid recumbency at least 30-60 minutes after pill ingestion.

SYMPATHETIC SYSTEM	PARASYMPATHETIC SYSTEM
NOREPINEPHRINE ("fight or flight")	**ACETYLCHOLINE** ("rest or digest")
Alpha-1: • **Vasoconstriction** • **Decreased urination** (↑bladder outlet resistance) • **↓GI motility** • **Pupillary dilation** **Beta receptors:** • **B1: Increased heart rate & contractility** • **B2: bronchodilation, skeletal muscle contraction**	**Alpha-1**: • **Vasodilation** • **Increased urination** • Increased GI motility • **Pupillary constriction** **Beta receptors** • **B1: Decreased heart rate & contractility** • **B2: bronchoconstriction**
Anti "SLUDD-C"	**Increased SLUDD-C**: increased **S**alivation, **L**acrimation, **U**rination, **D**igestion, **D**efecation; **C**onstriction of the pupil.

CHOLINERGIC TOXICITY

ETIOLOGIES

- **Insecticides (eg, Organophosphates, Carbamates), Medications [eg, Acetylcholinesterase inhibitors (eg, Pyridostigmine, Neostigmine)], Sarin gas.**
- These substances inhibit acetylcholinesterase, resulting in increased acetylcholine.
- Toxicity occurs following cutaneous exposure, inhalation, or ingestion.

CLINICAL MANIFESTATIONS

- **Muscarinic effects: Increased SLUDD-C: increased S**alivation and **S**weating, **L**acrimation, **U**rination, **D**igestion (eg, vomiting, GI cramps), **D**efecation (diarrhea), **C**onstriction of the pupil (pupillary miosis).** The most common cause of death is respiratory failure.
- **Beta receptors (muscarinic): bradycardia, bronchorrhea, bronchospasm,** muscle fasciculations.
- **Nicotinic effects: fasciculations, muscle weakness, paralysis due to neuromuscular blockade** (similar to succinylcholine), seizures, **tachycardia,** hypertension.
- CNS: Nicotinic & muscarinic effects — central respiratory depression, lethargy, seizures, and coma.

DIAGNOSIS

- Clinical diagnosis. Direct measurement of plasma or RBC acetylcholinesterase (RBC AChE) activity helpful in confirming acute toxicity, but patients require treatment before results become available.

MANAGEMENT

- **All symptomatic patients should be decontaminated and receive therapy with oxygen, Atropine in large doses, and an oxime (eg, Pralidoxime).**

Decontamination & supportive:

- **Decontamination**: if topical exposure with potential dermal absorption, aggressive decontamination with complete removal of the patient's clothes and vigorous irrigation of the affected areas.
- **Supportive care and ABCs** — Isotonic solutions (eg, Normal saline & Lactated ringers). Patients with markedly depressed mental status or respiratory failure require 100% oxygen and immediate tracheal intubation & mechanical ventilation until sufficient cholinesterase has been regenerated.

Medical management:

- **Atropine**: **anticholinergic (antimuscarinic)** titrated to therapeutic endpoint of cessation of bronchoconstriction clearing of respiratory secretions. Does not block the nicotinic receptors.
- Epinephrine if no response to Atropine.
- **Organophosphates: Atropine plus Pralidoxime. Pralidoxime is given after or concurrent with Atropine. Pralidoxime treats both the nicotinic and muscarinic symptoms.** Pralidoxime (2-PAM) competitively inhibits binding of organophosphates to acetylcholinesterase (forms a complex with the bound acetylcholinesterase enzyme to cause the release of the organophosphate from the enzyme). This results in regeneration of its ability to metabolize acetylcholine.
- Organophosphate-induced seizures are treated with a Benzodiazepine.

ANTICHOLINERGIC TOXICITY

ETIOLOGIES
Anticholinergic medications
- **Antihistamines**
- **Anticholinergics**
- **Antipsychotics**
- **Antidepressants**
- Anti-Parkinson agents, antispasmodics, and mydriatics.

CLINICAL MANIFESTATIONS
ANTI "SLUDD-C":
- Dry as a bone: **dry mouth, anhidrosis, decreased sweat**
- **Decreased lacrimation**
- **Urinary retention**
- **Decreased bowel sounds**
- Blind as a bat: **nonreactive mydriasis (dilated pupils)**
- Red as a beet: **dry flushed skin (cutaneous vasodilation)**
- Hot as Hades: **fever**
- Mad as a hatter: **delirium, hallucinations**
- Beta 1: tachycardia
- CNS anticholinergic toxicity include anxiety, agitation, disorientation, confusion, delirium, visual, psychosis (eg, paranoia), hallucinations, coma, and seizures.

DIAGNOSIS
- Clinical diagnosis
- Laboratory and other testing: obtain fingerstick blood glucose (assess for glucose abnormalities), Acetaminophen, and salicylate serum concentrations, and an electrocardiogram (ECG) to evaluate for changes to the QRS or QTc intervals.

MANAGEMENT
- **Management includes supportive care, assessment and stabilization of the airway, breathing, and circulation, treatment of agitation and seizures with Benzodiazepines, and gastrointestinal decontamination if appropriate.**
- **Antidotal Physostigmine therapy may be used in severe cases** — coma, seizures, hypotension, and agitation are refractory to conventional therapy.
- Physostigmine is a centrally acting parenteral acetylcholinesterase inhibitor used as an antidote for anticholinergic toxicity and delirium, but it is frequently unavailable due to manufacturing shortages. Rivastigmine may be used in times of shortage.

TOXINS	CLINICAL EXAM	WORKUP	ANTIDOTES/MGMT
ACETAMINOPHEN	Toxicity overwhelms the enzyme capability of the liver ⇨ ↓ glutathione ⇨ **hepatic necrosis** • Anorexia, N/V, diaphoresis ⇨ RUQ pain, jaundice, coagulation abnormalities.	• APAP levels Follow nomogram • LFTs • PT/PTT/INR • UA, ECG	• <u>N-acetylcysteine antidote</u> (glutathione substitute). • **Activated charcoal** especially within 1 hour of ingestion.
SALICYLATES - **Aspirin** - **Pepto Bismol** - Ben Gay - Oil of Wintergreen	• **Respiratory alkalosis** due to respiratory stimulation ⇨ **high anion gap metabolic acidosis** occurs later. Fever. • <u>CNS:</u> seizures, coma, encephalopathy. • Renal failure, pulmonary edema.	• Salicylates levels • Metabolic acidosis • *Hypokalemia* (from ↑ urinary K+ loss)	• Resuscitation (ABCs) • <u>GI decontamination:</u> Activated charcoal, gastric lavage • Alkalinization: sodium bicarbonate • Glucose helps with CNS sx • IV fluids • Hemodialysis (if severe).

BASES
  - **Oven cleaner**
  - **Drain cleaner**
  - **Bleach**
	• Esophageal or gastric perforation, epiglottitis.
	
	• Respiratory distress.
	
	• Irritated mucous membranes.
		• EGD to assess for damage.	• Supportive care
			• Emesis prevention
			• ±small amount of H_2O or milk as a diluent.
			• *Gastric lavage or acids contraindicated* (will worsen symptoms).

HYDROCARBONS - Gasoline - Benzene - Petroleum - Kerosene, Motor oil	• **Aspiration pneumonitis** • Tachycardia, fever • CNS depression • Mucosal irritation • Vomiting, bloody diarrhea	• CXR: ± pneumonia, pneumothorax of pleural effusion). • UA • ECG	• Supportive treatment • ±antibiotics if pneumonia • *Avoid emetics or lavage*
ANTICHOLINERGICS - **Antihistamines** - Atropine - **Tricyclic antidepressants (TCA's)** **Anticholinergics have antimuscarinic effects**	<u>**Sympathetic Stimulation:**</u> • **Hyperthermia (no sweating)** • **Tachycardia, HTN** • **Hot, flushed, dry skin & mucous membranes.** • <u>**Mydriasis,**</u> visual changes • Urinary retention, ileus <u>**CNS**</u> • Confusion, seizure, coma, respiratory depression,	• <u>ECG with TCA: **wide QRS, prolonged QT,**</u> heart block, asystole, brady & tachyarrhythmias, ventricular arrhythmia (due to <u>**Na channel blocker effects of TCA's**</u>)	• Activated charcoal • Whole bowel irrigation • **Physostigmine** (acetylcholinesterase inhibitor) <u>**TCA toxicity:**</u> supportive. • <u>**Sodium bicarbonate** is the antidote for cardiac toxicity & hypotension.</u> • Benzodiazepine for seizures.

CHOLINERGICS
- **Organophosphates**
 	
- **Insecticides & Pesticides**
  Chlorthion, Diazinon, Malathion
 	
- Sarin gas
	<u>Muscarinic S/E: "SLUDD-C":</u>
	↑**salivation, lacrimation, urination,** ↑**GI: diarrhea, emesis, miosis.**
	<u>CV:</u> bradycardia, hypotension,
	<u>Respiratory:</u> bronchospasm and rhinorrhea.
	<u>Nicotinic S/E:</u> mydriasis, tachycardia, weakness, HTN, fasciculations. **Children usually present with nicotinic adverse effects.**
	"Garlic" breath (also seen with arsenic).
		• RBC cholinesterase levels
		
		• Blood glucose levels
			• Remove contaminated clothes.
			
			• <u>**Atropine + Pralidoxime**</u>
			  - Atropine (anticholinergic)
			  - Pralidoxime reactivates the cholinesterase enzyme

IRON	**GI:** nausea, vomiting, abdominal pain, shock, coagulopathy, red urine.	• RBC indices. LFTs • Metabolic acidosis • UA: assess for renal damage	• Emesis with gastric lavage • Whole bowel irrigation • **Deferoxamine** • Hemodialysis

POISONS	TREATMENT	NOTES
Tricyclic antidepressants	**Sodium bicarbonate** may be used for cardiotoxicity.	Cardiotoxicity = prolonged QT interval, wide QRS complexes.
Amphetamines	Ammonium chloride	
Opioids	**Naloxone, Naltrexone**	May be needed if severe (eg, **respiratory depression**).
Benzodiazepines	Flumazenil	Only used in severe cases.
Beta blockers	Glucagon	Usually given as an IM injection.
Theophylline	**Beta blockers**	Overdose symptoms usually due to ↑ sympathetic activity.
Digitalis	**Digibind**	May need IV Magnesium.
Methemoglobin	Methylene blue, Vitamin C	
tPA, streptokinase	Aminocaproic acid	
Warfarin	**Vitamin K & Fresh frozen plasma** Cryoprecipitate if continued bleeding	Especially if INR >10
Heparin	**Protamine sulfate**	
Ethylene glycol (Antifreeze)	**IV Ethanol infusion** Fomepizole	

INFECTIOUS ESOPHAGITIS

RISK FACTORS
- **Immunocompromised states** eg, HIV, post-transplant, malignancy, chemotherapy, high-dose steroid use; However, they can occur in immunocompetent patients.
- **Candida is the most common cause.** In patients with classic symptoms, empiric treatment with Fluconazole can be initiated with upper endoscopy reserved if no response to initial therapy.

CLINICAL MANIFESTATIONS
- The three classic symptoms of esophagitis are [1] odynophagia (hallmark), [2] dysphagia, and [3] retrosternal chest pain.

DISEASE	ENDOSCOPIC FINDINGS	BIOPSY FINDINGS	MANAGEMENT
CANDIDA	**Linear yellow-white plaques or patches adherent to the mucosa**	**Yeast cells & pseudohyphae** invading mucosal cells	First-line: • **PO or IV Fluconazole** Second line: • Voriconazole • Caspofungin
CMV	**Large superficial shallow ulcers may be linear.** Ulcers are deeper vs. HSV	Eosinophilic intranuclear, basophilic intracytoplasmic inclusions with a peripheral halo (**owl's eye appearance**).	First-line: • **IV Ganciclovir** Second line: • Valganciclovir • Foscarnet
HSV	**Small vesicles or deep "punched out" ulcers "volcano-like" appearance.**	**Cowdry bodies:** eosinophilic intranuclear inclusions. **Multinucleated giant cells.**	First-line: • **Oral or IV Acyclovir** Second line: • Foscarnet

ESOPHAGEAL CANDIDIASIS

- *Candida* infections involving the mucous membranes of the esophagus.
- ***Candida albicans* most common strain.** Part of normal flora that becomes pathogenic.
- Other species (*Candida glabrata* or *Candida krusei*) may be occasionally seen.

EPIDEMIOLOGY
- **Most common cause of infectious Esophagitis** (HSV #2 & CMV #3). 88% of infectious Candidiasis are from *Candida albicans*, 10% are from Herpes simplex virus, and 2% are from Cytomegalovirus.

RISK FACTORS
- **Immunocompromised states** — eg, **advanced HIV with CD4 count <100 cells/microL**, post-transplant, malignancies, chemotherapy, glucocorticoid therapy, radiation to the neck, Diabetics.
- Can occur in immunocompetent patients — eg, use of inhaled corticosteroids, Proton-pump inhibitors.

CLINICAL MANIFESTATIONS
- **Odynophagia (hallmark symptom), dysphagia, & retrosternal chest discomfort** (similar findings in all types of Esophagitis).
- Other symptoms: heartburn, nausea, vomiting, abdominal pain, weight loss, diarrhea, & melena.
- Physical examination: The only finding may be associated oropharyngeal disease (thrush) on exam.

DIAGNOSIS:
- **Upper endoscopy: diagnostic test of choice** — **white-yellow mucosal plaque-like lesions or exudates adherent to the mucosa (may be linear)** with friability.
- **Biopsy: Budding yeasts, pseudohyphae, and hyphae invading mucosal cells** seen with Hematoxylin and eosin stain of biopsy tissues.
- Fungal culture: Less specific than histology because a positive culture alone can be indicative of colonization rather than infection.
- Empiric therapy: **An alternative diagnostic approach in immunosuppressed patients (especially with Thrush) in addition to symptoms of odynophagia or dysphagia, is empiric treatment with a 14–21-day course of oral Fluconazole**. If there is no improvement after 72 hours of treatment, upper endoscopy with biopsy should be performed to rule out causes other than or in addition to *Candida* esophagitis. The threshold for performing an upper endoscopy is lower in patients without evidence of oral thrush since other etiologies may cause the symptoms.

MANAGEMENT
- **Systemic antifungals: Fluconazole is the first-line agent** (200-400 mg/day orally for 14-21 days) due to its lower cost, lower toxicity, reduced risk of drug interactions, and ease of administration compared to the other antifungals. Intravenous therapy may be required initially in patients with severe disease who cannot take oral therapy (IV Fluconazole 400 mg daily can be used and then de-escalated to oral Fluconazole when the patient can tolerate oral medications). Odynophagia due to Candidiasis should improve within several days.
- Adverse effects of azole therapy include gastrointestinal upset and prolonged administration can cause hepatotoxicity.
- **Topical agents should not be used for esophageal Candidiasis**.
- Second-line agents: Voriconazole, Itraconazole oral solution, Posaconazole oral suspension, Isavuconazole, echinocandins (eg, Caspofungin, Micafungin, Anidulafungin), Amphotericin B.
Refractory to Fluconazole:
- For documented esophageal candidiasis due to *C. albicans* refractory to Fluconazole after 1 week of treatment, the dose should be increased.
- If symptoms still persist after several days, repeat endoscopy should be performed to obtain cultures and sensitivity and to make sure the symptoms are not secondary to another disease.
- If another disease is not found, a different antifungal agent should be used, pending culture results.

HERPES SIMPLEX VIRUS (HSV) ESOPHAGITIS

- **Herpes simplex virus (HSV) type I is the second most common cause of Infectious esophagitis (Candida #1, CMV #3).** 10% of Infectious esophagitis is due to HSV.

RISK FACTORS:
- **Immunocompromised states: Most commonly seen in immunocompromised patients** — eg, HIV, post-transplant (eg, solid organ and bone marrow), malignancy, chemotherapy, corticosteroid therapy, immunosuppressive medications.
- Herpes simplex can also occur in healthy hosts, in which case the infection is generally self-limited.

PATHOPHYSIOLOGY
- Reactivation: HSV esophagitis may result from reactivation of HSV with spread of virus to the esophageal mucosa via the vagus nerve or by direct extension of oral–pharyngeal infection.
- Primary infection HSV esophagitis may also occur during primary herpes infection.

CLINICAL MANIFESTATIONS
Similar findings in all causes of Esophagitis:
- **Odynophagia (hallmark) and/or dysphagia are the most common symptoms.**
- Retrosternal chest pain, fever.
- Weight loss.

HSV:
- Coexisting oral ulcers (Herpes labialis) or oropharyngeal ulcers may be seen.

DIAGNOSIS
- **The diagnosis of HSV esophagitis is usually based on endoscopic findings confirmed by histopathological examination of the observed lesions.**

Upper endoscopy:
- **Test of choice — multiple small, deep, discrete, well-circumscribed erosions and ulcers with a punched out or "volcano-like" appearance,** raised edges, & friable mucosa.
    Think of the S in HSV for small & submarine (deep).
- **Exudates,** plaques, or diffuse erosive esophagitis may also be seen.
- The earliest changes are vesicles but, this early stage is rarely seen on endoscopy.

Biopsy:
- **Eosinophilic intranuclear inclusions (Cowdry's Type A inclusion bodies)** that occupy up to 50% of the nuclear volume, **multinucleated giant cells**, and ground glass nuclei.
- In patients who do not respond to Acyclovir, viral culture of suspicious lesions should be performed during endoscopy, if possible, to confirm the diagnosis and to identify resistant viral isolates.

MANAGEMENT:
Immunocompromised host:
- **Acyclovir is the first-line agent for immunosuppressed individuals** (400 mg orally five times a day for 14–21 days). **Adjunctive therapy: high-dose proton pump inhibitor or Sucralfate.**
- Famciclovir (500 mg orally three times a day), or Valacyclovir (1 g orally three times a day).
- Foscarnet if unresponsive to first-line antivirals.
- Severe odynophagia or dysphagia — Patients with severe odynophagia may require hospitalization for parenteral antiviral therapy (Intravenous Acyclovir, 5 mg/kg every 8 h for 7–14 days), pain management, and hydration or alimentation.

Immunocompetent hosts:
- **Spontaneous resolution usually occurs in immunocompetent hosts after 1-2 weeks (self-limited), although patients may respond more quickly if treated with a short course of oral Acyclovir** (200 mg orally five times a day for 7–10 days).

CYTOMEGALOVIRUS (CMV) ESOPHAGITIS

- **Cytomegalovirus,** a member of the Herpesviridae family [human herpesvirus-5 (HHV5)]. A double stranded virus (largest virus that causes human infections).

EPIDEMIOLOGY
- **CMV is present in most people (60-70% in the US and almost universal in developing countries).** CMV is the most common viral opportunistic infection in people with AIDS.

RISK FACTORS
- **Immunocompromised states:** eg, **AIDS,** organ transplant recipients receiving immunosuppressive medication to avoid rejection, chemotherapy, high-dose glucocorticoid therapy; however, CMV esophagitis can occasionally occur in immunocompetent patients.
- **Most cases of CMV disease occur in the setting of advanced immunosuppression, with CD4 cell counts <50 cells/microL.**

CLINICAL MANIFESTATIONS
- **Odynophagia (hallmark and most common symptom), dysphagia,** & retrosternal chest pain/burning or mid-epigastric discomfort (similar findings in all causes of Esophagitis).
- May be accompanied by fever or nausea.

DIAGNOSIS
- **Upper endoscopy** test of choice: **CMV esophagitis and gastritis classically reveals large (sometimes >10 cm^2) superficial, shallow erosions or "punched-out" ulcers** that are well-demarcated and may be serpiginous. Think of the M in CMV for Mega (large).
- CMV Esophagitis: CMV most commonly causes multiple esophageal ulcers near the mid-lower part of the esophagus (eg, lower esophageal sphincter), but diffuse esophagitis may occur less commonly.
- CMV Colitis: The appearance of CMV colitis can range from punctate and superficial erosions to deep ulcerations and necrotizing colitis.
- Biopsy: **Histology — mucosal inflammation and large CMV infected cells (cytomegaly) with enlarged nuclei surrounded by clear zone (halo) extending towards the cell membrane's nucleus & the classic "owl's eye" inclusion bodies (typically basophilic intranuclear inclusions** at least half the diameter of the cell, eosinophilic cytoplasmic inclusions may be seen).
- Ophthalmologic evaluation: **screening for retinitis is recommended in all patients with extraocular CMV disease** because concurrent CMV retinitis is often present, even if asymptomatic.

MANAGEMENT
- **Treatment of CMV gastrointestinal disease includes induction therapy (eg, Ganciclovir), initiation of antiretroviral therapy (ART) in patients with HIV,** and maintenance therapy in selected patients.
- **IV Ganciclovir first-line treatment of choice.** CMV gastrointestinal disease should be treated with induction therapy with intravenous (IV) Ganciclovir at a dose of 10-15 mg/kg per day in 2-3 divided doses daily for 3-6 weeks, depending on clinical circumstances or until resolution of signs and symptoms.
- **Oral therapy (eg, Valganciclovir) may be used once the patient can absorb and tolerate oral agents and/or in patients with mild disease.**

- Second line: Foscarnet, Cidofovir, Valganciclovir. **Foscarnet is used as an alternative therapy in Ganciclovir resistant CMV infections or in patients with contraindications to Ganciclovir.** Foscarnet has a different mode of action as it directly inhibits polymerase function by blocking the pyrophosphate binding site of pUL54.

CAUSTIC (CORROSIVE) ESOPHAGITIS

- Ingestion of corrosive substances: alkali (drain cleaner, lye, bleach) or acids.
- Clinical manifestations: odynophagia, dysphagia, hematemesis, dyspnea.
- Diagnosis: Endoscopy is used to determine the extent of damage & look for complications.
- Management: Supportive, analgesia, IV fluids. No role for emetics, neutralizing agents, or corticosteroids

HIATAL HERNIA

- Herniation of structures from the abdominal cavity through the esophageal hiatus of the diaphragm.
- **Sliding:** Type I — GE junction "slides" into the mediastinum (increases reflux). **Most common type (95%).**
- **Paraesophageal:** Type II — **"rolling hernia"** – fundus of stomach protrudes through diaphragm with the GE junction remaining in its anatomic location.

CLINICAL MANIFESTATIONS

- Usually an asymptomatic incidental finding; may develop intermittent epigastric or substernal pain, postprandial fullness, retching, or nausea.

DIAGNOSIS

- Often discovered incidentally on upper endoscopy, manometry, or imaging done for other reasons.

MANAGEMENT

- **Sliding: management of GERD — PPIs first-line therapy; weight loss (if indicated).**
- Paraesophageal: surgical repair reserved for complications (eg, volvulus, obstruction, strangulation, bleeding, perforation, etc.).

ESOPHAGEAL ATRESIA

- Complete absence or closure of a portion of the esophagus.
- **Most commonly associated with a tracheoesophageal fistula,** polyhydramnios.
- Clinical manifestations: **Presents immediately after birth with excessive oral secretions that leads to choking, drooling, inability to feed, respiratory distress, and coughing** (especially when attempting to feed). Gastric distention may occur. Aspiration pneumonia common.

DIAGNOSIS

- Inability to pass a nasogastric tube further than 10-15 cm (coiling in the esophagus).
- Fluoroscopy: small amount of water-soluble contrast may reveal it (but must be removed promptly to prevent aspiration). Barium should not be used if Esophageal atresia is suspected.

MANAGEMENT

- Surgery: Surgical ligation of the fistula with primary anastomosis of the esophageal segments may be done in stages if the distance between the 2 segments is large.

BARRETT'S ESOPHAGUS

- **Esophageal squamous epithelium replaced by precancerous metaplastic columnar cells from the cardia of the stomach** (precursor to Esophageal adenocarcinoma).

Diagnosis: Upper endoscopy with biopsy

Barrett's esophagus only (metaplasia)	PPIs & rescope every 3-5 years; Long segments (≥3 cm) every 3 years; shorter segments (<3 cm) every 5 years.
Low-grade dysplasia	PPIs and rescope every 6 months for 1 year, then annually until reversion to nondysplastic Barrett.
High-grade dysplasia	Ablation with endoscopy, photodynamic therapy, endoscopic mucosal resection, radiofrequency ablation.

GASTROESOPHAGEAL REFLUX DISEASE (GERD)

- **Gastroesophageal reflux disease (GERD) is a condition that develops when the reflux of stomach contents causes troublesome symptoms and/or subsequent complications.**

CLASSIFICATION
- Nonerosive reflux GERD symptoms without visible esophageal mucosal injury on endoscopy (60-70%).
- Erosive esophagitis: endoscopically visible breaks in the distal esophageal mucosa.
- Barrett esophagitis: 6-12%.

RISK FACTORS
- **Hiatal hernia frequently associated with GERD and may exist without causing any symptoms.**
- **Obesity is a significant risk factor for the development of GERD.**
- Pregnancy — estrogens lower LES pressure. Postprandial supination
- Nicotine or tobacco use (smoking); Alcohol consumption. Gastric outlet obstruction.
- Connective tissue disorders (eg, Scleroderma). Age ≥50 years.
- Medications that decrease LES pressure — Calcium channel blockers, Beta Adrenergic agonists (including inhalers), anticholinergics, alpha-adrenergic antagonists, Tricyclic antidepressants, Diazepam, Estrogens, Progesterone. Narcotics, Theophylline. Medications that cause direct mucosal injury — Bisphosphonates, Aspirin, NSAIDs. Tetracycline, Potassium chloride tablets, and Iron salts.

PATHOPHYSIOLOGY
- **Incompetent LES:** reflux of gastric contents into the esophagus due to an [1] incompetent lower esophageal sphincter (LES) [hypotensive LES] or [2] pathological transient LES relaxations.

CLINICAL MANIFESTATIONS:
Typical symptoms:
Classic symptoms of GERD are [1] heartburn (pyrosis) and/or [2] regurgitation.
- **[1] Heartburn (pyrosis) hallmark — often described as a burning sensation in the retrosternal area, especially in 30-60 minutes postprandial period, increased with the supine (reclined) position or bending, and may be relieved with antacids.** May complain of belching.
- **[2] Regurgitation sour or bitter taste (acid)** or perception of the retrograde migration of acidic gastric contents into the mouth or hypopharynx.
- Symptoms can also be aggravated by ingestion of certain foods or beverages, such as tomato sauce, peppermint, chocolate, coffee, tea, and alcohol.

Atypical symptoms:
- **GERD-related chest pain** can mimic Angina pectoris. **GERD is the most common cause of noncardiac chest pain in patients with a negative cardiac workup.**
- Extraesophageal symptoms (eg, **chronic cough, wheezing, hoarseness**) due to reflux of acidic material into the lungs, acidic exposure leading to chronic laryngitis, or exacerbation of Asthma.
- Water brash (hypersalivation) foam at the mouth due to hypersecretion of saliva in response to reflux.
- Globus sensation is the almost persistent perception of a lump in the throat.

"Alarm" features:
- **The presence of alarm features may be suggestive of complications of GERD or Gastrointestinal malignancy and require Upper endoscopy.**
Alarm features include:
- **Dysphagia &/or odynophagia, anorexia, or unexplained weight loss.**
- **Evidence of GI bleeding** — eg, occult blood in stool, melena, hematemesis, hematochezia.
- Persistent vomiting, symptoms or findings of **Iron deficiency anemia, age ≥60 years,** GI cancer in a first-degree relative.

COMPLICATIONS

4 main complications often present with alarm features:

- **Esophagitis** due to inflammation from acid. **GERD is the most common cause of Esophagitis.**
- **Esophageal stricture**: narrowing from chronic acid exposure. Often presents with dysphagia.
- **Barrett's esophagus**: **esophageal squamous epithelium replaced by precancerous metaplastic columnar cells** from the cardia of the stomach. Precursor to Esophageal adenocarcinoma.
- **Esophageal adenocarcinoma** as a result of Barrett's esophagus.

DIAGNOSIS

- **Clinical diagnosis GERD can be presumptively diagnosed in most patients based upon history with classic symptoms (heartburn and/or regurgitation) without alarm features & empirical Proton pump inhibitor therapy can be initiated in this setting without additional studies.**
- A classic presentation does not usually require GI workup but may require ruling out cardiac etiology.
- Esophageal Manometry: May be performed in patients with suspected GERD with chest pain and/or dysphagia & a normal upper endoscopy. Decreased LES pressure is the classic finding of GERD.
- **24-hour ambulatory pH monitoring: Criterion standard for GERD. Used to confirm GERD in individuals with persistent symptoms (either typical and/or atypical symptoms), especially if medically refractory (persistent after a trial of twice-daily PPI),** and if inconclusive EGD. PPIs should be stopped 96 hours prior to ambulatory pH monitoring.
- Upper endoscopy: **Upper endoscopy is not required to establish the diagnosis of classic GERD.** The primary use of Upper endoscopy is to look for complications of GERD & to rule out malignancy.

Diagnosis if persistent or alarm features:

- **Upper endoscopy: with biopsy first-line diagnostic test if (1) persistent symptoms, (2) GERD with dysphagia**, (3) a complication of GERD is suspected **(eg, alarm features, malignancy etc.),** (4) new-onset of dyspepsia >60 years of age, and (5) in patients with suspected GERD who have not responded to an empirical 4–8-week trial of twice-daily Proton pump inhibitor (PPI).

MANAGEMENT

[1] Mild and intermittent GERD symptoms: <2 episodes/week:

- **"Step up therapy": in patients naïve to treatment, lifestyle and dietary modifications are the initial management — as needed low-dose histamine 2 receptor antagonists (H2RAs);** concomitant antacids &/or sodium alginate as needed if symptoms occur <once weekly.
- **Lifestyle modifications: considered to be the cornerstone of any GERD therapy** — avoidance of a supine position after meals and avoidance of meals 2-3 hours before bedtime or after eating, elevation the head of the bed 6-8 inches in patients with nocturnal symptoms, avoidance of food that delay gastric emptying (eg, fatty or spicy foods, citrus juice, chocolate, peppermint, tomato-based products, caffeinated products, carbonated beverages), avoidance of large meals at bedtime, smoking cessation, decreased alcohol intake, and weight loss in patients who are overweight or have had recent weight gain. Assess symptomatic response in 4 weeks.
- "as needed" pharmacologic therapy: **antacids with or without sodium alginate and low-dose H2 receptor antagonists "as needed".** If symptoms persist on low-dose H2RA, increased H2RA to standard dose, twice daily and reassess in 2 weeks.

[2] Moderate, severe, or frequent GERD:

≥2 episodes/week:

- **PPI trial: Trial of standard dose Proton pump inhibitor (PPI) once daily for 8 weeks in addition to lifestyle & dietary modifications.** Adults with upper GI symptoms who have completed a minimum 4-week course of PPI treatment, resulting in resolution of upper GI symptoms, can decrease the daily dose or discontinue and change to on-demand use.
- If there are no associated alarm symptoms (eg, dysphagia, odynophagia, anemia, weight loss, hematemesis), most patients with moderate or frequent GERD can be initiated on empiric medical therapy with Proton pump inhibitors (PPIs) without further investigations with a response to treatment confirming the diagnosis of GERD.
- **Definitive management: Surgical fundoplication (eg, laparoscopic) if refractory.**

ESOPHAGEAL NEOPLASMS

MAJOR TYPES

[1] Adenocarcinoma of the esophagus:
- **Most common type in the US** (50-80%). Seen in younger patients. **Common in White males.**
- **Most common in the distal esophagus & esophagogastric junction.**

[2] Squamous cell carcinoma of the esophagus:
- **Most common cause worldwide** (90-95%). Peaks 50-70 years of age.
- In the US, it is associated with **increased incidence in Black males.**
- **Most common in the mid to upper third of the esophagus.**

RISK FACTORS for **Adenocarcinoma:**
- **Major risk factors in the US are Barrett's esophagus (a complication of chronic GERD), smoking, & high body mass index. Unlike Squamous cell, alcohol is NOT a risk factor for Adenocarcinoma.**

RISK FACTORS for **Squamous cell carcinoma:**
- **Major risk factors in the US are smoking & alcohol.**
- Worldwide: poor nutritional status, low intake of fruits & vegetables, drinking hot beverages (thermal injury), HPV infection (especially 16 & 18), N-nitroso compounds, Atrophic gastritis, Achalasia, Tylosis.

PROTECTIVE FACTORS
- Aspirin or NSAIDs may have protective effect, particularly in the setting of Barrett's esophagus.

CLINICAL MANIFESTATIONS
- Patients often have extensive disease by the time they become symptomatic (eg, dysphagia & weight loss).
- **Progressive dysphagia:** hallmark — solid food dysphagia **progressing** to include fluids, odynophagia (20%).
- **Weight loss,** anorexia. Iron deficiency anemia (chronic blood loss).
- Chest pain, anorexia, cough, hematemesis, reflux, hoarseness (recurrent laryngeal nerve).
- Horner's syndrome, tracheal-esophageal fistula. Hypercalcemia with Squamous cell carcinoma.

DIAGNOSIS
The diagnosis of Esophageal cancer requires a histologic examination of tumor tissue, usually obtained by upper endoscopy or, if metastases are present, image-guided biopsy of the site.
- **Upper endoscopy with biopsy: diagnostic study of choice.** Appearance — early lesions may appear as superficial plaques, nodules, or ulcerations. Advanced lesions may appear as strictures, ulcerated masses, circumferential masses, or large ulcerations.
  Squamous cell: keratinocyte-like cells with intercellular bridges or keratinization.
  Adenocarcinoma: well or moderately differentiated intestinal-type mucosa cells.
- Double-contrast Barium esophagogram may be part of a workup to evaluate for dysphagia.
- Pretreatment staging: **Endoscopic ultrasound is the preferred method for locoregional staging.** Preoperative bronchoscopy with biopsy and brush cytology indicated for locally advanced lesions. CT neck chest abdomen, PET/CT scan.

MANAGEMENT
- Esophageal resection if early: T1N0 esophageal or esophagogastric junction AC or SCC, surgery, or endoscopic resection rather than initial chemotherapy or concurrent chemoradiotherapy (CRT).
- T3N0, T4aN0, and clinically node-positive thoracic esophageal cancer, regardless of histology, may be treated with combined therapy, rather than surgery alone.
- Radiation therapy; chemotherapy (eg, 5-FU).
- Palliative stenting to improve dysphagia may be needed in advanced cases.
- For patients with localized esophageal or esophagogastric junction cancer who have residual disease in the surgical specimen after initial chemoradiotherapy, Nivolumab for 1 year may be used.

ACHALASIA

- Idiopathic motility disorder characterized by **[1] impaired relaxation of the lower esophageal sphincter** (LES) & **[2] loss of peristalsis** in the distal two-thirds (smooth muscle) of the esophagus.

PATHOPHYSIOLOGY
- **Idiopathic progressive degeneration & loss of ganglion cells in the myenteric (Auerbach's) plexus** in the esophageal wall leads to impaired lower esophageal sphincter (LES) relaxation (increased LES pressure), accompanied by loss of peristalsis in the distal esophagus.
- LES hypertrophy, & esophageal dilation results from loss of vasoactive intestinal peptide (VIP) & nitric oxide–producing inhibitory neurons in the myenteric plexus.

CLINICAL MANIFESTATIONS
- **Dysphagia for solids and/or liquids simultaneously and regurgitation of undigested food or saliva are the most common presenting symptoms of Achalasia.** Heartburn, substernal pain.
- **Weight loss, chest pain.** Malnutrition & dehydration. Most common in adults 25-50 years of age.

DIAGNOSIS
- **Barium esophagogram:** may be normal in up to 1/3 of patients but classic findings are **[1] dilation of the proximal esophagus, [2] smooth tapering of the distal esophagus (LES and esophagogastric junction narrowing) with "bird-beak" appearance** caused by the persistently contracted LES; **[3] lack of peristalsis distally,** or [4] delayed emptying of Barium.
- **Manometry:** **most accurate test to confirm the diagnosis — increased LES pressure; lack of peristalsis & impaired LES relaxation after swallowing.**
- **Endoscopy: usually performed in Achalasia prior to initiating treatment to rule out Esophageal squamous cell carcinoma** (Achalasia increased the risk factor for cancer by 7-fold).

MANAGEMENT
- (1) mechanical disruption of the muscle fibers of the LES — eg, pneumatic dilation, surgical myotomy, or peroral endoscopic myotomy [POEM] or
- (2) therapy to reduce LES pressure — eg, injection of botulinum toxin or use of oral nitrates.
- (3) Laparoscopic Heller myotomy most common surgical procedure, often with partial fundoplication.

ZENKER DIVERTICULUM

- **Pharyngoesophageal pouch (false diverticulum — involves the mucosa** & possibly submucosa).
- Most common in males. Usually presents >60 years of age (often in the 70s).
- Outpouching occurs due to weakness at the junction of Killian's triangle (between the fibers of the **cricopharyngeal muscle** & lower inferior pharyngeal constrictor muscle).

CLINICAL MANIFESTATIONS
- **Dysphagia, regurgitation of undigested food, halitosis** (food retention in the pouch), cough, feeling as if there is a lump in neck (neck mass), throat discomfort, choking sensation, nocturnal choking or cough, gurgling in the throat. Complications: aspiration pneumonia, bronchiectasis, & lung abscess.

DIAGNOSIS
- **Barium Esophagogram with video fluoroscopy initial test of choice** — collection of dye behind the esophagus at the pharyngoesophageal junction. Upper endoscopy performed for surgical evaluation.

MANAGEMENT
- **Asymptomatic + small diverticula <1 cm: observation** — small asymptomatic diverticula that are <1 cm in size do not warrant treatment. Patients can be managed expectantly until symptoms occur.
- **Symptomatic or >1 cm: The definitive treatment of symptomatic ZD is surgical.** Open or transoral approach (rigid endoscope or a flexible endoscope). **Diverticulectomy with cricopharyngeal myotomy is the preferred open approach in good surgical candidates.**

DISTAL (DIFFUSE) ESOPHAGEAL SPASM (DES)

- Esophageal motility disorder characterized by **simultaneous, nonperistaltic (uncoordinated), or rapidly propagating esophageal contractions of normal amplitude.**

PATHOPHYSIOLOGY
- **Defective propagation of food bolus**: DES is thought to be a consequence of impaired inhibitory myenteric plexus innervation, resulting in premature and rapidly propagated contractions in the distal esophagus. **Commonly associated with psychiatric disorders.**

CLINICAL MANIFESTATIONS
- **Intermittent dysphagia to both solids and liquids simultaneously** (most prominent symptoms), sensation of "object stuck in the throat".
- **Chest pain**: stabbing, nonexertional, noncardiac pain **worse with hot or cold liquids or food**.

DIAGNOSIS
- **Esophagram:** Severe non-peristaltic spastic contractions of the circular muscle in the esophageal wall with a **"corkscrew "or "rosary bead" appearance of the esophagus** (not specific to DES).
- **Manometry: (definitive)** — **[1] premature contractions the presence of ≥2 premature contractions with short distal latency** (<4.5 seconds) relative to the time of pharyngeal contraction (uncoordinated spastic activity); **[2] uncoordinated (premature or simultaneous) contractions alternating with normal peristalsis in >20% of wet swallows** with amplitude of contraction >30 mmHg in the distal three-fifths of the esophagus.
- Manometry often combined with Esophagogram and Endoscopy to rule out malignancy.

MANAGEMENT
- PPI for patients with DES or HE and who have GERD symptoms. Peppermint oil as a muscle relaxant.
- **Smooth muscle relaxants**: antispasmodic agent **(eg, Hyoscyamine, Isosorbide dinitrate, Calcium channel blockers (eg, Nifedipine). Low-dose TCAs (eg, Nortriptyline) second line**.
- **Endoscopy-guided botulinum toxin injection**; Pneumatic esophageal dilation.
- Surgical therapy: Myotomy (eg, peroral endoscopic myotomy or long myotomy) if refractory to above.

HYPERCONTRACTILE (JACKHAMMER, NUTCRACKER) ESOPHAGUS

- Esophageal motility disorder characterized by increased pressure during peristalsis (hypercontractility) where esophageal smooth muscle contractions are in a **normal sequence but at excessively high amplitudes (hypercontractility) or excessive duration.**

CLINICAL MANIFESTATIONS
- **Chest pain** similar to Distal (diffuse) esophageal spasm. **Dysphagia to both liquids & solids.**

DIAGNOSIS
- **Manometry: (definitive)** — **increased pressure during peristalsis >180 mmHg or duration of contraction >7.5 seconds** but normally sequential contractions in the smooth muscle esophagus.
- Upper endoscopy and Esophagram are usually normal.

MANAGEMENT
- Same as DES: PPIs for GERD; **smooth muscle relaxants** — eg, Calcium channel blockers, Nitrates (eg, Isosorbide dinitrate), Botulinum toxin injection. Tricyclic antidepressants second line.
- Surgical therapy: Myotomy (eg, peroral endoscopic myotomy or long myotomy) if refractory to above.

- **Exam tip**
- Distal (Diffuse) esophageal spasm and Hypercontractile esophagus have a similar presentation, but manometry will show different peristaltic patterns to be able to distinguish between the two.

ACHALASIA:

Barium esophagogram:

- **(1) dilation of the proximal esophagus** that terminates in a "beak-like narrowing.
- **(2) smooth tapering of the distal esophagus (LES and esophagogastric junction narrowing) with "bird-beak" appearance** caused by the persistently contracted LES;

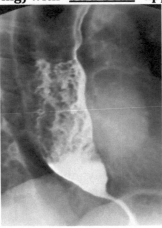

ZENKER DIVERTICULUM

- **Barium Esophagogram:** collection of dye behind the esophagus at the pharyngoesophageal junction.

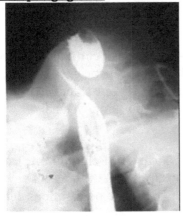

DISTAL (DIFFUSE) ESOPHAGEAL SPASM

- **Esophagogram:** Severe non-peristaltic spastic contractions of the circular muscle in the esophageal wall with a **"corkscrew "or "rosary bead" appearance of the esophagus** (not specific to DES).

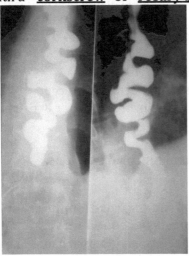

ESOPHAGEAL RUPTURE & BOERHAAVE SYNDROME

- **Full thickness rupture, most commonly affecting the left posterolateral wall of the lower esophagus** 3-5 cm above the gastroesophageal junction. Effort rupture = Boerhaave syndrome.

ETIOLOGIES:
- **Iatrogenic perforation of the esophagus during endoscopy most common cause** (~65%).
- **Trauma: repeated, forceful retching or vomiting (eg, Bulimia, alcoholism).**

PATHOPHYSIOLOGY
- A tear results from a sudden increase in intraluminal pressure combined with negative intrathoracic pressure (eg, severe straining, vomiting). Leak of gastric contents may lead to mediastinitis.

CLINICAL MANIFESTATIONS
- **Severe pleuritic retrosternal chest pain or upper abdominal (thoracic esophagus), worse with deep breathing or swallowing**; neck pain. **Dyspnea**, hematemesis, odynophagia, hoarseness.
- **Mackler triad: [1] lower chest pain + [2] vomiting + [3] subcutaneous emphysema.**

PHYSICAL EXAMINATION:
- **Crepitus on chest auscultation or palpation (subcutaneous emphysema).**
- **Hamman's sign: mediastinal "crackle or crunch" accompanying every heartbeat,** especially in the left lateral decubitus position, due to the heart beating against air-filled tissues.

DIAGNOSIS
- **Contrast esophagogram: initial diagnostic test of choice — leakage of contrast material. Water-soluble contrast (eg, Gastrografin) preferred** because Barium is caustic if it extravasates.
- **Chest CT scan: most sensitive test to detect mediastinal air** — left-sided hydrothorax (most common), **pneumomediastinum**, esophageal edema, subcutaneous emphysema.

MANAGEMENT
- Initial: **surgical consult, IV broad-spectrum antibiotics (eg, Ticarcillin-clavulanate),** avoidance of oral intake, IV Proton pump inhibitor, parenteral nutritional support, & drainage of any collections.
- Small & stable: conservative medical management as above for contained perforations detected early.
- Large or severe: endoscopic therapy or surgical repair as per surgical consult.

MALLORY-WEISS SYNDROME (TEARS)

- **Longitudinal superficial mucosal lacerations** at the gastroesophageal junction or the gastric cardia.
- Sudden rise in intraabdominal pressure or gastric prolapse into the esophagus (eg, **persistent retching or vomiting after ETOH binge, vigorous cough**). May be associated with Hiatal hernias.

CLINICAL MANIFESTATIONS
- **Upper GI bleeding   bright red hematemesis,** melena, hematochezia preceded by retching or vomiting (5-10% of all UGIB). Syncope if severe. Abdominal pain, back pain, or hydrophobia.

DIAGNOSIS
- **Upper endoscopy test of choice — superficial longitudinal mucosal erosions.**

MANAGEMENT
- **Not actively bleeding: supportive mainstay of treatment** (eg, **acid suppression with PPIs** promotes healing). **Most cases stop bleeding spontaneously without intervention.**
- Severe bleeding: options include thermal coagulation, hemoclips, endoscopic band ligation (with or without epinephrine), & balloon tamponade (eg, Sengstaken-Blakemore tube or Minnesota tube).

ESOPHAGEAL WEB

- **Noncircumferential thin diaphragm-like membrane in the mid-upper esophagus.** Esophageal webs are covered with squamous epithelium and most commonly occur anteriorly in the cervical esophagus, resulting in focal narrowing in the postcricoid area.
- May be congenital or acquired (eg, associated with Zenker's diverticulum, dermatologic and immunologic disorders, and Iron deficiency anemia).
- **Most cases associated with a Hiatal hernia** and reflux symptoms are common.
- <u>Plummer-Vinson Syndrome:</u> **triad of [1] dysphagia, [2] cervical esophageal webs, and [3] iron deficiency anemia.** May also be associated with **atrophic glossitis**, angular cheilitis, koilonychias & splenomegaly. Most common in Caucasian women 30-60y. Patients with Plummer-Vinson syndrome are at increased risk for Esophageal or pharyngeal squamous cell carcinoma.

CLINICAL MANIFESTATIONS

- Most esophageal rings and webs are asymptomatic.
- **Intermittent dysphagia to solids especially hard solids** (eg, meat or bread), not progressive.

DIAGNOSIS

- <u>Barium esophagogram (swallow):</u> **diagnostic test of choice & more sensitive than endoscopy** — webs often missed on upper endoscopy due to proximity to the upper esophageal sphincter.

MANAGEMENT:

- **Endoscopic dilation** of the area if severe symptoms (eg, large bougie dilator a balloon dilator).
- **PPI therapy after dilation** may decrease the risk of recurrence and reduce heartburn symptoms.

ESOPHAGEAL (SCHATZKI) RING

- Smooth, circumferential (2-5 mm) diaphragm of tissue that protrudes into the esophageal lumen.
- **Most commonly at the lower esophagus at the squamocolumnar (gastroesophageal) junction.**

RISK FACTORS

- **Hiatal hernia present in most patients**
- **Corrosive esophageal injury (eg, acid reflux)**
- Eosinophilic esophagitis.

CLINICAL MANIFESTATIONS

- Most Esophageal rings and webs are asymptomatic.
- <u>Intermittent dysphagia to solids</u> **especially hard solids (eg, meat or bread);** not progressive. Large poorly chewed boluses of food may get stuck in the lower esophagus (Steakhouse syndrome).

DIAGNOSIS

- **Barium esophagogram (swallow): best to visualize the rings, more sensitive than endoscopy** — circumferential ridge a few cm above the hiatus of the diaphragm with symmetric narrowing.
- <u>Upper endoscopy:</u> less sensitive than Barium esophagogram; often performed in patients with rings to biopsy the esophagus for associated Eosinophilic esophagitis. Endoscopically, an esophageal ring appears as a thin membrane with a concentric smooth contour that projects into the lumen.

MANAGEMENT

- <u>Symptomatic:</u> **single dilation via passage of endoscopic bougie or endoscopic balloon dilators to disrupt the lesion or endoscopic electrosurgical incision of the ring** [large bougie dilator at least 50 French or balloon dilator (18 to 20 mm)] in patients without associated Eosinophilic esophagitis; obliteration with biopsy forceps. Antireflux surgery if reflux is present. Acid-suppressive therapy with PPIs if heartburn symptoms.
- Graded dilation if associated with Eosinophilic esophagitis.

ESOPHAGEAL VARICES

- **Dilation of the gastroesophageal collateral submucosal veins as a complication of portal vein hypertension** (including the left gastric vein). 50% of Cirrhotic patients have varices.
- Varices divert pressure from the portal circulation to systemic circulation, but dilation may increase the risk of upper GI bleed.

RISK FACTORS:
- **Cirrhosis most common cause of Portal hypertension & varices in adults.** Signs of liver disease: palmar erythema, shifting dullness, spider angiomas, jaundice, caput medusae, gynecomastia.
- Portal vein thrombosis is the most common cause of Esophageal varices in children.

CLINICAL MANIFESTATIONS
- **Upper GI bleed: hematemesis, coffee-ground emesis, melena, hematochezia.** Signs & symptoms of hypovolemia or shock if severe. 30% of patients with varices develop UGI bleeding.

DIAGNOSIS:
- **Upper endoscopy: test of choice — can be both diagnostic and therapeutic.**

MANAGEMENT OF ACUTE VARICEAL BLEED:
- **Stabilize the patient: 2 large bore IV lines, IV fluids.** May need packed red blood cells if low hematocrit.
- **Combination of medical therapy (Octreotide) & endoscopic therapy (ligation or sclerotherapy) is superior to either therapy alone** in controlling acute bleeding and decreasing rebleeding.

Pharmacologic vasoconstrictors:
- **Octreotide first-line medical management — can be used alone or as an adjunct to endoscopic treatment.** Octreotide is a somatostatin analog that causes vasoconstriction of the portal venous flow, decreasing portal pressure and reducing bleeding.
- Second line: Vasopressin decreases portal venous pressure. Adverse effects: vessel constriction in other areas (eg, coronary artery vasospasm, myocardial infarction), & bowel ischemia.

Endoscopic interventions:
- **Endoscopic variceal ligation initial treatment of choice** — banding achieves lower rates of rebleeding, complications, & death than sclerotherapy (banding is endoscopic treatment of choice).
- Sclerotherapy: seldom used due to higher complication and rebleed potential.
- If unconscious with active bleeding, endotracheal intubation may protect against aspiration.

Other management:
- Balloon tamponade is used as a temporizing measure only in patients with rapid bleeding that cannot be controlled with pharmacologic or endoscopic techniques until more definitive decompressive therapy (eg, TIPS) can be provided.
- Surgical decompression: Transjugular intrahepatic portosystemic shunt (TIPS) is indicated if persistent or recurrent bleeding (≥2 episodes) despite endoscopic &/or pharmacologic treatment and in some advanced cases.

Adjunctive management:
- **Antibiotic prophylaxis: Fluoroquinolones (eg, Norfloxacin) or Ceftriaxone given to prevent infectious complications** (eg, Spontaneous bacterial peritonitis) & decrease in-hospital mortality.
- Vitamin K (10 mg intravenously) administered in cirrhotic patients with abnormal Prothrombin time.
- Lactulose may be administered in patients with Encephalopathy.

PREVENTION OF REBLEED
- **Nonselective beta blockers (eg, Nadolol or Propranolol) prevent rebleeding once the patient has been stabilized — decrease portal pressure.** The combination of Beta blockers & endoscopic ligation is more effective than either alone in reduction of recurrent esophageal variceal bleeding.
- Prevention is important because 70% rebled within the 1st year of the initial bleed (especially in the first 6 weeks) and 33% of those rebleeds are fatal.

UPPER GASTROINTESTINAL BLEEDING (UGIB)

- **Bleeding from a proximal source to the ligamental of Treitz.**
- Risk factors: history of use of NSAIDs, Aspirin, anticoagulants, antiplatelet agents; Alcohol consumption, cigarette smoking, previous GI bleed, liver disease, coagulopathy, vomiting.

MAJOR ETIOLOGIES
- **Peptic ulcer disease most common cause of UGIB overall.** *H. pylori* & NSAIDs are contributive.
- **Esophagogastric or gastric varices most common cause of UGIB in patients with Cirrhosis.**
- Erosive gastritis, Esophageal (Mallory-Weiss) tear, tumor, arteriovenous malformation.

CLINICAL FEATURES
- **Hematemesis or "coffee ground" emesis, passing melena/tarry stool** (stool may be frankly bloody or maroon with massive or brisk upper GI bleeding); Abdominal pain.

Physical examination:
- Tachycardia; orthostatic blood pressure changes suggest moderate to severe blood loss; hypotension suggests life-threatening blood loss (hypotension may be late finding in healthy younger patients).
- **Rectal exam & fecal occult test** to assess stool color (melena, hematochezia, maroon, or brown).
- Perforation: significant abdominal tenderness, involuntary guarding, rebound tenderness, rigidity.

DIAGNOSTIC TESTING
- Obtain type and crossmatch for hemodynamic instability, severe bleeding, or high-risk patient; obtain type and screen for hemodynamically stable patient without signs of severe bleeding.
- Labs including BMP, CBC (hematocrit measurement may be inaccurate with acute severe blood loss), platelet, coags (PT/INR/PTT), liver studies. BUN:creatinine ratio ≥30 suggests an upper GI source.
- **Nasogastric aspirate & lavage helpful to diagnose UGIB if source of bleeding is unclear** (upper or lower GI tract), decompress the stomach, and is helpful to clean the stomach prior to endoscopy.
- **Upper endoscopy definitive study to confirm UGIB; can also be therapeutic (for hemostasis).**

MANAGEMENT
- Closely monitor airway, clinical status, vital signs, cardiac rhythm, urine output, nasogastric output (if nasogastric tube in place). **IV Proton pump inhibitor with suspected or known severe bleeding.**
- Do **NOT** give patient anything by mouth; Establish two large bore IV lines (16 gauge or larger).
- **IV fluid resuscitation** rapid, bolus infusions of isotonic crystalloid — eg, 500-1,000 mL per bolus; smaller boluses and lower total volumes used patients with decreased cardiac function.
- Provide supplemental oxygen: goal oxygen saturation ≥94% for patients without COPD.
- **Endotracheal intubation to protect the patient's airway is usually performed for patients with hemodynamic instability, altered mental status, and/or ongoing hematemesis.** Extubation should be performed when possible after endoscopy to reduce complications.

Transfusion:
- For severe, ongoing bleeding, immediately transfuse blood products in 1:1:1 ration of RBCs, plasma, and platelets, as indicated in trauma patients.
- If hemodynamically unstable despite IV crystalloid resuscitation, transfuse 1-2 units RBCs
- For hemoglobin <8 g/dL in high-risk patients (eg, older adult, coronary artery disease), transfuse 1 unit RBCs and reassess the patient's clinical status.
- For hemoglobin <7 g/dL in low-risk patients, transfuse 1 units RBCs and reassess the patient's clinical patient's clinical condition. Avoid over-transfusion with possible variceal bleeding.
- Coagulopathy: reverse coagulopathy when possible. Give plasma for coagulopathy or after transfusing 4 units of RBCs; give platelets for thrombocytopenia (platelets <50,000) or platelet dysfunction (eg, chronic aspirin therapy) or after transfusing 4 units of RBCs.
- Obtain immediate consultation with gastroenterologist, surgery, and others, as indicated.
- Known or suspected Esophageal varices &/or Cirrhosis: Somatostatin analog (eg, Octreotide), IV antibiotics (eg, Ceftriaxone or Ciprofloxacin), and endoscopic therapy (eg, rubber band ligation).

PEPTIC ULCER DISEASE (PUD)

- Defect in the gastric or duodenal mucosa that extends through the muscularis mucosa (gastric erosion >0.5 cm in diameter on imaging).

	DUODENAL ULCERS (DU)	GASTRIC ULCERS (GU)
CAUSATIVE FACTORS	↑ DAMAGING factors: Gastric acid, pepsin, *H. pylori*, NSAIDs	↓ MUCOSAL PROTECTIVE factors: ↓mucus, bicarb, prostaglandins, & blood flow to the mucosa (eg, **NSAID use**).
INCIDENCE	• **90% occur in the duodenal bulb** • **Almost always benign** • DU 4 times more common than GU	• **Most common in the antrum of stomach.** • **4% malignant:** most gastric ulcers need repeat endoscopy to document healing.
PAIN	• **Better with meals.** • **Worse 2-5 hours after meals**	• **Worse with meals** (especially **1-2 hours after meals**)
AGE	• MC in **younger patients:** 30-55 years.	• MC in **older patients:** 55-70 years.

ETIOLOGIES

The 2 major factors: *H. pylori* infection & use of nonsteroidal anti-inflammatory drugs (NSAIDs).
- ***Helicobacter pylori*: Most common cause of gastritis and PUD (both GUs and DUs).**
- **NSAIDs & Aspirin: NSAID-induced mucosal damage second most common cause (especially with gastric ulcers).** 10–20% prevalence of GUs & 2–5% prevalence of DUs in chronic NSAID users. NSAIDs can cause ulcers via inhibition of prostaglandins because inhibition decreases the stomach's ability to protect itself from gastric acids (decreased mucus, bicarbonate, and mucosal blood flow).
- Zollinger-Ellison Syndrome: Gastrin producing tumor. Causes 1% of all cases of PUD.
- Other factors: Alcohol use, cigarette smoking, stress (burns, trauma, surgery, severe medical illness); males, elderly, corticosteroid use, Gastric cancer (uncommon cause).

CLINICAL MANIFESTATIONS
- Asymptomatic: ~70% of Peptic ulcers are asymptomatic. Patients with silent peptic ulcers may later present with ulcer-related complications such as hemorrhage or perforation.
- **Dyspepsia hallmark — burning, gnawing, dull, aching, "hunger-like" epigastric pain or discomfort** seen in 80-90%. May localize to the upper quadrants or radiate to the back.
- Nausea, fullness, and early satiety. Significant vomiting and weight loss are not common and may suggest gastric outlet obstruction or gastric malignancy.
- **"Classic" Duodenal ulcer: dyspepsia classically relieved with food, antacids, or acid suppressants. Worse before meals, 2-5 hours after meals** (when acid is secreted in the absence of a food buffer), **and at night, often awakening the patient out of sleep (between about 11 PM and 2 AM** when the circadian pattern of acid secretion is highest).
- **"Classic" Gastric ulcer: Food-provoked dyspepsia — symptoms that worsen with eating, especially 1-2 hours after meals** (due to decreased barrier protection). Often associated with postprandial belching and epigastric fullness, early satiety, fatty food intolerance, nausea. Weight loss may be seen. Vomiting may occasionally occur.

PHYSICAL EXAMINATION
- The physical examination is often normal in uncomplicated Peptic ulcer disease.
- Mild, localized epigastric tenderness to deep palpation may be present.
- Guaiac test is positive in one-third of patients.

COMPLICATIONS
- Ulcer complications present without antecedent symptoms in 10–20% of patients ("silent ulcers").
- **Bleeding ulcer: Acute upper gastrointestinal hemorrhage is the most common complication of Peptic ulcer disease. PUD is the most common cause of upper GI bleeding** & may occur without any preceding symptoms. Clinical manifestations: May present with nausea, **hematemesis (red blood or coffee-ground emesis), or melena (black, tarry stool).**

- **Perforated ulcer:** Most common with peripyloric gastric ulcerations followed by duodenal bulb ulcers. **A classic triad of sudden onset of severe diffuse abdominal pain, tachycardia, and abdominal rigidity is the hallmark of peptic ulcer perforation.** Clinical manifestations: sudden onset of severe diffuse abdominal pain (may radiate to the shoulder). Physical examination: **tachycardia, peritonitis (rebound tenderness, guarding, & abdominal rigidity).**
- **Penetration:** Peptic ulcers may penetrate through the bowel wall without free perforation or leakage of luminal contents into the peritoneal cavity. DUs tend to penetrate posteriorly into the pancreas, leading to Pancreatitis, whereas GUs tend to penetrate into the left hepatic lobe.
- **Gastric outlet obstruction:** Relative obstruction secondary to ulcer related inflammation and edema in the peripyloric region; Especially seen with ulcers located in the pyloric channel or duodenum. Clinical manifestations: symptoms of mechanical obstruction, include bloating, indigestion, early satiety, anorexia, nausea, vomiting, postprandial epigastric pain, & weight loss.

DIAGNOSIS
- **Upper endoscopy: Diagnostic test of choice in most patients — most accurate diagnostic test for direct visualization of PUD and allows tissue biopsy to test for *H. pylori* and malignancy.**
- Biopsy: Duodenal ulcers are virtually never malignant and do not need require biopsy. However, because up to 5% of Gastric ulcers are malignant & documentation of complete healing 12 weeks after the start of therapy is necessary to exclude gastric malignancy in Gastric ulcers.
- *H. pylori* testing: **All patients diagnosed with PUD should undergo testing for *H. pylori* infection.**

MANAGEMENT
H. pylori-positive PUD:
- **Bismuth quadruple therapy: Bismuth subsalicylate + Tetracycline + Metronidazole + PPI x14 days,** especially if previous macrolide exposure or if Penicillin allergic (>90% eradication rate).
- **Concomitant therapy: "CAMP"** — Clarithromycin + Amoxicillin + Metronidazole + PPI for 10-14 days.
- Triple therapy: Clarithromycin + Amoxicillin + PPI for 10-14 days "CAP" (Metronidazole if Penicillin allergic). Alternative is Bismuth subsalicylate + Tetracycline + Metronidazole (<80% eradication).
- Vonoprazan 20 mg, Amoxicillin 1000 mg, and Clarithromycin 500 mg, all taken twice daily for 14 days; or Vonoprazan 20 mg twice daily, and Amoxicillin 1,000 mg three times daily for 14 days.
- Rifabutin triple therapy: Omeprazole, Rifabutin, and Amoxicillin. Used as a salvage regimen.
- PPI use results in faster control of symptoms, higher ulcer healing rates, & more effective healing of NSAID-related ulcers as compared with H2RA due to stronger acid suppression with PPIs. PPIs inhibit >90% of 24-hour acid secretion (65% for H2 receptor antagonists) in standard doses.
- Long-term acid suppression (maintenance therapy) may be indicated in "high-risk" patients — eg, persistent ulcer on endoscopy after management, large ulcers (>2 cm), frequently recurrent ulcers (2 documented episodes/year), and conditions requiring long-term Aspirin/NSAID use.
- **Confirm eradication of *H. pylori* at least 4 weeks after completion of antibiotic treatment.**
H. pylori negative PUD:
- **Antisecretory therapy: Proton pump inhibitors (usually preferred) or Histamine-2 receptor antagonists (H2RA).** Rabeprazole, Omeprazole, Lansoprazole, Dexlansoprazole, Pantoprazole.
- Histamine-2 receptor antagonists (H2RA): Nizatidine, Famotidine, Cimetidine.
- **Initial PPI therapy for 4 weeks for uncomplicated duodenal ulcers, and 8 weeks for a gastric ulcer** or complicated ulcers before repeating endoscopic evaluation to assess for ulcer healing.
- **PPIs result in faster control of symptoms, higher ulcer healing rates, and more effective healing of NSAID-related ulcers as compared with H2RA due to stronger acid suppression with PPIs.**
NSAID-associated ulcers:
- PPI (eg, Omeprazole 20-40 mg daily) for 4-8 weeks based on ulcer size.
- In patients with PUD who must remain on NSAIDs or Aspirin, maintenance antisecretory therapy with a PPI (eg, Omeprazole 20 mg daily) can decrease the risk of ulcer recurrence of complications.

REFRACTORY
- Parietal cell vagotomy. Bilroth II (associated with Dumping syndrome).

FOLLOW-UP
Duodenal ulcers:
- **Patients with Duodenal ulcers who have been treated <u>do not</u> need further endoscopy unless symptoms persist at 4 weeks or with recurrence.**

Gastric ulcers:
- **Surveillance endoscopy (with biopsies of the ulcer if still present) often performed after 8-12 weeks of antisecretory therapy in patients with Gastric ulcers with increased risk or any one of the following** — unclear etiology, symptoms despite medical therapy, giant gastric ulcer (>2 cm), ulcers appear suspicious for malignancy (eg, mass lesion, elevated irregular ulcer borders, or abnormal adjacent mucosal folds), biopsy samples were not performed or inadequate, bleeding ulcers at initial presentation who show signs of continued bleeding, or risk factors for Gastric cancer.

4 TESTS FOR *H. PYLORI*:
- **<u>(1) Endoscopy with biopsy:</u> gold standard in diagnosing *H pylori* infection.** A rapid urease test and direct staining can be performed on the biopsy specimen.

Noninvasive testing:
- Noninvasive assessment for *H. pylori* with fecal antigen assay or urea breath testing may be done in patients with a history of PUD to diagnose active infection or in patients following its treatment to confirm successful eradication. Both tests have a sensitivity and specificity of 92–95%.
- **<u>(2) Urea breath test:</u>** Noninvasive. *H. pylori* converts labeled urea into labeled carbon dioxide. Breathing out labeled CO_2 = presence of *H. pylori*. PPIs may cause false-negative urea breath tests and fecal antigen tests and should be withheld for at least 14 days before testing.
- **<u>(3) *H. Pylori* stool antigen (HpSA):</u>** Useful for diagnosing *H. pylori* & confirming eradication.
- <u>(4) Serologic antibodies:</u> only useful in confirming *H. pylori* infection NOT eradication (antibodies can stay elevated long after eradication of *H. pylori*). Because of its lower sensitivity (85%) and specificity (79%), serologic testing should not be performed unless fecal antigen testing, or urea breath testing is unavailable.
- **Eradication can be confirmed with a urea breath test, stool antigen testing, or endoscopy.**

MEDICAL MANAGEMENT OF PEPTIC ULCER DISEASE (PUD)

MEDICATION	COMMENTS
PROTON PUMP INHIBITORS "AZOLES" - **Omeprazole** - **Lansoprazole** - **Pantoprazole** - **Rabeprazole** - **Esomeprazole** - **Dexlansoprazole**	<u>Mechanism of action (MOA):</u> **Most potent inhibitors of gastric acid secretion by irreversibly binding & inactivating the parietal cell H+/K+ATP-ase (proton pump)** primarily responsible for producing stomach acid (diminish daily acid production by 80%–95%). **Usually taken 30 minutes prior to the first meal in the morning** (the amount of H-K-ATPase in the parietal cells is greatest after a prolonged fast). <u>Indications:</u> **most effective drug to treat PUD.** Gastritis, GERD, ZES. - 90% healing of duodenal ulcers after 4 weeks & gastric ulcers after 6 weeks. Maintenance therapy if long-term therapy required (eg, patients who require long-term therapy with Aspirin or NSAID). <u>Adverse effects:</u> few – nausea, diarrhea, constipation, abdominal pain, flatulence & headache occur infrequently. **Long-term use: B$_{12}$ and iron deficiencies, Hypocalcemia, and Hypomagnesemia.** Small increased risk of respiratory and enteric infections (eg, *C. difficile*). Omeprazole associated with *C. difficile* infections & hip fractures. **PPIs may inhibit conversion of Clopidogrel** (at the level of CYP2C19) **to the active anticoagulating form, but this is controversial.** <u>DI:</u> Omeprazole causes **CP450 inhibition** ⇨ ↑levels of Theophylline, Warfarin, Phenytoin, & other drugs.

H₂ RECEPTOR ANTAGONISTS "TIDINES" - Famotidine - Nizatidine - Cimetidine	**MOA: Reversibly block histamine's action on the histamine-2 receptors on gastric parietal cells (indirectly inhibits the proton pump), reducing acid & pepsin secretion** (especially nocturnal, when the basal acid output is the highest), so **best taken at night.** Indications: Peptic ulcer disease, uncomplicated GERD, reflux gastritis. Adverse effects: Diarrhea, headache, drowsiness, fatigue, muscular pain, and constipation. **B12 deficiency** — B12 is normally absorbed in acidic environment so decreased acid production via H2RA can impair vitamin B12 absorption. Famotidine can prolong QT interval. Uncommon: elevated transaminases (LFTs), Famotidine and Nizatidine may cause blood dyscrasias (pancytopenia, neutropenia, anemia, and thrombocytopenia). CNS: confusion, dizziness, headache. **Caution of renal or hepatic dysfunction.** Neuropsychiatric symptoms can occur in the elderly patient being treated with Cimetidine, especially those with reduced renal function. Therefore, **assessment of renal function is advised before beginning Cimetidine therapy, especially in the older patient population.** **Cimetidine only:** **Antiandrogenic effects: Cimetidine, but not other H2 blockers, is a weak antiandrogenic agent (may cause reversible gynecomastia, decreased libido, erectile dysfunction).** **CP450 enzyme inhibitor** so careful monitoring of drugs such as Warfarin, Phenytoin, and Theophylline is indicated with long-term usage (↑levels of these & other drugs).
MISOPROSTOL	**MOA: Prostaglandin E1 analogue that [1] increases mucus & bicarbonate secretion (protection) and [2] inhibits acid secretion.** **May be used for preventing NSAID-induced ulcers** in high-risk patients but not for healing already existing ulcers. Multiple daily dosing. Adverse effects: **diarrhea (most common),** abdominal cramping. Contraindications: premenopausal women (**abortifacient,** causes intrauterine contractions, and cervical ripening).

ANTACIDS	MOA: neutralize acid, prevents conversion of pepsinogen to pepsin.
	 Systemic: Calcium carbonate (Tums).
	    Adverse effects: acid rebound, milk alkali syndrome.
	 Nonsystemic: **Milk of Magnesia** (± cause **diarrhea**)
	      Amphogel (AlOH) (± cause **constipation**, hypophosphatemia)
	      Mg + ALOH + Simethicone (less adverse effects).

BISMUTH COMPOUNDS Colloidal bismuth subcitrate (CBS) Bismuth subsalicylate	MOA: **antibacterial, cytoprotective,** & inhibits peptic activity. Indications: limited role (used in quadruple therapy for *H. pylori*). Adverse effects: **darkening of tongue/stool, constipation,** neurotoxicity in high doses. Salicylate toxicity in overdose. Cautious use with renal insufficiency.
SUCRALFATE	**MOA: cytoprotective - forms viscous adhesive ulcer coating that promotes healing, protects the stomach mucosa.** Indications: usually used as an ulcer prophylactic measure than as for treatment of ulcers. Must be taken 4 times daily & on empty stomach. Adverse effects: constipation (most common), metallic taste, nausea. Antacids may interfere with its action. Take at least 2 hours before meds. Drug Interactions: **may reduce the bioavailability of H₂RAs, PPIs, & Fluoroquinolones,** when given simultaneously.

GASTROPATHY & ACUTE GASTRITIS

- Gastritis: inflammatory process — superficial inflammation or irritation of the stomach mucosa with mucosal injury (histologically documented inflammation of the gastric mucosa).
- Gastropathy: **gastric mucosal injury & pathology (epithelial or endothelial damage without inflammation);** minimal to no inflammation.

GASTROPATHY
- **Most commonly seen in alcoholic or critically ill patients** (stress due to severe medical or surgical illness), **medications, especially NSAIDs,** or portal hypertension ("portal gastropathy").
- **Reactive (chemical): Alcohol. Medications: NSAIDs, bile reflux, Iron salts, Alendronate.**
- **Stress-related mucosal disease**: **Ischemic: mucosal ischemia due to shock, sepsis, massive burns, hypovolemia, severe trauma, mucosal prolapse, cocaine.** Stress-related injury (superficial mucosal damage) and stress ulcers (focal deep mucosal damage).
- Most commonly observed in the acid producing (fundus and body) portions of the stomach.

GASTRITIS
- **Infectious: Gastritis is usually caused by infectious agents (most commonly, *H. pylori*),** which If not treated, may progress to chronic gastritis. Other bacteria, viral, parasitic, fungal.
- **Immune-mediated**: Autoimmune gastritis, Granulomatous disease (eg, Crohn disease, Sarcoidosis), Eosinophilic. Most commonly asymptomatic.

CLINICAL MANIFESTATIONS
Gastropathy:
- Erosive gastropathy is usually asymptomatic. If symptoms do occur, they may be similar to Peptic ulcer disease (eg, anorexia, epigastric pain, nausea, vomiting).
- Erosive gastritis: upper gastrointestinal bleeding — hematemesis, "coffee grounds" emesis, or as melena. Because erosive gastritis is superficial, hemodynamically significant bleeding is rare.

DIAGNOSIS
- **Upper endoscopy and gastric mucosal biopsy diagnostic tests of choice** — allows for visualization, biopsy, histology, and *H. pylori* testing.

Upper endoscopy:
- Gastropathy: Endoscopic findings include subepithelial hemorrhages, petechiae, and erosions. These lesions are superficial, vary in size and number, and may be focal or diffuse.
- Gastritis: endoscopic features include erythema, mucosal erosions, the absence of rugal folds, and the presence of visible vessels.

Histology:
- **Gastropathy: no significant inflammation on histologic examination & no evidence of *H. pylori*.**
- **Gastritis: inflammation** — histologic findings can vary, such as epithelial hyperplasia with minimal inflammation to extensive epithelial cell damage, mucosal erosions, & inflammatory infiltration.

MANAGEMENT
Gastropathy:
- **Prophylaxis suppression of gastric acid with H2 receptor antagonists (intravenous) or Proton pump inhibitors (oral or intravenous)** reduce the incidence of clinically overt and significant bleeding in critically ill patients with risk factors for significant bleeding.
- **Bleeding: Once bleeding occurs, patients should receive continuous infusions of a Proton pump inhibitor** (Esomeprazole or Pantoprazole, 80 mg intravenous bolus, followed by 8 mg/h continuous infusion) **as well as Sucralfate** suspension, 1 g orally every 4 to 6 hours. Endoscopy should be performed in patients with clinically significant bleeding to look for treatable causes, especially stress related.

Gastritis:
- Similar to Peptic ulcer disease — *H. pylori* eradication, acid suppression therapy (PPIs or H2 receptor antagonists), avoidance of causative factors (eg, alcohol, NSAIDs), & treat the underlying cause.

AUTOIMMUNE METAPLASTIC ATROPHIC GASTRITIS (AMAG)

- **Immune-mediated form of chronic gastritis denotes replacement of the normal oxyntic mucosa in the gastric corpus by atrophic and metaplastic mucosa (Type A gastritis).**

TYPES OF CHRONIC GASTRITIS

Chronic atrophic gastritis is considered a precursor lesion for Gastric cancer.
- Type B Gastritis (antral predominant): Multifocal Atrophic Gastritis (MAG) — chronic inflammation, mostly due to *H. pylori,* leads to a gradual loss of glandular oxyntic mucosa. This starts in the body and antrum (antral predominant) and then spreads throughout the stomach.
- **Type A Gastritis (antral sparing):** Autoimmune-mediated chronic gastritis, restricted to **oxyntic (acid-producing) mucosa in the corpus (anatomic body & fundus) of the stomach.**

PATHOPHYSIOLOGY
- T-cell (CD4+)-mediated destruction of the normal oxyntic mucosa due to autoantibodies & subsequent replacement by atrophic and metaplastic mucosa, such as intestinal-like epithelium (epithelial metaplasia). **Metaplasia is an important predisposing factor for Gastric cancers.**
- **Autoantibodies against [1] intrinsic factor (IF) &/or [2] parietal cells (antibody is directed against H+,K+ATPase) impair B12 absorption & lead to severe vitamin B12 deficiency (Pernicious anemia)** & its sequelae (megaloblastic anemia & neurologic dysfunction).
- **Achlorhydria:** The loss of parietal cells can lead to reduced pepsin & hypochlorhydria, prompting antral G cells to continuously produce gastrin (hypergastrinemia & G cell and EC hyperplasia).

CLINICAL MANIFESTATIONS
- May be asymptomatic but many patients experience dyspepsia, especially postprandial.
- **Pernicious anemia (PA):** B12 deficiency — **neurological (eg, symmetric paresthesias or numbness, gait disturbances), cognitive, or psychiatric changes; glossitis** (pain, swelling, tenderness, & loss of papillae of the tongue), **anemia** (eg, fatigue, irritability, cognitive decline).

DIAGNOSIS
The presence of [1] anti-intrinsic factor and anti-parietal cell antibodies + elevated fasting gastrin levels supports the diagnosis of AMAG in patients with [2] early/evolving histologic features.
- **Elevated fasting serum gastrin** — due to parietal cell atrophy and hypochlorhydria & achlorhydria. Gastrin levels can be markedly elevated (>500 pg/mL) in patients with Pernicious anemia.
- **Parietal cell antibodies** sensitive but not specific — have been detected in >90% of patients with Pernicious anemia and in up to 50% of patients with type A gastritis.
- **Intrinsic factor antibodies** are more specific than parietal cell antibodies for type A gastritis, being present in ~40% of patients with pernicious anemia and 50-70% of patients with AMAG.
- Decreased serum pepsinogen I/II ratio: atrophy of chief cells result in reduced serum pepsinogen I.
- **Iron deficiency anemia** often precedes Pernicious anemia onset due to hypochlorhydria because gastric acid is required for the absorption of inorganic iron.
- **Vitamin B12 deficiency:** Low serum B12 level, anemia, macrocytosis (high MCV), elevated methylmalonic acid, pancytopenia, hypersegmented neutrophils.
- **Upper endoscopy:** In patients with PA, an upper endoscopy should be performed to identify lesions (eg, carcinoid tumors and gastric cancer)** at diagnosis & to stage the severity of AMAG.
- **Gastric biopsies:** In patients with AMAG, the metaplasia, glandular atrophy, and inflammation are confined to the oxyntic mucosa of the gastric body and fundus** (spares the antrum).

MANAGEMENT
- **There is no specific treatment for Metaplastic (chronic) atrophic gastritis.** No surveillance if mild. Severe atrophic changes **or** intestinal metaplasia in both antrum and corpus — **endoscopic surveillance** (eg, every 3 years; every 1-2 years if family history of Gastric cancer).
- Pernicious anemia: **Patients with Pernicious anemia will require parenteral vitamin B12 supplementation on a long-term basis.**

GASTRIC CANCER

- **<u>Adenocarcinoma</u> most common (90%) and arises from gastric mucosal epithelial cells.** Most gastric cancers arise in the lesser curvature at body & antrum. 2 main types: (1) well differentiated (intestinal type), which is more common, and (2) undifferentiated (diffuse type).
- <u>Linitis plastica</u> **(infiltrative) is a rare variant of diffuse type,** accounting for ~5% of primary gastric cancers. **In Linitis plastica, a broad region of the gastric wall or even the entire stomach is extensively infiltrated by malignancy, resulting in a rigid thickened stomach.** More common in younger age groups and **has a worse prognosis than the intestinal type.** Men = women.
- <u>Other types:</u> 4% Lymphoma. Carcinoid tumors, stromal, sarcomas and other rare tumors.

RISK FACTORS
- **<u>*Helicobacter pylori*</u> infection (90%) & family history of Gastric cancer are the 2 strongest risk factors for Gastric cancer.** Smoking, heavy alcohol use, blood type A, non-White race, male sex.
- <u>Dietary:</u> High intake of salted, smoked, or pickled foods. <u>Nitroso compounds</u> — food containing nitrites or nitrates (eg, cheeses, cured meats). Diets high in fried food, processed meat, fish, and alcohol as well as low in vegetables, raw fruits, milk, & vitamin A. **Obesity.**
- <u>Abnormally high gastric pH:</u> **Pernicious anemia, chronic Atrophic gastritis, previous gastric surgery, and achlorhydria.** 25% of patients have a history of **Gastric ulcer.**

POSSIBLE PROTECTIVE FACTORS
- **Increased intake of fruits, raw vegetables, and fiber; chronic Aspirin & NSAID use.**

CLINICAL MANIFESTATIONS
- Most patients with Gastric cancer in the US are symptomatic (up to 80% in early stages) until late.
- **Weight loss and abdominal pain are most common symptoms, and most have advanced** (80-90% have stage III or IV), **incurable disease at the time of presentation.** Early satiety, anorexia.

PHYSICAL EXAMINATION
- A palpable abdominal mass although uncommon, is the most common physical finding and usually denotes long-standing, advanced disease.
- Paraneoplastic dermatologic manifestations include diffuse Seborrheic keratosis (Leser-Trélat sign) or Acanthosis nigricans (velvety and darkly pigmented patches on skin folds).
- <u>Nonspecific signs of Metastasis:</u> supraclavicular lymph nodes (Virchow's node), umbilical LN (Sister Mary Joseph's node), ovarian METS (Krukenberg tumor), palpable nodule on rectal exam (Blumer's shelf), left axillary lymph node (LN) involvement (Irish sign); all are associated with other GI tumors.

DIAGNOSIS
- **<u>Upper endoscopy with biopsy:</u> initial test of choice for most Gastric cancers.**
- <u>Upper GI series</u> (Barium studies): has a high false-negative rate, especially with early Gastric cancer. **Linitis plastica is the one exception where Upper GI series (Barium studies) may be superior to upper endoscopy for initial diagnostic evaluation.**
- CT scan is often used for staging. Iron deficiency anemia is a common finding.
- <u>Histologic examination</u> of tumor tissue is required for diagnosis (commonly acquired endoscopically).

MANAGEMENT
- <u>Early local disease (node negative):</u> Endoscopic resection. Recurrence is common.
- Gastrectomy + systemic chemotherapy and/or radiation therapy. Radiation for Lymphoma.

PROGNOSIS
- **<u>Poor prognosis</u> — patients usually present late; tumor recurrence is high, even with treatment,**
- 2 important factors influencing survival in resectable Gastric cancer are depth of cancer invasion through the gastric wall and presence or absence of regional lymph node involvement.

GASTRINOMA (ZOLLINGER-ELLISON SYNDROME) [ZES]

- An ectopic neuroendocrine gastrin-secreting tumor that stimulates the acid-secreting cells of the stomach, leading to severe gastric acid hypersecretion: [1] Peptic ulcer disease that is often severe and atypical & [2] chronic diarrhea. 0.1% - 1% of patients with Peptic ulcer disease.
- Most common in the duodenal wall, especially the first part (45%), pancreas (25%), lymph nodes (5-15%). 2/3 are malignant. Most are sporadic; 25% occur with Men 1 syndrome.

PATHOPHYSIOLOGY
- **Excessive gastrin secretion** results in acid hypersecretion. Gastrinomas result in high gastric acid output via the trophic effect of gastrin on parietal cells & gastric enterochromaffin-like (ECL) cells.
- **Chronic secretory diarrhea** in ZES results from the inability to completely reabsorb the high volume of gastric acid secretion, inactivation of the pancreatic digestive enzymes by the low pH, acid damage to the intestinal epithelial cells and villi, and inhibition of the absorption of sodium and water.

CLINICAL MANIFESTATIONS
- The most common manifestations of ZES include abdominal pain (75%), followed by chronic diarrhea (73%), and heartburn (GERD symptoms).
- **Severe Peptic ulcer disease:** abdominal pain most common symptom, heartburn; ulcers are usually solitary but may be multiple, severe, or refractory. Symptoms may relate to a complication of Peptic ulcer disease — eg, bleeding (eg, melena, hematemesis), perforation.
- **Chronic diarrhea** multifactorial (see above), steatorrhea, and weight loss.

DIAGNOSIS
- **Screening (fasting Gastrin):** elevated fasting serum gastrin levels best initial test in patients with suspected ZES (most sensitive test for the diagnosis of ZES). A serum gastrin value >10 times the upper limit of normal (>1,000 pg/mL) + the presence of a low gastric pH <2 is diagnostic of ZES (pH >3 excludes Gastrinoma). PPIs should be stopped for 6 days before testing.
- **Confirmatory (Secretin test):** Secretin stimulation test used to differentiate patients with Gastrinomas from other causes of hypergastrinemia, especially in patients with intermediate gastrin levels (150-1,000 pg/mL). Increased fasting serum gastrin release (≥200 pg/ml) after secretin administration indicates Gastrinomas. Normally, gastrin release is inhibited by secretin. Other causes of hypergastrinemia are usually inhibited by secretin.
- **Basal acid output:** increased Basal acid output (BAO) >10 mEq/h.
- Chromogranin A: non-specific tumor marker that is increased in neuroendocrine tumors.
- Upper endoscopy: Multiple ulcers, ulcers on the opposite sides of bowel wall (kissing ulcers), ulcers distal to the duodenum, ulcers in unusual locations, recurrent ulcers, and prominent gastric folds.
- **Tumor localization:** After the diagnosis of ZES is made, tumor localization begins with an upper endoscopy if not already performed, Somatostatin receptor-based imaging, or Cross-sectional imaging with helical, contrast-enhanced, triple-phase CT, or MRI. If CT/MRI and somatostatin receptor-based imaging are negative, and surgery is being considered, an endoscopic ultrasound (EUS) should be performed because of its greater sensitivity. Ga-PET scans combined with CT scan.
- **Somatostatin receptor scintigraphy:** most sensitive noninvasive test for localizing the primary tumors, secondary tumors, & metastases. Gastrinomas have increased somatostatin receptors.

MANAGEMENT
- **Medical therapy** Proton pump inhibitors are the current standard of care for most patients with Zollinger-Ellison syndrome (ZES), including MEN 1 syndrome due to the multiplicity of tumors, extra-pancreatic location, co-existent metastatic disease, and low chance of surgical cure.
- **Surgical resection:** Surgical resection is the only curative treatment for Gastrinomas because it is associated with increased survival (+ PPIs). Exploratory laparotomy & resection with curative intent indicated in sporadic Gastrinoma without evidence of metastatic spread of disease.
- Liver metastases & extent of liver involvement are the most important prognostic factors for survival.

GASTROPARESIS

- **Gastroparesis is <u>delayed gastric emptying and decreased peristalsis</u> resulting in food & liquid in the stomach for prolonged periods in the absence of a mechanical obstructing lesion.**
- This can result in impaired absorption of nutrients, inadequate nutrition, and poor glycemic control.

ETIOLOGIES

- **<u>Idiopathic</u>: most common**, GERD, Medications. Gastroparesis occurs more commonly in women;
- <u>Endocrine disorders</u>: **Diabetes mellitus most common systemic cause**, Hypothyroidism.
- <u>Postsurgical</u>: vagotomy, partial gastric resection, fundoplication, bariatric & gastric surgery, Whipple procedure. <u>Rheumatologic</u>: eg, Systemic sclerosis. <u>Infections</u> eg, postviral, Chagas disease.
- <u>Neurologic conditions</u>: eg, Parkinson disease, autonomic dysfunction, Multiple sclerosis.

CLINICAL MANIFESTATIONS

- **Symptoms of Gastroparesis typically include postprandial nausea & vomiting (1-3 hours after meals), bloating, early satiety, postprandial fullness, & heartburn. Abdominal pain is not usually the predominant symptom**, and if it is, a search for other causes should be performed.
- Weight loss, electrolyte abnormalities, vitamin deficiencies, small bowel intestinal overgrowth.
- **<u>Physical examination:</u> may reveal a succussion splash** (excessive gastric fluid from delayed emptying or outlet obstruction). Significant abdominal tenderness & peritoneal findings are uncommon.

DIAGNOSIS

- **<u>Upper endoscopy</u> to rule exclude mechanical obstruction** (eg, Peptic ulcer disease or gastric outlet obstruction). **CT or MR enterography to exclude mechanical obstruction**. In patients with suspected Gastroparesis with no evidence of mechanical obstruction on Upper endoscopy or imaging, a gastric motility study to assess delayed gastric emptying of solids establishes the diagnosis of Gastroparesis.
- **<u>Gastric emptying scintigraphy</u> with low-fat solid meal remains the preferred method for assessing 3–4-hour gastric emptying.** Alternative assessments of gastric emptying include wireless motility capsule testing & ^{13}C breath test with octanoate or spirulina within a solid meal.

MANAGEMENT
Supportive management:

- **<u>Dietary modification</u> is the initial management** (eg, small, frequent meals that are low in fat and contain only soluble fiber), hydration; optimization of glycemic control in Diabetic gastroparesis.
- <u>Avoid things that delay emptying</u>: foods that slow gastric emptying (eg, fatty, acidic, spicy food). Diet should be low in fat and indigestible (insoluble) fiber [eg, fresh fruits, salads, and leafy vegetables]. Avoid carbonated beverages (may worsen gastric distention). Avoid alcohol and smoking.
- For patients who are unable to tolerate solid food, meals should be homogenized, as gastric emptying of liquids is often normal even when emptying of solids is delayed & prolonged.

Medical therapy:

- **<u>Prokinetic agents</u>: Metoclopramide is the first-line medical therapy to increase the rate of gastric emptying in patients with continued symptoms despite supportive management & dietary modification.** Administered 10-15 minutes before meals. Another dose can be given at bedtime if additional dosing needed. Metoclopramide is a dopamine 2 receptor antagonist, a 5-HT4 agonist, and weak 5-HT3 receptor antagonist that decreases nausea, provides analgesia, and acts as a prokinetic. <u>Adverse effects</u>: anxiety, depression, restlessness, increased prolactin, prolonged QT.
- **In patients who fail to respond to Metoclopramide, a trial of Domperidone (a peripherally selective dopamine D2 receptor antagonist), and subsequently oral liquid Erythromycin** (motilin receptor agonist) are used. Cisapride (5HT4 agonist), if available, can be used if refractory.
- **<u>Antiemetics</u> — in patients with persistent nausea and vomiting despite prokinetics, antihistamines (eg, Diphenhydramine) or 5-HT3 antagonists (eg, Ondansetron) may be used.**
- Gastroparesis medically refractory to prokinetics and antiemetics may be treated with jejunostomy for enteral nutrition and venting gastrostomy tube for decompression with subsequent use of TCA (eg, low-dose Nortriptyline) if they remain symptomatic.

REFEEDING SYNDROME

- **Classic medical complications that occur due to fluid & electrolyte shifts during rapid or excessive nutritional rehabilitation of significantly malnourished patients.** Associated with enteral or parenteral refeeding, often occurring within the first 4 days of initiating caloric repletion.
- **Refeeding syndrome is characterized by Hypophosphatemia, Hypokalemia, Decompensated heart failure, peripheral edema, Rhabdomyolysis, seizures, hemolysis, and respiratory insufficiency.** Refeeding syndrome is a potentially a life-threatening metabolic complication.

RISK FACTORS
- **Anorexia nervosa,** chronic alcoholism, cancer cachexia, and other wasting syndromes.
- Severe weight loss in obese patients, severe long-standing malnutrition (eg, starvation), severe illness, major surgery, chronic alcoholism, and patients with renal failure on hemodialysis.
- The greater the degree of weight deficit & rapidity of replenishment increase the risk.

PATHOPHYSIOLOGY
Pathogenesis of Hypophosphatemia:
- **Hypophosphatemia is the hallmark and the predominant cause of the Refeeding syndrome.**
- During the fasting state, the body switches its main fuel source from carbohydrates to fatty acids and amino acids as its main energy sources, depleting many of the intracellular minerals. Insulin secretion is suppressed as the counterregulatory hormones are increased (eg, glucagon).
- During refeeding, stores of phosphate are depleted because nutrition replenishment and increased blood glucose from nutrition repletion shifts metabolism from fat to carbohydrate substrate. Glucose in the replenishment causes insulin release, resulting in increased cellular uptake of electrolytes (eg, phosphate used to produce ATP, potassium, calcium, magnesium, and thiamine).
- The increased metabolic rate & demand (1) require the use of phosphate, magnesium, and potassium, which are already depleted, using up remaining stores; (2) strains the heart, resulting in Heart failure, and (3) uses up a large amount of oxygen, which may lead to strain on the lungs.

CLINICAL MANIFESTATIONS
- Most fatalities due to Refeeding syndrome result from cardiac complications induced by Hypophosphatemia, including impaired contractility, decreased stroke volume, Decompensated heart failure, arrhythmias, Rhabdomyolysis, hemolysis, seizures, &/or respiratory insufficiency.

EVALUATION
- **The Refeeding syndrome is marked by Hypophosphatemia and volume overload,** so monitoring of electrolytes (eg, phosphate, magnesium, potassium, calcium levels), albumin, prealbumin, vital signs, and frequent physical examinations are essential for early detection of Refeeding syndrome.

MANAGEMENT
- **If the Refeeding syndrome occurs, slow &/or reduce nutritional replenishment & aggressively correct Hypophosphatemia and other electrolyte abnormalities, frequent monitoring of vital signs, daily weights, input, and outputs.**
- Thiamine is administered at least 30 minutes before the initiation of dextrose-based solutions & replenishment to prevent neurological complications. Multivitamins (including Vitamin B complex).
- ICU admission: Moderately to severely ill patients with marked edema or a serum phosphorous <2 mg/dL should be hospitalized to intravenously correct electrolyte and volume deficits. Patients should be admitted to the ICU for close monitoring.

PREVENTION
- The Refeeding syndrome can almost always be avoided by instituting slow caloric repletion, cautiously avoiding very rapid increases in the number of daily calories ingested, correcting phosphate levels ≤2.0 mEq/dL prior to beginning parenteral nutrition, and close monitoring of the patients and their laboratory tests (especially phosphate and other electrolytes), fluid balance, & vital signs, during the first few weeks of refeeding. Any deficits should be corrected as they develop.

INFANTILE HYPERTOPHIC PYLORIC STENOSIS (IHPS)

- **Hypertrophy & hyperplasia of the pyloric muscles causing a functional gastric outlet obstruction** (preventing gastric emptying), leading to forceful nonbilious vomiting, dehydration, and alkalosis in infants < 12 weeks.
- The exact etiology of Infantile hypertrophic pyloric stenosis is unknown.

RISK FACTORS
- **Most common in the first 3-12 weeks of life. Caucasians, Male predominance** 4:1, **first born infants** (30-40% of cases), maternal smoking during pregnancy.
- **Macrolide antibiotics** — **both Erythromycin & Azithromycin, particularly when administered to infants <2 weeks of age,** are associated with increased risk of IHPS.

PATHOPHYSIOLOGY
- The hallmark of IHPS is marked hypertrophy and hyperplasia of both the circular & longitudinal muscular layers of the pylorus (most common cause of intestinal obstruction in infancy).

CLINICAL MANIFESTATIONS
- Symptoms usually begin between 3-6 weeks of age and very rarely occur after 12 weeks of age.
- **Nonbilious, forceful (projectile) vomiting, especially after feeding.** Vomiting may be intermittent or occur after each feeding.
- **Strong appetite: Infants are usually hungry and nurse avidly,** often demanding to be refed soon afterwards (a "hungry vomiter").

PHYSICAL EXAMINATION
- **Olive sign: palpable pylorus ("olive-shaped" nontender, mobile firm 1 - 2 cm mass to the right of the epigastrium at the lateral edge of the rectus abdominis muscle [RUQ], especially after emesis.**
- May have hyperperistalsis, weight loss, or malnutrition. **May have signs of dehydration:** depressed fontanelles, dry mucous membranes, decreased tearing, poor skin turgor, lethargy.

DIAGNOSIS
- **Ultrasound is the initial imaging test of choice for infants presenting with typical symptoms of IHPS** (new onset of nonbilious vomiting in infants up to 3 months of age). Findings include an **elongated, thickened pylorus** (Hypoechoic muscle ring > 4 mm thickness with a hyperdense center & pyloric channel length > 15 mm). Classic "target" sign on transverse view. Ultrasound is highly sensitive & specific, easily performed, and no radiation risk.
- **Upper GI series: string sign: narrowed elongated pyloric channel** with a double track of barium.
Laboratory evaluation:
- **Hypochloremic metabolic alkalosis from vomiting** (due to the loss of large amounts of gastric hydrochloric acid). **Hypokalemia** with prolonged symptoms. Hyperbilirubinemia. Dehydration may elevate hemoglobin and hematocrit, cause hyper- or hyponatremia, or Acute kidney injury.

MANAGEMENT
- **Definitive management of IHPS is surgical Pyloromyotomy, often after initial fluid and electrolyte replacement.**
- Fluid and electrolyte management: Rehydration (IV fluids) & electrolyte repletion (eg, potassium replacement) before surgical treatment, even if it takes 24–48 hours.
- **Pyloromyotomy is the treatment of choice (definitive)** and consists of incision down to the mucosa along the pyloric length and the pyloric muscle is divided down to the submucosa. The surgery can be performed open or laparoscopically, depending on the expertise of the surgeon.
PROGNOSIS
- Surgery is curative and has a low morbidity, though patients may show as much as a four times greater risk for development of chronic abdominal pain of childhood.

CARCINOID TUMORS

- **Rare, well-differentiated neuroendocrine tumors (NET) that arise from enterochromaffin cells.**
- **55% occur in the GI tract**; 30% in the lungs.

CLINICAL MANIFESTATIONS
- Asymptomatic in many (incidental finding on endoscopy). Local symptoms depend on tumor location.
- **Carcinoid syndrome: periodic episodes of diarrhea (serotonin release), flushing, tachycardia, & bronchoconstriction** (histamine release), & hemodynamic instability (eg, hypotension).

DIAGNOSIS
- **24-hour urinary 5-hydroxyindoleacetic acid/5-HIAA excretion** (end product of serotonin metabolism), most useful initial test for Carcinoid syndrome. Not useful in foregut NETs.
- Tumor localization: Radiolabeled somatostatin analogs.
- Contrast-enhanced, triple-phase CT scans of the abdomen and pelvis. Contrast-enhanced MRI.

MANAGEMENT: Depends on the site. Options include surgical resection.

AUTOIMMUNE HEPATITIS

- Idiopathic chronic, inflammation of the liver characterized by [1] circulating autoantibodies and [2] elevated serum globulin levels.

EPIDEMIOLOGY
- **Most common in young to middle-aged women;** May occur with other autoimmune disorders.
- **Type I: most common type in the US.** May be associated with HLA-DR3 or HLA-DR4 (especially *B8-DRB1*03).
- Type II: is more commonly seen in children (2-14y) and Mediterranean populations.

CLINICAL MANIFESTATIONS
- Asymptomatic (25%) — may be picked up based on abnormal liver function laboratory tests.
- Nonspecific symptoms: (25%) — fatigue, nausea, malaise, abdominal pain, arthralgia, weight loss.
- Physical examination: normal or findings Cirrhosis/liver failure (eg, jaundice, ascites, splenomegaly).

DIAGNOSIS
- **Liver function tests — In acute presentations, elevations in aminotransferases (ALT & AST) may be >10-20 times the upper limit of the reference range.** Chronic symptoms or those with Cirrhosis may have normal serum bilirubin, alkaline phosphatase, with minimal transaminitis.
- **Hypergammaglobulinemia:** elevation in gamma globulins, especially IgG (associated with circulating autoantibodies) on Serum protein electrophoresis.

Autoantibodies
- **Type I (classic): positive Antinuclear antibodies (ANA) most common &/or anti-smooth muscle autoantibodies [(SMA) more specific], seen in ~65%** (titers ≥1:40). Rheumatoid factor positivity.
- Type II: anti-liver-kidney microsomal-1 antibodies (>1:10) alone or accompanied by anti-liver cytosol antibody-1 (ALC-1). Anti-mitochondrial antibodies (AMA) may be seen.

Liver biopsy:
- Liver biopsy: definitive diagnosis (not always necessary) — bridging necrosis or multiacinar necrosis, bridging fibrosis, & inflammatory lymphoplasmacytic infiltrate (cytotoxic T cells & plasma cells).

MANAGEMENT
- **Glucocorticoids: In adults, initial treatment with glucocorticoid monotherapy (eg, Prednisone 60 mg daily, Prednisolone) is the mainstay of treatment.** Azathioprine may be added.
- Lower-dose glucocorticoid for monotherapy (eg, 30 mg) or in combination with either Azathioprine (often started 2 weeks after Prednisone) or its prodrug, 6-Mercaptopurine, may be used.

NEONATAL HYPERBILIRUBINEMIA & JAUNDICE

- **Yellowish discoloration of the skin, sclera, & conjunctiva due to elevated plasma bilirubin in a newborn.** 65% of newborns develop jaundice with total serum bilirubin >6mg/dL in first week of life.
- **Usually, a transient & mild condition but in severe or rapid cases, may lead to Chronic bilirubin encephalopathy (kernicterus), characterized by cerebral dysfunction & encephalopathy.**
- Mechanism of neonatal hyperbilirubinemia: Hyperbilirubinemia from increased bilirubin load either due to [1] decrease in bilirubin clearance (decreased conjugation), [2] increased enterohepatic circulation of bilirubin, [3] an increase in bilirubin production, or a combination.

TYPES OF JAUNDICE
BENIGN (NONPATHOLOGIC) HYPERBILIRUBINEMIA (FORMERLY KNOWN AS PHYSIOLOGIC JAUNDICE):

- **Transient jaundice presenting after 24 hours of age,*** often days 2-5 of life due to normal newborn conditions** caused by 3 main causes: **[1] shortened RBC lifespan:** higher hematocrit + increased fetal RBC turnover rates increase bilirubin production, **[2] decreased activity of the enzymes of conjugation within the liver:** delayed clearance of bilirubin due to relative transient uridine diphosphate glucuronosyltransferase (UGT) deficiency, which increases with time; the sterile newborn gut results in decreased bilirubin clearance (normally, intestinal flora convert bilirubin to urobilinogen) & **[3] increased enterohepatic recirculation of bilirubin.**
- **Mild unconjugated (indirect) hyperbilirubinemia: Total bilirubin (TB) rises <5 mg/dL per day, peak occurs at 3-5 days of age, & TB ≤15mg/dL.** Mean TB levels peak at 7-9 mg/dL in White & Black infants; often higher in Eastern Asian infants, 10-14 mg/dL.
- In Benign jaundice, bilirubin levels fall in about 50% of the neonates during the first week of life & within 2 weeks, as mechanisms for bilirubin disposition mature, such as increased RBC lifespan, increased liver enzyme production, development of intestinal flora, and stooling patterns.

Increased enterohepatic recirculation of bilirubin:
(1) Breast milk jaundice:

- Etiologies: not fully understood but the infant liver is not mature enough to process lipids & increased enterohepatic recirculation play a role. **Seen in thriving breast-fed infants without hemolysis.**
- **Onset around the latter half of the first week of life (4th-7th day), with a peak bilirubin level around 2 weeks after birth, and progressively declines to normal levels within 3-12 weeks.**
- Management: The mother should continue to breastfeed as it will decline slowly over the next several months. Continued monitoring of the total bilirubin to ensure it remains within a safe range.

(2) Breastfeeding (lactational) failure jaundice (inadequate milk intake):

- **Breastfeeding (lactation) failure jaundice is due to prolonged inadequate (suboptimal) milk intake (fluid and caloric intake) during the first seven days of life,** resulting in **significant weight loss, hypovolemia,** and in severe cases, Hypernatremia.
- Decreased amounts of bowel movements to excrete bilirubin from the body, slower bilirubin elimination, and prolonged transit time increases enterohepatic circulation of bilirubin.
- These infants have prolonged duration of meconium stools (tarry and black) or transitional stools (turns from dark green to lighter green before transitioning to classic yellow "breastfeeding" stools).
- **May be associated with dark green stools, persistent 3 wet diapers in 24 hours** (normally the amount increases as infants grow) **and weight loss >10% from birth weight** (up to 10% weight loss is normal in neonates as long as the infant appears hydrated).

PATHOLOGIC

- **Pathologic causes may occur in the first 24 hours of life,*** persists >10-14 days, bilirubin increase >5 mg/dL/day, associated with a bilirubin >12 mg/dL in a term infant**; conjugated bilirubin >2 mg/dL or >20% of total bilirubin.
- **(1) Decreased clearance (conjugation):** Crigler-Najjar, Gilbert, or Dubin-Johnson syndromes.
- **(2) Overproduction of bilirubin: due to hemolytic anemia most common** (eg, ABO or Rh[D] incompatibility, Hereditary spherocytosis, G6PD deficiency. **TB often >5 mg/dL before 24h of age.**

CLINICAL MANIFESTATIONS
- **Jaundice:** yellowing of the skin, sclera, and the conjunctiva. In neonates, jaundice usually progresses from head to toe with increasing bilirubin levels. **Associated with bilirubin levels >5 mg/dL.**
- <u>Chronic bilirubin encephalopathy (kernicterus)</u> — **cerebral dysfunction & encephalopathy** due to bilirubin deposition in brain tissue (bilirubin crosses an immature blood-brain barrier, precipitating in the basal ganglia & other brain areas). May manifest as seizures, lethargy, irritability, hearing loss, & mental developmental delays. **Associated with total bilirubin >20-25 mg/dL.**

WORKUP
- <u>Liver function tests</u>, blood smear if hemolysis. <u>Coombs test</u> distinguishes between immune-mediated (eg, ABO incompatibility) from non-immune-mediated hemolytic disorders.
- Jaundice on day 1 may be worked up for sepsis, hemolysis, Rubella, Toxoplasmosis, occult hemorrhage, Erythroblastosis fetalis.

MANAGEMENT
- **No management needed in Physiologic jaundice.** Often resolves by 1 week in the full-term infant and by 2 weeks in the preterm infant.

[1] Phototherapy:
- <u>**Phototherapy**</u> is the initial intervention used to reduce total bilirubin (TB) levels **when TB exceeds a threshold level. Goal is to keep TB <20 mg/dL.** Phototherapy converts bilirubin into water-soluble photoisomers that are excreted directly into bile. Different thresholds in preterms.
- For term infants (≥38 weeks GA) without risk factors, phototherapy is initiated based on total bilirubin: 24 hours of age >12 mg/dL, 48 hours of age >15 mg/dL or 72 hours of age >18 mg/dL.

[2] Exchange transfusion
- <u>**Exchange transfusion**</u> **usually reserved for severe cases** (eg, hemolysis, ABO incompatibility. Rh isoimmunization), symptomatic infants, severe hyperbilirubinemia (increasing TB), rapidly rising TB levels (rate of raise >0.2 mg/dL per hour), or at risk for severe hyperbilirubinemia with failure to respond adequately to intensive phototherapy. IVIG in some cases of iso-immune hemolysis.

PATTERNS OF LIVER INJURY

❶ **HEPATOCELLULAR DAMAGE:** ↑ALT & AST primarily. ALT more sensitive for liver disease than AST.

❷ **CHOLESTASIS:** <u>↑levels of alkaline phosphatase with ↑GGT,</u> ↑bilirubin greater than ↑ALT & AST.

❸ **LIVER "SYNTHETIC" FUNCTION:**
<u>PROTHROMBIN TIME (PT):</u> depends on synthesis of vitamin K-dependent coagulation factors 2,7,9,10. **PT is an earlier indicator of severe liver injury/prognosis than albumin.** Prolonged PT is seen when 80% of the liver's protein synthesizing ability is lost.
<u>ALBUMIN:</u> useful marker of overall liver protein synthesis. Levels decreases with liver failure.

DISORDERS	LABORATORY PATTERN OF LIVER INJURIES
(1) ALCOHOL (ETOH) HEPATITIS	A<u>S</u>T:ALT>2:1 ⇨ alcohol hepatitis "S = Scotch" **(AST levels usually <500).** AST is found primarily in the mitochondria. ETOH causes direct mitochondrial injury ⇨ ↑AST
(2) VIRAL/TOXIC/INFLAMMATORY PROCESSES	• ALT > AST ⇨ usually. Think A<u>L</u>T for <u>L</u>iver. • <u>AST & ALT >1,000</u> ⇨ usually **acute viral hepatitis** (A, B, & rarely C) • Chronic viral hepatitis B, C, D ⇨ mildly ↑ALT & AST (<400)
(3) BILIARY OBSTRUCTION OR INTRAHEPATIC CHOLESTASIS	• ↑alkaline phosphatase (ALP) ⇨ <u>↑ALP with ↑GGT suggests hepatic source or biliary obstruction.</u> • GGT most sensitive indicator of biliary injury (nonspecific). • **If ↑ALP without ↑GGT, look for sources other than the liver (eg, bone**, gut**).**
(4) TRUE HEPATIC FUNCTION	Decreased hepatic protein production: • **Decreased albumin, increased PT** (later increased aPTT)

DUBIN-JOHNSON SYNDROME

- Hereditary conjugated (direct) hyperbilirubinemia due to decreased hepatocyte excretion of conjugated bilirubin (gene mutation MRP2). Think Ds: **D**ubin, **Direct** bilirubinemia, **Dark liver**

CLINICAL MANIFESTATIONS
- **Most are asymptomatic**. May present with generalized constitutional symptoms. **Mild icterus.**
- **Dark urine may be seen due** to bilirubinuria resulting from a rise in conjugated bilirubin.

DIAGNOSIS
- **Mild, isolated conjugated (direct) hyperbilirubinemia** (at least 50% of the total bilirubin is the direct fraction, often between 2–5 mg/dL but can increase as high as 20-25 mg/dL with concurrent illness, pregnancy, or oral contraceptive pill use. **LFTs otherwise normal** as are routine lab testing.
- The total urinary coproporphyrin is normal in Dubin-Johnson syndrome, but >80% of it is coproporphyrin I (compared to 75% of coproporphyrin III in normal subjects).
- Biopsy: **grossly black liver & dark granular pigment in the hepatocytes.**

MANAGEMENT
- Dubin-Johnson syndrome is a benign condition, and no treatment is required.

Rotor's syndrome: similar to Dubin-Johnson but milder in nature, associated with **conjugated & unconjugated hyperbilirubinemia but is not associated with grossly black liver on biopsy.**

CRIGLER-NAJJAR SYNDROME

- **Rare autosomal recessive disorder — Hereditary unconjugated (indirect) hyperbilirubinemia.**
- Pathophysiology: **decreased activity of the glucuronosyltransferase (UGT) enzyme** needed to convert indirect bilirubin to direct bilirubin. Can result in bilirubin-induced neurologic dysfunction.

TYPES:
- **Type I: no UGT activity** (or trace). High risk of developing bilirubin-induced neurologic dysfunction.
- **Type II (Arias Syndrome): markedly reduced UGT activity** (≤10% of normal activity).

CLINICAL MANIFESTATIONS
- **Type I: neonatal jaundice with severe progression in the second week (severe & persistent elevations of unconjugated bilirubin) that may lead to kernicterus (bilirubin-induced encephalopathy)** — hypotonia, deafness, lethargy, oculomotor palsy. Potentially fatal.
- **Type II: usually asymptomatic.** Often an incidental finding on routine lab testing or after an acute episode of jaundice, often triggered by fasting, an intercurrent illness, or general anesthesia.

DIAGNOSIS:
- **Isolated indirect (unconjugated) hyperbilirubinemia + otherwise normal liver function tests.**
- **Type I:** striking unconjugated hyperbilirubinemia **(indirect bilirubin often 20-50 mg/dL).**
- **Type II: serum indirect bilirubin often 7-10 mg/dL** (<20). May increase during illness or fasting.
- Molecular testing for mutations in the bilirubin-UGT1 A1 gene. Normal hepatic histology on biopsy.

MANAGEMENT OF TYPE I:
- **Chronic daily phototherapy mainstay of treatment** + oral calcium. Liver transplant definitive.
- Plasmapheresis may be used in acute exacerbations & elevations of bilirubin levels (eg, crisis).

MANAGEMENT OF TYPE II:
- **Treatment usually not needed** but if required, **Phenobarbital is an enzyme inducer, increasing UGT activity** (decreases bilirubin by 30-80%). Type I not responsive to Phenobarbital.

GILBERT SYNDROME

- **Hereditary <u>mild isolated unconjugated (indirect) hyperbilirubinemia</u>.**
- Relatively common (5–10% of the US population) — Most common inherited disorder of bilirubin glucuronidation. Due to a mutation on the UGT1A1 gene on chromosome 2 (2q37).
- More common in males.

PATHOPHYSIOLOGY
- **Reduced uridine diphosphoglucuronate-glucuronosyltransferase 1A1 (UGT1A1) activity (10-35% of normal)** & decreased bilirubin uptake, leading to increased indirect bilirubin. UGT is the enzyme responsible for the conjugation of bilirubin with glucuronic acid.

CLINICAL MANIFESTATIONS
- Other than episodic jaundice, most patients are usually asymptomatic with a normal physical exam.
- **May develop <u>transient &/or recurrent episodes of jaundice</u> triggered during periods of stress, fasting, illness, dehydration, menstruation, alcohol use, & physical exertion.**

DIAGNOSIS
<u>Mild isolated unconjugated (indirect) hyperbilirubinemia:</u>
- <u>Usually an incidental finding</u>: **slight increase in isolated Indirect (unconjugated) bilirubin level with otherwise normal LFTs.**
- **Total bilirubin levels are usually <3mg/dL** (although wide variation can be seen). May be <u>transiently</u> higher in the context of increased bilirubin production during "stress" as described above.

<u>Liver biopsy:</u>
- Not usually needed — usually normal hepatic histology; mild increased lipofuscin pigment in some.

MANAGEMENT
- **<u>Supportive care & reassurance</u>: no treatment needed in most as it is a mild, benign disease.**
- Phenobarbital normalizes both the serum bilirubin concentration and hepatic bilirubin clearance. Phenobarbital is an enzyme inducer, increasing UGT activity.

UNCONJUGATED (INDIRECT) HYPERBILIRUBINEMIA		CONJUGATED (DIRECT) HYPERBILIRUBINEMIA	
GILBERT SYNDROME	**CRIGGLER NAJJAR**	**DUBIN-JOHSNON**	**ROTOR SYNDROME**
• **<u>UGT activity</u> 10-35% of normal**	• **<u>UGT activity</u> ≤10% of normal Absent in Type 1**	**3 Ds:** • **(1) Direct bili: Isolated mild conjugated (direct) bilirubinemia**	• **Direct bili**
• **Mild unconjugated hyperbilirubinemia (<4 mg/dL)**	• **Unconjugated hyperbilirubinemia (>4 mg/dL)**		• Normal liver
		• **(2) Dark urine**	Total urinary coproporphyrin excretion is substantially increased in RS, in contrast to the normal levels seen in DJS.
• Normal AST, ALT, & alkaline phosphatase	• Normal AST, ALT, & alkaline phosphatase	• **(3) Dark liver** on biopsy	
• Normal CBC, blood smear, reticulocytes	• Normal CBC, blood smear, reticulocytes		

ACUTE CALCULOUS CHOLECYSTITIS

- Inflammation and infection of the gallbladder due to obstruction of the cystic duct by gallstones.

ETIOLOGIES:
- **_E. coli_ most common** & other Gram-negative enteric organisms (eg, _Klebsiella_ spp., and _Enterobacter_).
- _Enterococcus_ (12%).

CLINICAL MANIFESTATIONS
Triad: [1] RUQ pain, [2] fever, and [3] ↑WBC count. May have **nausea, vomiting**, and anorexia.
- **Right upper quadrant, epigastric pain** — **usually severe, steady, & continuous (prolonged >4-6 hours), progressive, may radiate to the right shoulder, interscapular area, right scapula, or back, may be aggravated by movement, and is often precipitated by fatty foods or large meals** (release of CCK after meals causes gallbladder contraction).

PHYSICAL EXAMINATION
- **Fever** often low-grade and associated with tachycardia. Chills and rigors are not common. **Enlarged, palpable gallbladder.** Voluntary and involuntary guarding. **Jaundice is <u>not</u> usually seen.**
- **⊕ Murphy's sign: RUQ pain or inspiratory arrest with palpation of the gallbladder fossa.**
- **⊕ Boas sign: referred pain to right shoulder subscapular area** (right phrenic nerve irritation).

DIAGNOSIS
- **Acute cholecystitis should be suspected in a patient presenting with the triad of:**
  [1] right upper quadrant or epigastric pain (often continuous), [2] fever, and [3] leukocytosis.
- **Increased WBCs** — leukocytosis with neutrophilia. WBC often 12,000-15,000/mcL.
- **LFTs:** Because the obstruction is limited to the gallbladder, (1) **significant increase in LFTs is not common if uncomplicated** (only 25% have modest serum transaminase elevations, usually <5-fold elevation), & (2) **cholestatic labs (increased alkaline phosphatase & GGT) are not usually seen**.
- **Transabdominal ultrasound: initial test of choice to see gallbladder inflammation** — gallbladder wall thickening (>4-5 mm) or edema (double wall sign), gallbladder distention, pericholecystic fluid, sonographic Murphy's sign. Gallbladder calculi seen in 90–95%.
- **Radionuclide Cholescintigraphy (HIDA scan): criterion standard** (most sensitive). **HIDA used if the diagnosis remains unclear despite Ultrasound.** Findings: Cholecystitis = nonvisualization of the gallbladder (failure of the gallbladder to fill) due to the stone blocking the cystic duct.

MANAGEMENT
- **Nonoperative management followed by early cholecystectomy (laparoscopic preferred when possible) as early as possible, ideally within 72 hours of admission to the hospital.**
Nonoperative management
- **Supportive management — eg, NPO, IV fluids, pain control with NSAIDs** (eg, Ketorolac) or **opioids** (eg, Morphine, Hydromorphone, Meperidine), electrolyte correction, **and IV antibiotics.**
- **Antibiotic regimens: — Metronidazole plus EITHER Cephalosporin (eg, Ceftriaxone, Cefazolin, Cefuroxime, Cefotaxime) or Fluoroquinolone** (eg, Ciprofloxacin or Levofloxacin). High-risk patients (eg, septic or critically ill): Metronidazole plus EITHER Cefepime or Cefotaxime; or single-agent Imipenem-Cilastatin, Meropenem, Doripenem, or Piperacillin-tazobactam.

Operative management:
- **Early cholecystectomy: laparoscopic cholecystectomy preferred over open cholecystectomy.**
- **Emergent cholecystectomy is indicated if there is a complication** (eg, perforation, gangrene, or emphysematous cholecystitis), progressive symptoms (eg, high fever, hemodynamic instability).
- Gallbladder drainage: in conjunction with IV antibiotics are often indicated in patients with a high surgical risk (eg, septic or critically ill patients, inoperable patients), or noncritical patients who fail to respond after 1-3 days of antibiotic therapy. Drainage options include Percutaneous cholecystostomy and Endoscopic transpapillary or Transmural drainage.

ACUTE CHOLECYSTITIS

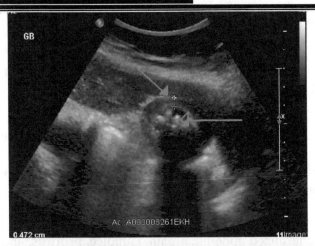

Transabdominal ultrasound:

- Gallbladder wall thickening (closed arrow) or edema (double wall sign)

- Gallbladder distention, pericholecystic fluid, sonographic Murphy's sign.

- Gallbladder calculi in 90–95% (open arrow).

ACUTE ACALCULOUS CHOLECYSTITIS

- **Acute necroinflammatory disease of the gallbladder not due to gallstones.**
- Accounts for 10% of Acute cholecystitis. **Associated with high morbidity & mortality**.

PATHOPHYSIOLOGY
- **Gallbladder stasis and ischemia** leading to a local inflammatory reaction in the gallbladder wall; leads to concentration of bile salts, gallbladder distention, secondary infection, perforation, or necrosis of gallbladder tissue. Multiorgan failure is often present.

RISK FACTORS
- **Current hospitalization, critically ill patients with no oral intake for a prolonged period**, within 2-4 weeks of major surgery.

CLINICAL MANIFESTATIONS
- **Fever, leukocytosis, jaundice, sepsis, vague abdominal discomfort.** May be septic.
- Because of gradual presentation, gallbladder necrosis, gangrene, & perforation often present.

DIAGNOSIS
Based on clinical symptoms in the setting of supportive imaging & exclusion of an alternative diagnosis.
- <u>Ultrasound</u> **initial test of choice — distended gallbladder with thickened walls and pericholecystic fluid without calcifications.**
- <u>Abdominal CT scan</u> (contrast-enhanced) if the diagnosis remains uncertain after Ultrasound.
- <u>HIDA scan</u> performed if diagnosis remains uncertain after CT scan.
- <u>Laboratory evaluation:</u> leukocytosis and/or elevated liver function tests

MANAGEMENT
- **Supportive care** — IV fluids, bowel rest, analgesia, electrolyte correction, broad-spectrum antibiotics.
- **Definitive treatment with either cholecystectomy or cholecystostomy.** Indications for emergent cholecystectomy include emphysema, gallbladder perforation, or gallbladder necrosis.

CHRONIC CHOLECYSTITIS

- Fibrosis and thickening of the gallbladder due to chronic inflammatory cell infiltration of the gallbladder evident on histopathology.
- The presence of Chronic cholecystitis does not correlate with symptoms.
- Almost always associated with gallstones.

ACUTE ASCENDING CHOLANGITIS

- **Biliary tract inflammation & infection secondary to obstruction of the common bile duct.**

MICROBIOLOGY
- Most due to Gram-negative enteric organisms ascending from the duodenum — *E. coli* **most common,** *Klebsiella* (second most common), *Enterobacter, B. fragilis.* Anaerobes or Enterococcus.

ETIOLOGIES
- **Choledocholithiasis is the most common cause,** with infection-causing stones in the common bile duct leading to partial or complete obstruction of the biliary system.
- Other causes include benign or malignant strictures of biliary ducts, pancreatic cancer, ampullary adenoma or cancer, parasites, roundworm (*Ascaris lumbricoides)*, tapeworm (*Taenia).*

CLINICAL MANIFESTATIONS
- Symptoms include fever, chills, malaise, rigors, generalized abdominal pain, jaundice, pruritus, and pale stools.
- **Charcot's triad: [1] spiking fever with chills, [2] RUQ pain, and [3] jaundice** (50-70%).
- **Reynold's pentad addition of [4] hypotension or shock + [5] altered mental status.**
- Elderly patients may have minimal abdominal pain and may only present with hypotension.

PHYSICAL EXAMINATION
- **Fever, right upper quadrant tenderness, jaundice**, abdominal distension.
- Severe: altered mental status or hemodynamic instability.

DIAGNOSIS
- **Leukocytosis with neutrophil predominance; may have left shift.**
- **Liver function tests: Cholestatic pattern — increased alkaline phosphatase & gamma-glutamyl transpeptidase (GGT), increased bilirubin ≥2 mg/dL (mostly conjugated).** Aminotransferases (AST, ALT) may be mildly or significantly elevated.
- **RUQ Ultrasound: initial imaging of choice — common bile duct dilatation or stones, thickening of the walls of the bile ducts, pyogenic material.**
- Abdominal CT scan: **performed in patients with abdominal pain with a normal abdominal US.**
- Magnetic resonance imaging (MRI/MRCP) if both US and CT scan are normal & diagnosis is unclear.
- **Cholangiography: Criterion standard via ERCP or PTC (percutaneous transhepatic cholangiography)** — usually performed once the patient has been afebrile/stable for 48 hours after IV antibiotics.

INITIAL MANAGEMENT
- **IV antibiotics followed by biliary drainage with CBD decompression & stone extraction once stable [eg, Endoscopic retrograde cholangiopancreatography (ERCP)] within 24-48 hours.**
- **Antibiotics:** Options include Ampicillin/sulbactam; Piperacillin/tazobactam; Ceftriaxone + Metronidazole; Fluoroquinolone + Metronidazole; Ampicillin + Gentamicin.

Common bile duct decompression & stone extraction:
- **ERCP (endoscopic sphincterotomy) with stone extraction &/or stent insertion** (depending on the cause of the obstruction) **is the treatment of choice for establishing biliary drainage in Acute cholangitis — usually performed once the patent has been afebrile/stable for 48 hours after IV antibiotics.**
- Percutaneous transhepatic cholangiogram (PTC) catheter drainage or Percutaneous cholecystostomy tube in unstable patients, if unable to do ERCP, or if ERCP drainage is unsuccessful.
- Open surgical decompression + T-tube insertion is reserved for patients in whom other methods of biliary drainage cannot be performed or have failed.

CHOLELITHIASIS

- **Gallstones in the biliary tract (usually in the gallbladder) without inflammation.**
- Complications include Choledocholithiasis, Acute cholangitis, & Acute cholecystitis.

TYPES OF GALLSTONES
- **Cholesterol most common (mixed & pure) 90%;** Pigmented 10%.
- Black stones: hemolysis or Alcohol-related Cirrhosis.
- Brown stones: increased in the Asian population; parasitic or bacterial infections.

RISK FACTORS
- More common in female patients, pregnancy, OCP use, older patients, patients with high serum lipid levels, increased triglycerides, Native Americans, chronic hemolysis, Cirrhosis, IBD, Fibrate use.

CLINICAL MANIFESTATIONS
- Most individuals with gallstones are asymptomatic (detected incidentally on abdominal imaging).
- **Biliary "colic": episodic, abrupt RUQ** or epigastric pain, resolves slowly, **lasting 30 minutes to <6 hours.** May be associated with **nausea & precipitated by fatty foods or large meals.**

DIAGNOSIS
- **Uncomplicated gallstone disease is characterized by transient biliary colic (<4-6 hours), a normal physical examination, and normal laboratory tests** [complete blood count, LFTs (aminotransferases, bilirubin, alkaline phosphatase), amylase, and lipase].
- **Ultrasound: initial test of choice** — gallstones appear as echogenic foci that cast an acoustic shadow.
- CT or MRI may also be used.

MANAGEMENT
- **Asymptomatic: Observation** — many found incidentally will remain asymptomatic.
- **Symptomatic: elective Laparoscopic cholecystectomy is the standard of care, and most patients are managed as outpatients.** Ursodeoxycholic acid can be used but not as helpful.

CHOLEDOCHOLITHIASIS

- **Gallstones in the common bile duct,** which can lead to cholestasis due to blockage.
- More common in female patients, pregnancy, older patients, and those with high serum lipid levels.
- The 2 major complications of Choledocholithiasis are (1) Acute pancreatitis and (2) Acute cholangitis.

CLINICAL MANIFESTATIONS
- **Prolonged biliary colic: The RUQ or epigastric pain is usually more prolonged (>6 hours) than is classically associated with typical biliary colic** (which typically resolves within 6 hours) due to the presence of the stone blocking the bile duct. Nausea, and vomiting.
- Physical examination: RUQ or epigastric tenderness. **Jaundice** may be accompanied with a history including clay-colored stools and urine turning tea-colored.

DIAGNOSIS
- Labs: elevated AST and ALT. **Cholestatic pattern: increased alkaline phosphatase + GGT.**
- **Ultrasound: often initial imaging test ordered — dilated common bile duct is suggestive.**
- **ERCP (Endoscopic retrograde cholangiopancreatography) diagnostic test of choice.** ERCP can be diagnostic as well as therapeutic (allows for stone extraction). Often obtained after ultrasound.
- Magnetic resonance cholangiopancreatography (MRCP) and endoscopic ultrasound (EUS) may be used in patients with intermediate risk (determined by labs & Transabdominal ultrasound).

MANAGEMENT
- **ERCP stone extraction preferred** over laparoscopic cholecystectomy or choledocholithotomy.

ACUTE HEPATITIS

ACUTE VIRAL HEPATITIS
CLINICAL MANIFESTATIONS
- <u>Prodromal phase</u>: malaise, arthralgia, fatigue, URI symptoms, anorexia, **decreased desire to smoke,** nausea, vomiting, abdominal pain, loss of appetite, acholic stools.
- **Hepatitis A is associated with spiking fever.**
- <u>Icteric phase</u>: **jaundice** (most don't develop this phase). If present, jaundice usually develops once the fever subsides.
- <u>Fulminant</u>: **encephalopathy, coagulopathy**, hepatomegaly, jaundice, edema, ascites, asterixis, hyperreflexia.

LABORATORY VALUES
- Increased ALT and AST (both usually >500 if acute & <500 if chronic); May have hyperbilirubinemia.

OUTCOMES
- Clinical recovery usually within 3-16 weeks; 10% of adults with HBV & 80% of HCV become chronic.
- **Chronic Hepatitis:** disease >6 months duration. **Only HBV, HCV, & HDV associated with chronicity.** Chronic may lead to End stage liver disease (ESLD) or Hepatocellular carcinoma (HCC).

FULMINANT HEPATITIS
- **Acute hepatic failure in patients with Acute Hepatitis.**
ETIOLOGIES
- **Acetaminophen toxicity most common cause in the US.**
- **Viral hepatitis,** Autoimmune hepatitis, drug reactions (eg, Tolcapone), sepsis. **Reye syndrome.**

CLINICAL MANIFESTATIONS
- **Encephalopathy:** vomiting, coma, AMS, seizures, **asterixis (flapping tremor of the hand with wrist extension), hyperreflexia.** Cerebral edema & increased intracranial pressure (ICP).
- **Coagulopathy:** increased prothrombin time (PT), INR ≥1.5, and eventually increased PTT, due to decreased hepatic production of coagulation factors.
- Edema, hepatomegaly. Jaundice (not usually seen in Reye syndrome; mild if present).
Reye syndrome:
- **An uncommon, rapidly progressive, noninflammatory encephalopathy associated with altered mental status, cerebral edema, & liver dysfunction (fulminant hepatitis).**
- Reye syndrome often begins **several days (3-5 days)** <u>after recovery from a viral illness</u> (most common with Varicella or Influenza A), <u>especially with ingestion of Salicylates (Aspirin)</u> **during the viral illness.** Liver damage, hepatomegaly, and multi-organ failure may occur.
- <u>Encephalopathy</u>: **behavioral changes, intractable vomiting, and confusion, which may progress to seizures and coma;** dilated pupils with minimal response to light.
- <u>Physical examination</u>: **Hepatomegaly common.** May have a rash on the hands & feet. Jaundice rare.

DIAGNOSIS
- **Combination of symptoms of encephalopathy, marked elevation in aminotransferase, coagulopathy [increased prothrombin time (PT), increased INR ≥1.5], Hypoglycemia common** (results from impaired hepatic gluconeogenesis), **increased ammonia** (encephalopathy), and metabolic acidosis. Fatty liver may be seen on imaging in Reye syndrome.
- Labs to determine potential etiologies: eg, Acetaminophen levels, viral serologies.

MANAGEMENT
- <u>Supportive</u>: IV fluids electrolyte repletion, Mannitol if ICP elevation, PPI stress ulcer prophylaxis. Blood products of platelets or cryoprecipitate reserved for active bleeding coagulopathy.
- **Liver transplant definitive.**

HEPATITIS E VIRUS (HEV)

- Acute viral infection of the liver due to Hepatitis E virus (HEV) infection.
- HEV is a 27-34 nm RNA hepevirus (in the Hepeviridae family).
- **Hepatitis E virus (HEV) is the most common cause of acute viral hepatitis in the world.**

TRANSMISSION:
- **Fecal-oral (similar to HAV) — consumption of contaminated food or water, especially with international travel to endemic areas.**
- Blood transfusions. Mother-to-child transmission.
- Uncommon routes of transmission: secondary person-to-person spread from infected persons to their close contacts. Fecal shedding uncommon.

CLINICAL MANIFESTATIONS
- Incubation period of Hepatitis E is from 14-60 days (mean 5–6 weeks).
- **Most patients are asymptomatic or mildly symptomatic self-limited illness** — eg, nausea, vomiting, RUQ abdominal pain, fatigue, malaise, myalgia, poor appetite, anorexia, and fever.
- Prodrome of anorexia, nausea, vomiting, malaise, and aversion to smoking.
- Malaise, myalgia, arthralgia, easy fatigability, upper respiratory symptoms, and anorexia.
- **Fulminant hepatitis is rare (1–2% of all cases), however Fulminant hepatitis E and death are seen with increased incidence in pregnant women (up to 20% of cases in pregnant women), malnourished individuals, or patients with preexisting liver disease.**

PHYSICAL EXAMINATION
- **Physical findings may include jaundice, scleral icterus, hepatomegaly, & right upper quadrant tenderness to palpation.** A low-grade fever [38°-39°C (100°–102°F)] more often HAV & HEV.
- Jaundice phase: occurs after 5–10 days but may appear at the same time as the initial symptoms. Patients may develop dark urine (bilirubinuria) and pale, acholic stools (lacking bilirubin pigment) within a week, followed by jaundice, icteric (yellow-tinted) sclera, and pruritus (40-70% of cases). The early signs & symptoms usually diminish with jaundice onset.

DIAGNOSIS
- **Liver function testing: Strikingly elevated ALT or AST levels occur early (often >1,000 international units/dL) with serum ALT usually higher than AST**, followed by elevations of bilirubin (typically ≤10 mg/dL) and alkaline phosphatase (up to 400 U/L).
Serologic testing:
- **Acute infection: serum IgM anti-HEV antibodies.** Diagnosis is confirmed by measuring HEV-specific immunoglobulin (IgM) antibodies in the blood.
- **Past exposure & immunity: IgG HEV Ab with negative IgM.** Immunoglobulin G (IgG) anti-HEV emerges soon after infection and remains present for the person's lifetime, denoting lifelong protective immunity.
- Additional testing can include reverse transcriptase-polymerase chain reaction to detect the viral RNA.

MANAGEMENT
- **Supportive care only: No specific treatment needed in most patients with acute uncomplicated HEV infection** — similar to HAV, HEV is self-limiting and not associated with a chronic state after acute HEV infection, except in immunocompromised patients such as transplant recipients.
- **Clinical recovery is generally complete within 3 months.**

PREVENTION:
- Improved public hygiene reduces the risk of HEV infection in endemic areas.

HEPATITIS A VIRUS (HAV)

- Acute viral infection of the liver due to Hepatitis A virus (HAV) infection.
- HAV is an RNA hepatovirus (picornavirus family) that causes epidemics or sporadic cases of hepatitis.

TRANSMISSION
- **Fecal-oral (similar to HEV) — either via person-to-person contact or consumption of contaminated food or water, especially with international travel.**
- **Globally, sanitation has the greatest impact on HAV.** Endemic rates are high in developing countries with poor sanitation.
- High-risk groups in low endemic areas include injection-drug users, men who have sex with men, people traveling to endemic areas, and day care workers.
- **There is no chronic carrier state; therefore, HAV does not cause chronic liver disease.**

CLINICAL MANIFESTATIONS
- The incubation period usually ranges from 14-28 days but can last up to 50 days.
- Clinical illness is more common (>70%) and more severe in adults compared to children, in whom it is usually asymptomatic (especially <6 years of age).
- **Most patients are asymptomatic or develop a mildly symptomatic self-limited illness —** eg, nausea, vomiting, RUQ or epigastric abdominal pain, fatigue, malaise, myalgia, poor appetite, anorexia, and fever; **HAV may be associated with spiking fever.**
- **Prodrome of anorexia, nausea, vomiting, malaise, and aversion to smoking.**
- Cholestatic hepatitis: Jaundice, dark urine (bilirubinemia), clay-colored stool, and pruritus may occur, with elevated alkaline phosphatase and bilirubin.
- Fulminant hepatitis (rare <1%) — hepatic encephalopathy, abnormal LFTs, and increased INR ≥1.5.

PHYSICAL EXAMINATION
- **Physical findings may include hepatomegaly (80%), right upper quadrant tenderness to palpation, jaundice, or scleral icterus.** Splenomegaly in 15%.
- **Jaundice phase:** occurs after 5–10 days but may appear at the same time as the initial symptoms. **Patients may develop dark urine (bilirubinuria) and pale, acholic stools (lacking bilirubin pigment) within a week, followed by jaundice, icteric (yellow-tinted) sclera, and pruritus** (40-70% of cases). The early signs & symptoms usually diminish with jaundice onset.

DIAGNOSIS
- **Liver function testing: Strikingly elevated ALT or AST levels occur early (often >1,000 IU/dL) with serum ALT usually higher than AST,** followed by elevations of bilirubin (typically ≤10 mg/dL) & alkaline phosphatase (up to 400 U/L). Serum aminotransferases peak ~4 weeks after exposure onset of symptoms and then decrease by ~75% per week.
- Complete blood count (CBC): The white blood cell count is normal to low, especially in the preicteric phase, but may reveal a mild lymphocytosis. Large, atypical lymphocytes are sometimes noted.

Serologic testing:
- **Acute:** ⊕ **serum IgM anti-HAV antibodies.** Diagnosis is confirmed by measuring HAV-specific immunoglobulin (IgM) antibodies in the blood. IgM anti-HAV & IgG-HAV appear early in the illness.
- **Past exposure & immunity: IgG HAV Ab with negative IgM.** Immunoglobulin G (IgG) anti-HAV develops soon after infection & remains present for the person's lifetime (lifelong immunity).
- Additional testing can include reverse transcriptase-polymerase chain reaction to detect HAV viral RNA.

MANAGEMENT
- **Supportive management only:** **no specific treatment needed in most patients with acute uncomplicated HAV infection beyond supportive care** — similar to HEV, HAV is self-limiting and not associated with a chronic state or chronic liver disease.
- In the rare case of fulminant HAV hepatitis, liver transplantation may be a life-saving measure.

PROGNOSIS
- **Excellent prognosis** — **HAV infection does not become chronic, and individuals do not become reinfected after recovering from infection (long term immunity is common).** HAV not associated with Cirrhosis because there is no chronic state.
- However, relapse may occur. Full clinical recovery generally occurs within 3 months.
- The most important prognostic factor is age; the older the individual, the increased risk for an adverse reaction or event. Long term sequelae are very rare.

PREVENTION
- **Handwashing & improved sanitation has the greatest impact to reduce transmission; food safety and HAV immunization also reduces the risk.**

HAV VACCINE
- Vaccination against Hepatitis A is available as inactivated, single-antigen vaccines or in combination with Hepatitis B.
- **Standard adult dosing** recommends administration of **2 doses of the vaccine 6-12 months apart.**
- Efficacy: Hepatitis A vaccine is very effective in preventing the infection with effectiveness rates 82%-95%. However, the effectiveness wanes after 15 years. Vaccines with booster doses are estimated to be effective for 25 years.

HAV vaccine indications include:
- **international travelers 6 months of age or older.**
- routine immunization for children, beginning at age one year old (12-23 months) following routine vaccine schedules; persons >40 years of age, patients, chronic liver disease; men who have sex with men, persons with HIV infection; animal handlers, persons who use injection or non-injection drugs, persons; experiencing homelessness, persons who are incarcerated; close personal contacts of international adoptees, persons living in group settings for those with developmental disabilities, and individuals who request HAV vaccination.

POSTEXPOSURE PROPHYLAXIS
(1) Healthy individuals 1-40 years old:
- **HAV vaccine preferred** over immunoglobulin, **within 2 weeks of exposure.** Vaccination is superior to immune globulin to produce antibody concentrations and durability of immune response.

(2) Healthy individuals > 40 years old:
- **HAV vaccine (with or without immune globulin, depending on risk)** within 2 weeks of exposure, rather than immunoglobulin alone. The HAV and immune globulin should be given at different sites.

(3) Immunocompromised or chronic liver disease >1 year old:
- **HAV vaccine + HAV immunoglobulin,** within 2 weeks of exposure.

(4) Immunoglobulin only:
- **Children <12 months** and individuals for whom HAV vaccine is contraindicated (eg, who are allergic to the vaccine).

HEPATITIS D VIRUS (HDV)

- **Defective RNA virus that requires Hepatitis B virus surface antigen (HBsAg) to cause coinfection or superimposed infection.** It is cleared when surface antigen (HBsAg) is cleared.

PATHOPHYSIOLOGY
- Although HDV can replicate autonomously, the simultaneous presence of HBV is required for complete virion assembly and secretion because HDV uses the HBsAg as its envelope protein.
- Therefore, individuals with **Hepatitis D are <u>always</u> dually infected with HDV and HBV.**

Coinfection:
- Coinfection of HBV and HDV in an individual susceptible to HBV infection (eg, anti-HBs-negative) results in acute hepatitis B + D.
- It is clinically indistinguishable from classical acute Hepatitis B alone and is usually transient and self-limited. However, a high incidence of liver failure has been reported among injection drug users.
- The rate of progression to chronic infection is similar to acute Hepatitis B alone since persistence of HDV infection is dependent upon persistence of HBV infection.

Superinfection:
- HDV superinfection of a chronic HBsAg carrier may present as a severe acute hepatitis in a previously unrecognized HBV carrier, or as an exacerbation of preexisting chronic Hepatitis B.
- Progression to chronic HDV infection occurs in almost all patients. However, HBV replication is usually suppressed by HDV. **Increased risk for decompensation & Hepatocellular carcinoma.**
- **In chronic Hepatitis B, superimposed infection by HDV appears to carry a worse short-term prognosis, often resulting in acute liver failure or severe chronic hepatitis that progresses rapidly to Cirrhosis** due to the direct cytopathic effect of HDV.

TRANSMISSION
- **Primarily parenteral**: eg, percutaneous exposure via injection drug use, blood, or blood products.

CLINICAL MANIFESTATIONS
- Most are asymptomatic. <u>Symptomatic</u> — fatigue, myalgia, nausea, RUQ pain, jaundice, dark urine.

DIAGNOSIS
- <u>Screening:</u> **Detection of antibody to hepatitis D antigen (anti-HDV) and, where available, hepatitis D antigen (HDAg) or HDV RNA in serum.**
- Confirmed by immunochemical staining of liver biopsies for HDAg or RT-PCR for **HDV RNA in serum.**
- **Hepatitis B serologies: Due to the dependence of HDV on Hepatitis B virus (HBV), the presence of Hepatitis B surface antigen (HBsAg) is necessary for the diagnosis of HDV infection.**
- <u>HBV/HDV coinfection:</u> The additional presence of IgM antibody to Hepatitis B core antigen (IgM anti-HBc) is necessary for the diagnosis of acute HBV/HDV coinfection.
- <u>Acute HDV superinfection:</u> HBsAg is present in both situations, but IgM anti-HBc should be negative in acute HDV superinfection.

MANAGEMENT
- <u>Pegylated Interferon alfa 2b</u> has been used in the management of Chronic HDV, which may normalize serum aminotransferase levels, result in histologic improvement, and elimination of HDV RNA from serum in 20–50% of patients, but relapse may occur, and tolerance is low.
- Nucleoside and nucleotide analogs are generally not effective in treating chronic hepatitis D.
- Liver transplant definitive management.

PREVENTION
- **Hepatitis B vaccination protects against both Hepatitis B and D.**

HEPATITIS B VIRUS (HBV)

TRANSMISSION
- **Percutaneous, sexual, parenteral, & perinatal** — inoculation of infected blood or blood products or by sexual contact and can be found in saliva, semen, and vaginal secretions. Vertical transmission.

CLINICAL MANIFESTATIONS OF ACUTE
- Subclinical (anicteric): most are asymptomatic or mildly symptomatic (eg, malaise, arthralgia, fatigue, URI symptoms, nausea, vomiting, abdominal pain, anorexia, and **aversion to smoking in smokers**).
- **Icteric: jaundice** (only seen in 30%) — **dark urine, pale, acholic stools, jaundice, & pruritus.**
- Fulminant: acute hepatic failure (eg, encephalopathy, coagulopathy, jaundice, edema, ascites).
- Physical findings: jaundice, scleral icterus, hepatomegaly, splenomegaly, RUQ tenderness to palpation.

CLINICAL MANIFESTATIONS OF CHRONIC
- Chronic hepatitis: persistent symptoms, elevated LFTs, and increased viral load.
- Chronic (carrier) state: asymptomatic, normal LFTs, low viral load, and undetectable HBeAg.
- **Chronic Hepatitis B increases the risk for Cirrhosis and Hepatocellular carcinoma.**

DIAGNOSIS
- **Serologies: HB surface antigen (HBsAg), surface antibody(anti-HBs), core antibody (anti-HBc).**

Diagnosis	HBsAg	anti-HBs	anti-HBc	HBeAg	Anti-HBe
WINDOW PERIOD	Negative	Negative	IgM	Negative	Negative
ACUTE HEPATITIS	POSITIVE	Negative	IgM	±	±
RECOVERY (RESOLVED)	Negative	POSITIVE	IgG	Negative	Negative
IMMUNIZATION	Negative	POSITIVE	Negative	Negative	Negative
CHRONIC HEPATITIS (REPLICATIVE)	POSITIVE	Negative	IgG	POSITIVE	Negative
CHRONIC HEPATITIS (NONREPLICATIVE)	POSITIVE	Negative	IgG	Negative	POSITIVE

Chronic hepatitis = surface antigen positivity and failure to produce surface antibodies > 6 months
- LFTs: acute: AST and ALT in the thousands range; chronic: ALT and AST in the hundreds range or normal. Increased bilirubin especially in the icteric phase.
- **HBV DNA: best way to assess viral replication activity**; often parallels the presence of HBeAg.
- Liver biopsy can be used to determine the extent of damage.

MANAGEMENT OF ACUTE HBV
- **Supportive is the mainstay of treatment; most will not progress to chronic infection.**

MANAGEMENT OF CHRONIC HBV
- Antiviral therapy may be indicated if persistent, severe symptoms, marked jaundice (bilirubin >10 mg/dL), inflammation on liver biopsy, ↑ALT, or ⊕ Hepatitis B envelope antigen persistence.
- **Entecavir or Tenofovir first line.** Adefovir, Telbivudine, Lamivudine. Entecavir is rarely associated with resistance unless a patient is already resistant to Lamivudine.
- Treatment can be stopped after 2 consecutive tests 4 weeks apart show clearance of HBsAg.

HEPATITIS B VACCINATION
- Recombinant HB vaccine (non-adjuvanted) derived from yeast most commonly used for vaccination.

Vaccination schedule:
- Infant: usually administered at birth, 1-2 months, and at 6-18 months of age.
- Adult (no prior vaccination): 3 doses at 0, 1, and 6 months.
- HBV vaccine is contraindicated if history of allergy to Baker's yeast.

HEPATITIS B SEROLOGIES

There are 5 variations of Hepatitis B you must know:

1. <u>Window period:</u> positive core IgM (IgM anti-HBc) may be the only positive serologic marker.
2. <u>Successful vaccination:</u> positive surface antibody (anti-HBs) only positive serologic marker.
3. <u>Acute hepatitis:</u> positive surface antigen + positive core IgM antibody (HBsAg + anti-HBc IgM).
4. <u>Chronic hepatitis:</u> positive surface antigen + positive core IgG antibody (HBsAg + anti-HBc IgG).
5. <u>Distant resolved infection (recovery):</u> positive surface antibody + positive core IgG antibody.

<u>ANTIBODY INTERPRETATION</u>

- **Positive HB surface Ag is a marker of infection and infectivity, either (1) acute infection or (2) chronic infection.** *HbsAg is usually the first positive serologic marker in acute Hepatitis.* The core antibody determines if acute or chronic (core IgM = acute, core IgG = chronic).
- **Positive HB surface Ab is a marker of immunity and noninfectivity, either due to (1) recovery from HBV infection or (2) successful vaccination.**
- **HB core Ab IgM**: seen in either (1) the window period or (2) acute hepatitis.
- **HB core Ab IgG**: seen in either (1) resolved infection or (2) chronic hepatitis.
- **HBeAg: found only in HBsAg-positive serum and indicates viral replication and infectivity.**

HEPATITIS B SEROLOGIES – 3 STEP APPROACH

STEP 1 – look at **Surface antigen** - if surface Ag is positive:

•⊕ = **acute** OR **chronic**

STEP 2 - if surface Ag (step 1) is positive, look at **Core antibody**:

•if **IgM** is ⊕ ⇨ **acute.** if **IgG** is ⊕ ⇨ **chronic.**

Step 3 is only needed if Surface antigen was negative in step 1

STEP 3 – If surface Ag was negative, look at **surface Ab**. If positive:

•Either **Vaccination** OR **recovery** (distant infection)

•If **surface Ab** is the **only thing positive** ⇨ **vaccination**

•If **core IgG Antibody** is **positive** ⇨ **recovery** (distant/resolved infection)

Another hack: If Envelope Ag is positive in either acute or chronic hepatitis, it doesn't help determine their status. Positive HBeAg = high viral replication; HBeAg = not highly replicative. Useful only if the initial testing reveals Acute or chronic Hepatitis.

In evaluating a patient, the following labs are obtained:

HB surface antigen: positive
HB surface antibody: negative
HB core antibody: positive IgG
Which of the following is the most likely diagnosis?

    a. Window period
    b. Successful vaccination
    c. Acute Hepatitis B
    d. Chronic Hepatitis B
    e. Distant resolved infection (recovery)

<u>STEP 1</u>

Look at surface antigen (positive), so the answer has to be either acute or chronic.

<u>STEP 2</u>

Look at core antibody. If positive, it will either be IgG or IgM
Since it is IgG+, the answer is chronic hepatitis. You're done! ☺

HEPATITIS C VIRUS (HCV)

- HCV is a single-stranded RNA virus (hepacivirus).
- **HCV is the most common infectious cause of chronic liver disease, Cirrhosis, & liver transplantation in the US. 85% of patients with HCV develop chronic infection.**

TRANSMISSION:
- **Parenteral:** **IV drug use** most common in US **(>50%)** and both reinfection and superinfection of HCV are common in people who actively inject drugs. <u>Needlestick injuries</u> the average incidence of HCV seroconversion to be 1.8% (range, 0-7%) after a needle stick or sharps exposure from a source with HCV infection. <u>Other blood transfer:</u> tattoos, body piercings, and hemodialysis. Increased risk if received blood transfusion before May 1992.
- <u>Low risk:</u> The risk of sexual transmission and maternal–neonatal transmission is low and may be greatest in a subset of patients with high circulating levels of HCV RNA. Transmission via breastfeeding has not been documented.

CLINICAL MANIFESTATIONS
- The incubation period for Hepatitis C averages 6–7 weeks.
- Most patient with HCV usually remain asymptomatic for most of the course of the disease until they complications of Cirrhosis develops (eg, ascites, esophageal varices, & portal hypertension).
- **Clinical illness is often mostly asymptomatic or mild, and characterized by waxing and waning aminotransferase elevations and a high rate (>80%) of chronic hepatitis.**
- <u>Acute:</u> fatigue, myalgia, nausea, RUQ pain, jaundice, dark urine, clay-colored stools.

DIAGNOSIS
- <u>Liver function testing:</u> <u>Increased LFTs:</u> waxing and waning aminotransferase elevations.
Screening test:
- **HCV antibodies (via ELISA or RIBA) indicate acute or chronic hepatitis & usually becomes positive within 6 weeks. Anti-HCV is <u>not</u> protective & does <u>not</u> imply recovery** (may become negative after recovery). Anti-HCV without HCV RNA in the serum suggests past recovery from HCV.
- **After the detection of antibodies to HCV (anti-HCV), the infection can be confirmed by NAAT for HCV RNA by qualitative and quantitative methods.**
Confirmatory:
- **HCV RNA more sensitive than HCV antibody (may be positive in patients with negative antibody testing).**
- Genotyping is used to determine effective treatment options.

MANAGEMENT
- <u>Oral direct-acting agents:</u> Newer options can achieve a cure rate, which yield >90% sustained virologic response (SVR) rates after 12 weeks of treatment. Options include: <u>Ledipasvir-Sofosbuvir</u> (6-week course) has been shown to prevent chronic hepatitis in patients with acute genotype-1 hepatitis C; Elbasvir-Grazoprevir; Ombitasvir-Paritaprevir-Ritonavir plus Dasabuvir with or without Ribavirin; Simeprevir plus Sofosbuvir & Daclatasvir plus Sofosbuvir.
- <u>Older treatment:</u> <u>Interferon-based therapy:</u> Pegylated interferon alpa-2b AND Ribavirin. Adverse effect of interferon include psychosis & depression.

PROGNOSIS
- Newer treatments may possibly reactivate Hepatitis B so perform HBV testing prior to initiating.
- **Chronic hepatitis, which may be slowly progressive, develops up to 85% of individuals with acute hepatitis C. Chronic HCV is associated with increased risk for Cirrhosis (20% over 20-30 years), Hepatocellular carcinoma (1-5%/year), and liver failure.**

COAGULOPATHY IN LIVER DISEASE

- **Decreased production of coagulation factor proteins associated with advanced liver disease.**
- In the liver, the hepatocyte is the site of production most of the numbered coagulation factors including fibrinogen (factor I), thrombin (factor IIa), V, VII, IX, X, and XI. Important exceptions are factor VIII, which is produced in endothelial cells, and the factor XIII A-subunit, which is produced in megakaryocytes.

CLINICAL MANIFESTATIONS
- **Bleeding is the classic presentation** (eg, GI bleeding). May have signs of underlying liver disease.

DIAGNOSIS
- **Coagulopathy: Increased Prothrombin time (PT), international normalized ratio (INR), & low albumin.** As the disease advances, **increased activated partial thromboplastin time (aPTT) will occur.** The coagulopathy corrects with mixing studies.
- **Decreased fibrinogen**: if low, adequate repletion could prevent bleeding episodes in Cirrhosis.
- **CBC:** May have normal platelet counts (eg, ≥150,000/microL) or varying degrees of thrombocytopenia & platelet dysfunction (impaired platelet function). Peripheral smear may show target cells.

MANAGEMENT
- In most patients, no intervention is needed in the setting of asymptomatic laboratory changes (eg, elevations in the PT/INR or aPTT, decreased platelet count) due to underlying liver disease.
- **Active or poorly controlled bleeding: Cryoprecipitate may be administered** (eg, one bag per 10 kg of body weight). Cryoprecipitate corrects decreased or abnormally functioning fibrinogen (replaces fibrinogen, factor VIII, & VWF). Prior to receiving the results of the fibrinogen level, administer a source of fibrinogen [preferably Cryoprecipitate, which creates a smaller volume load than Fresh frozen plasma (FFP)] to maintain a fibrinogen level ≥100-120 mg/dL.
- For individuals with possible Vitamin K deficiency (eg, suspected poor nutrition, cholestatic disease, diarrheal illness, antibiotic use), Vitamin K can be administered.

HEPATOCELLULAR CARCINOMA (HCC)

- Primary neoplasm of the liver derived from parenchymal cells (>85% of primary liver cancers).
- Risk factors: **The main risk factor for HCC is Cirrhosis (especially macronodular) and associated chronic liver damage (eg, HBV, HCV, HDV).** Aflatoxin B1 exposure (*Aspergillus* spp).

CLINICAL MANIFESTATIONS
- Many are asymptomatic. Malaise, weight loss, jaundice, abdominal pain, hepatosplenomegaly.

DIAGNOSIS
- **Multiphasic helical CT and MRI with contrast enhancement are the preferred imaging studies.**
- Increased serum α-fetoprotein (AFP) levels in up to 70%. Liver biopsy definitive.

MANAGEMENT
- Surgical resection if confined to a lobe & not associated with Cirrhosis.
- Advanced disease: The combination of Atezolizumab & Bevacizumab has been shown to be superior to Sorafenib and is now standard first-line therapy. Tremelimumab; Darvulumab.
- Primary prevention of HCC: vaccination against HBV & effective treatment of HBV and HCV infection.

SURVEILLANCE
- **Ultrasonography every 6 months,** with or without serum α-fetoprotein (AFP) levels — performed in high-risk patients (eg, active Hepatitis B with high AST and/or high viral load).

CIRRHOSIS

- **Mostly irreversible liver fibrosis with nodular regeneration** secondary to hepatocellular injury.

PATHOPHYSIOLOGY
- Hepatic cell dysfunction, portosystemic shunting, and nodules lead to portal hypertension.

ETIOLOGIES
- **<u>Chronic hepatitis C infection</u> most common cause of Cirrhosis in US. Alcohol.** Chronic HBV, HDV.
- Nonalcoholic fatty liver disease (eg, obesity, DM, & hypertriglyceridemia), medication toxicity.
- Hemochromatosis, autoimmune hepatitis, Primary biliary cirrhosis, Primary sclerosing cholangitis.

CLINICAL MANIFESTATIONS
- <u>General symptoms:</u> fatigue, weakness, weight loss, muscle cramps, anorexia, abdominal pain.
- Upper GI tract bleeding may occur from varices, portal hypertensive gastropathy, or peptic ulcers.
- **<u>Physical Exam:</u> ascites, hepatosplenomegaly, gynecomastia, spider angiomata, telangiectasias, caput medusa,** muscle wasting, bleeding, palmar erythema, jaundice, Dupuytren's contractures.
- **<u>Ascites:</u> positive fluid wave test and shifting fullness.**
- <u>Hepatic encephalopathy:</u> **confusion & lethargy (increased ammonia levels** toxic to the brain).
  <u>PE:</u> **asterixis (flapping tremor** with wrist extension) & fetor hepaticus. Esophageal varices.

DIAGNOSTIC STUDIES
- <u>Hepatic ultrasound:</u> fibrosis nodularity; increased echogenicity atrophy or hypertrophy of liver lobes.
- <u>Transient elastography</u> measures liver stiffness — hepatic fibrosis and increased stiffness.
- <u>Liver biopsy</u> may be indicated in patients who cannot undergo elastography or for definitive diagnosis.

CIRRHOSIS STAGING CHILD-PUGH CLASSIFICATION

PARAMETERS	1 POINT	2 POINTS	3 POINTS
Total Bilirubin (mg/dL)	<2	2-3	>3
Serum albumin (g/dL)	>3.5	2.8 – 3.5	<2.8
PT INR	<1.7	1.71 – 2.30	>2.30
Ascites	None	Mild	Moderate to severe
Hepatic Encephalopathy	None	Grade I-II (or suppressed with medication)	Grade III-IV or refractory

POINTS	CLASS	1 YEAR SURVIVAL	2 YEAR SURVIVAL
5-6	A	100%	85%
7-9	B	81%	57%
	C	45%	35%

MODEL FOR END STAGE LIVER DISEASE : slightly more accurate way to measure 3-month mortality.
MELD = 3.78×ln[serum bilirubin (mg/dL)] + 11.2×ln[INR] + 9.57×ln[serum creatinine (mg/dL)] + 6.43

MANAGEMENT
- Avoidance of alcohol and hepatotoxic medications, weight reduction, sodium restriction, vaccination for HAV, HBV, and 23-valent pneumococcal vaccine. Treat the underlying cause when possible.
- <u>Liver transplant:</u> definitive management. Screening for HCC (ultrasound, alpha-fetoprotein).

<u>Ascites & edema:</u>
- **Sodium restriction (first line). Diuretics (Spironolactone, generally with Furosemide)** if no response to salt restriction. Large-volume paracentesis if no response to diuretics or if massive.

<u>Pruritus:</u>
- **<u>Cholestyramine</u> is a bile acid sequestrant** that reduces bile salts in the skin, reducing irritation.

<u>Hepatocellular carcinoma surveillance:</u>
- **Ultrasonography every 6 months (with or without alpha-fetoprotein).**
- <u>Complications:</u> end stage liver disease, Hepatocellular carcinoma, esophageal or gastric varices, spontaneous bacterial peritonitis, hepatic hydrothorax.

SPONTANEOUS BACTERIAL PERITONITIS (SBP)

- **Spontaneous bacterial peritonitis (SBP)** is an acute infection of ascitic fluid that is not attributed to any other intrabdominal infection. **Often, there is a history of chronic liver disease or Cirrhosis.**

EPIDEMIOLOGY
- ~20–30% of cirrhotic patients with ascites develop Spontaneous peritonitis; however, the incidence is >40% in patients with ascitic fluid total protein <1 g/dL, due to decreased opsonic activity.

MICROBIOLOGY
- Translocation of enteric bacteria from the gut wall or mesenteric lymphatics into the ascitic fluid.
- Most cases of Spontaneous bacterial peritonitis are caused by a monomicrobial infection.
- The most common pathogens are **enteric gram-negative bacteria (*Klebsiella pneumoniae, E coli*)** or gram-positive bacteria (*Streptococcus pneumoniae*, viridans streptococci, *Enterococcus* species). A positive culture is not needed to establish the diagnosis of SBP.

CLINICAL MANIFESTATIONS
- **Fever, chills, and abdominal pain are the most common symptoms (present in two-thirds).**
- New-onset or worsening Encephalopathy (eg, altered mental status); worsening of kidney function.

PHYSICAL EXAMINATION
- Signs of chronic liver disease with ascites — eg, shifting dullness, fluid wave test.
- Abdominal tenderness. Peritoneal signs are not common findings.

DIAGNOSIS
Abdominal paracentesis: analysis of the ascitic fluid
- **A peritoneal fluid absolute polymorphonuclear neutrophil count ≥250 cells/mm³,** culture results are positive, and secondary causes of peritonitis are excluded. The percentage of PMNs is >50–70% of the ascitic fluid WBCs and is often close to 100%. **pH <7.34.**

MANAGEMENT
- **Early administration of empiric antibiotics:** **third-generation Cephalosporin (eg, Cefotaxime or Ceftriaxone)** or Ampicillin-sulbactam for 5 days (or longer if more virulent organisms) or until the ascitic fluid PMN count decreases to <250 cells/mcL. **Ciprofloxacin is an alternative.**
- **Adjunctive IV Albumin (25%): is given within 6 hours of diagnosis in patients with increased risk of hepatorenal failure** (eg, baseline creatinine >1 mg/dL, BUN >30 mg/dL, or bilirubin >4 mg/dL). Kidney injury develops in ≤40% of patients and is a major cause of death. Albumin increases effective arterial circulating volume & renal perfusion, decreasing kidney injury & mortality.
- **Discontinuing nonselective Beta blockers** because nonselective Beta blocker use in SBP has been associated with increased rates of hepatorenal syndrome, more days of hospitalization, and decreased transplant-free survival compared with patients not receiving nonselective Beta blockers. They should be discontinued permanently due to their adverse impact on cardiac output, renal perfusion, and long-term survival in advanced Cirrhosis.

PREVENTION
- Up to 70% of patients who survive an episode of spontaneous bacterial peritonitis will have another episode within 1 year.
- Therefore, certain high-risk patients may benefit from antibiotic prophylactic therapy with Ciprofloxacin 500 mg, Norfloxacin, or Trimethoprim-sulfamethoxazole one double-strength tablet to decrease the rate of recurrent infections to <20%.
- High-risk individuals may include prior episode of SBP, or ascitic fluid with either a low protein count (< 1 g/dL) or association with a GI bleed.

HEPATIC ENCEPHALOPATHY

- **Neuropsychiatric abnormalities resulting from accumulation of neurotoxic substances (eg, ammonia) in the brain due to failure of the liver to detoxify noxious chemicals of gut origin.**

PRECIPITANTS
- Under normal conditions, ammonia produced by gut bacteria is metabolized and cleared by the liver.
- In liver disease, ammonia crosses the blood-brain barrier and is converted to glutamine, an osmolyte that promotes cerebral edema.
- Triggers include Hyponatremia, GI bleeding (increases protein in the bowel), constipation, alkalosis, dehydration, sedatives, hepatic or systemic infection; and portosystemic shunts (including TIPS).

CLINICAL MANIFESTATIONS
- **CNS symptoms**: **due to CNS toxicity from increased ammonia levels** in different grades: (1) mild confusion, slurred speech (eg, dysarthria), abnormal sleep (eg, day-night sleep reversal disturbance); (2) drowsiness, (3) stupor, and (4) coma. Mood changes, bradykinesia, & ataxia.
- Physical examination: **asterixis (flapping tremor with wrist extension),** hyperreflexia, positive Babinski sign, Parkinsonian symptoms (eg, tremor, rigidity), and fetor hepaticus.

DIAGNOSIS
- Laboratory evaluation: **elevated ammonia**; abnormal LFTs; Hyponatremia or Hyperkalemia possible.
- The diagnosis is based primarily on detection of characteristic symptoms and signs (eg, asterixis).

MANAGEMENT
- **Management includes correcting any predisposing conditions** (eg, nutritional support, correcting electrolyte abnormalities) **& lowering blood ammonia levels (eg, Lactulose, Lactitol, or Rifaximin).** Neomycin (rarely used) or Metronidazole. Protein intake generally not restricted.
- **Lactulose or Lactitol: often first-line — bacterial flora converts lactulose into lactic & fatty acids, neutralizing ammonia in patients with Hepatic encephalopathy** and changes the bowel flora to fewer ammonia-producing organisms. Adverse effects: bloating, flatulence, and diarrhea.
- **Rifaximin is an alternative if no improvement of mental status within 48 hours of Lactulose** or if unable to take Lactulose or Lactitol. Rifaximin is a nonabsorbable antibiotic that reduces risk of rehospitalization for Hepatic encephalopathy over a 24-month period, with or without Lactulose.

NONALCOHOLIC FATTY LIVER DISEASE (NAFLD)

- Hepatic steatosis in the absence of other causes of hepatic fat accumulation (eg, alcohol use).
- **Most common cause of mildly abnormal liver function tests in the US.**
- **May be seen with obesity (40%), Diabetes mellitus, hypertriglyceridemia.**
- Most patients are asymptomatic; mild right upper quadrant discomfort. **Hepatomegaly (75%).**

2 TYPES
- **Nonalcoholic fatty liver (NAFL): relatively benign accumulation of triglycerides within hepatocytes (isolated steatosis).** Not associated with fibrosis or malignant potential.
- **Nonalcoholic steatohepatitis (NASH) is associated with** liver cell injury and death, **inflammation, and fibrosis,** with the potential to progress to Cirrhosis & Hepatocellular carcinoma.

DIAGNOSIS
- Laboratory tests: mild elevation in serum aminotransferase and ferritin but may be normal.
- **Ultrasound** — hyperechoic texture or a bright liver as a result of diffuse fatty infiltration.
- **Biopsy: most accurate test** — microvesicular fatty deposits similar to alcoholic liver disease.

MANAGEMENT
- **Lifestyle changes remove or modify offending factors** (eg, weight loss, fat restriction, & exercise).
- NAFLD is currently the leading indication for liver transplantation in the United States.

PRIMARY BILIARY CHOLANGITIS/CIRRHOSIS (PBC)

- **Idiopathic autoimmune disorder of <u>intrahepatic small bile ducts</u>** that may lead to the gradual destruction of the small intrahepatic bile ducts, resulting in periportal inflammation and cholestasis due to decreased bile salt excretion.
- **Most common in women (90-95%), especially aged 30-60 years (middle-aged women).**

<u>RISK FACTORS</u>
- **<u>Autoimmune disease</u>**: PBC may be associated with Sjögren syndrome, autoimmune thyroid disease, Raynaud syndrome, Systemic sclerosis (scleroderma), Hypothyroidism, and Celiac disease.
- Genetic predisposition & environmental triggers (eg, cigarette smoking, urinary tract infections).

<u>PATHOPHYSIOLOGY</u>
- PBC is a chronic disease of the liver characterized by **(1) T-cell mediated autoimmune destruction of the small intrahepatic intralobular bile ducts and (2) cholestasis.**

<u>CLINICAL MANIFESTATIONS</u>
- **Most are asymptomatic** (50-60%) — **incidental finding of <u>high alkaline phosphatase</u>**.
- **<u>Symptomatic:</u> fatigue (usually first symptom) & pruritus are most common.** RUQ discomfort.
- <u>Physical examination:</u> None early. **Hepatomegaly,** skin findings (eg, hyperpigmentation, xanthelasma, xanthomas), osteoporosis. Jaundice or signs of Cirrhosis may occur late in the disease.

<u>DIAGNOSIS</u>
<u>Laboratory evaluation:</u>
- **<u>Cholestatic pattern:</u> <u>increased alkaline phosphatase</u>** (compared to transaminases) **& GGT.**
- **⊕ <u>Antimitochondrial antibody (AMA)</u> hallmark** (95% sensitivity). ⊕Antinuclear antibodies (ANA).
- **<u>Hypercholesterolemia:</u> especially high-density lipoprotein** & lipoprotein X (hepatic dysfunction).

<u>Imaging:</u>
- **<u>Ultrasound</u>: often initial imaging test — <u>intrahepatic</u> biliary obstruction with no extrahepatic biliary obstruction.**
- MRCP or ERCP: performed to rule out the extrahepatic biliary obstruction.

<u>Liver biopsy:</u>
- **<u>Liver biopsy:</u> definitive diagnosis** (not always necessary). **The florid duct lesion: granulomatous destruction of the bile duct with a bile duct in the middle of a dense lymphocytic infiltrate, is the histological hallmark of PBC** (nonsuppurative destructive cholangitis), interlobular bile duct destruction & lymphocytic infiltration.

<u>MANAGEMENT</u>
- **<u>Ursodeoxycholic acid</u> (UDCA) first-line medical treatment for PBC because it delays the progression to end-stage liver disease, enhances survival, and is well tolerated.** UDCA reduces the risk of recurrent Colorectal adenomas in patients with PBC. <u>Mechanism of action:</u> UDCA is a hydrophilic bile salt, which stabilizes hepatocyte membranes against toxic bile salts and inhibits apoptosis and fibrosis.
- Obeticholic acid (OBCA) may be indicated in patients with no response to Ursodeoxycholic acid. OBCA is a farnesoid X receptor agonist that increases bile salt excretion and has choleretic and antifibrotic properties. OBCA reduces ALP, GGT, and transaminase levels; however, it does not improve survival or disease-related symptoms.
- <u>Pruritus:</u> Cholestyramine & UV light for pruritus.
- **<u>Liver transplant</u> is the definitive management of PBC.**

<u>COMPLICATIONS</u>
- Cirrhosis, Hepatocellular carcinoma, malabsorption & steatorrhea, and Metabolic bone disease.

PRIMARY SCLEROSING CHOLANGITIS (PSC)

- **Uncommon autoimmune, chronic progressive cholestasis leading to inflammation, diffuse fibrosis, and stricturing of medium and large intra- and extra-hepatic biliary ducts.**

RISK FACTORS:
- **Inflammatory bowel disease** — majority of patients with PSC have IBD (predominantly **Ulcerative colitis in ~80%** and Crohn disease in 20%). **70% of PSC occur in men.**

CLINICAL MANIFESTATIONS
- ~50% are asymptomatic at the time of diagnosis, often detected by abnormal LFTs.
- **Progressive obstructive jaundice: pruritus and fatigue most common.** Anorexia and indigestion.
- Physical examination: normal in ~50%. **Hepatomegaly, splenomegaly, jaundice,** or excoriations.
- Sporadic bacterial cholangitis: episodic RUQ pain, fever, chills, and night sweats may occur.

DIAGNOSIS
- Cholestatic pattern: **increased alkaline phosphatase & GGT.** Increased ALT, AST, bilirubin, & IgM.
- ⊕ **P-ANCA Perinuclear antineutrophil cytoplasmic antibodies hallmark** (30-80%).
- **MRCP, ERCP: Most accurate tests — "beaded" appearance:** irregularity and multifocal stricturing of both intrahepatic and extrahepatic ducts, segmental dilations alternating normal segments.
- Liver biopsy: rarely used — PSC is the only cause of Cirrhosis where liver biopsy isn't the most accurate test. **The key feature on histology is periductal or onion skin fibrosis (concentric and circumferential laminations).** Bile duct wall thickening.
- Workup for IBD: because the majority of patients with PSC have underlying ulcerative colitis (UC).

MANAGEMENT
- Stricture dilation for symptomatic relief. Cholestyramine for pruritus. Liver transplant definitive.

COMPLICATIONS
- Cirrhosis, Hepatocellular carcinoma (secondary to Cirrhosis), Liver failure. PSC is a premalignant disease (eg, **Cholangiocarcinoma, Gallbladder cancer),** Colon cancer (patients with UC).

	PRIMARY SCLEROSING CHOLANGITIS (PSC)	PRIMARY BILIARY CHOLANGITIS (PBC)
PATHOPHYSIOLOGY	• Diffuse inflammation, **fibrosis,** cholestasis, and stricturing of medium and large ducts in the **intrahepatic and/or extrahepatic** biliary tree.	• **Granulomatous inflammation** destroying the **small intrahepatic* biliary ducts.**
ASSOCIATION	• **Ulcerative colitis* 80%,** Crohn (20%)	• Other autoimmune diseases
EPIDEMIOLOGY	• **Males:** 30-40 years of age (mean 40y)	• **Females** (95%), age 30-60 years
KEY MICROSCOPIC FEATURES	• **Concentric "onion skin"** fibrosis around the bile ducts.	• **Florid duct lesions:** granulomas & lymphocytic infiltrates around the bile ducts.
IMAGING	• **MRCP or ERCP: beaded appearance** (multifocal stricturing and dilation) **intrahepatic & extrahepatic.**	• **Ultrasound:** intrahepatic biliary **obstruction** without extrahepatic biliary obstruction
LABS	• **P-ANCA positivity.*** • ASCA antibodies	• **Anti-mitochondrial (AMA) antibody positivity.***
COMPLICATIONS	• Increased risk Cirrhosis • Cholangiocarcinoma	• Increased risk Cirrhosis.

HEPATIC VEIN OUTFLOW OBSTRUCTION (BUDD-CHIARI SYNDROME)

- **Noncardiac hepatic venous outflow blockage,** leading to decreased liver drainage with subsequent Portal hypertension & Cirrhosis.

TYPES
- **Primary:** obstruction from a primary venous process (eg, **hepatic vein thrombosis or phlebitis).**
- Secondary: hepatic vein or inferior vena cava occlusion due to compression or external lesion.

ETIOLOGIES
- **Hereditary & acquired hypercoagulable states** eg, myeloproliferative neoplasms (50%) including Polycythemia vera and Essential thrombocythemia, malignancy (10%), pregnancy and oral contraceptives (20%), clotting disorders, & idiopathic.

EPIDEMIOLOGY
- Most common in the third & fourth decade of life, predominantly in females.
- **Most common cause of Portal hypertension in children.**

CLINICAL MANIFESTATIONS
- **Acute: classic triad: [1] ascites, [2] hepatomegaly, & [3] RUQ abdominal pain and tenderness** developing rapidly. Jaundice, hepatomegaly, renal failure, Hepatic encephalopathy.
- Subacute presentation — fever, abdominal distension (progressive ascites), lower extremity edema, GI bleeding (from varices or portal hypertensive gastropathy), hepatic encephalopathy.
- Physical examination: **ascites, tender, painful hepatic enlargement,** jaundice, splenomegaly.

DIAGNOSIS
- **Doppler ultrasonography: initial screening test of choice — findings may include a prominent caudate lobe (venous drainage occlusion);** hepatic vein wall irregularity, thickening, stenosis, thrombosis, or dilation; hyperechoic cord replacing a normal hepatic vein.
- **CT or MRI** usually performed if US nondiagnostic — **occlusion/absence of hepatic vein or IVC flow.**
- Venography criterion standard. Not commonly performed because it is invasive.
- **Liver biopsy: usually not needed** — findings include sinusoidal dilation, necrosis, hemorrhage, and **congestive hepatopathy in the central zone classically described as "nutmeg liver" (centrilobular congestion with a mottled pattern of contrast enhancement with decreased enhancement in the periphery).**

MANAGEMENT
- **Initial management includes managing any underlying disorders, and management of the complications of Portal hypertension** [eg, Ascites is treated with salt restriction and diuretics (eg, Spironolactone ± Furosemide)].
- **Thrombotic: anticoagulation mainstay of treatment — Low molecular weight heparins are preferred** (LMWH) over unfractionated Heparin because of a lower rate of Heparin-induced thrombocytopenia; After 3-5 days & once the INR is 2-3 on Warfarin, Heparin is discontinued.
- Other options: thrombolysis, balloon angioplasty with placement of an intravascular metallic stent.
- Defibrotide is an adenosine receptor agonist that increases endogenous tissue plasminogen activator levels, which can be used for treatment and prevention of sinusoidal obstruction syndrome.

Refractory cases:
- Shunt decompression of the liver: TIPS placement may be attempted in patients with Budd-Chiari syndrome and persistent hepatic congestion or failed thrombolytic therapy and possibly in those with sinusoidal obstruction syndrome. When TIPS is technically not feasible because of complete hepatic vein obstruction, ultrasound-guided direct intrahepatic portosystemic shunt is an alternative approach.
- Liver transplantation: option for patients who fail all therapies or develop acute liver failure.

HEPATOLENTICULAR DEGENERATION (WILSON'S DISEASE)

- **Rare autosomal recessive disorder of copper metabolism, leading to <u>copper accumulation in the body [eg. liver, brain (especially the basal ganglia), cornea, kidney, and joints</u>].**

EPIDEMIOLOGY
- Usually occurs in individuals <40 years of age but symptom onset after 40 years is common.

PATHOPHYSIOLOGY
A defect in the *ATP7B* gene, the copper transport protein on chromosome 13, leads to:
- **[1] <u>decreased biliary copper excretion</u> due to <u>low circulating levels of ceruloplasmin</u>,** the main copper transporting protein, and
- **[2] <u>excessive absorption of copper</u> from the small intestine, resulting in increased tissue deposition, especially in the liver, brain, cornea, kidney, and joints.**

CLINICAL MANIFESTATIONS
- **<u>Liver</u>: initial site of copper accumulation** — fatigue, anorexia, vomiting, weakness, jaundice, hepatitis, hepatosplenomegaly, edema, ascites, pruritus, portal hypertension, cirrhosis, liver failure.
- **<u>CNS</u>: neurological manifestations due to basal ganglia dysfunction** — <u>early changes</u>: **asymmetric tremor, dysarthria (speech difficulty),** excessive salivation, gait ataxia, hand clumsiness. <u>Later changes</u>: dystonia, Parkinson-like symptoms (bradykinesia, tremor, rigidity), spasticity, hallucinations, hemiballismus, choreiform movement, dysgraphia, cognitive impairment, dementia.
- **<u>Psychiatric</u>: personality & behavioral changes,** emotional lability (eg, irritability, anger), mood disorder (eg, depression, anxiety), delusions, hallucinations. Mask-like facies.
- **<u>Joints</u>: arthralgias from copper deposition,** arthropathy especially involving the spine and large appendicular joints (eg, knees, wrists, hips). Various skeletal abnormalities — eg, Osteoporosis, Osteomalacia, Rickets, spontaneous fractures, polyarthritis.
- Skin pigmentation and a bluish discoloration at the base of the fingernails. Decreased fertility.
- <u>Renal tubular dysfunction</u> in Wilson's disease leads to abnormal losses of amino acids, electrolytes, calcium, phosphorus, and glucose. Urolithiasis and hematuria.
- <u>Hemolytic anemia</u> due to the direct toxic effects of copper on red blood cell membranes is usually associated with release of massive quantities of hepatic copper into the circulation.

PHYSICAL EXAMINATION
- **<u>Kayser-Fleischer ring</u>: brown or green pigmented rings due to copper deposition in the Descemet membrane in the limbus of the cornea** with the unaided eye or slit lamp. KF ring is not specific; the only other disease with KF ring is Primary biliary cholangitis.

DIAGNOSIS
- **<u>Decreased serum ceruloplasmin</u> <20 mg/dL (<14 more specific); decreased serum copper.**
- **<u>Increased 24-hour urinary copper excretion</u> >100 µg/24 h.** Also useful for monitoring treatment.
- Elevated transaminases. Aminoaciduria. Hemolytic anemia (Coombs negative). MRI of brain.
- <u>Molecular genetic testing</u> for ATP7B
- **<u>Liver biopsy</u>: definitive — increased hepatic copper concentration >250 mcg/g of dry liver tissue.**

MANAGEMENT
- **<u>Copper-chelating agents</u>: D-Penicillamine or Trientine (Trientine has less adverse effects).** D-Penicillamine increases urinary excretion of copper. Pyridoxine (Vitamin B6) is often given with D-Penicillamine to prevent B6 deficiency. Tetrathiomolybdate is another chelating agent.
- **<u>Zinc supplementation</u>** interferes with intestinal copper absorption; promotes fecal copper excretion.
- **<u>Diet low in copper-containing foods</u>** may be helpful. Foods high in copper include shellfish, organ foods such as liver, nuts, mushrooms, and chocolate; intakes of these food should be limited.
- <u>Liver transplantation</u> is a consideration for Wilson's disease in advanced stages and/or if refractory to medical therapy and dietary changes.

ACUTE PANCREATITIS

- Acinar cell injury ⇨ **intracellular activation of pancreatic enzymes** ⇨ **autodigestion of pancreas.**

ETIOLOGIES
- **Gallstones & heavy alcohol use** are the 2 most common causes — Gallstones most common cause of Pancreatitis (40%); heavy alcohol use is the second most common cause (35%).
- Medications: eg, **Thiazides, Protease inhibitors, Valproic acid, GLP-1 agonists (eg, Exenatide), DPP-4 inhibitors,** Sulfa drugs, NRTIs including Didanosine, Estrogens, Statins, and many others.
- Iatrogenic (ERCP), malignancy, scorpion sting, trauma, Cystic fibrosis, **Hypertriglyceridemia** (>1,000 mg/dL), Hypercalcemia, infection. Abdominal trauma or Mumps in children. Idiopathic.

CLINICAL MANIFESTATIONS
- **Epigastric pain** — steady, boring, deep pain that often <u>radiates to the back</u> or other quadrant. Pain exacerbated if supine & eating; relieved with leaning forward, sitting, or fetal position.
- **Fever, nausea, vomiting, & abdominal distention** (GI hypomotility) **common.**
- Physical examination: **epigastric tenderness,** abdominal distention, tachycardia, fever. Decreased bowel sounds may be seen secondary to Adynamic ileus. Dehydration or shock if severe.
- Necrotizing, hemorrhagic: **ecchymosis — Cullen's sign (periumbilical); Grey Turner sign (flank).**

DIAGNOSTIC CRITERIA
The presence of <u>2 of the following 3 criteria</u> establishes the diagnosis of Acute pancreatitis:
- **[1] Severe epigastric pain often radiating to the back** that is acute in onset and persistent,
- **[2] Elevation in serum lipase or amylase** ≥3 times the upper limit of normal,
- **[3] Imaging suggestive of pancreatitis:** characteristic findings on imaging (eg, CT, MRI, US).
No imaging is required if the patient meets the first 2 criteria.

DIAGNOSTIC LABS
- **Increased amylase & lipase:** best initial tests. Lipase more specific than amylase. Levels don't equal severity (not specific).
- ALT increase of 3-fold is highly suggestive of gallstone pancreatitis.
- **Hypocalcemia:** necrotic fat binds to calcium, lowering serum calcium levels (saponification).
- Leukocytosis; elevated glucose, bilirubin, & triglycerides may also be seen.

DIAGNOSTIC IMAGING
- **Abdominal CT: diagnostic imaging of choice.** Also recommended in patients who fail to improve or worsen after 48 hours of management to assess extent of necrosis. MRI alternative. Findings may include enlarged pancreas, indistinct margins, necrotic peripancreatic fluid, pseudocyst, or abscess.
- **Transabdominal US: recommended to assess for gallstones and bile duct dilatation.**
- Abdominal radiograph: **"sentinel loop" = localized ileus** of a segment of small bowel in the LUQ. **Colon cutoff sign:** abrupt collapse of the colon near the pancreas. Pancreatic calcification (chronic).
- MRCP may also be useful to detect stones, stricture, or tumor.
- Chest radiograph: left-sided, exudative pleural effusion in moderate to severe cases.

MANAGEMENT
- **"Rest the pancreas": withhold food & liquids by mouth (NPO) until tolerated;** NG suction if severe vomiting. Most cases are mild and 90% recover without complications in 3-7 days.
- **Supportive: moderate IV fluid resuscitation — Lactated ringers preferred** (LR is associated with decreased systemic inflammatory response compared to Normal saline) eg, bolus of 10 mL/kg in patients with no hypovolemia followed by no more than 1.5 mg/kg/hr; **Analgesia (eg, NSAIDS, Meperidine;** Morphine is an alternative). Electrolyte repletion.
- **Antibiotics are not routinely used.** If severe infected pancreatic necrosis is seen (eg, >30% necrosis on CT or MRI), broad spectrum antibiotics (eg, Imipenem) may be used.

RANSONS CRITERIA: used to determine prognosis. APACHE II score also used.

ADMISSION		WITHIN 48 HOURS	
Glucose	>200 mg/dL	**C**alcium	<8.0 mg/dL
Age	>55 years	**H**ematocrit fall	↓ by >10%
LDH	>350 IU/L	**O**xygen	P_{O2} <60 mmHg
AST	>250 IU/dL	**B**UN	↑ by >5 mg/dL after IV fluids
WBC	>16,000/µL	**B**ase deficit	>4 mEq/L
		Sequestration of fluid	> 6L

Interpretation of Ranson's Criteria   Score 0 to 2 = 2% mortality
  If the score ≥ 3, severe pancreatitis likely.   Score 3 to 4 = 15-20% mortality
  If the score < 3, severe pancreatitis is unlikely   Score 5 to 6 = 40% mortality
      Score 7 to 8 : 100% mortality

CHRONIC PANCREATITIS

- Progressive irreversible **inflammatory changes to the pancreas that lead to <u>loss of pancreatic endocrine and exocrine function,</u>** resulting in abnormal insulin secretion and digestive dysfunction respectively.

ETIOLOGIES

- **<u>Heavy alcohol use</u> most common cause of Chronic pancreatitis in the US (70%).**
- **<u>Smoking</u>** — (25%) and may be synergistic with concurrent alcohol use.
- **Hypertriglyceridemia.**
- Idiopathic, underlying genetic predisposition. **Cystic fibrosis most common cause in children.**
- Hypocalcemia, Dyslipidemia, islet cell tumors, familial, trauma, iatrogenic. Autoimmune (eg, SLE).
- <u>Ductal obstruction</u> (eg, malignancy, stones, trauma). Gallstones not significant cause as in Acute Pancreatitis.

CLINICAL MANIFESTATIONS

- **<u>Abdominal pain:</u> most common symptom** — epigastric &/or back pain; **may be atypical or absent.**
- **<u>Triad</u> of ❶ calcifications, ❷ steatorrhea, & ❸ Diabetes mellitus is hallmark** (only in 1/3 of patients).
- <u>Fat maldigestion:</u> steatorrhea (oily or floating stool). ± weight loss or diarrhea.

DIAGNOSIS

- <u>Serum pancreatic enzyme levels:</u> serum amylase and lipase levels are usually not strikingly elevated in Chronic pancreatitis and may even be low.

Imaging:

- **<u>Abdominal CT (often initial)</u> or MRCP initial imaging modalities of choice** — findings include **calcification of the pancreas,** dilated pancreatic or biliary ducts, or an atrophic pancreas. Abdominal CT often performed to rule out other causes of abdominal pain.
- **<u>Abdominal radiographs:</u> calcified pancreas is pathognomonic of Chronic pancreatitis.**
- Endoscopic ultrasound , MRCP, or pancreatic function testing (eg, secretin) if inconclusive imaging.

Pancreatic function testing:

- <u>Indirect pancreatic function testing</u> — **<u>Random fecal elastase 1</u> sensitive & specific to confirm exocrine pancreatic insufficiency.** Performed on a formed stool specimen.
- <u>Direct pancreatic function testing</u> — Pancreatic stimulation with secretin or CCK (not usually done). Hormone stimulation test using secretin is the test with the best sensitivity. The Secretin test becomes abnormal when ≥60% of the pancreatic exocrine function has been lost.

MANAGEMENT

- Alcohol abstinence, pain control, low fat diet, vitamin supplementation. Oral pancreatic enzyme replacement.
- Pancreatectomy only if retractable pain despite medical therapy.

COMPLICATIONS

- Exocrine insufficiency most common — Chronic pancreatitis–related Diabetes >80%. Osteoporosis and osteopenia. The cumulative risk of Pancreatic ductal adenocarcinoma is 4% after 20 years.

PANCREATIC CARCINOMA

- **70% are found in the head of pancreas,** 20% body, 10% tail.
- Fourth leading cause of cancer death in the US among men and women.

TYPES
- **Adenocarcinoma (ductal) most common >85%.** Pancreatic adenocarcinoma begins in the pancreatic ductal epithelium. >95% of malignant neoplasms arise from the exocrine elements.
- Islet cell 5-10%. Ampullary & duodenal carcinomas; cystadenoma & cystocarcinoma.

RISK FACTORS
- **Smoking** (>25%), **>55 years of age, heavy alcohol consumption** (≥4 drinks per day).
- Pancreatic disorders: Chronic pancreatitis, Diabetes mellitus.
- Obesity — Body mass index ≥30 kg/m^2, physical inactivity, males, Blacks > Whites, *H. pylori.*
- Family history, *BRCA1* or *BRCA2* gene carrier, Peutz-Jeghers syndrome, Lynch syndrome, MEN I.

CLINICAL MANIFESTATIONS
- **Most symptomatic patients with PC have advanced, incurable disease at diagnosis,** with metastases often present at presentation (eg, regional lymph node and liver involvement).
- Common bile duct obstruction: **Painless jaundice classic. Pruritus** due to increased bile salts in skin, anorexia, acholic stools, & dark urine. Obstructive symptoms because most PC occurs at the head.
- **Abdominal pain** radiating to the back. May be relieved with sitting up & leaning forward. Tumors in body or tail produce symptoms later than in the head, so usually more advanced at diagnosis.
- Nonspecific symptoms: **weight loss** (90%), anorexia, early satiety, nausea, dyspepsia, generalized fatigue, lack of energy, depression.

PHYSICAL EXAMINATION
- **Courvoisier's sign palpable, nontender, distended gallbladder** due to common bile duct **obstruction,** especially seen with cancer at the head of the pancreas.
- **Pancreatic head tumors most commonly present with jaundice [most frequent sign (55%)] and weight loss.** Steatorrhea due to exocrine insufficiency or blockage of the main pancreatic duct.
- Liver involvement: hepatomegaly, RUQ or epigastric mass, abdominal tenderness, jaundice, cachexia.
- **Trousseau's malignancy sign: migratory phlebitis** associated with malignancy (nonspecific).

DIAGNOSIS
- **Transabdominal ultrasound: often the initial imaging study in patients with jaundice.**
- **CT scan: initial imaging study and standard for the diagnosis and staging of suspected Pancreatic cancer, especially in patients with epigastric pain & weight loss without jaundice.**
    - If CT is negative: the next step is an Endoscopic ultrasound with biopsy of the pancreatic lesion.
    - If CT is positive: the next step is simultaneous surgical removal/biopsy.
- Tumor markers: **Carbohydrate (cancer) antigen (CA) 19-9 often used to monitor after treatment and predict prognosis and recurrence after resection** (not specific). CEA.

MANAGEMENT
- Surgical: **Whipple procedure (Pancreaticoduodenectomy) if confined to the head or duodenal area.** Tail (distal resection). Post-op chemotherapy (eg, 5-FU, Gemcitabine) or radiotherapy.
- Advanced or inoperative: (>80%) — ERCP with stent placement palliative for intractable itching. Chemotherapy — FOLFIRINOX (Leucovorin/5-Fluorouracil + Oxaliplatin + Irinotecan) first line for metastatic/locally advanced unresectable disease with good performance. Gemcitabine-based chemotherapy (eg, Gemcitabine + Cisplatin and FOLFOX; Gemcitabine plus Nabpaclitaxel).

PROGNOSIS
- Only 20% are resectable at the time of diagnosis.
- Overall, 5-year survival rate is 5-15%. Fourth leading cause of cancer-related deaths in the US.

APPENDICITIS

- Obstruction of the lumen of the appendix, resulting in inflammation & bacterial overgrowth.
- **Obstruction due to fecalith or lymphoid hyperplasia most common,** inflammation, malignancy, or foreign body. **Lymphoid hyperplasia due to infection most common cause in children.**

EPIDEMIOLOGY:
- Occurs most commonly between 10-30 years. **Most common abdominal surgical emergency.**
- Appendicitis is the most common cause of acute abdomen in children 12-18 years.

CLINICAL MANIFESTATIONS
- Classic: **Early: anorexia & colicky periumbilical or epigastric pain worse with movement, with later migration to the right lower quadrant** (within 12-18 hours), **anorexia, nausea, & vomiting (vomiting usually occurs after onset of pain).** Appendiceal inflammation stimulates nerve fibers around T8-T10, causing vague periumbilical pain. Once the parietal peritoneum becomes irritated, it radiates to the RLQ. If untreated, gangrene and perforation may develop within 36 hours.
- A retrocecal appendix may present with an atypical pattern (eg, diarrhea, positive Psoas sign) and positive rectal or gynecologic examination. Pelvic location associated with Obturator sign.

PHYSICAL EXAMINATION
- Localized rebound tenderness, rigidity, & guarding. Retrocecal appendix may have atypical findings.
- Low-grade fever (38-38.5°C) is common. Examination findings to assess for Appendicitis include:
   McBurney's point tenderness: point $1/3$ the distance from the anterior sup. iliac spine & navel.
   Rovsing sign: Right lower quadrant (RLQ) pain elicited with palpation of the LLQ.
   Obturator sign: RLQ pain with internal & external right hip rotation with a flexed knee (pelvic).
   Psoas sign: RLQ pain on external rotation or passive extension of the right hip (if retrocecal).

DIAGNOSIS
The diagnosis is often based on clinical presentation & may be supported with imaging.
- Laboratory: **Moderate leukocytosis** (10,000–20,000/mcL) **with neutrophilia is common.**
Imaging:
- **In adults, CT scan is the preferred imaging of choice (more accurate). Ultrasound (preferred) or MRI reserved for radiosensitive populations (eg, pregnant women & children).** Positive findings include wall thickening (>2 mm), periappendiceal fat stranding, appendiceal wall enhancement, appendicolith, and enlarged appendiceal double-wall thickness (>6 mm).
- **Ultrasound: preferred imaging in children and pregnant women** due to its lack of ionizing radiation and IV contrast and can be performed at bedside. Positive findings include focal pain over appendix with compression, noncompressible appendix with enlarged double-wall thickness (>6 mm), increased echogenicity of inflamed periappendiceal fat, and fluid in the right lower quadrant.
- In children, a surgical consult is often obtained prior to imaging to determine if imaging is needed, depending on the risk.

MANAGEMENT
[1] Non-perforated early uncomplicated appendicitis:
- **Appendectomy (laparoscopic preferred when possible** or open laparotomy) should be performed within 24 hours of diagnosis. **Recommended preoperative IV antibiotics (eg, Cefoxitin or Cefotetan; Ampicillin-sulbactam or Ertapenem).** NPO & IV crystalloid fluids.
- **Conservative management with antibiotics alone may be used.** Up to 80–90% of patients with uncomplicated Appendicitis treated with antibiotics alone for 7 days have resolution of symptoms.
[2] Perforated appendicitis with hemodynamic instability, sepsis, free perforation, or peritonitis:
- **Emergency appendectomy,** irrigation and drainage of peritoneal cavity, bowel resection if needed.
[3] Stable perforated appendicitis:
- **Initial nonoperative management, IV antibiotics.** Percutaneous drainage of abscess if present. Rescue appendectomy for patients who do not respond to antibiotics.

SPLENIC INJURY (RUPTURE OR LACERATION)

- The spleen is the most common organ injured during trauma (liver most common cause of bleeding).
- Associated with left-sided rib fractures, blunt abdominal trauma, Epstein-Barr infection ("Mono").

CLINICAL MANIFESTATIONS
- May have abdominal pain (left upper quadrant). May have signs of hypotension and shock.
- **Kehr sign: referred left shoulder pain due to irritation of the diaphragm and the phrenic nerve.**

DIAGNOSIS: **sonography for trauma (FAST)**; CT shows the extent of injury; exploratory laparotomy.

MANAGEMENT
- Incomplete rupture: endovascular embolization. Surgical exploration if hemodynamically unstable.
- Complete rupture or intractable bleeding: splenectomy.

SMALL BOWEL OBSTRUCTION (SBO)

- **Partial or complete MECHANICAL obstruction (blockage) of the small intestine,** disrupting the normal flow of intraluminal contents and products of digestion.
- Decreased absorption, vomiting, & reduced intake lead to volume depletion with hemoconcentration.

ETIOLOGIES
- **3 most common causes of mechanical obstruction: [1] postsurgical intraabdominal adhesions (most common), [2] hernias, & [3] neoplasms.** Crohn disease, malignancy, intussusception.

TYPES
- Closed loop vs. open loop: in closed loop, the lumen is occluded at two points, which can reduce the mesenteric blood supply, causing strangulation, necrosis, & peritonitis.
- Complete vs. partial: complete associated with severe obstipation (inability to pass stool or gas).
- Distal vs. proximal: abdominal distention more common with distal; vomiting seen more in proximal.

CLINICAL MANIFESTATIONS
- 4 hallmark symptoms "CAVO" — **C**rampy abdominal pain, **A**bdominal distention (esp. if distal), nausea & **V**omiting (bilious esp. if proximal), & **O**bstipation (inability to pass flatus or stool).

PHYSICAL EXAMINATION
- **Abdominal distention** varies based on the site. Distention may be absent with proximal SBO.
- Bowel sounds: **high-pitched tinkles on auscultation & visible peristalsis (early obstruction).** In late obstruction, hypoactive bowel sounds are a common finding.

DIAGNOSIS
- **Abdominal radiograph — multiple air-fluid levels ("stepladder" appearance), dilated bowel loops** >3 cm, & visualization of the valvulae conniventes. Minimum colonic gas if complete obstruction.
- **CT scan of the abdomen with IV contrast: imaging of choice* — more accurate to assess etiology, site of obstruction, severity, & complications. Transition zone** from dilated loops of bowel with contrast to an area of bowel with no contrast.
- Abdominal ultrasound: more sensitive than Plain radiographs; advantage of no radiation exposure.

MANAGEMENT
- Nonstrangulated: **Supportive — bowel rest (NPO), volume resuscitation (IV fluids), analgesia, treatment of nausea, electrolyte repletion, & gastrointestinal decompression via nasogastric tube placement with intermittent suction (if significant abdominal distention or vomiting).**
- Abdominal radiograph with water soluble contrast challenge may be performed in patients who fail to improve after 48 hours of conservative treatment for both diagnostic and therapeutic purposes.
- Strangulated: surgical options include adhesiolysis and/or bowel resection if severe or refractory.

PARALYTIC (ADYNAMIC, FUNCTIONAL) ILEUS

- **FUNCTIONAL obstruction:** Paralytic (Adynamic) ileus due to a neurogenic failure of peristalsis to propel intestinal contents **without** mechanical obstruction.
- An ileus usually becomes evident on the third to the fifth day after surgery and usually lasts 2-3 days with the small bowel returning to function (0-24 hours), stomach (24-48 h), and colon (48-72 h).

ETIOLOGIES
- **Postoperative state,** especially intra-abdominal surgery; most common within the first few days.
- Medications — eg, **opioids,** antimuscarinics (anticholinergics), & anesthesia decrease GI motility.
- Electrolyte abnormalities — **Hypokalemia, Hypercalcemia,** Hypomagnesemia, Hypophosphatemia.
- Severe medical illness, metabolic (eg, **Hypothyroidism,** Diabetes mellitus), spinal cord injury.

CLINICAL MANIFESTATIONS
- Symptoms similar to Small bowel obstruction but slower in onset — mild abdominal pain, nausea, vomiting, obstipation, abdominal distention, bloating, increased flatus, inability to tolerate oral diet.

PHYSICAL EXAMINATION
- **Decreased or absent bowel sounds** (unlike early SBO, which is associated with high-pitched sounds).
- **Abdominal distention and tympany,** no tenderness (or mild if present). No peritoneal signs.

DIAGNOSIS
- Laboratory evaluation: CBC, electrolytes (look for Hypokalemia & Hypercalcemia), LFT, amylase, lipase.
- **Plain radiographs: diffuse dilated loops of bowel without a transition zone, paucity of air (gas) in the colon and rectum** (unlike mechanical SBO, which has a transition zone).
- **CT of the abdomen: criterion standard if further imaging needs to be performed** to differentiate between functional or mechanic obstruction, etiologies, possible complications, or other etiologies.

MANAGEMENT
- **Supportive care: bowel rest (NPO) or dietary restriction with clear fluids with progression to liquid diet, electrolyte & IV fluid repletion,** removal of any inciting factors, and serial abdominal examination. Treat underlying cause (eg, remove offending medications, electrolyte management).
- Bowel decompression with NG suction if persistent nausea, vomiting, or severe abdominal distention.
- Prognosis is generally good (postop ileus typically resolves within 1-3 days with supportive care.
- **Reduction of incidence: minimally invasive (laparoscopic) surgery, use of patient-controlled or epidural analgesia, early ambulation, gum chewing, & initiation of clear liquid diet.**

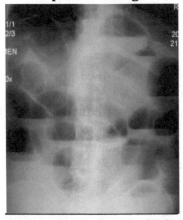

SMALL BOWEL OBSTRUCTION
- **Multiple air-fluid levels in a "stepladder" appearance, dilated bowel loops.**

Photo: James Heilman, MD (Wikimedia commons)

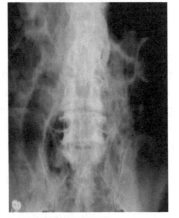

PARALYTIC ILEUS
- **Dilated loops of bowel with no transition zone.**

Photo: Nevit Dilmen (Wikimedia Commons)

INTUSSUSCEPTION

- **Telescoping (invagination) of an intestinal segment into the adjoining distal intestinal lumen, leading to bowel obstruction.** Usually involves the small bowel.
- **Ileocolic junction intussusception (90%)** — terminal ileum telescopes into proximal large bowel.

EPIDEMIOLOGY:
- **Most common cause of bowel obstruction in children 6 months–36 months of age** (80–90% occur in children <2 years of age). More common in **males; commonly seen after viral infections.**

ETIOLOGIES:
- **Idiopathic most common cause in children (75%).**
- **Luminal lead points** drag one portion of bowel into another (25%) — Meckel diverticulum, enlarged mesenteric lymph nodes, hyperplasia of Peyer's patches, tumors, Henoch-Schönlein purpura.

CLINICAL MANIFESTATIONS
- **Classic triad: [1] vomiting + [2] abdominal pain + [3] passage of blood per rectum — "currant jelly" stools (stool mixed with blood & mucus)** only seen in 1/3 of patients. Sudden onset of intermittent, severe, crampy, progressive abdominal pain, accompanied by crying & drawing up of the legs toward the abdomen to relieve the pain, often with pallor; appears well in between episodes.
- Vomiting is not usually present at first but may develop over 6 to 12 hours and may be bilious.
- **Lethargy** or altered consciousness alone, without pain, rectal bleeding. Fever is not a common finding.
Physical examination:
- **Sausage-shaped mass may be palpated in the mid abdomen or right upper quadrant or hypochondrium + Dance's sign right lower quadrant that is scaphoid (empty)** due to telescoping of the bowel. Occult blood (positive stool guaiac).
- No abdominal tenderness or focal tenderness, especially in the right mid or upper abdomen.

DIAGNOSIS
- **Ultrasound: best initial test** (high accuracy & lack of radiation). **Findings include the donut, target, or bull's eye sign — concentric alternating echogenic and hypoechoic bands.** The echogenic bands are formed by mucosa and muscularis whereas the hypoechoic bands are the submucosa.
- **Air or contrast enema: both diagnostic & therapeutic. Air enema more commonly used than hydrostatic enema,** especially if peritonitis is present. Water-soluble contrast enema preferred over barium. **Findings include occluding mass prolapsing into the lumen, known as the "coiled spring" appearance** (barium in the lumen of the intussusceptum and in the intraluminal space).
- Children with a high suspicion of Intussusception should undergo immediate Air-contrast enema.

MANAGEMENT
Non-surgical management
- **IV fluid & electrolyte replacement most important initial steps, followed by decompression if clinically and hemodynamically stable with no evidence of bowel perforation or shock.**
- **Pneumatic (air) decompression enema preferred over hydrostatic (saline- or contrast-based) enemas,** using fluoroscopic or sonographic guidance.
- Hydrostatic decompression enema (saline or contrast) both diagnostic and therapeutic.
- Admission for observation for 24 hours after successful reduction to monitor for recurrence or complications. 10% have recurrence within 24 hours after treatment.
Surgical intervention
- Surgical reduction indicated when pneumatic or hydrostatic enema fails to relieve obstruction. Resection of gangrenous/necrotic segments. The appendix is usually removed to prevent confusion in evaluating the abdominal pain in the future.
- Peritonitis or shock: Children with peritonitis, with free air on plain radiographs, or in shock should not undergo air-contrast enema and require emergent surgical reduction.

INTUSSUSCEPTION

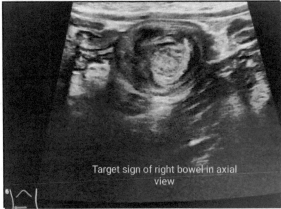

Target sign of right bowel in axial view

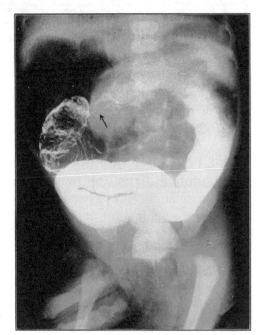

- **Ultrasound:** donut, target, or bull's eye sign — concentric alternating echogenic and hypoechoic bands. The echogenic bands are formed by mucosa & muscularis; the submucosa (hypoechoic bands).

Cerevisae, CC BY-SA 4.0 <https://creativecommons.org/licenses/by-sa/4.0>, via Wikimedia Commons

LARGE BOWEL OBSTRUCTION (LBO)

- **MECHANICAL** large bowel obstruction occurs when normal flow of intraluminal contents is blocked.

ETIOLOGIES
- **Colorectal cancer** most common cause of LBO (60%) especially if left-sided, **Volvulus [15-20%]** (sigmoid more common in elderly and cecal in young adults)], **Diverticular disease (10%) are the most common causes of LBO.**
- Inflammatory bowel disease, stricture formation, fecal impaction (elderly).

CLINICAL MANIFESTATIONS
- **Crampy abdominal pain, obstipation**; **chronic: progressive change in bowel habits**; Vomiting is less common in LBO. Diarrhea due to overflow from bacterial liquefaction of entrapped fecal matter.
- Physical examination: **significant abdominal distension**, tympany with percussion, decreased or absent bowel sounds. If perforation, guarding, rigidity, and rebound tenderness may be seen.
- The digital rectal examination may reveal an empty rectum or hard stool in the rectal vault.
- Large bowel obstruction usually presents as an emergency with dehydration, sepsis, or hemodynamically compromised state.

DIAGNOSIS
- **Abdominal CT:** highly sensitive and specific for detecting large bowel obstruction (imaging of choice for LBO) and can accurately distinguish between other causes of obstruction.
- **Plain radiographs:** dilated colon, a cutoff at obstruction site, & a paucity of gas in the rectum.

MANAGEMENT
- **Initial supportive care:** bowel rest (NPO), IV fluid therapy, correction of electrolyte abnormalities. NG decompression with intermittent suction if severe vomiting, antibiotics.
- **Further treatment** depends upon the etiology and location of the obstruction, as well as the medical comorbidities of the patient. **Most LBOs require surgical intervention.**
- Malignant obstruction: surgery for definitive management (open or laparoscopic). Endoscopic stenting for decompression as a bridge to surgery if immediate surgery is not required.
- Patients with impending perforation, fecal peritonitis, or cecal ischemia often require an emergency laparotomy and resection of the perforated colon as well as the obstructing lesion.

ACUTE COLONIC PSEUDO-OBSTRUCTION (OGILVIE SYNDROME)

- **FUNCTIONAL obstruction:** neurogenic decrease or absence of peristalsis due to inhibition of GI motility, causing acute colonic dilation **in the absence of any mechanical obstruction**.
- Usually involves cecum & proximal ascending colon (right hemicolon), with transition near splenic flexure.

ETIOLOGIES

- Similar to Adynamic (paralytic) ileus — **postoperative state**, medications (eg, **opioids**, anticholinergics), metabolic (eg, **Hypokalemia**, **Hypercalcemia**), severe medical illness, metabolic (eg, **Hypothyroidism**, Diabetes mellitus), chronic constipation, bedridden, and older adults.

CLINICAL MANIFESTATIONS

- **Abdominal distention main feature** (over 3-5 days). Abdominal discomfort, nausea, vomiting, constipation. May have paradoxical diarrhea. Minimal or mild abdominal tenderness.
- Physical examination: abdominal distention & abdominal tympany. Bowel sounds usually present.

DIAGNOSIS

- **CT scan with oral and intravenous (IV) contrast is the preferred modality for diagnosis.**
- Contrast enema (water-soluble) alternative if CT is unavailable & no peritonitis. Avoid colonoscopy.
- Abdominal radiographs: dilated right colon often from the cecum with cutoff at the splenic flexure.

MANAGEMENT

- **Conservative:** IV fluid & electrolyte repletion is the first step if colon dilation <12 cm & absence of severe symptoms or peritonitis. A nasogastric tube and a rectal tube should be placed.
- **Medical decompression:** Neostigmine in patients at risk for perforation (eg, cecal diameter >12 cm) or if failed 48-72 hours of conservative therapy. Not used if pulse <60/m or SBP <90.
- **Colonoscopic decompression:** if symptoms despite conservative treatment & Neostigmine.
- **Surgical decompression:** (cecostomy or colectomy) if other therapies fail, ischemia, or if perforation.

TOXIC MEGACOLON

- **Nonobstructive, extreme colon dilation >6 cm + signs of systemic toxicity.**
- ETIOLOGIES: **complications of IBD (eg, Ulcerative colitis), infectious colitis (eg, *C. difficile*, CMV).** Other causes: Ischemic colitis, Volvulus, Diverticulitis, radiation, or obstructive Colorectal cancer.

CLINICAL MANIFESTATIONS

- **Profound bloody diarrhea hallmark,** abdominal pain & distention, nausea, vomiting, tenesmus.

Physical examination:
- **Lower abdominal tenderness & distention** with or without peritonitis.
- **Signs of toxicity:** altered mental status, fever, tachycardia, hypotension, dehydration. May have signs of peritonitis (eg, rigidity, guarding, rebound tenderness), especially if perforation occurs.

DIAGNOSIS

- **Radiologic evidence of colon >6 cm:** abdominal radiographs &/or CT scan usually the initial imaging tests of choice. CT scan may be used to assess for complications. **Avoid Colonoscopy.**
- At least 3: fever >38°C, pulse >120/min, neutrophilic leukocytosis >10,500/microL, anemia PLUS
- At least 1: hypotension, dehydration, electrolyte abnormalities, or altered mental status.

MANAGEMENT

- **Supportive mainstay of treatment** — IV fluids, bowel rest, fluid & electrolyte replacement, **broad-spectrum antibiotics (eg, Ceftriaxone + Metronidazole),** bowel decompression with NG tube if needed, and avoidance of antimotility agents (eg, opioids, anticholinergics).
- Management of the underlying cause — **Ulcerative colitis:** IV glucocorticoids; **CMV colitis:** IV Ganciclovir; *C. difficile:* **Oral Vancomycin or oral Fidaxomicin.**

CONGENITAL AGANGLIONIC MEGACOLON (HIRSCHSPRUNG DISEASE)

- **Congenital megacolon** due to an **absence of ganglion cells** in the mucosal & muscular layers of the colon, leading to a **functional obstruction** (failure of colonic muscles to relax).
- **Rectum & part of the sigmoid colon most common** (80%) with short-segment disease.
  15-20% extend proximal to the sigmoid colon (long-segment disease), or entire colon.
- Risk factors: Males: females 4:1, Down syndrome, Chagas disease, MEN 2, RET gene mutation.

PATHOPHYSIOLOGY
- **Failure of neural crest cells migration** neural crest cells (precursors of enteric ganglion cells) **fail to completely migrate craniocaudally during intestinal development during fetal life, leading to an absence of enteric ganglion cells (Auerbach & Meissner plexuses)**. This results in deficient nitric oxide synthesis & failure of the colonic muscles to relax (constant contraction), leading to a localized functional obstruction. An imperforate anus may coexist.

CLINICAL MANIFESTATIONS
- **[1] Neonatal large bowel obstruction (LBO): meconium ileus (failure of meconium passage in the first 48 hours of life) in a full-term infant or failure to pass stools, followed by bilious vomiting, progressive abdominal distention,** poor feeding, poor weight gain, failure to thrive.
- **[2] Enterocolitis** sepsis-like presentation with associated foul-smelling watery diarrhea, abdominal distention, vomiting, lethargy, and poor feeding, which may progress to Toxic megacolon.
- **[3] Chronic progressive constipation may be seen with milder disease** (short-segment or ultrashort-segment) and present later in infancy or childhood.

Physical examination:
- **No stool in the rectal vault:** On digital rectal examination, **tight anal sphincter and the anal canal and rectum are devoid of fecal material despite retained stool. Abdominal distention.**
- **Squirt or blast sign**: explosive gush of flatus and liquid stool as the finger is withdrawn during rectal examination if the aganglionic segment is short, which may relieve the obstruction temporarily.

DIAGNOSIS
- **Barium contrast enema: best initial test.** Findings include **funnel-shaped transition zone (caliber change)** between normal and agalionic affected bowel. Avoided if enterocolitis is suspected.
- Anorectal manometry: may be used as a screening test if mild to moderate suspicion — increased anal sphincter pressure & lack of relaxation of the internal anal sphincter upon balloon rectal distention.
- **Rectal biopsy: definitive & confirmatory (required for the diagnosis) — findings include absence of ganglion cells in both the submucosal and muscular layers of involved bowel.** On rectal suction biopsy samples, special stains may show nerve trunk hypertrophy and **increased acetylcholinesterase staining (activity). Rectal suction biopsy usually performed**, with full thickness biopsy reserved for if rectal suction biopsy is nondiagnostic.
- Plain abdominal radiographs: not helpful in excluding the diagnosis of HD, except if there is low suspicion. Findings — decreased/absent air in the rectum + dilated proximal colon bowel loops.

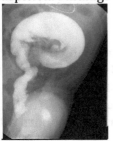

Barium contrast enema: funnel-shaped transition zone (caliber change).

Case courtesy of Frank Gaillard, Radiopaedia.org, rID: 7846

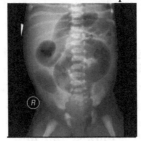

- Plain radiographs: decreased/absent air in the rectum + dilated proximal colon bowel loops.

MANAGEMENT
- **Surgical resection: removal of affected bowel section is the mainstay of treatment.**
- Enterocolitis: nothing by mouth, IV fluid resuscitation, IV antibiotic therapy including anaerobic coverage via (eg, Metronidazole), rectal irrigations, and, in rare cases, an emergency colostomy for decompression. Once bowel has returned to normal, definitive treatment can be performed.

VOLVULUS

- **Twisting of any part of the bowel about its mesenteric attachment site & axis of its blood supply.**
- **The sigmoid colon is involved in up to 90% of cases, but Volvuli can involve the cecum (<20%)** or transverse colon. **Midgut (intestinal malrotation) and ileum common in children.**
- Sigmoid volvulus presents most commonly in patients who are less mobile, bed bound and institutionalized, usually with a background of chronic constipation (chronic distention).
- Complications of Volvulus include [1] obstruction of the intestinal lumen and [2] impairment of vascular perfusion occur when the degree of torsion exceeds 180° & 360° respectively.

CLINICAL MANIFESTATIONS

- **Obstruction: slowly progressive crampy abdominal pain, abdominal distension, nausea, vomiting, and constipation.** Vomiting usually occurs several days after the onset of pain.
- **Neonates: bilious vomiting within the first week of life & colicky abdominal pain.**
- Impaired vascular supply: fever, tachycardia, peritonitis (rigidity, guarding, rebound tenderness).
- Loss of appetite and reduced oral intake, increasing abdominal distension, and cessation of bowel output may require hospital admission.

Physical examination:
- **Distended & tympanitic abdomen.** Abdominal tenderness to palpation may be seen.
- Impaired vascular supply: fever, tachycardia, peritonitis (abdominal rigidity, guarding, rebound tenderness), and rarely sepsis. Fever & leukocytosis if gangrene and/or perforation.

DIAGNOSIS

- **Abdominal CT: establishes the diagnosis of sigmoid Volvulus** & can rule out other causes of abdominal pain — **dilated sigmoid colon, "bird-beak" appearance at site of the Volvulus.**
- **Plain radiographs: Sigmoid:** "bent inner tube" or "coffee bean" sign — U-shaped appearance of the air-filled closed loop of distended colon with loss of haustral markings. Ordered if CT not available. **Cecal Volvulus: embryo sign; Midgut volvulus: "double bubble:" sign with distal gas present.**

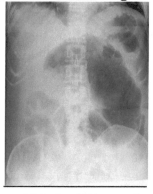

Sigmoid Volvulus	Cecal Volvulus
• "bent inner tube" or "coffee bean" sign • Arises in the LLQ & pelvis; extends towards the RUQ. • Ahaustral in appearance Case courtesy of Wael Nemattalla, Radiopaedia.org, rID: 10633	• Arises in the RLQ, extends up to the epigastrium or LUQ, similar to an **embryo** (**"embryo sign"**) • Colonic haustral pattern still seen. Case courtesy of Vikas Shah, Radiopaedia.org, rID: 54998

- Intestinal malrotation in children: Abdominal ultrasound. **Limited Upper GI series: corkscrew sign.**
- Gastrografin contrast enema: Rarely performed and not indicated if peritonitis is present.

MANAGEMENT

- **Endoscopic decompression (Proctosigmoidoscopy) initial treatment of choice for Sigmoid volvulus without evidence of perforation, gangrene, or peritonitis. Often, a rectal tube is left in place post decompression** to decrease acute recurrence & decrease distention.
- **Definitive management: Decompression is often followed by elective surgery** (eg, sigmoid colectomy or resection with primary anastomosis) **during admission or 24-72 hours after to prevent recurrence after endoscopic detorsion** due to high rate of recurrence (up to 40%).
- Immediate surgical management (laparotomy): peritonitis, gangrene, or if endoscopic decompression is unsuccessful. Sigmoid resection with primary anastomosis or Hartmann's procedure.
- **Children with midgut Volvulus (malrotation): surgical management (eg, Ladd procedure).**
- **Cecal Volvulus requires emergent surgery** (eg, detorsion & cecopexy, right hemicolectomy).

MECKEL'S (ILEAL) DIVERTICULUM

- **Persistent remnant of a portion of embryonic vitelline duct (yolk stalk, omphalomesenteric duct),** located on the antimesenteric border of the small intestine (ileum).
- Most common congenital anomaly (malformation) of the GI tract.
- **Rule of 2s:** 2% of population; within 2 feet from the ileocecal valve, 2% symptomatic, 2 inches in length, 2 types of ectopic tissue (**gastric most common** or pancreatic), 2 years most common age at clinical presentation, 2 times more common in males.

PATHOPHYSIOLOGY
- Ectopic gastric or pancreatic tissue may secrete digestive hormones, leading to ulcers & bleeding.

CLINICAL MANIFESTATIONS
- **Usually asymptomatic** — often an incidental finding during abdominal surgery for other causes.
- **Painless rectal bleeding or ulceration.** If painful, it is usually periumbilical (similar to appendicitis).
- May cause Intussusception, Volvulus, or Obstruction. May cause Diverticulitis in adults.

DIAGNOSIS
- **Technetium-99m pertechnetate (Meckel) scan: looks for ectopic gastric tissue in the ileal area.**
- Mesenteric arteriography or abdominal exploration.

MANAGEMENT
- Surgical resection of the Meckel's diverticulum if symptomatic.

DUODENAL ATRESIA

- Complete absence or closure of a portion of the duodenum, leading to a **gastric outlet obstruction.**
- **Risk factors: polyhydramnios** (increased amniotic fluid), Trisomy 21 (Down syndrome).
- Associated with other congenital defects.

CLINICAL MANIFESTATIONS
- **Neonatal intestinal obstruction: shortly after birth (within the first 24-48 hours of life) with abdominal distention and bilious vomiting** (may be nonbilious).

DIAGNOSIS
- Abdominal radiographs: **double bubble sign — distended air-filled stomach + smaller distended duodenum separated by the pyloric valve. Distal gas is absent (unlike in malrotation).**
- Upper GI series: often performed preoperatively to assess the GI tract.

MANAGEMENT
- GI tract decompression & electrolyte and fluid replacement. **Duodenoduodenostomy (definitive).**

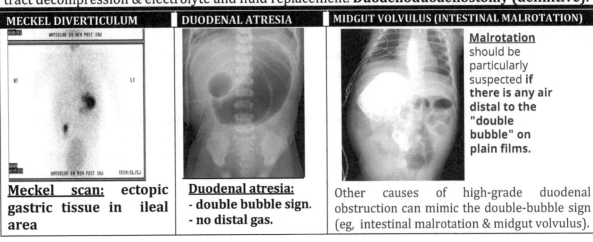

MECKEL DIVERTICULUM	DUODENAL ATRESIA	MIDGUT VOLVULUS (INTESTINAL MALROTATION)	
Meckel scan: ectopic gastric tissue in ileal area	**Duodenal atresia:** - double bubble sign. - no distal gas.	Other causes of high-grade duodenal obstruction can mimic the double-bubble sign (eg, intestinal malrotation & midgut volvulus).	**Malrotation** should be particularly suspected **if there is any air distal to the "double bubble" on plain films.**

CELIAC DISEASE (CELIAC SPRUE)

- **Autoimmune-mediated inflammation of the <u>small bowel due to reaction with alpha-gliadin in gluten-containing foods</u> (eg, wheat, rye, barley).** May have variant HLA-DQ2 or HLA-DQ8 alleles.
- Increased incidence in females, European descent (Irish & Finnish). May have autoimmune history.

PATHOPHYSIOLOGY
- Autoimmune damage leads to loss of villi with subsequent malabsorption.

CLINICAL MANIFESTATIONS
- **Malabsorption: diarrhea,** abdominal pain/distention, bloating, flatulence, **steatorrhea (bulky, foul-smelling, oily. or floating stool).** Growth delays in children. Weight loss or failure to gain weight. **Vitamin deficiencies (eg, Vitamins A, D, E, K), Calcium &/or iron deficiencies.**
- **<u>Dermatitis herpetiformis</u>: pruritic, papulovesicular rash most common on extensor surfaces, neck, trunk, & scalp due to IgA deposits** (anti-epidermal transglutaminase) in the upper dermis.
- Repeated infections may be seen if IgA deficient.

PHYSICAL EXAMINATION
- Physical examination may reveal abdominal distension pallor, mouth ulcers, and short stature.

DIAGNOSIS
- Clinical diagnosis: symptom improvement with a trial of gluten-free diet.

Screening:
- **<u>Transglutaminase IgA antibodies</u> preferred initial test of choice.** Endomysial IgA antibodies.
- Total IgA levels to assess for IgA deficiency. For patients with IgA deficiency (low levels), deamidated gliadin peptide (DGP) IgG testing is available. HLA-DQ2/DQ8 typing if equivocal tests.

Definitive & confirmatory:
- **<u>Upper endoscopy with small bowel biopsy</u> — atrophic mucosa with loss of the villi (most accurate),** increased intraepithelial lymphocytes and plasma cells, or crypt hyperplasia.

MANAGEMENT
- **<u>Gluten-free diet</u> — avoid wheat, rye, barley.** Limit oat consumption. Rice, wine, & corn are safe.
- Steroids or immunosuppressant (eg, Azathioprine) considered in patients with refractory disease.
- Vitamin supplementation.

LACTOSE INTOLERANCE

- **Inability to digest lactose due to low levels of lactase enzyme in the small intestine.**
- Lactase enzyme production normally declines in adulthood, especially in African Americans, Asian Americans, South Americans, and Native Americans.
- Intestinal bacteria ferment & convert malabsorbed lactose into hydrogen gas, causing symptoms.

CLINICAL MANIFESTATIONS
- Abdominal pain, bloating, flatulence, gassiness, loose stools, diarrhea, borborygmi, nausea, vomiting, after ingestion of milk or milk-containing products. Stools may be bulky, frothy, or watery.

DIAGNOSIS
- **Clinical diagnosis — symptom improvement after a trial of lactose-free diet.** ↑Stool osmotic gap.
- **<u>Hydrogen breath test:</u> test of choice.** Hydrogen is produced when colonic bacteria ferment the undigested lactose. Usually performed after a trial of a lactose-free diet if the diagnosis is uncertain.

MANAGEMENT
- **Dietary lactose restriction or use lactase enzyme preparations + Calcium & Vitamin D intake.**
- Lactaid or other prehydrolyzed milk may be used as a substitute for milk.

DIVERTICULOSIS

- Diverticula are outpouchings due to herniation of the mucosa and submucosa into the weakened walls of the colon along natural openings at the vasa recta of the colon due to increased luminal pressure.
- Left colon most common in incidence; Right colon most common location for bleeding (due to wider neck, longer vasa recta, and thinner walls).
- Risks: **low dietary fiber, constipation, obesity,** increases with age (prevalence >50% by age 60y).

CLINICAL MANIFESTATIONS

- **Asymptomatic (70-80%)** — discovered incidentally at endoscopy or on barium enema.
- **Painless rectal bleeding: Diverticulosis is the most common cause of <u>acute</u> lower GI bleeding (brisk hematochezia) in adults.** Hypertensive, atherosclerosis, & regular use Aspirin & NSAIDs ↑ risk.

DIAGNOSIS

- **Colonoscopy test of choice (diagnostic and therapeutic) once** upper GI bleed has been ruled out.
- Radionuclide imaging (eg, technetium-99 tagged red blood cell scan) usually followed by arteriography is the next step if the bleeding is not visualized on colonoscopy. CT angiography.

MANAGEMENT

- **Supportive management: in most cases, the bleeding stops spontaneously.** Asymptomatic Diverticulosis can be followed on a high fiber diet, use of Bran, or psyllium, and risk reduction.
- Severe bleeding: Resuscitation (2 large bore IVs, fluids &/or blood products), coagulopathy correction.
- Active bleeding: Endoscopic therapy to control bleeding (eg, Epinephrine injection, tamponade).
- Angiography and embolization for unstable patients or failure of endoscopic therapy.

ACUTE DIVERTICULITIS

- Microscopic perforation or macroperforation of a diverticulum leads to inflammation & focal necrosis.
- **Sigmoid colon most common area** (due to high intraluminal pressure). Onset usually >40y of age.

CLINICAL MANIFESTATIONS

- **LLQ abdominal pain (most common due to sigmoid location),** LLQ tenderness, **low-grade fever.** May have nausea, vomiting, constipation, diarrhea, flatulence, bloating, or changes in bowel habits.
- Increased incidence of right-sided (cecal) involvement in Asians, which may cause R-sided symptoms.
- Physical examination: often normal. A tender mass may be present due to inflammation or abscess.

DIAGNOSIS

- **CT scan initial imaging test of choice** — localized bowel wall thickening (>4 mm), pericolic fat stranding, increase in soft tissue density within pericolonic fat, presence of colonic diverticula.
- Labs: **leukocytosis.** Colonoscopy & Barium enema not used (perforation risk).

MANAGEMENT

- **Uncomplicated: treated as an outpatient with analgesics & clear liquid diet (or diet as tolerated); oral antibiotics only in select patients (eg, Metronidazole + either Ciprofloxacin or Levofloxacin)** for 7-10 days. Trimethoprim-sulfamethoxazole + Metronidazole is an alternative.
- **Abscess: <3-4 cm: IV Antibiotic therapy; >3-4 cm: consider CT-guided percutaneous drainage.**
- Surgery: indicated if refractory to medical therapy, frequent recurrences, perforation, or strictures.

Criteria for admission:
- Patients with complicated Diverticulitis (perforation, abscess, obstruction, or fistula). CT-guided percutaneous drainage may be needed for resolution in Acute diverticulitis with abscesses >3 cm.
- Uncomplicated Diverticulitis with high-risk — high fever >102.5°F, sepsis, immunosuppression, increased age, unable to tolerate oral intake etc.

Follow up after Acute diverticulitis:
- **Follow-up colonoscopy indicated 4-6 weeks after recovery from Acute diverticulitis to rule out Colorectal cancer.** Low fiber intake during the acute stage; High fiber long-term prevention.

INFLAMMATORY BOWEL DISEASE (IBD)

- Repetitive episodes of inflammation of the gastrointestinal tract caused by an abnormal immune response to gut microflora, resulting in dysregulation in mucosal immunity.
- Includes both [1] Ulcerative colitis (UC) and [2] Crohn disease (CD).

RISK FACTORS
- **Race & Ethnicity:** more common in the Jewish population (especially **Ashkenazi Jews**), increased incidence in Whites compared to Blacks & Hispanics.
- **Age & Gender: classic onset is most common in adolescents & young adults between 15-35 years.** UC seen slightly more common in males; CD seen slightly more common in females.
- Genetics: 10-30% patients have a first-degree relative with IBD.
- **Smoking: Cigarette smoking increases the incidence of Crohn disease,** resistance to medical therapy, and early disease relapse. **Cigarette smoking may be protective in UC** (smokers who stop smoking who have a history of UC have increased incidence of flares).
- **Diet:** Western style diet is associated with increased incidence of IBD.
- Infections: alteration in bowel microbes (eg, during viral or bacterial infections) may trigger an inflammatory process that goes unchecked.
- Medications: NSAIDs, oral contraceptives, or hormone replacement therapy may be associated with an increased risk.

EXTRA-INTESTINAL MANIFESTATIONS
These manifestations can be seen with Crohn disease & Ulcerative colitis:
- **Rheumatologic: Arthritis is the most common extraintestinal manifestation of IBD** (21%), musculoskeletal pain, Ankylosing spondylitis, Osteoporosis, and bone loss.
- **Dermatologic: Erythema nodosum most common derm manifestation**; Pyoderma gangrenosum.
- **Ocular: Anterior uveitis/iritis** (ocular pain, headache, blurred vision, headache) **& Episcleritis most common ocular manifestations of IBD.** Conjunctivitis, mild ocular burning.
- Hepatobiliary: fatty liver, Primary sclerosing cholangitis. **Aphthous stomatitis.**
- Hematologic: vitamin B12 & Iron deficiency, especially with CD. Increased risk of thromboembolism.
- Renal stones: calcium oxalate stones and urate stones from diarrhea and steatorrhea.

	ULCERATIVE COLITIS (UC)	CROHN DISEASE (CD)
AREA AFFECTED	• **Limited to colon (begins in rectum** with CONTIGUOUS SPREAD PROXIMALLY to colon. • **RECTUM ALWAYS INVOLVED**	• **ANY SEGMENT OF THE GI TRACT** from mouth to anus. • **MC in TERMINAL ILEUM ⇨ RLQ pain**
DEPTH	• Mucosa & submucosa only	• **TRANSMURAL**
CLINICAL MANIFESTATIONS	• Abdominal pain: **LLQ MC,** colicky. • **Tenesmus, urgency** • **BLOODY DIARRHEA hallmark** (stools with mucus/pus), hematochezia	• Abdominal pain: **RLQ pain MC** (crampy) & weight loss more common with Crohn • Diarrhea with no visible blood usually (may be Guaiac positive).
COMPLICATIONS	• Primary Sclerosing Cholangitis, Colon ca, Toxic megacolon (more common in UC). • **Smoking decreases risk for UC.**	• **Perianal disease:** fistulas, strictures, abscesses, GRANULOMAS. • Malabsorption: Fe & **B12 deficiency** • **Smoking increases risk for CD.**
COLONOSCOPY	• **Uniform inflammation** • ± ulceration in the rectum and/or colon. • **PSEUDOPOLYPS.**	• **"SKIP LESIONS"** = normal areas interspersed between inflamed areas, COBBLESTONE **appearance.**
BARIUM STUDIES	**"STOVEPIPE SIGN"** - loss of haustral markings.	• **"STRING SIGN":** barium flow through narrowed inflamed/scarred area due to transmural strictures.
LABS	• ⊕ **P-ANCA (more common in UC)**	• ⊕ **ASCA (antibodies vs Saccharomyces cerevisiae)**
SURGERY	• May be curative in some	• Noncurative

Corticosteroids:
- Indications: **symptom flare-ups while patients transition to more effective therapies.**
- **Budesonide** adverse effects diarrhea, nausea, arthralgias, headache, URI, sinusitis.
- **Prednisone** adverse effects: Hypertension, fluid retention, weight gain, hypernatremia, elevated blood glucose, osteoporosis, mood disorder, increased risk of infection, narrow angle glaucoma
- Triamcinolone acetonide may be used topically for local symptom relief of aphthous ulcers.

MAINTENANCE THERAPY FOR CD & UC

6-Mercaptopurine (6-MP) & Azathioprine
- Mechanism purine analogues that inhibit the immune response. Azathioprine is converted to 6-MP.
- Indications: May be used adjunctively for their **steroid-sparing effects** (limited use as monotherapy).
- Azathioprine: adverse effects include gastritis, nausea, vomiting, Lymphoma, fever, pancreatitis, leukopenia, anemia, thrombocytopenia. Chronic immunosuppression increases risk for neoplasia.
- 6-Mercaptopurine adverse effects include myelosuppression, hepatic toxicity, immunosuppression, hepatic encephalopathy, pancreatitis, rash, hyperpigmentation, Lymphoma, fever.

Methotrexate
- Mechanism: anti-inflammatory that decreases interleukin (IL) production.
- Indications: used to induce remission & to reduce the use of corticosteroids.
- **Adverse reactions: bone marrow suppression (eg, leukopenia) & hepatic fibrosis** (evaluate with periodic CBCs & LFTs), **pneumonitis & lung fibrosis,** alopecia, photosensitivity, rash, diarrhea, anorexia, nausea, vomiting, stomatitis. Hyperuricemia, GI hemorrhage, renal failure, infections.

Cyclosporine: immunomodulator that reduces interleukin production by T cells & inhibits calcineurin (a chemical messenger that activates macrophages). Used for UC refractory to IV glucocorticoids.
   Adverse effects: Nephrotoxicity, hypertension, liver toxicity.
Tacrolimus: macrolide antibiotic with immunomodulatory properties. Used in refractory disease.

Biologic anti-Tumor necrosis factor (TNF) agents:
Infliximab: CD and UC; **Adalimumab** CD and UC; **Certolizumab** CD; Golimumab (UC)
- Anti-TNFs induce and maintain remission in moderate- to high-risk patients, or in patients with inadequate response to corticosteroids & immunomodulators. Biologics have improved effectiveness & tolerability compared to immunomodulators. Adverse effects: **All monoclonal antibodies increase risk of certain cancers & infections, including reactivation of Tuberculosis.** Lupus-like syndrome.
- Adalimumab adverse effects: injection site reactions, infection, tuberculosis, Lymphoma.
- Certolizumab adverse effects: injection site reactions, URI, headache, hypertension, rash, infections.
- **Infliximab: infusion-related reactions,** delayed reaction (eg, serum sickness, myalgia, arthralgia), increased infections (fungal, bacterial, sepsis, pneumonia, cellulitis, abscess), skin ulceration.

Vedolizumab and Natalizumab are anti-integrin agents that target leukocyte trafficking.
- **Vedolizumab is preferred because of its specificity to leukocyte trafficking in the gut (less systemic effects),** & very effective in achieving clinical response & corticosteroid-free remission.
- Vedolizumab adverse effects include nasopharyngitis, headache, arthralgias, nausea, pyrexia, upper respiratory infection and other infections, hypersensitivity reactions, lupus-like syndrome.
- Natalizumab adverse effects: headache, fatigue, upper or lower respiratory infections, nausea, arthralgia, depression, infusion-related reaction. Progressive multifocal leukoencephalopathy (only be used in patients who are not seropositive for anti–John Cunningham virus antibody).

Biologic Anti-interleukin:
- **Ustekinumab** — Anti-interleukin 12/23p40 antibody therapy is a treatment option for patients with Crohn disease when standard therapies have been ineffective.
- Adverse effects include vomiting, nasopharyngitis, injection site erythema, infections, pruritus.

Janus kinase inhibitor (Tofacitinib): Moderate to severe UC. Adverse effects: increased risk of Herpes zoster, increased lipids, increased risk of thrombosis and pulmonary embolism, Lymphoma.

CROHN DISEASE (CD)

CHARACTERISTICS

- **Transmural inflammation that affects any part of the GI tract** (from the mouth to the anus). Transmural inflammation may lead to **fistulas, bowel strictures, perianal disease, abscesses,** fissures, fibrosis, & bowel obstruction. Cigarette smoking increases the risk of flares of CD.
- **Skip areas of involvement** — segments of normal-appearing bowel interrupted by areas of disease.
- **Terminal ileum most commonly involved segment** — ~80% have small bowel involvement, often distal ileum, with 1/3 of patients having terminal ileum (ileitis) exclusively. **~50% ileocolitis** (ileum & proximal ascending colon), & ~20% limited to the colon. 50% of colitis in CD spares the rectum.

CLINICAL MANIFESTATIONS

- **The cardinal symptoms of Crohn disease (CD) include crampy abdominal pain, chronic but intermittent diarrhea often without gross blood** (with or without gross bleeding), **fatigue, and weight loss** (due to malabsorption and decreased oral intake).
- Malabsorption — Patients with small bowel CD and bile salt malabsorption may present with watery diarrhea and steatorrhea, resulting in protein calorie malnutrition, vitamin deficiency (eg, vitamins B12 and D), metabolic bone disease, and Hypocalcemia. Aphthous ulcers.
- **Ileocolitis: crampy abdominal pain (especially right lower quadrant), diarrhea (not usually grossly bloody and often intermittent), fatigue, weight loss, fever, anorexia.**
- Jejunoileitis: malabsorption, steatorrhea, nutritional deficiencies, & electrolyte disorders.
- Colitis & perianal disease: diarrhea, rectal bleeding, perirectal abscess or ulcer, phlegmon/abscess. Anorectal fistula & fissure formation, perianal skin tags, bowel obstruction.
- **In severe cases, perianal abscess, perianal Crohn disease, and cutaneous fistulas can be seen.**

DIAGNOSIS

- **Small bowel imaging: Enterography MRI with small bowel enterography (MRE) preferred** because it avoids radiation & has comparable diagnostic accuracy compared to CT enterography.
- **Ileocolonoscopy with biopsy**: segmental "skip areas" (normal-appearing mucosa in between inflamed mucosa), **cobblestoning** of the mucosa; aphthoid, linear, or stellate ulcerations; strictures. **Biopsy findings: transmural inflammation,** microscopic skip areas, focal lesions with or without **noncaseating granulomas.** Creeping fat on gross dissection is pathognomonic of CD.
- Labs: ⊕ **anti-Saccharomyces cerevisiae antibodies,** ↑ESR & CRP. Deficiencies in iron, vitamin B12, and vitamin D if severe.
- **Upper GI series: not usually performed unless MR or CT enterography are unavailable.** Findings: **string sign** (barium flowing through narrowed inflamed/scarred areas), fistula.

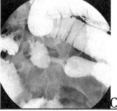
Crohn disease: string sign (narrowing of the lumen).

MANAGEMENT

- **Limited ileocolonic disease: "Step-up" approach: oral Glucocorticoids [Prednisone or Prednisolone preferred for diffuse or left colon disease; Budesonide for ileum &/or proximal colon]** or oral 5-aminosalicylates (eg, Mesalamine) in patients who prefer to avoid Glucocorticoids.
- **Ileal & proximal colon disease: Glucocorticoids** (eg, **enteric coated Budesonide**, Prednisone).
- Severe & refractory: **"Top-down" approach with more potent therapies with immunomodulators (eg, Azathioprine, 6-Mercaptopurine, Methotrexate), and/or biologic therapy (eg, the anti-TNF agents such as Adalimumab, Infliximab)** relatively early in the course of the disease. Indications: **high-risk patients with moderate to severe Crohn disease.**
- Surgical indications: refractory to medical therapy, intestinal obstruction, massive bleeding, symptomatic refractory internal or perianal fistulas, intra-abdominal abscess.

ULCERATIVE COLITIS (UC)

- **Chronic, intermittent inflammation of the colon limited to the mucosal & submucosal layers.**
- **Usually involves the rectum & may extend proximally to the colon in a continuous, circumferential pattern** — 40–50% is limited to the rectum & rectosigmoid area; 30–40% disease extends proximal to the sigmoid (left sided colitis); 20% involves the entire colon (pancolitis).
- **Smokers & persons who have had an appendectomy are less likely to develop Ulcerative colitis.**

CLINICAL MANIFESTATIONS

- **UC typically presents with hematochezia, diarrhea which may be associated with blood &/or mucus (bloody diarrhea main symptom), & abdominal pain.** Bowel movements are frequent & small in volume as a result of rectal inflammation. Triggers include smoking cessation & NSAID use.
- **Crampy abdominal pain especially involving the left lower quadrant.**
- **Urgency, tenesmus,** & constipation periods. <u>Systemic symptoms</u> fever, fatigue, malaise, weight loss.

DIAGNOSIS

- **<u>Flexible sigmoidoscopy</u> key to the diagnosis of UC.** <u>Nonspecific findings</u> — **uniform mucosal erythema, granularity, & ulceration (eg, friable mucosa involving the distal rectum and may extend proximally in a symmetric, continuous, & circumferential pattern). Non-neoplastic pseudopolyps,** erosions, & loss of vascular pattern. Colonoscopy avoided in hospitalized patients with severe colitis because of the potential to precipitate Toxic megacolon or colonic perforation.
- **<u>Endoscopic biopsy histologic findings:</u>** Nonspecific — crypt abscesses & atrophy, inflammation, basal plasmacytosis, and goblet depletion. Infiltrates of the mucosal layer of the colon — eg, lymphocytes, plasma cells, and granulocytes. **Diffuse and contiguous rectal involvement of the mucosa and submucosa only.**
- <u>Double-contrast Barium enema:</u> **<u>Stovepipe or lead pipe sign</u> — cylindrical bowel with loss of Haustral markings.** Narrowing of the luminal caliber & pseudopolyps. **Barium enema should be avoided in patients who are severely ill since it may precipitate Toxic megacolon & ileus.**
- <u>Labs:</u> **positive P-ANCA.** Increased ESR, CRP, leukocytosis; Anemia of chronic disease. **Fetal lactoferrin & calprotectin are sensitive markers of acute inflammation.**

MANAGEMENT

[1] Mild to moderate distal colitis:

- **<u>Topical 5-aminosalicylic acid</u> (ASA) [eg, rectal Mesalamine (Mesalazine) suppository or enema] is the first-line treatment for inducing remission in low-risk patients with mild to moderate ulcerative proctitis or proctosigmoiditis.** Adverse effects of topical 5-ASAs are minimal. May include headache, interstitial nephritis, nausea, and vomiting.
- For patients who tolerate topical Mesalamine but who do not experience sufficient improvement in symptoms after 4-8 weeks of therapy, options include [1] adding a topical glucocorticoid (eg, suppository, enema); [2] adding an oral 5-ASA agent; &/or [3] initiating an oral glucocorticoid (eg, Budesonide multi-matrix or Prednisone).
- **<u>Topical glucocorticoids</u> can be added to topical 5-ASA or in patients who can't tolerate 5-ASA.**

[2] Left-sided or extensive colitis:

- **<u>Combination therapy</u> with oral 5-ASA (eg, standard or high-dose Mesalamine, Sulfasalazine, or Balsalazide) + topical (rectal) ASA (eg, Mesalamine enema) for left-sided or extensive colitis.**
- For patients who do not respond to combination therapy, topical Mesalamine can be replaced with topical glucocorticoid therapy (enema, foam, or suppository daily); oral 5-ASA agents are continued.
- For patients who do not respond to a combination of oral 5-ASA and topical Mesalamine (or topical glucocorticoids), Budesonide MMX can be added to the existing regimen.

[3] Severe:

- For ambulatory patients with moderate to severe UC, initial induction therapy options include — Anti-TNF therapy with or without an immunomodulator (eg, Azathioprine or 6-Mercaptopurine), Anti-integrin therapy (eg, Vedolizumab), or Anti-interleukin 12/23 therapy (eg, Ustekinumab).
- **<u>IV glucocorticoids</u> backbone of therapy for hospitalized, acute severe UC (eg, fulminant colitis).**

CHRONIC MESENTERIC ISCHEMIA (INTESTINAL ANGINA)

- **Reduced blood flow to the small bowel due to atherosclerotic narrowing of at least 2 of 3 major splanchnic vessels** (celiac axis, superior mesenteric artery, &/or inferior mesenteric artery).
- **Episodic intestinal hypoperfusion related to eating** (increased demand during eating + decreased blood supply). **Most patients either have [1] atherosclerotic disease** (eg, history of MI, Peripheral arterial disease) &/or **[2] atherosclerotic risk factors** (eg, DM, Hypertension, smoking).

CLINICAL MANIFESTATIONS
- **Intestinal angina:** chronic dull, crampy abdominal pain worse after meals, lasting 1-3 hours.
- Anorexia **aversion to eating, leading to weight loss** (eating triggers the abdominal pain).
- Abdomen examination: usually normal or mildly tender. **Abdominal bruit in up to 50% of patients.**

DIAGNOSIS
- Clinical diagnosis. **CT angiography** initial imaging study. Conventional angiography (definitive).

MANAGEMENT
- **Asymptomatic:** Modification of risk factors (eg, smoking cessation) & anti-platelet therapy.
- **Symptomatic:** Revascularization (open or endovascular) is the definitive management (eg, angioplasty with stenting or bypass).

ACUTE MESENTERIC ISCHEMIA

Acute occlusion (abrupt reduction) of small intestinal blood flow from either:
- **[1] Acute arterial occlusion: progressive thrombus or embolism from Atrial fibrillation (most common 50%)** or Atherosclerosis (25%). **Superior mesenteric artery occlusion most common.**
- **[2] Nonocclusive mesenteric arterial ischemia (NOMI)**: 25%: Low-flow state, most commonly due to splanchnic hypoperfusion (eg, shock, vasopressor, MI, CHF) or arterial vasospasm (eg, cocaine).
- **[3] Mesenteric venous thrombosis**: obstruction of intestinal venous outflow tract — usually idiopathic (**hypercoagulable states most common**) or secondary to malignancy, prior abdominal surgery, or Inflammation. Main cause in younger patients with no known cardiovascular disease.

CLINICAL MANIFESTATIONS
- **Arterial embolus or thrombus: severe abdominal (periumbilical) pain "out of proportion" to physical findings** — minimal exam findings & no peritoneal signs. Pain is usually poorly localized. 50% with thrombosis have chronic ischemia history (abdominal pain worse with eating, food aversion).
- May develop nausea, vomiting, diarrhea. Venous or NOMI have variable presentations.
- Advanced disease: peritonitis (eg, rigidity, guarding & rebound tenderness), guaiac positive, shock.

DIAGNOSIS
- **CT angiography: often initial test to assess ischemia if stable.** Done <u>without</u> oral contrast.
- **Catheter-based arteriography definitive diagnosis (can be both diagnostic and therapeutic)** allows lesion visualization & facilitates interventions (eg, vasodilators, angioplasty, thrombolytics).
- Labs: **leukocytosis, lactic acidosis,** ↑ hematocrit (hemoconcentration), ↑ amylase & LDH.

MANAGEMENT
Revascularization: The goal of AMI treatment is rapid surgical restoration of intestinal blood flow, with excision of necrotic bowel if necessary. Hemodynamic stabilization & anticoagulation.
- **Embolism: early surgical laparotomy with embolectomy** (or thrombolytics in some).
- **Arterial thrombosis: options include surgical revascularization with aortomesenteric bypass grafting or endovascular balloon dilation angioplasty with stenting.**
- **Venous thrombosis: systemic anticoagulation (mainstay of therapy)** or thrombolytics.
- Perforation or peritoneal signs: **Patients with peritoneal signs or clinical suspicion of perforation or gangrene require emergent surgical exploration (laparotomy),** after hemodynamic stabilization, to immediately restore mesenteric blood flow & surgically resect nonviable bowel.

ISCHEMIC COLITIS

- **Ischemic injury to the colon usually as a consequence of a sudden and transient reduction in blood flow, resulting in a low-flow state** — 75% of all intestinal ischemia, primarily in the elderly.

LOCATION
- <u>Watershed areas</u>: Although it may occur anywhere, **colonic ischemia most commonly affects the "watershed areas" with limited collateral blood supply** (eg, between 2 arteries with decreased collaterals, such as the splenic flexure and the left colon at the rectosigmoid junction).
- Ischemia is usually mucosal & rarely transmural.

ETIOLOGIES
- **[1] Nonocclusive colonic ischemia most common (95% of cases): low-flow states leading to transient colonic hypoperfusion** & systemic hypotension or atherosclerosis of the superior & inferior mesenteric arteries. Prolonged nonocclusive ischemia can lead to transmural necrosis.
- [2] Embolic arterial occlusion — spontaneous emboli from a proximal source to the mesenteric vessels or iatrogenically from aortic instrumentation.
- [3] Thrombotic arterial occlusion Thrombotic secondary to atherosclerotic disease.

RISK FACTORS
- **Elderly (>90% are >60y of age),** dehydration, Diabetes mellitus, cardiovascular disease, aortoiliac surgery or instrumentation, cholesterol emboli, cardiac catheterization, Myocardial infarction, constipation-inducing medications, hypercoagulable states, constipation-inducing medications.

CLINICAL MANIFESTATIONS
- **[1] Mild abdominal pain: rapid onset of mild crampy abdominal pain over the affected bowel (left-sided and left lower quadrant most common) often felt laterally** (rather than periumbilically in Acute mesenteric ischemia), **abdominal tenderness, often followed by**
- **[2] Bloody diarrhea or hematochezia (bright or maroon blood) within 24 hours of the onset of abdominal pain** (due to colonic sloughing from ischemia). Increased urge to defecate.
- May develop bowel gangrene (associated with lactic acidosis & leukocytosis).

DIAGNOSIS
- **CT of the abdomen: is often the first imaging test for acute colonic ischemia**. Findings — **wall edema & "thumbprinting" (segmental bowel wall thickening and edema in a nonsegmental pattern) are nonspecific**; mucosal and submucosal hemorrhage, and pericolic fat stranding, and occasionally bowel wall pneumatosis. <u>Double halo or target sign</u>: two continuous thickened layers — higher-attenuation outer ring (muscularis propria) surrounding a lower-attenuation inner ring (edematous submucosa) also nonspecific.
- **Sigmoidoscopy or Colonoscopy: confirms the diagnosis and should be performed in all patients when colonic ischemia is suspected, if possible** with no signs of peritonitis or bowel perforation. Findings include segmental ischemic changes, in areas of low perfusion (eg, splenic flexure) such as edematous, pale, and friable mucosa; erythema, petechial bleeding, and interspersed pale areas. Bluish hemorrhagic nodules (submucosal bleeding).
- Catheter-based arteriography: rarely needed but may be useful when the diagnosis is unclear.

MANAGEMENT
- **Supportive care: restore perfusion** with maintenance of blood pressure and perfusion until collateral circulation becomes well established, **bowel rest, IV fluids, & observe for signs of perforation is the management for most patients** (most cases are mild and usually spontaneously resolve without specific therapy). May need empiric broad-spectrum antibiotics to cover bowel flora.
- Abdominal surgical exploration: **Surgical exploration if colon infarction & necrosis suspected** (eg, ongoing pain that is persistent or out of proportion to clinical examination, hemodynamic instability, peritoneal signs), evidence of bowel necrosis.

COLORECTAL CANCER (CRC)

- **Histopathologically, >90% of cancers arising in the colon and rectum are adenocarcinomas that arise from an adenomatous polyp.** 70% sporadic; familial clustering (20%), inherited (10%).
- The progression of normal colonic epithelium to a precancerous lesion (eg, adenoma) and eventually an invasive carcinoma requires an accumulation of genetic mutations in a ~10 to 15-year period.

EPIDEMIOLOGY:
- CRC is the 3rd most common non-skin cancer in the US after Lung cancer in both sexes.
- CRC is the 2nd most common cause of cancer deaths (8% of cancer-related deaths in the US). In the US, both the incidence & mortality have been slowly decreasing but rising rates in the <50y population.

RISK FACTORS
- **Major factors: age (risk increases 40-50 years), personal or family history of CRC, hereditary forms of CRC, Inflammatory bowel disease, and a history of abdominal irradiation.**
- **IBD:** The risk begins to rise 8 years after disease onset in patients with Ulcerative colitis & Crohn's.
- **African Americans have the highest CRC rates of all ethnic groups** in the US (occur at younger age and higher mortality). Male gender, polyps, Endocrine (eg, Diabetes mellitus, Insulin resistance).
- Diet & lifestyle: diet (low fiber, high in red or processed meat, animal fat), obesity, smoking, ETOH.
- **Familial adenomatous polyposis:** genetic mutation of the APC gene. Adenomas begin in childhood. Diffuse pancolonic adenomatous polyposis (**up to several thousand polyps**). Almost all will develop Colon cancer by age 45 years. **Prophylactic colectomy is the best method for survival.**
- Gardner's syndrome: Variant of FAP with associated soft tissue tumors — eg, epidermoid cysts, osteomas, lipomas, fibromas, desmoids, thyroid cancer.
- Turcot syndrome: FAP-like syndrome + CNS tumors (eg, medulloblastoma & glial tumors).
- **Lynch syndrome (Hereditary nonpolyposis colorectal cancer):** autosomal dominant. Due to loss-of-function in DNA mismatch repair genes (MLH1, MSH2/6, PMS3). Has 40% risk of Colon cancer (type I especially seen on the right side). Type II has increased risk of extra-colonic cancers: **endometrial** (especially), ovarian, small intestine, brain, & skin. Mean age is in the late 40s but can develop cancer in their 20s.
- **Peutz-Jeghers Syndrome:** autosomal dominant. Associated with **hamartomatous polyps, mucocutaneous hyperpigmentation** (lips, oral mucosa, hands), risk of breast & pancreatic cancer.

PROTECTIVE FACTORS
- Physical activity, regular use of Aspirin, and regular NSAID use are associated with decreased risk.

CLINICAL MANIFESTATIONS
- Usually present in 3 ways: [1] suspicious symptoms and/or signs (80%), [2] asymptomatic individuals found to have CRC by routine screening (11%), & [3] emergency complications of CRC (eg, intestinal obstruction, perforation, or uncommonly, an acute gastrointestinal bleed) 7%.
- **Symptoms from the local tumor — rectal bleeding (eg, hematochezia or melena), change in bowel habits, otherwise unexplained Iron deficiency anemia** (fatigue, weakness), **and/or abdominal pain.** Less common presenting symptoms include large bowel obstruction (eg, abdominal distention, and/or nausea and vomiting) or perforation.
- **Large bowel obstruction:** CRC is the most common cause of large bowel obstruction in adults.
- **Right-sided (proximal): chronic occult bleeding (eg, Iron deficiency anemia, positive Guaiac) and diarrhea is more common with right-sided CRCs.** Cecal and ascending colon tumors have a 4-fold higher mean daily blood loss. **Iron-deficiency anemia is more commonly associated with advanced Colorectal cancer than with early disease.**
- **Left-sided (distal): Bowel obstruction, changes in stool diameter, change in bowel habits, and blood-streaked stools are more common presenting symptoms for left-sided than right-sided CRCs** (because the fecal contents are more solid in the distal colon and lumen caliber is smaller)
- Rectal cancer associated with hematochezia and rectal tenesmus, as well as rectosigmoid cancers.
- May develop *Streptococcus bovis* endocarditis.

DIAGNOSIS
- **Colonoscopy with biopsy: diagnostic test of choice & most accurate test (criterion standard).**
- CT colonography a sensitive, less invasive alternative, but unable to perform biopsy if positive.
- Barium enema: **apple core lesion classic** (filling defect). Lesions seen on barium enema require a follow up colonoscopy or CT colonography.
- Laboratory: **Iron deficiency anemia (CRC is the most common cause of occult GI bleed in adults).**
- Staging: CT of the chest, abdomen, and pelvis with contrast + Carcinoembryonic antigen (CEA)
- **Carcinoembryonic antigen: CEA is the most commonly monitored tumor marker** (not specific). A preoperative CEA >5 ng/mL is a poor prognostic indicator. CEA should normalize after resection.

MANAGEMENT
- **Localized (stages I-III): Surgical resection (eg, right, left, or total colectomy) is the only curative modality for localized Colon cancer**; may be used even in some cases of metastatic disease.
- In stage III, postoperative adjuvant chemotherapy (eg, FOLFOX) increases disease-free survival.
- Stage IV: Palliative systemic chemotherapy an option in non-surgical candidates, unresectable locally advanced disease, or high metastatic burden to improve quality of life & prolong life expectancy.

COLON POLYPS

- A polyp of the colon refers to a protuberance into the lumen above the surrounding colonic mucosa.
- Colon polyps are usually asymptomatic but may ulcerate and bleed, cause tenesmus if in the rectum, and, when very large, produce intestinal obstruction.
- Colonic polyps may be (1) neoplastic (eg, adenomas) or (2) non-neoplastic (eg, inflammatory polyps).

Pseudopolyps/Inflammatory polyps:
- **Non-neoplastic** stromal & epithelial components as well as inflammatory cells.
- Pseudopolyps are a result of the mucosal ulceration and regeneration in response to localized or diffuse inflammation **[Inflammatory bowel disease — Ulcerative colitis or Crohn disease].**
- Management — because they do not undergo neoplastic transformation, inflammatory pseudopolyps do not require excision unless they cause symptoms (eg, bleeding, obstruction).

Hyperplastic polyp:
- **Most common non-neoplastic polyp.** They are a type of serrated polyps (saw tooth pattern).
- Asymptomatic; usually incidental finding at colonoscopy; rarely >5 mm.
- **Low risk of malignant potential.** No treatment required but may be removed if necessary.

Hamartomatous polyps
- Sporadic juvenile polyp: relatively more common during childhood. An isolated (solitary) juvenile polyp is not associated with increased cancer risk.
- Juvenile polyposis syndrome: autosomal dominant condition associated with multiple hamartomatous polyps. Associated with increased risk of colorectal & gastric cancer, so resected.
- Peutz-Jeghers polyps: usually associated with Peutz-Jeghers syndrome (STK11 mutation). Usually benign but may undergo malignant transformation so they are usually resected.

Adenomatous polyps: Most common neoplastic polyp (2/3 of all colonic polyps). Average is 10-20 years before becoming cancerous (especially >1cm). **Adenomas should be resected completely.**
- **Tubular adenomas**: >80% of colonic adenomas (branching adenomatous epithelium). Associated with the least risk of all the 3 types of adenomatous polyps. Overall risk of malignant degeneration correlates with size (<2% if <1.5 cm in diameter; >10% if >2.5 cm in diameter) and is higher in sessile polyps; 65% found in rectosigmoid colon; Endoscopic resection (surgery if polyp large or inaccessible by colonoscopy); follow-up surveillance by colonoscopy every 2–3 years.
- Tubulovillous (mixture) account for 5-15% of colonic adenomas. Intermediate risk.
- **Villous adenoma: Highest risk of becoming cancerous** (up to 30% when >2 cm); more prevalent in left colon; occasionally associated with potassium-rich secretory diarrhea. Generally larger than tubular adenomas at diagnosis; often sessile.

COLON CANCER SCREENING GUIDELINES

	Fecal Occult Blood test	COLONOSCOPY
Average Risk	Annually at 50 years	Colonoscopy every 10 years (or flexible sigmoidoscopy every 5 years) up to 75 years of age.
1st-degree relative ≥60y	Annually at 40 years (or 10 years before the age the relative was diagnosed).	Colonoscopy every 10 years up to 75 years of age.
1st degree relative <60y	Annually at 40 years (or 10 years before the age the relative was diagnosed).	Colonoscopy every 5 years up to 75 years of age.

AVERAGE RISK

- **A colonoscopy has the best sensitivity and specificity for a screening test, with a reduction of cancer mortality as high as 53%.**
- **Colonoscopy:** In May 2021, the U.S. Preventive Services Task Force (USPSTF) issued new recommendations for Colorectal cancer stating that **people at average risk should start screening at age 45 (Grade B),** which will allow health insurance companies to cover the cost of the test at a younger age, **while maintaining its strongest recommendation (Grade A) for initiating at age 50 through age 75 years for average-risk patients as long as their life expectancy is 10 years or greater, with colonoscopy intervals every 10 years for most patients at average risk for CRC** who are willing to undergo this procedure.

OTHER TESTING OPTIONS

- **Fecal immunochemical testing — FIT for occult blood annually on a single sample for patients unable or unwilling to have a colonoscopy as initial screening,** Patients with positive FIT results should undergo prompt colonoscopy.
- **Multitarget stool DNA testing** — MT-sDNA, also known as FIT-DNA and multitarget fecal DNA, combines fecal markers for hemoglobin and DNA mutation and methylation. **It is available as Cologuard in the US.** The test is **performed every 1 to 3 years on one stool collection sample.** MT-sDNA testing has a higher single-application sensitivity and a lower specificity than FIT for CRC and advanced precancerous lesions, but it is more expensive than FIT.
- **Computed tomography colonography** — "virtual colonoscopy" is an option that is performed **every 5 years.** CTC is more sensitive than any test other than colonoscopy to detect adenoma polyps, although data are limited on other outcomes. Patients with abnormal CTC findings (eg, polyps or CRC) should undergo prompt colonoscopy for evaluation.
- **Sigmoidoscopy + FIT (or sensitive gFOBT)** — The combination of sigmoidoscopy with FIT or guaiac-based FOBT (gFOBT) theoretically enhances lesion detection by offering direct visualization up to 60 cm as well as by detecting colon lesions beyond the reach of a sigmoidoscope by testing for occult blood. FIT is preferred over sensitive gFOBT. **USPSTF recommends sigmoidoscopy every 10 years if done with annual FIT.**
- **Sigmoidoscopy alone** — screening with **sigmoidoscopy every 5-10 years may be offered alone.** A sigmoidoscopy can only identify lesions up to the distal 60 cm of the bowel (women and older patients because they have a higher frequency of more proximal lesions).
- **Guaiac-based fecal occult blood test** — **If this method is chosen, the sensitive gFOBT is preferred. gFOBT is done annually on three samples as a take-home test** that the patient mails back, rather than on stool obtained during a digital rectal examination (DRE). Stool obtained by DRE is not sensitive for CRC screening. Stool guaiac tests (gFOBT) have low sensitivity for polyps and relatively low specificity for clinically important disease.
- **Capsule colonoscopy** — Capsule colonoscopy every 5 years is a third-tier option, although it is not among the tests included in several other screening guidelines.

Inflammatory bowel disease:
- The risk of adenocarcinoma of the colon begins to rise 8 years after disease onset in patients with Ulcerative colitis and Crohn colitis. For this reason, **initiation of surveillance with colonoscopy is recommended at 8–10 years after onset of Inflammatory bowel disease symptoms.**

Lynch syndrome (HNPCC):
- Colonoscopy beginning at 20-25 years of age with colonoscopy every 1-2 years; OR 2-5 years prior to the earliest age of CRC diagnosis in the family (whichever comes first).
- For carriers of *MSH6* and *PMS2* mutations, screening can potentially start later (at age 30 to 35 or two to five years prior to the earliest CRC in the family) and conducted evert 1-2 years, unless an early-onset CRC has been diagnosed in a given family.

Familial adenomatous polyposis (FAP):
- In individuals at risk for classic FAP, CRC screening around age 10-12 years with colonoscopy or sigmoidoscopy every 1-2 years. If attenuated FAP, screen every 1-2 years starting at age 18-20y.

RECTAL PROLAPSE (RECTAL PROCIDENTIA)

- Rectal procidentia (Rectal prolapse) & Intussusception (occult Rectal prolapse) are pelvic floor disorders most common in adults >40y (esp. >60y), women, h/o vaginal delivery or pelvic surgery.
- Women with Rectal prolapse have increased incidence of associated pelvic floor disorders, including urinary incontinence, rectocele, cystocele, and enterocele. Cystic fibrosis may be a cause in children.

- <u>Complete rectal procidentia</u> (full-thickness rectal prolapse) is the protrusion of all layers of the rectum through the anus, as evident by concentric (circumferential) rings of rectal mucosa.
- <u>Partial procidentia</u> (rectal mucosal prolapse) involves prolapse of the mucosa only.
- <u>Occult rectal prolapse</u> (rectal intussusception): "telescoping" of the bowel on itself internally, without protruding through the anal verge. Not a true rectal prolapse.

CLINICAL MANIFESTATIONS
- <u>Local symptoms:</u> bleeding per rectum, bowel dysfunction (eg, constipation, fecal incontinence, or seepage), poor perianal hygiene, and mild abdominal discomfort.
- Mucous &/or stool discharge, altered bowel habits, incomplete evacuation, "mass" that prolapses through the anus that may reduce spontaneously after defecation or require manual reduction.

Physical examination:
- **Erythematous mass with concentric rings of the rectal mucosa (stacked coins) protruding through the anus hallmark of Rectal prolapse, especially with Valsalva;** may be intermittent.

DIAGNOSIS
- Rectal prolapse is diagnosed by the presence of rectal protrusion on physical examination or Defecography.
- Because Rectal prolapse is associated with pelvic floor disorders in women (eg, urinary incontinence, rectocele, cystocele, vaginal vault prolapse, and enterocele), diagnostic studies to evaluate for pelvic floor disorders may include Cystoproctography, Colonoscopy as per screening guidelines, Defecography, and Anorectal physiology studies.

MANAGEMENT
- **<u>Surgical repair</u> is the mainstay of therapy for patients with rectal prolapse** via transabdominal or transperineal approaches. Surgical indications include the sensation of a Rectal prolapse and fecal incontinence and/or constipation associated with the prolapse.
- **<u>Supportive management</u>:** For patients with comorbid illness in which surgery is not an option or for patients who refuse surgery, supportive management includes increased fluid, fiber supplementation, stool-bulking agents, & pelvic floor muscle exercises (eg, Kegel) for symptoms.

ANORECTAL ABSCESS

- **Bacterial infection of obstructed anal ducts or anal crypt glands.** May be seen in Crohn disease.
- <u>4 types</u>: perianal (40-50%), ischiorectal (20-25%), intersphincteric (2-5%), & supralevator (2.5%).

EPIDEMIOLOGY
- More common in <u>immunocompromised patients</u> [eg, Diabetes, HIV, chronic corticosteroid use, hematologic disorders]; Crohn disease.

PATHOPHYSIOLOGY
- Anorectal abscesses and Fistulas are believed to be 2 consequential phases of one anorectal infectious condition: Abscess (acute phase); fistula (chronic phase of suppuration and fistulization).
- <u>Complications</u> include the formation of an Anal fistula, systemic infection, & spread to adjacent areas.

MICROBIOLOGY
- **Often polymicrobial:** ***Staphylococcus aureus* most common**, *E. coli, Bacteroides, Streptococcus, Proteus.* **Posterior rectal wall most common site (often located at the anal verge).**
- If left untreated, the abscess can extend into the ischioanal space, intersphincteric space, or cause systemic infection. More common in men.

CLINICAL MANIFESTATIONS
- **Perianal or perirectal pain and fever are hallmark.**
- **Local anorectal swelling, severe anal or rectal pain (often dull or throbbing), that is worse with sitting, coughing, & defecation.**
- **May be associated with fever, chills, malaise, constipation, or diarrhea.** Purulent discharge.

PHYSICAL EXAMINATION
- **<u>Superficial (eg, perianal abscess)</u>: focal edema, induration, fluctuant mass, or a patch of erythematous, indurated skin overlying the perianal skin.** May be associated with Cellulitis.
- <u>Deeper (eg, supralevator) abscess</u> may not have external examination findings, and are diagnosed by a tender, often fluctuant mass felt on digital rectal examination or by performing imaging studies.
- Purulent rectal drainage may be noted if the abscess has begun to drain spontaneously.

DIAGNOSIS
- **A superficial abscess can be diagnosed on physical examination with findings without imaging.**
- Although imaging is generally not required for the diagnosis for most cases, imaging may be required for deeper abscesses. Therefore, **patients with a suspicion of an abscess but no obvious physical exam findings should either be imaged [eg, MRI (preferred) or CT or Endoanal ultrasound] or taken to the operating room for an examination under anesthesia (EUA).**

MANAGEMENT
[1] Surgical drainage:
- **<u>Incision & drainage</u>: mainstay of treatment of abscess, followed by WASH — <u>W</u>arm-water** cleansing, <u>A</u>nalgesics, <u>S</u>itz baths, <u>H</u>igh-fiber diet.
- Superficial abscess may be drained in the office/ED. More extensive, deeper, or complicated abscesses may require the operating room under anesthesia for adequate examination.

[2] Antibiotics:
- **Antibiotics are not usually required in <u>simple cases</u>.** Routine wound culture not usually necessary.
- **The American Society of Colorectal Surgery (ASCRS) guidelines suggest a course of empiric antibiotics after drainage of an anorectal abscess if Cellulitis** (significant surrounding perianal/perineal Cellulitis), **<u>signs of systemic infection</u>** (eg, fever); **immunocompromised** (eg, chemotherapy, **Diabetic patients**), IBD, septic patients; history of valvular heart disease, prosthetic heart valves, or artificial joints.
- **<u>Empiric antibiotics</u>: [1] Amoxicillin-clavulanate or [2] Ciprofloxacin + Metronidazole** (4-5 days).

ANORECTAL FISTULA (FISTULA IN ANO)

- Abnormal open tract between 2 epithelium-lined areas (perianal skin & anorectal canal epithelium).
- **~50% of Anorectal abscesses (especially deeper abscesses) will result in the development of a chronic fistula** that connects the causative anal gland with the skin overlying the drainage site.
- <u>Other etiologies</u>: Crohn disease (due to penetrating inflammation), malignancy, infection.

CLINICAL MANIFESTATIONS
- **[1] Anal or perirectal pain and/or [2] constant purulent drainage (discharge), with a firm mass** (drainage & pain may be augmented with defecation). Poor perianal hygiene, itching.

<u>Physical examination:</u>
- **Perirectal skin lesion: small surface opening, occurring with or without drainage.**
- Inflammatory papule or pustule in the perianal or buttock area may be seen.

DIAGNOSIS
- Simple Fistulas don't require imaging to guide treatment; often visualized or seen with gentle probing.
- When needed, MRI and Endosonography (EUS) are the preferred imaging studies to determine the anatomy of the fistula tract and the extent of anal sphincter involvement. CT-fistulogram.

MANAGEMENT
- **Surgical management mainstay of treatment of Anal fistulas (eg, fistulotomy**; fistulectomy).

ANAL FISSURES

- **Painful linear tear/crack in the lining of the anal canal distal to the dentate line.**

ETIOLOGIES
Primary: usually posterior midline.
- **Anal trauma most common (eg, constipation or diarrhea);** anal intercourse, vaginal delivery.

Secondary: due to underlying medical condition, especially if <u>lateral:</u>
- Crohn disease, granulomatous disease (eg, TB), Malignancy, infection (eg, HIV, Syphilis).

CLINICAL MANIFESTATIONS
- **[1] <u>recurrent anal pain</u>:** — **severe anal/rectal pain & bowel movement provoked by defecation (often lasts hours afterwards), causing patient to refrain from defecating (constipation).**
- **[2] <u>hematochezia</u> bright red blood per rectum**.

PHYSICAL EXAMINATION & DIAGNOSIS
- **Visible longitudinal tear** in the anoderm that usually extends no more proximally than the dentate line. **Anal pain reproduction with gentle digital palpation** of the posterior (or anterior) midline anal verge. **90% located in the posterior midline of the anal canal.** Anterior midline (8-25%).
- **Chronic fissure:** hypertrophied anal papilla at the proximal end of the fissure and a **sentinel pile or skin tag at the distal end.**
- **Lateral fissures are atypical & systemic disorders should be ruled** out if a lateral fissure is noted.

MANAGEMENT
- **Supportive measures first line management: "WASH"** — **W**arm-water cleansing, **A**nalgesics/anesthetics (eg, topical Lidocaine), **S**itz baths, **H**igh-fiber diet. **Increased water, stool softeners if constipated, laxatives, and mineral oil. >80% resolve spontaneously.**

<u>Second-line treatment:</u>
- **Topical vasodilators: (eg, Nifedipine or Nitroglycerin ointment)** promote healing by increasing local blood flow & reducing pressure in the internal anal sphincter. **Nifedipine ointment** has fewer adverse effects; <u>Adverse effects of Nitroglycerin ointment</u>: headache & dizziness due to hypotension.
- <u>Botulinum toxin type A injection</u> for typical anal fissure patients who fail 8 weeks of initial medical treatment. Reduces spasm of the internal sphincter (more effective than topical dilators).
- <u>Surgery (eg, Lateral internal sphincterotomy)</u>: reserved for refractory/chronic cases.

HEMORRHOIDS

* Engorgement of venous plexuses.

Internal hemorrhoids
* Originate from superior hemorrhoid vein cushion & are proximal to (above) the dentate line.
* **Internal hemorrhoids tend to bleed & are usually painless.**
    Based on the degree (grade) of prolapse from the anal canal:

I	does not prolapse (confined to anal canal on anoscopy). May bleed with defecation.
II	prolapses with defecation or straining but reduces spontaneously.
III	prolapses with defecation or straining, and requires manual reduction.
IV	Irreducible & may strangulate.

External hemorrhoids
* Originate from the inferior hemorrhoid vein plexus & are distal to (below) the dentate line.
* **External hemorrhoids tend to be painful when thrombosed and don't usually bleed.**

RISK FACTORS
* Increased venous pressure: straining during defecation (eg, constipation), pregnancy, obesity, prolonged sitting, Cirrhosis with portal hypertension. Western diet (low-fiber, high-fat).

CLINICAL MANIFESTATIONS
Internal hemorrhoids:
* **Intermittent rectal bleeding most common — painless bright red blood per rectum (hematochezia)** seen on toilet paper, upon wiping, coating the stool, or dispersed in toilet water.
* May have rectal or perianal pruritus (itching) & fullness, mucus discharge, or fecal soilage.
* Uncomplicated Internal hemorrhoids are usually not tender and not palpable (unless they are thrombosed). Rectal pain with Internal hemorrhoids suggests a complication.

External hemorrhoids:
* **Perianal pain aggravated with defecation is associated with a thrombosed hemorrhoid.** It is often a mild dull ache.
* May have tender palpable dusky/purple mass if thrombosed. May have skin tags.

DIAGNOSIS
* Visual inspection, digital rectal examination, fecal occult blood testing.
* Anoscopy for internal hemorrhoids allows for direct visualization and diagnosis.
* Proctosigmoidoscopy or Colonoscopy may be indicated in patients with hematochezia to rule out proximal sigmoid disease.

MANAGEMENT
Conservative:
* **High-fiber diet, increased fluid intake, warm Sitz baths, topical rectal corticosteroids,** analgesics (eg, lidocaine) for pruritus & discomfort. Reduce fat intake.
Procedures:
Internal hemorrhoids:
* Options after conservative management include **[1] rubber band ligation (most commonly used treatment of bleeding internal hemorrhoids),** [2] sclerotherapy, or [3] infrared coagulation.
External hemorrhoids:
* **Within the first 72 hours of symptoms: office-based excision may be used for acute Thrombosed external hemorrhoids.**
* **>2-3 days of symptoms (thrombosed): expectant management** (usually lasts 7-10 days).
* Hemorrhoidectomy: stage IV or if not responsive to above therapies.

LOWER GASTROINTESTINAL BLEEDING (LGIB)

- Lower gastrointestinal bleeding (LGIB) refers to blood loss of recent onset originating from a site distal to the ligament of Treitz. UGIB is most common source of blood detected in the lower GI tract.

ETIOLOGIES OF ESTABLISHED LOWER GI SOURCES
- **Diverticulosis is the most common cause of <u>acute</u> LGIB** (60%). Although left-sided diverticula are more common, right-sided diverticular are more prone to cause bleeding.
- **Inflammatory (colitis): second most common cause** — Inflammatory bowel disease (Crohn, Ulcerative colitis, Ischemic colitis, infectious); Meckel diverticulum.
- **Benign anorectal disease: Hemorrhoids,** Anal fissure, Fistula-in-ano.
- Neoplastic polyps or neoplasms of the small intestine, colon, rectum, and anus.
- Vascular: angiodysplasia, ischemic, radiation-induced, AV malformations, coagulopathies.

CLINICAL MANIFESTATIONS
- **Hematochezia (passage of maroon or bright red blood or blood clots per rectum).** Blood originating from the left colon tends to be bright red in color, whereas bleeding from the right colon usually appears dark or maroon colored & may be mixed with stool. Fever may be seen in infection.
- **Melena** usually indicates an upper GI source but may represent slow bleeding from the right side of the colon (eg, Colorectal cancer). **Colorectal cancer is the most common cause of chronic occult GI bleeding in older adults.**
- Significant bleeding may be associated with orthostatic hypotension (which suggests a ≥15% loss of blood volume), tachycardia, tachypnea, or altered mental status.

EVALUATION
- Laboratory evaluation: CBC, serum electrolytes, coagulation panel, type and cross matching.
Imaging:
- If an upper GI source is suspected, Upper endoscopy should be performed first; Upper endoscopy may also be performed if Colonoscopy fails to determine the source of bleeding.
- Colonoscopy first-line for patients who are hemodynamically stable. **Colonoscopy can be both diagnostic of the source and therapeutic** [may permit hemostasis, such as ablation of bleeding sites with various endoscopic hemostasis methods (injection sclerotherapy, electrocoagulation, heater probe therapy, banding, and clipping)]. May be performed within the first 24 hours.
- Radionuclide scan: Technetium-labeled red cell scans can also localize the site of bleeding in obscure hemorrhage.
- Mesenteric angiography with or without preceding CT angiography may be necessary for massive bleeding in hemodynamically unstable patients who cannot be stabilized for colonoscopy or when colonoscopy is unrevealing.

MANAGEMENT
- **General supportive measures** (eg, oxygen, establishment of adequate intravenous access with 2 large-bore IVs lines), appropriate volume replacement (crystalloid fluids), and correction of coagulopathies or anticoagulants. ~80% of episodes of LGIB resolve spontaneously.
- Blood product resuscitation (eg, transfusion) if continued active bleeding not responsive to crystalloid resuscitation, if hemoglobin <7 g/dL, or any other indication (lower threshold in older patients).
Treatment of the bleeding source:
- The treatment of lower GI bleeding depends on the source of the bleeding. In many cases, the bleeding can be controlled with therapies employed at the time of Colonoscopy or Angiography.
- Surgical intervention may rarely be indicated in cases of LGIB that persist despite attempts to stop the bleeding with endoscopic or interventional radiology intervention, in hemodynamically unstable patients that are refractory to resuscitation, or if there is persistent or recurrent bleeding.

FECAL INCONTINENCE

- <u>Fecal incontinence</u>: involuntary passage of fecal material (solid or liquid feces) for at least 1 month.
- <u>Anal incontinence</u>: involuntary passage of fecal material (solid or liquid feces) or flatus.
- <u>Fecal urge incontinence</u> desire to defecate, but incontinence occurs despite efforts to retain stool.
- <u>Passive fecal incontinence</u> lack of awareness of the need to defecate prior to the incontinent episode.

PATHOPHYSIOLOGY
- The majority of patients are women and >65 years of age.
- Loss of continence is often multifactorial, resulting from a combination of dysfunction of the anal sphincters, decreased rectal sensation, &/or abnormal rectal compliance.

CLINICAL MANIFESTATIONS
- <u>Minor incontinence</u> includes incontinence to flatus and occasional seepage of liquid stool.
- <u>Major incontinence</u> frequent inability to control solid waste. Poor perianal hygiene.

EVALUATION
- Evaluation should include a thorough history and physical examination including digital rectal examination (DRE). Weak sphincter tone on DRE may indicate neurogenic dysfunction.
- Endoscopic evaluation may be needed to rule out colonic inflammation or malignancy.
- In patients with diarrhea, laboratory studies to determine the underlying etiology may be performed.
- Anorectal manometry, Endorectal ultrasound, or MRI may be indicated in patients who do not respond to conservative measures. Defecography is reserved for refractory symptoms.

MANAGEMENT
- **Supportive management:** including avoiding foods or activities known to worsen symptoms [eg, avoidance of incompletely digested sugars (eg, fructose, lactose) and caffeine].
- <u>Improving perianal skin hygiene</u>: Perianal skin should be kept clean and dry; a premoistened pad or tissue can be used for wiping. Application of a barrier cream (eg, Zinc oxide) to the perianal skin if needed. Incontinence pads may shield both the skin and clothing from fecal soiling.

Medical therapy:
- No specific medication has been proven to be beneficial for Fecal incontinence, except for antidiarrheal drugs in patients with liquid stools. Treat the underlying cause.
- **Strategies to bulk up the stool to increasing fecal sensation — fiber supplementation with a bulking agent (eg, Psyllium or Methylcellulose 1 to 2 tablespoons per day) to improve stool consistency. Antidiarrheals (eg, Loperamide, Diphenoxylate) and Bile acid binders (eg, Cholestyramine) reduce Fecal incontinence and minimize fecal urgency.** These agents harden the stool and delay frequency of bowel movements. In patients with Fecal incontinence due to diarrhea, Bismuth subsalicylate may be used if no response to Loperamide or Bile acid sequestrants.
- <u>Fecal impaction</u>: disimpaction. Constipation should be treated to prevent recurrent episodes.
- <u>Overflow incontinence</u>: Evacuation of the rectum by using suppositories or enemas in patients with neurogenic bowel dysfunction due to spinal cord injury.

Refractory:
- Referral to a gastroenterologist or colorectal surgeon should be considered in patients unresponsive to initial management for additional evaluation (eg, Anorectal manometry, Endorectal ultrasound, or Magnetic resonance imaging) to detect functional and structural abnormalities.
- For patients who fail to respond to initial management, options include biofeedback, surgery (including anal overlapping sphincteroplasty), Sacral nerve stimulation if there is an intact but weak anal sphincters, & Collagen-enhancing injectable anal bulking agent (eg, stabilized hyaluronic acid),
- Fecal diversion with a colostomy or ileostomy should be reserved for patients with intractable symptoms who have failed nonsurgical management and who are not candidates for minimally invasive surgical interventions.

IRRITABLE BOWEL SYNDROME (IBS)

- Chronic (>3 months) functional disorder characterized by abdominal pain with alterations in bowel habits with <u>NO</u> organic cause (idiopathic). Symptoms begin in late teens to early 20s. MC in women.

PATHOPHYSIOLOGY OF IBS

- **Abnormal motility:** chemical imbalance in the intestine (including serotonin & acetylcholine) causing abnormal motility & spasm ⇨ abdominal pain. Altered gut microbiota.
- **Visceral hypersensitivity** patients have lowered visceral pain thresholds to intestinal distention associated with abdominal pain at lower volumes of colonic gas insufflation, increased visceral sensitivity, increased gas production, impaired intestinal gas transit, or impaired rectal expulsion.
- **Psychosocial interactions**: (1) >50% of patients with irritable bowel who seek medical attention have underlying depression, anxiety, or somatization, which may influence how the patient perceives or reacts to minor visceral sensation & (2) altered CNS pain processing.

CLINICAL MANIFESTATIONS

- <u>Hallmark:</u> **abdominal pain associated with altered defecation/bowel habits** (diarrhea, constipation, or alternation between the two). **Pain often relieved with defecation.**
- Abnormal stool frequency; abnormal stool form (lumpy or hard; loose or watery); abnormal stool passage (straining, urgency, or feeling of incomplete evacuation); abdominal bloating or distention.

Alarm symptoms in IBS:
- <u>Evidence of GI bleeding</u>: occult blood in stool, more than minimal rectal bleeding, anemia.
- Anorexia or weight loss, fever, nocturnal symptoms, family history of GI cancer, IBD or Celiac disease.
- Persistent diarrhea causing dehydration; severe constipation or fecal impaction; Onset >45y.

DIAGNOSIS

- Diagnosis of exclusion after workup (eg, colonoscopy & abdominal CT rule out other etiologies).
- A CBC (for Iron deficiency anemia), CRP, Fecal calprotectin level (screen for IBD); serum TG IgA for Celiac disease (TG IgA), & stool specimen.
- **Rome IV Criteria**: **recurrent abdominal pain** on average at least 1 day/week in the last 3 months associated with at least 2 of the following 3:
    - ❶ **related to defecation** (relief or worsening)
    - ❷ onset associated with **change in stool frequency**
    - ❸ onset associated with **change in form (appearance) of stool.**

MANAGEMENT

- **Lifestyle & dietary changes** **first-line management - low fat, high fiber, & unprocessed food diet,** increased sleep, smoking cessation, exercise, peppermint oil. Avoid beverages containing sorbitol or fructose (eg, apples, raisins), avoid gas-producing food (eg, beans, some cruciferous vegetables).

CONSTIPATION SYMPTOMS (IBC-C):
- <u>Prokinetics</u>: **fiber, Psyllium trial. Polyethylene glycol, an osmotic laxative, may be added after Psyllium trial if no relief.** Bulk-forming or saline laxatives.
- **Lubiprostone (chloride channel activator) or Linaclotide (guanylate cyclase agonist) are usually reserved for people with no response to osmotic laxatives.** Through different mechanisms, they stimulate increased intestinal chloride and fluid secretion, resulting in accelerated colonic transit. Tenapanor is a secretagogue.

DIARRHEA SYMPTOMS (IBS-D):
- **Loperamide first line for diarrhea-dominant IBS-D.** Loperamide is an opioid receptor agonist.
- **Bile acid sequestrants second line for IBS-D** (eg, Cholestyramine, Colesevelam, Colestipol).
- **Alosetron (selective 5-HT3 agonist)** if no response to above regimens. Rifaximin; TCAs
- Eluxadoline (opioid antagonist) not as effective (reserved for selective few; may cause Pancreatitis).
- **Abdominal pain: Anticholinergics/antispasmodics** eg, **Dicyclomine, Hyoscyamine, Methscopolamine as needed.** Anticholinergic effects common (constipation, dry mouth). Low-dose TCAs (eg, Amitriptyline); Rifaximin.

CONSTIPATION

INITIAL MANAGEMENT

- **Dietary and lifestyle changes:** **first-line management of constipation in most** — high-fiber diet (20-35g daily), adequate fluid intake, regular exercise, appropriate bowel habits and training.

DRUG/INTERVENTION	COMMENTS
FIBER	Mechanism of action: **retains water in the stool & improves GI transit. Daily fiber intake of 20-35 g/day is generally recommended, along with increased fluid intake as first line management.**
BULK FORMING LAXATIVES **Psyllium** **Methylcellulose** **Polycarbophil** **Wheat Dextran**	• Mechanism: **absorb water & increase fecal mass.** Increase stool frequency & soften the consistency of stool with minimal side effects. • **Indications: Dietary fiber & bulk forming laxatives are the most physiologic & effective approach to constipation, often used if no response to dietary and lifestyle modification.** Onset 12-72 hours. • Adverse effects: bloating (most common), flatulence.
OSMOTIC LAXATIVES **Polyethylene Glycol (PEG)**	• MOA: causes H_2O retention in stool (osmotic effect pulls H_2O into gut). • **Osmotic laxatives used if no response to bulk-forming laxatives.** • Adverse effects: flatulence, bloating, nausea, cramping.
Lactulose	Synthetic disaccharide (sugar) not absorbed (pulls water into the gut). Also used in Hepatic encephalopathy. Adverse effects: bloating, flatulence.
Sorbitol	Synthetic sugar (cheap). Adverse effects: bloating, flatulence.
Saline Laxatives - **Milk of Magnesia** - **Magnesium Citrate**	Adverse effects of Saline laxatives: • **Diarrhea** most common • Hypermagnesemia (especially with chronic renal disease).
STIMULANT LAXATIVES **Bisacodyl** **Senna**	• Mechanism: **increases acetylcholine-regulated GI motility (peristalsis)** & alters electrolyte transport in the mucosa. • **Stimulant laxatives are frequently recommended in patients who do not respond to Osmotic laxatives.** • Adverse effects: nausea, vomiting, abdominal cramp, diarrhea. Bisacodyl not used for >10 days (can cause atonic colon).

FECAL IMPACTION

- Copious amount of an immovable solid bulk of stool in the rectum.
- Due to decreased mobility & inability to sense and respond to the presence of stool in the rectum.
- **May cause chronic constipation, abdominal pain & distention, or overflow fecal incontinence.**

DIAGNOSIS

- **Digital rectal examination — copious amounts of stool.**
- Abdominal radiographs if digital rectal examination is nondiagnostic.

MANAGEMENT

Disimpaction and colon evacuation, followed by a routine bowel regimen to reduce recurrence:

- **Digital (manual) disimpaction followed by warm-water enema washout with mineral oil** — disimpaction allows for manual fragmentation of the fecal bolus to ease passage through the anal canal. Warm-water enema with mineral oil is used to soften the impaction and facilitate passage.
- **Polyethylene glycol (PEG) can be employed after disimpaction of the distal colon and warm water enema.** PEG can be given either orally or via nasogastric tube.
- If disimpaction is unsuccessful, options include water-soluble contrast enema (under fluoroscopy), Local anesthesia to relax the anal canal & pelvic floor muscles + abdominal massage or Colonoscopy with a snare to fragment the fecal bolus (after preparation with mineral oil enemas).
- Identify and reduce or eliminate causes of constipation.

MANAGEMENT OF DIARRHEA

❶ FLUID REPLETION

> <u>**Mainstay of management of gastroenteritis.**</u> **Oral hydration preferred** — sports drinks, broths, Pedialyte, Ceralyte. IV saline may be used if severe of if patient cannot tolerate oral fluids.

❷ DIET

- **Bland low-residue diet** usually best tolerated (eg, crackers, boiled vegetables, yogurts, soup). "BRAT" diet <u>B</u>ananas, <u>A</u>pplesauce, <u>R</u>ice, <u>T</u>oast.

❸ ANTI-MOTILITY AGENTS

- <u>Indications:</u> Patients <65 years of age with moderate to severe signs of volume depletion.
- <u>CI:</u> **DO NOT give anti-motility drugs to patients with invasive diarrhea (may cause toxicity).**

ANTI-DIARRHEALS	COMMENTS
BISMUTH SUBSALICYLATE Pepto-Bismol Kaopectate	<u>MOA:</u> **antimicrobial properties** against bacterial & viral pathogens, **Salicylate: anti-secretory & anti-inflammatory properties.** Bismuth also relieves cramps and nausea. <u>Ind:</u> safe in patients with dysentery (eg, significant fever, bloody diarrhea). <u>Adverse effects:</u> **dark colored stools, darkening of tongue.** CNS side effects, hearing loss, and tinnitus. <u>CI:</u> children with viral illness (salicylate associated with ↑risk of Reye syndrome).
OPIOID AGONISTS **Diphenoxylate/Atropine**	<u>MOA:</u> binds to gut wall opioid receptors, inhibiting peristalsis (subtherapeutic Atropine added to discourage opioid overdose or misuse). <u>Adverse effects:</u> **CNS (central opiate effects), constipation,** anticholinergic side effects (eg, nausea, dry mouth, blurred vision).
Loperamide	<u>Ind:</u> **noninvasive diarrhea** [no fever (or low grade) & non bloody]. <u>MOA:</u> **binds gut wall mu opioid receptors, inhibiting peristalsis.** ↑'es anal sphincter tone. <u>S/E:</u> **avoid in patients with acute dysentery** or colitis. <u>Adverse effects:</u> constipation, paralytic ileus.
ANTICHOLINERGICS **Phenobarbital/Hyoscyamine/** **Atropine/ Scopolamine**	<u>MOA:</u> **anticholinergics** (Hyoscyamine, Atropine, Scopolamine) inhibit acetylcholine-related GI motility, relax GI muscles (**antispasmodic**), decrease gastric secretions; Phenobarbital slows down GI motility.

❹ ANTIEMETICS vomiting usually due to imbalance of serotonin, acetylcholine, dopamine, or histamine

Ondansetron **Granisetron** **Dolasetron**	<u>MOA:</u> **blocks serotonin receptors** (5-HT3) both peripherally & centrally in the chemoreceptor trigger zone. <u>Adverse effects:</u> <u>neurologic:</u> headache, fatigue, sedation, lightheadedness. <u>GI</u> bloating, diarrhea, constipation. <u>Cardiac:</u> prolonged QT interval, cardiac arrhythmias.
DOPAMINE ANTAGONISTS **Prochlorperazine** **Promethazine** **Metoclopramide**	<u>MOA:</u> **blocks CNS <u>dopamine receptors</u> ($D_1 D_2$).** Mild antihistaminic & antimuscarinic effects. Metoclopramide is also a prokinetic agent (increases GI motility). <u>Adverse effects:</u> **QT prolongation, anticholinergic & antihistaminic adverse effects (eg, drowsiness),** hypotension, hyperprolactinemia. **Extrapyramidal symptoms (EPS):** **rigidity, bradykinesia, tremor, akathisia** (restlessness) include: 1. **Dystonic Reactions (Dyskinesia):** reversible EPS hours-days after initiation → intermittent, spasmodic, sustained involuntary contractions (trismus, protrusions of tongue, forced jaw opening, facial grimacing, difficulty speaking, torticollis). **Mgmt:** Diphenhydramine IV or add anticholinergic agent (eg, Benztropine). 2. Parkinsonism: (due to ↓dopamine in nigrostriatal pathways) – rigidity, tremor

	NON-INVASIVE DIARRHEAS	INVASIVE DIARRHEAS
Pathophysiology:	**Enterotoxins** increase GI secretion of electrolytes ⇨ **secretory diarrhea** **No cell destruction/mucosal invasion.**	**Cytotoxins** cause mucosal invasion & cell damage.
Affected area:	**Small bowel** ⇨ **large voluminous** stool	**Large bowel** ⇨ many small-volume stools, high fever.
Vomiting	**Vomiting predominant symptom.**	Vomiting not as common.
Fecal Blood/WBC/mucus:	Absent	⊕ **Fecal blood/WBCs & mucus.**
Examples	Viral, S. Aureus, B. cereus, V. cholera, Enterotoxigenic E coli	Enterohemorrhagic E coli, Shigella, Salmonella, Campylobacter Yersinia.

NONINVASIVE (ENTEROTOXIN) INFECTIOUS DIARRHEA

- NONINVASIVE: vomiting, watery, voluminous (involves small intestine), no fecal WBCs or blood.

NOROVIRUS GASTROENTERITIS
- **Most common overall cause of gastroenteritis & foodborne disease in adults in the US and most common cause of viral gastroenteritis worldwide** and in children vaccinated for Rotavirus.
- Peak incidence in the winter but can occur at any time of the year.

TRANSMISSION
- Fecal-oral route, contaminated food & water, fomite contamination, and direct person-person contact.
- **Outbreaks: Norovirus is often associated with outbreaks — eg, cruise ships, healthcare settings, restaurants, military barracks, resorts, schools, catered food, etc.**

CLINICAL MANIFESTATIONS
- 24-48-hour incubation period. Symptoms usually last 2-3 days. Generalized symptoms.
- Characterized by one or more of the following symptoms: **nausea and vomiting (nonbloody, nonbilious, and may be the predominant symptom, especially in children), watery diarrhea (nonbloody), and abdominal pain.** Headache, myalgias, chills.
- Diagnosis: Stool testing not needed; reverse transcription PCR assay and diagnostic immunoassays.

MANAGEMENT
- **Oral rehydration therapy mainstay** — oral rehydration solutions with electrolytes and glucose. If severe dehydration develops, IV fluid therapy is indicated. The disease is self-limited.
- Adjunctive: anti-motility agents and antiemetics may provide symptomatic relief.

Prevention:
- **Hand hygiene — soap and water rather than alcohol-based hand rubs** (Norovirus is not killed by alcohol), surface cleaning, & prevention of body fluid exposure are mainstays of infection control.
- Norovirus is not eliminated by disinfection with standard cleaning products. Contaminated surfaces should be disinfected with bleach (5-25 tablespoons per gallon of water) or other disinfectant.

ROTAVIRUS
- **Most commonly seen in young unimmunized children** between 6 months–2 years of age.
- Transmission: fecal-oral route. IP <48 hours. In the US, vaccination has reduced the incidence.

CLINICAL MANIFESTATIONS
- Children: vomiting & watery (nonbloody) diarrhea, accompanied by fever in at least 50% of cases.
- Adults: symptoms are usually less severe.

DIAGNOSIS: Rotavirus antigen in the stool by specific ELISA, latex agglutination, or PCR assays.

MANAGEMENT: **Oral hydration mainstay of management.** Illness usually lasts from 4-7 days.

STAPHYLOCOCCUS AUREUS GASTROENTERITIS
- **Infection due to preformed heat-stable enterotoxin B.** Common cause of food poisoning.

SOURCES
- **Food contamination** most common source — eg, **dairy products, eggs, mayonnaise, cream, salty processed meats, egg salad, especially at room temperature.** No person-to-person spread.

CLINICAL MANIFESTATIONS
- **Short incubation period within 6 hours of ingested foodstuffs containing sufficient toxin.**
- **Prominent nausea, vomiting,** & abdominal cramps are the usual symptoms.
- Fever, headache, & diarrhea are seen in a small number of cases.

DIAGNOSIS
- The diagnosis is best established by isolating *Staphylococcus aureus* or enterotoxin

MANAGEMENT
- **Fluid replacement (oral preferred).** IV if unable to tolerate oral.
- **Duration of symptoms rarely exceeds 24 hours, and quick recovery is standard.**
- Prevention: washing hands thoroughly prior to food preparation; ensuring proper refrigeration for storage (prevents proliferation and enterotoxin production).

BACILLUS CEREUS GASTROENTERITIS
Bacillus cereus, a gram-positive, spore-forming bacillus, can produce 2 distinct types of food poisoning:
- (1) some strains produce a performed heat-stable enterotoxin in vitro that induces vomiting;
- (2) other strains produce a preformed heat-labile enterotoxin that causes diarrhea.
- Sources: contaminated starchy food, **especially fried rice (toxins can survive brief reheating** or if left at room temperature); previously cooked meats, vegetables, dried fruits, fish, and milk.

CLINICAL MANIFESTATIONS
- **Short incubation period within 6 hours (similar to *S. aureus*).** Meats, sauces, and dairy product associated with a longer incubation following ingestion of contaminated food (6–18 hours).
- **Prominent nausea and vomiting associated with abdominal cramping,** which may be associated with mild watery nonbloody diarrhea. Fever headache.

MANAGEMENT
- **Fluid replacement (oral preferred).** IV fluids if unable to tolerate oral. Antiemetics if needed.
- The illness is self-limited, averaging about 8 hours, often resolving within 24 hours of symptom onset.

ENTEROTOXIGENIC E. COLI (ETEC)
- **Most common cause of Traveler's diarrhea at any age.**

RISK FACTORS
- **Contaminated food and water.** Contaminated water includes unpeeled fruits washed in the water and untreated drinking water/ice (large inoculum is required).
- Produces heat-stable toxins & heat-labile toxins. Incubation period 24-72 hours.

CLINICAL MANIFESTATIONS
- **Abrupt onset of watery non-bloody diarrhea**, nausea, abdominal cramping. Vomiting & fever.

DIAGNOSIS: Gram stain & cultures. DNA probes to assess for toxin genes.

MANAGEMENT
- **Oral rehydration is the cornerstone of therapy.** Usually a self-limited illness.
- **Antidiarrheals**: eg, Loperamide, Bismuth subsalicylate for mild disease.
- Severe diarrhea: Short courses of antibiotics (eg, Fluoroquinolones, Azithromycin, Rifaximin) shorten the duration about a day or so, are not usually used, & usually reserved for severe diarrhea.

CLOSTRIDIOIDES DIFFICILE INFECTION (CDI)

- *Clostridioides difficile* (formerly Clostridium): Gram ⊕ spore-forming, toxin-producing, anaerobe.
- Transmission of *C. difficile* and colonization of the intestinal tract due person-to-person contact via the fecal-oral route or by direct exposure to a contaminated environment; precipitated by disruption of normal intestinal flora (often due to antimicrobial therapy).

Risk factors:
- **Recent antibiotic use: Although any antimicrobial agent may cause *C. difficile* infection, the antibiotics most frequently associated with CDI include Clindamycin (most common),** Beta-lactams (eg, Cephalosporins, Penicillins; Amoxicillin in children), and Fluoroquinolones.
- **Advanced age (>65 years), gastric acid suppression therapy (PPIs, H$_2$ blockers).**
- ***C. difficile* is the major cause of hospital-acquired & healthcare associated infectious diarrhea.**

PREVENTION & CONTROL
- Infection control includes the use of contact precautions, good hand hygiene, environmental cleaning & disinfection, & patient showering. Contact precautions. Antibiotic stewardship. Sporicidal agents.
- **Hand hygiene: hands should be cleaned with soap and water, which is preferred over alcohol-based products** (more effective at reducing *C. difficile* colony-forming unit).

PATHOPHYSIOLOGY
- Organism overgrowth secondary to alteration of the normal GI flora, most commonly seen after a course of antibiotics or chemotherapy. Community or healthcare associated infection.
- Toxin-mediated colonic damage: *C. difficile* colonizes the large intestine and releases two potent exotoxins that lead to inflammation and diarrhea. Toxins A (enterotoxin) and B (cytotoxin) may result in inflammation, leading to mucosal injury, intestinal fluid secretion, diarrhea, & superficial ulcerations on the intestinal mucosa. Toxigenic *C. difficile* produces either both or only toxin B.

CLINICAL MANIFESTATIONS
- *C. difficile* infection (CDI) can be asymptomatic (carrier) or associated with a variety of symptoms, from mild or moderate diarrhea to severe complications.
- **Nonsevere disease: Watery diarrhea (≥3 loose stools in 24 hours) is the hallmark symptom of CDI.** Diarrhea may be associated with mucus or occult blood (minimal). Melena or hematochezia are rare. **Low-grade fever, lower abdominal pain or cramping decreased appetite (anorexia), nausea, and malaise may be present.** Lower abdominal tenderness. WBC ≤15,000 cells/microL.
- Severe: Diarrhea, lower quadrant or diffuse abdominal pain, abdominal distention, fever, hypovolemia, or labs consistent with marked leukocytosis, lactic acidosis, and elevated creatinine.
- **Fulminant colitis:** hypotension or shock, ileus (little or no diarrhea), megacolon, bowel perforation.
- Recurrent disease: resolution of CDI symptoms while on appropriate therapy, followed by symptom resurgence within 2-8 weeks after discontinuation of treatment.

DIAGNOSIS
Indications for testing:
- The Infectious Diseases Society of America (IDSA) and the Society for Healthcare Epidemiology of America recommend **limiting testing for *C. difficile* infection to patients with unexplained onset of ≥3 unformed stools in 24 hours while not taking laxatives,** since testing cannot distinguish between CDI and asymptomatic carriage which does not warrant treatment.
- The 2017 IDSA guidelines recommend testing in patients older than two years after antibiotic use, and in those with health care–associated diarrhea or persistent diarrhea in the absence of risk
- In children >12 months, testing is recommended only for those with prolonged diarrhea & risk factors.
- Laboratory testing warranted only in patients older than 2 years of age with clinically significant diarrhea with risk factors (eg, antibiotic use), since testing cannot distinguish between CDI and asymptomatic carriage (which does not warrant treatment).
- **Screening for *C. difficile* carriage not needed in asymptomatic individuals and asymptomatic carriage of *C. difficile* does not warrant treatment or contact precautions.**

Testing can be initiated with either:
- **Two-step algorithm:** [1] <u>Enzyme immunoassays (EIA)</u> for glutamate dehydrogenase (GDH) and stool toxins A and B, followed by [2] <u>Nucleic acid amplification testing (NAAT)</u> amplification of the tcdB gene if initial results are indeterminant OR
- <u>One step algorithm:</u> **NAAT may be done in patients with a high probability of CDI.** NAAT alone should not be performed in patients with a lower probability of *C. difficile* infection because a positive test may signify asymptomatic colonization (can't distinguish colonization vs. infection).
- **The EIA for GDH has high sensitivity, which makes it a useful screening test** because a negative result essentially rules out infection. GDH antigen is an essential enzyme produced by all *C. difficile* strains (however, its presence cannot distinguish between toxigenic and nontoxigenic strains). GDH antigen positive results followed by more specific tests (eg, toxin A & B EIA or NAAT).
- Enzyme immunoassays (EIA) can detect exotoxin B. The EIA for toxins A and B has the highest specificity, whereas NAAT is both sensitive and specific.

<u>Adjuvant laboratory testing:</u>
- **Leukocytosis:** CDI is commonly associated with average white blood cell count of 15,000 cells/mL
- **Peripheral leukocytosis, lactic acidosis, or hypoalbuminemia indicates more severe *C. difficile*.**

<u>Adjuvant imaging (not needed in most cases of CDI):</u>
- <u>CT abdomen & pelvis:</u> with oral and intravenous contrast is the preferred imaging modality; Plain abdominal radiographs may be useful if CT is not readily available.
- <u>Lower GI endoscopy:</u> not usually warranted in patients with typical clinical manifestations of CDI, a positive laboratory test, and/or clinical response to empiric treatment. Findings include bowel wall mucosal edema, erythema, friability, and inflammation with or without the **presence of pseudomembranes (elevated yellow or off-white plaques ≤2 cm in diameter scattered over the colonic mucosa that may coalesce to form the <u>pseudomembrane</u> appearance).**

MANAGEMENT
- **Discontinuing the offending antibiotic is the initial step in the management.**
- **<u>Contact precautions</u>** while performing diagnostic workup.
- **<u>Hand hygiene</u> with soap & water more effective than alcohol-based hand sanitizers in removing *C. difficile* spores — spores are resistant to killing by alcohol.**

Initial episode of CDI:
- **Either <u>oral Fidaxomicin</u> (preferred) OR <u>oral Vancomycin</u> is the first-line management of an initial episode of *Clostridioides difficile* infection (CDI), regardless of severity.**
- New guidelines on management of CDI issued by the Infectious Disease Society of America (IDSA) in June 2021 favor use of Fidaxomicin over Vancomycin.
- **<u>Metronidazole</u> is an alternative but less effective agent for treatment of nonsevere CDI if oral Fidaxomicin or oral Vancomycin are not available** (Metronidazole is no longer recommended as first-line therapy for adults); Metronidazole should be avoided in patients who are frail, age >65 years, or who develop CDI in association with Inflammatory bowel disease.
- <u>Fulminant colitis:</u> Vancomycin, orally or via NG tube, *plus* IV Metronidazole (especially with ileus).

<u>First recurrence:</u>
- Oral Vancomycin is preferred if Metronidazole was used for the initial episode OR Prolonged taper and pulsed Vancomycin regimen if standard Vancomycin regimen was used for the initial episode OR Fidaxomicin if Vancomycin was used for the initial episode.
- <u>Second or subsequent recurrence:</u> Standard- or extended-pulsed-regimen Fidaxomicin over a standard course of Vancomycin (prolonged taper & pulsed) for recurrent CDI episodes.
- <u>Bezlotoxumab:</u> **The IDSA guidelines favor use of adjunctive Bezlotoxumab (with a standard antibiotic regimen) for patients with recurrent CDI & prior episode within the last 6 months.**
- **<u>Third or subsequent CDI recurrence:</u> fecal microbiota transplantation (FMT) preferred** via capsule (cap-FMT) and colonoscopy (colo-FMT) whenever available. FMT consists of instillation of processed donor stool into the intestinal tract of a patient with recurrent CDI. FMT is usually avoided in patients with Inflammatory bowel disease or if immunocompromised.

VIBRIO CHOLERAE

- Gram-negative, comma-shaped rod transmitted via **contaminated food & water or fecal-oral route.**
- **Outbreaks may occur during poor sanitation & overcrowding conditions (especially abroad).**

PATHOPHYSIOLOGY

- **Exotoxin causes a secretory diarrhea** (inhibition of water, sodium, and chloride absorption), which **may cause profound dehydration & hypovolemia.** Short incubation period (1-2 days).
- *V. cholerae* **is a highly motile, comma-shaped (curved or spiral-shaped) gram-negative bacterial rod with a single polar flagellum** that grows best on special media.

CLINICAL MANIFESTATIONS

- Usually rapid onset, beginning with abdominal fullness and discomfort, rushes of peristalsis (borborygmi), and painless loose stools. Vomiting or abdominal cramping may occur.
- <u>Cholera:</u> **watery & voluminous stools — copious severe watery painless diarrhea with liquid that is gray and slightly cloudy, with flecks of mucus, & may have a "fishy odor" but no fecal odor, blood, or pus ("rice-water" stools** similar to water in which rice has been washed).
- <u>Noninvasive:</u> Fever uncommon. Absence of fecal RBCs or WBCs.
- <u>Dehydration:</u> The high rate of fluid loss (eg, up to 1 liter an hour) and high stool sodium concentration distinguishes Cholera from other causes of diarrhea. Severe cholera is characterized by profound fluid & electrolyte losses in the stool & rapid development of hypovolemic shock, often within 24h.

<u>DIAGNOSIS:</u> Clinical diagnosis. Stool cultures on specific media, PCR rapid testing.

MANAGEMENT

- **<u>Oral rehydration therapy & electrolyte replacement</u> mainstay of treatment.** Often self-limited. Patients with severe dehydration or profound vomiting require aggressive IV hydration initially.
- <u>Adjunctive antibiotics:</u> **Tetracyclines often used as first-line agents if moderate to severe; Macrolides or Fluoroquinolones are alternatives.** A single 1 g oral dose of Azithromycin is effective for severe cholera caused by strains with reduced susceptibility to Fluoroquinolones.
- <u>Prevention:</u> in areas where Cholera is endemic, use bottled water, wash hands often with soap and safe water, use chemical toilets, and cook food thoroughly.

VIBRIO PARAHAEMOLYTICUS & VIBRIO VULNIFICUS

- Gram-negative rods transmitted via **raw or undercooked shellfish consumption and seawater** (direct contact of water with wounds or shucking oysters), especially during warm summer months.
- *V. parahaemolyticus:* gastroenteritis. *V. vulnificus:* **gastroenteritis, necrotizing fasciitis, cellulitis. Most common cause of death from seafood consumption in the US** - thrives in warm salty water.

<u>Risk factors for bacteremia:</u>
- **<u>Underlying liver disease</u>**: eg, cirrhosis, moderate alcohol use, Hemochromatosis.
- **<u>Immunocompromised</u>**: eg, Diabetes mellitus. Chronic diseases.

CLINICAL MANIFESTATIONS

- <u>Gastroenteritis:</u> diarrhea, abdominal cramps, nausea, vomiting, and fever due to enterotoxins.
- <u>Cellulitis:</u> due to exposure of wound to seawater or estuarine (brackish) water.
- <u>Necrotizing fasciitis:</u> hemorrhagic bullae and may rapidly progress to shock.

<u>DIAGNOSIS:</u> Clinical, stool samples requires use of selective media; wound and blood cultures.

MANAGEMENT

- **<u>Gastroenteritis:</u> supportive and hydration therapy. <u>Cellulitis:</u> Tetracyclines;** FQ (Ciprofloxacin).
- <u>Severe disease:</u> Third-generation cephalosporin (eg, Cefotaxime or Ceftriaxone) plus either a Tetracycline (eg, Doxycycline or Minocycline) or a Fluoroquinolone (eg, Ciprofloxacin).

INVASIVE INFECTIOUS DIARRHEA

- **INVASIVE: high fever, ⊕ blood & fecal leukocytes,** not as voluminous (large intestine), **mucus.**
- **DO NOT give anti-motility drugs with invasive diarrhea (may cause increased toxicity).**
- Includes: Campylobacter, Shigella, Salmonella, Yersinia, Enterohemorrhagic *E coli*, Campylobacter.

YERSINIA ENTEROCOLITICA, YERSINIA PSEUDOTUBERCULOSIS

- Gram-negative coccobacillus with bipolar staining ("safety pin" appearance). 1–10-day IP.
- Sources: **contaminated pork (most common in the US),** fecally contaminated water, milk, & tofu.
- Increased iron stores (eg, Hemochromatosis, Thalassemia) increase susceptibility to infection.

CLINICAL MANIFESTATIONS

- Fever, diarrhea (±bloody); **RLQ abdominal pain & leukocytosis may mimic acute Appendicitis (mesenteric lymphadenitis may cause abdominal tenderness),** vomiting (symptoms last 2 weeks).
- Pharyngitis, Erythema nodosum (2-14 days after abdominal pain) and Reactive arthritis may occur.
- Diagnosis culture isolation from stool (preferred), mesenteric lymph nodes, or blood.

MANAGEMENT

- **Hydration mainstay of therapy, correction of any electrolyte abnormalities, no antibiotics.**
- Enterocolitis: oral Fluoroquinolone (Ciprofloxacin), Trimethoprim-Sulfamethoxazole, or Doxycycline.
- Severe illness: Ceftriaxone plus Gentamicin; Ciprofloxacin alternative to Ceftriaxone.

SHIGELLOSIS

- Diarrheal illness most commonly caused by gram-negative rods — *Shigella sonnei* **(most common in US),** *flexneri,* and *dysenteriae* (produces the most toxin). A small inoculum is needed.
- **High risk: children <5 years in childcare setting** (eg, daycare, preschool, crowded living condition).

TRANSMISSION

- Direct person-to-person spread (fecal-oral). Less commonly through contaminated food & water.
- **Highly virulent** infection of the colon, particularly the rectosigmoid portion of the colon.

PATHOPHYSIOLOGY

- *S. dysenteriae* produces a "Shiga" enterotoxin that is neurotoxic, cytotoxic, & enterotoxic. IP 1-7 days.

CLINICAL MANIFESTATIONS

- Colonic dysentery — **lower abdominal pain, abdominal cramps, explosive watery diarrhea (frequent, small-volume stools) that progresses to mucoid & bloody diarrhea with tenesmus, & systemic symptoms (eg, high fever,** chills, anorexia, malaise, headache), nausea, vomiting.
- **Neurologic manifestations especially in young children** — eg, **febrile seizures,** encephalopathy.
- Rare complications: Reactive arthritis, **Hemolytic uremic syndrome (especially children),** Toxic megacolon, proctitis, rectal prolapse, intestinal obstruction, & colonic perforation.

DIAGNOSIS

- **Stool studies: positive fecal WBCs & RBCs (inflammatory invasive diarrhea);** Stool cultures.
- CBC: **Leukocytosis. Leukemoid reaction (may be >50,000 WBCs/microL).**
- Sigmoidoscopy: in patients with dysentery reveal punctate areas of ulceration & inflammation.

MANAGEMENT

- **Oral hydration mainstay of treatment and electrolyte replacement.** Generally, it is self-limited, lasting no more than 7 days in an untreated immunocompetent host. Zinc helpful in children.
- **In general, anti-motility drugs should be avoided** (can worsen the illness due to retained toxins).
- Antibiotics may be indicated if severe (eg, considered if fever is high, documented infection [positive stool or blood cultures especially in infants and young children but also in adults], severe dysentery. **When needed, Fluoroquinolones is first-line in adults), Azithromycin is first-line in children;** third generation Cephalosporins, Trimethoprim-sulfamethoxazole, and Ampicillin are options.

CAMPYLOBACTER ENTERITIS

- ***Campylobacter jejuni*** **most common cause of** <u>**bacterial**</u> **enteritis in the US;** *C. coli.*
- **C. jejuni is the most common antecedent event in post-infectious Guillain-Barré syndrome.**
- Most commonly affects children & young adults. 3-day incubation period.

<u>Sources:</u>
- <u>Contaminated food</u> — <u>**raw or undercooked poultry**</u> **most common** (~50%), contaminated water, raw unpasteurized milk, or dairy cattle (beef, lamb, pork). Puppies an important source in children.

<u>CLINICAL MANIFESTATIONS</u>
- <u>**Crampy periumbilical abdominal pain**</u> **(may mimic acute appendicitis),** cramps, nausea, fever.
- <u>**Diarrhea**</u> **initially watery progressing to bloody; abdominal cramps.** Hematochezia (15–50%).
- <u>Complications:</u> **Reactive arthritis or Guillain-Barré syndrome may complicate** *C jejuni* **infection,** with a range of onset of 1 week to 2 months after the presentation with gastrointestinal symptoms.

<u>DIAGNOSIS</u>
- <u>Stool studies:</u> Stool culture (definitive). <u>Stool examination:</u> gram-negative, spiral-shaped ("S, comma or seagull shaped") rapidly motile organisms. Fecal WBCs & RBCs; Enzyme immunoassay or PCR.

<u>MANAGEMENT</u>
- <u>**Hydration**</u> **mainstay of treatment, with electrolyte replacement** (usually mild & self-limiting, with peak of illness lasting 24-48 hours). Antibiotics not needed in most cases of *C. jejuni* gastroenteritis.
- <u>**Severe disease or high-risk patients:**</u> **Macrolides first-line antibiotic of choice when needed (eg, Azithromycin).** Fluoroquinolones is an alternative. Doxycycline. Antibiotics shorten the duration of symptoms if given within 1-2 days of onset.
- **Avoid Loperamide & other anti-motility agents in invasive diarrhea.**

<u>PREVENTION</u>
- Proper food handling and handwashing can prevent spread. May cause Traveler's diarrhea.

ENTEROHEMORRHAGIC E. COLI (EHEC) O157:H7

- <u>**Foodborne**</u>**: ingestion of undercooked meat, especially** <u>**ground beef**</u>**, unpasteurized milk or apple cider, day care centers, & contaminated water.** Incubation period average 3-9 days.
- <u>**Animal contact:**</u> eg, occupational exposure to animals (eg, farms and petting zoos).

<u>PATHOPHYSIOLOGY</u>
- <u>**Shiga-like toxin**</u> (verotoxin) causes endothelial & vascular damage, leading to (bloody diarrhea) and predisposition to develop Hemolytic uremic syndrome (HUS), especially in children <10 years.
- **Most commonly seen in children & elderly.**

<u>CLINICAL MANIFESTATIONS</u>
- **Watery diarrhea early on before becoming visibly bloody 1-3 days afterwards (90%).** Severe cramps and abdominal pain are common, vomiting.
- **Fever is usually absent in most** (low-grade if present). May have right lower quadrant tenderness.
- <u>**Hemolytic uremic syndrome**</u> **may occur in children between days 5-15 of illness** — triad of (1) Hemolytic anemia, (2) thrombocytopenia, and (3) Acute kidney injury.

<u>DIAGNOSIS</u>
- Peripheral leukocytosis of 10,000–20,000/µL common. Stool cultures using sorbitol-MacConkey agar.

<u>MANAGEMENT</u>
- **Hydration mainstay of treatment & supportive measures.**
- **Avoid antibiotics in children due to** <u>**increased incidence of Hemolytic uremic syndrome**</u> (antibiotics have no benefit and may increase the release of Shiga-like toxins & HUS 3-fold).
- **Avoid anti-motility drugs** — their use is associated with increased complications.

TYPHOID (ENTERIC) FEVER

- ***Salmonella enterica* serotype Typhi (formerly *S. typhi*) & *S. enterica* serotypes Paratyphi** A, B, or C to a lesser extent. More common in children & young adults. 5–21-day incubation period.

Transmission:
- Fecal-oral route: **ingestion of contaminated food or water, history of travel to areas where sanitation is poor (eg, endemic areas in Latin America, Asia, and India). Contact with asymptomatic chronic carrier** if a patient with Typhoid has not traveled to an endemic area.
- The bacteria crosses intestinal epithelium barrier through M cells overlying the lymphoid follicles of Peyer's patches. May colonize the gallbladder in chronic carriers.

CLINICAL MANIFESTATIONS
- Enteric fever usually presents with chills, abdominal pain, & fever ~5-21 days after ingestion of Salmonella.
- **Week 1 (Prodromal stage): systemic symptoms (bacteremia) — headache, slow rising fever in a stepwise fashion** that may drop by the next morning, chills, malaise, cough, sore throat, anorexia.
- **Week 2 (Gastrointestinal stage): eg, abdominal pain, abdominal tenderness, and constipation initially** occur over the course of the first week of illness and last for the duration of the illness. Due to the hypertrophy of Payer patches from monocytic infiltration and inflammation, constipation (due narrowed bowel lumen) may predominate over diarrhea in some cases. **Mild to severe "pea soup" diarrhea (foul green-yellow liquid) with or without blood may occur.** Weight loss.

PHYSICAL EXAMINATION
- **Fever with relative bradycardia (temp-pulse dissociation)** classic but rare, abdominal tenderness.
- **Rose spots (faint pink or salmon-colored macular rash that spreads from trunk to extremities; blanches with pressure) occurs in the second week.**
- **Week 3: Hepatosplenomegaly**, GI bleeding, signs of dehydration, and delirium may be seen.

DIAGNOSIS: Blood culture best diagnostic tool. Culture of the stool may be negative with symptoms.

MANAGEMENT
- **Oral hydration first-line management & electrolyte replacement + antibiotics often given.**
- **Antibiotics: Fluoroquinolones first-line** (Ciprofloxacin, Ofloxacin), Macrolides, or Ceftriaxone.

NONTYPHOIDAL SALMONELLA

- Other Nontyphoid Salmonella species (eg, *S. enteriditis, S. typhimurium*).
- **One of the most common causes of foodborne disease in US (eg, poultry, eggs, & milk products, fresh produce) and contact with exotic pets, especially reptiles** (eg, turtles).

CLINICAL MANIFESTATIONS
- 8–72-hour incubation period — **nausea, vomiting, fever, abdominal cramping, and diarrhea that may become bloody.** Diarrhea may be "pea soup" (brown green) in color. Malaise, headaches.
- Salmonella is a common cause of Osteomyelitis in children with Sickle cell disease.

DIAGNOSIS
- Routine stool cultures. Stool studies: positive for fecal WBCs and RBCs.

MANAGEMENT
- **Oral rehydration mainstay of treatment & electrolyte replacement.** In most healthy adults, the disease is self-limited, with fever abating within 2–3 days and diarrhea lasting no more than 10 days.
- **Antibiotics if severe illness: Fluoroquinolones (eg, Ciprofloxacin) first line when needed (Azithromycin in children),** Trimethoprim-sulfamethoxazole an alternative — eg, severe illness (high or persistent fever, very frequent bowel movements, need for hospitalization), infants <12 months, adults >50 years, immunocompromised patients, individuals with chronic illness.

PROTOZOAN INFECTIONS

GIARDIASIS (GIARDIA LAMBLIA)
- *Giardia duodenalis* (also known as *G. lamblia* or *G. intestinalis*) is a protozoan parasite associated with sporadic or epidemic diarrheal illness. Most common protozoal infestation in the US.

SOURCES
- **Ingestion of contaminated water from remote streams, surface wells, or lakes: "Backpacker's diarrhea"** — travel to wilderness, drinking water not been adequately filtered, treated, or boiled. Water-dwelling mammals (eg, beavers) are reservoirs for the protozoa (Beaver fever).
- Outbreaks occur due to contaminated water, food, fecal-oral transmission, in daycare centers, and illness can occur in international travelers.

CLINICAL MANIFESTATIONS
- ~50% of individuals infested with *G lamblia* have no symptoms and can be asymptomatic.
- **Steatorrhea: frothy, greasy, foul-smelling diarrhea with no blood or pus for >1 week.**
- **Abdominal cramps, bloating, flatulence.** Malabsorption, malaise, weight loss, chronic diarrhea.

DIAGNOSIS:
- **Antigen & nucleic acid detection assays** are more sensitive than stool microscopy.
- **Stool microscopy: may reveal trophozoites & cysts on stool examination.**

MANAGEMENT
- **Oral rehydration mainstay of treatment.** If left untreated, most symptomatic patients recover spontaneously & eliminate the parasite within 3–4 weeks. Up to 25% may develop chronic infection.
- Individuals ≥3 yrs — **Tinidazole single dose (preferred).** Nitazoxanide, Albendazole, Furazolidone.
- Individuals 1-3 years old — **Nitazoxanide** 3-day course.
- Individuals <12 months old — **Metronidazole** (often 5-7 days)

AMEBIASIS
- *Entamoeba histolytica* — protozoan most commonly transmitted by ingestion of cysts from fecally contaminated food and/or water, institutionalized patients, and men who have sex with men.
- Not common in the US. Usually occurs in migrants from or travelers to endemic tropical areas.
- **May develop an amebic liver abscess.**

CLINICAL MANIFESTATIONS
- Most infections are asymptomatic.
- GI symptoms: 1–3-week subacute onset, varying from **mild diarrhea to severe dysentery** (abdominal pain, diarrhea, bloody stools, mucus in stools weight loss, fever). **Recurrent diarrhea.**
- **Amebic liver abscess: fever, RUQ pain, anorexia, weight loss, tender hepatomegaly.**

DIAGNOSIS
- *E histolytica*-specific antigen in the stool (eg, ELISA) **sensitive, easy to perform, and rapid.**
- Stool microscopy O&P (ova & parasites) — cysts with ingested RBCs. Because cysts are not constantly shed, at least 3 stool samples on different days should be examined. Not as sensitive as stool antigen.
- Stool PCR — detects parasitic DNA or RNA in the stool. Leukocytosis.
- Liver abscess: ultrasound, CT, or MRI. Increased LFTs with amebic liver abscess.

MANAGEMENT
- **Colitis: Metronidazole (first line) or Tinidazole, followed by an intraluminal agent (eg, Paromomycin,** Diloxanide furoate, or Diiodohydroxyquinoline).
- **Liver abscess:** Metronidazole or Tinidazole + intraluminal amebicide followed by Chloroquine. May need drainage (eg, needle aspiration) if no response to medications after 3 days.
- Asymptomatic infections should be treated with an intraluminal agent alone.

	SECRETORY DIARRHEA	OSMOTIC DIARRHEA
ETIOLOGIES	• **Hormonal:** serotonin & histamine (eg, Carcinoid syndrome), calcitonin (medullary cancer of thyroid), **gastrin (Zollinger-Ellison Syndrome);** VIP-producing tumors. • **Motility disorders:** eg, Scleroderma and Diabetic autonomic neuropathy, IBS • **Infections: Bacterial** (eg, *E. coli, Vibrio cholerae*), **viral, or parasitic.**	• **Medications:** Nonabsorbale solutes (eg, **Lactulose, Sorbitol**), Osmotic laxatives (eg, Mg, PO4) • Bacterial overgrowth: eg, Whipple's disease, Tropical sprue. • **Malabsorption:** Celiac disease, Pancreatic insufficiency, Lactase deficiency, short bowel syndrome.
DIARRHEA	• **Large volume of watery stools** **>200 ml/24h** • **No change in diarrhea with fasting (unaffected)**	• Smaller volumes of watery stools <200 ml/24h • **Improves or resolves with fasting.** • Deficiency in fat-soluble vitamins if malabsorption present.
STOOL STUDIES	• **Normal/low stool osmolal gap** <40 mOsm/kg • **Elevated stool Na+** (>70 mEq/L), K+, Cl- (>40 mEq/L), and pH >6	• **High stool osmolal gap** >40 mOsm/kg (often >75 mOsm/kg) • **Low stool Na⁺** (<70 mEq/L), Cl- (<35 mEq/L), and pH <5 • **Increased fecal fat if malabsorption.**

WHIPPLE'S DISEASE

- *Tropheryma whipplei:* a Gram-positive, non-acid-fast, periodic acid-Schiff-positive rod.

TRANSMISSION
- Contaminated soil (most commonly seen in farmers).
- Most commonly occurs in white males of European ancestry.

CLINICAL MANIFESTATIONS
4 cardinal manifestations (arthralgias, diarrhea, abdominal pain, and weight loss).
- **Arthralgias:** Joint symptoms (eg, migratory arthralgias of the large joints), generally precede other manifestations by many years.
- **Abdominal pain & diarrhea:** Later in the course of disease, intermittent diarrhea with colicky abdominal pain occur and ultimately can progress to a severe wasting syndrome (malabsorption).
- **Malabsorption:** chronic diarrhea, weight loss, steatorrhea, nutritional deficiency. Fever, lymphadenopathy, **nondeforming arthritis.**
- **CNS involvement:** Neurologic symptoms include memory impairment, cognitive dysfunction, & confusion. **Rhythmic motion of eye muscles while chewing.**

DIAGNOSIS
- **Upper endoscopy & biopsies** of the small intestine for *T. whipplei* testing — **Periodic acid-Schiff (PAS)-positive macrophages, non-acid-fast bacilli, dilation of lacteals.**
- For all patients diagnosed with Whipple's disease, *T. whipplei* PCR should be performed on the CSF, even if there are no neurological symptoms.

MANAGEMENT
- Prolonged antibiotic therapy (eg 1-2 years). Initial phase of an intravenous antibiotic that is active against *T. whipplei* with good penetration of the blood-brain barrier (eg, Penicillin or Ceftriaxone), followed by maintenance therapy with oral Trimethoprim-sulfamethoxazole (often for 12 months).
- Doxycycline + Hydroxychloroquine is an alternative.

PEANUT AND TREE NUT ALLERGY

- **Most are IgE mediated** but may be non-Ig-E mediated or mixed.

Risk factors:
- **Genetics:** siblings of children with peanut allergy are at increased risk of developing a peanut allergy. Family history of personal history of atopic disease. Family history of peanut allergy
- Timing of exposure — **delayed introduction of nuts until >3 years of age = increased risk.**

CLINICAL MANIFESTATIONS
- Skin: pruritus, flushing, diaphoresis, urticaria & angioedema, contact urticaria.
- Oropharyngeal: sneezing, nasal congestion, oral pruritus, rhinorrhea.
- Respiratory: wheezing, dyspnea, cough. Cardiovascular: arrhythmias.
- Eyes: conjunctival injection, lacrimation, pruritus, & periorbital edema
- GI: nausea, vomiting, abdominal pain, diarrhea. Neurologic: dizziness, syncope, sense of doom

MANAGEMENT
- Patient education on avoiding products containing or cooked with the associated foods
- Complete avoidance of foods and similar foods
- Epinephrine autoinjectors should be prescribed in case of accidental exposure and reaction.

MANAGEMENT OF AN ACUTE ATTACK
- **Antihistamines if mild. Intramuscular Epinephrine if severe.**

DUMPING SYNDROME

- Rapid gastric emptying & rapid fluid shifts with ingestion of large amounts of simple carbohydrates.
- **Often a complication of gastric surgery: bariatric surgery** with Roux-en-Y gastric bypass causes Dumping syndrome in as many as 50% of patients. Gastrectomy, Truncal vagotomy.

CLINICAL MANIFESTATIONS
- **Early dumping syndrome symptoms** occurs during or immediately after a meal (within 15 minutes) and is characterized by
  - **(1) GI symptoms: nausea, vomiting, bloating, flatus, abdominal pain, diarrhea, &**
  - **(2) vasomotor symptoms (eg, diaphoresis, dizziness, tachypnea, hypotension, flushing, fatigue).** Hyperosmolality food load in the small bowel causes rapid fluid shifts from the plasma into the bowel, resulting in hypotension & sympathetic nervous system response.
- **Late dumping symptoms:** occur 1-3 hours after a meal and is characterized by **hypoglycemia, weakness, sweating, dizziness, and possible syncope**. Secondary hypoglycemia occurs because a high carbohydrate content absorption into the small bowel evokes a strong insulin response.

DIAGNOSIS
- **Clinical diagnosis**, Modified oral glucose tolerance test.
- Dual-phase gastric radionuclide scintigraphy is the best diagnostic test to confirm rapid gastric emptying. If early dumping syndrome is suspected, an early peak will be noted, usually within 1 hour of ingestion. Barium fluoroscopy.

MANAGEMENT
- **Dietary modifications: decreased carbohydrate intake (minimize simple sugars), eat smaller, more frequent high-fiber, complex carbohydrate, and protein-rich meals.**
- **Avoid simultaneous fluid & solid intake (separate by 30 minutes);** and adding supplemental fiber (pectin, guar gum) to increase the viscosity of the ingested food and delay gastric emptying.
- Usually, early dumping is self-limiting and resolves within 7 to 12 weeks.

PHENYLKETONURIA (PKU)

- **Autosomal recessive inborn disorder of amino acid metabolism associated with phenylketone neurotoxicity** due to the accumulation of excessive phenylalanine in the urine and the blood.
- **Children often are blond and blue-eyed with light skin.**

PATHOPHYSIOLOGY
- **Phenylalanine hydroxylase deficiency:** Decrease in the hepatic enzyme phenylalanine hydroxylase that metabolizes the amino acid phenylalanine into tyrosine, resulting in **excessive phenylalanine**.
- Neurotoxicity is often irreversible if not detected by 3 years old.

CLINICAL MANIFESTATIONS
- Neonates appear normal at birth. After birth: **vomiting, mental delays**, irritability, convulsions, eczema, **increased deep tendon reflexes**. Intellectual disability, microcephaly.

DIAGNOSIS
- **Increased serum phenylalanine.** Molecular analysis. MRI may show white matter injury.
- **Urine with musty (mousy) odor** from phenylacetic acid.
- Newborn screening routinely performed in US. Can be monitored during pregnancy (eg, 24 weeks GA).

MANAGEMENT
- **Lifetime dietary restriction of phenylalanine** + **increase tyrosine supplementation.** Phenylalanine levels followed at regular intervals in neonates & less often in older children/adults. Some adults show improvement in behavior, symptoms, & sequelae when treated with a phenylalanine-restricted diet. Liberal fruits & vegetables. Enzyme therapy with Pegvaliase in adults.
- **Avoid foods high in phenylalanine:** eg, milk, cheese, nuts, fish, meats (eg, chicken, pork, beef), eggs, legumes, aspartame found in diet sodas. Limited carbohydrates.

VITAMIN C (ASCORBIC ACID) DEFICIENCY

RISK FACTORS
- **Diets lacking raw citrus fruits & green vegetables** (excess heat denatures vitamin C), smoking, illicit drug use, alcoholism, malnourished individuals, elderly. Uncommon in the US.
- Symptoms can occur after 1-3 months of deficient vitamin C intake.

CLINICAL MANIFESTATIONS
Scurvy 3 Hs
- The most specific symptoms, occurring as early as 1-3 months after deficient intake, are **follicular hyperkeratosis and perifollicular hemorrhage, with petechiae and coiled hairs.**
- **Hyperkeratosis:** hyperkeratotic follicular papules, often surrounded by hemorrhage. Coiled hairs.
- **Hemorrhage: vascular fragility** (abnormal collagen production) with **recurrent hemorrhages into the gums** (gingivitis with bleeding and receding gums, loose teeth, and dental caries), **skin (perifollicular hemorrhages, petechiae, ecchymosis), & joints (arthralgias** & musculoskeletal pain may be caused by hemorrhage into the muscles or periosteum). Hemorrhagic skin lesions are flat at onset, but may coalesce & become palpable, especially on the legs. **Impaired wound healing.**
- **Hematologic abnormalities:** anemia, glossitis, malaise, weakness. Increased bleeding time.
- Fractures and brittle bones due to disrupted endochondral bone formation.
- Generalized symptoms: malaise, weakness, anorexia, neuropathy, irritability, emotional lability.

DIAGNOSIS
- Clinical. Serum ascorbic acid levels. Leukocyte ascorbic levels more accurate.

MANAGEMENT
- **Ascorbic acid replacement.** Hematologic symptoms improve within weeks, generalized symptoms can improve within days.

VITAMIN D DEFICIENCY

- Low bone turnover + **decreased bone (osteoid) mineralization (Osteomalacia in adults, causing soft bones) and/or cartilage at the epiphyseal plates (Rickets in children).**

OSTEOMALACIA

ETIOLOGIES
- **Severe vitamin D deficiency most common** — leads to decreased serum calcium & phosphate with subsequent **demineralization of the bone osteoid only ("soft bones").** Phosphate deficiency.
- Malabsorption — eg, chronic liver or kidney disease, gastric bypass, Celiac disease etc..

CLINICAL MANIFESTATIONS
- **Diffuse bone pain & tenderness** eg, lower spine, pelvis, & lower extremities. Fatigue.
- **Proximal muscle weakness** **& pain,** ±muscle wasting, hypotonia, & discomfort with movement.
- Hip pain & **bowing of long bones may cause antalgic (waddling) gait.** Pathologic fractures.
- Hypocalcemia — muscle spasms, cramps, a positive Chvostek's sign, tingling/numbness.

DIAGNOSIS
- Classic **decreased calcium, phosphate, & 25-hydroxyvitamin D** (<20 ng/mL). Low urinary calcium.
- Increased alkaline phosphatase & **increased parathyroid hormone (PTH).**
- Radiographs: **Looser lines (zones) — transverse pseudo-fracture lines (narrow radiolucent lines** due to visible osteoid) bilateral & symmetrical seen at the femoral neck, shaft, or trochanter.

MANAGEMENT
- **Vitamin D supplementation first-line** (eg, **Ergocalciferol**). Maintain calcium intake of ≥1,000 mg/d.

RICKETS

- **Low bone turnover + decreased osteoid mineralization (Osteomalacia) and/or cartilage at the growth plates (Rickets).**
- Vitamin D deficiency most commonly seen between 3 months–3 years when growth (calcium) needs are high + **decreased sunlight exposure, prolonged exclusive breastfeeding** without vitamin D supplementation), heavy skin pigmentation, absence of fortified foods with Vitamin D (eg, dairy).

ETIOLOGIES
- **Calcipenic (calcium deficiency &/or vitamin D deficiency** including dietary deficiency, Celiac disease, Cystic fibrosis, or extensive bowel resection.
- Phosphopenic due to renal phosphate wasting (eg, Fanconi syndrome) or, less commonly, deficiency.

CLINICAL MANIFESTATIONS
- Initially manifests at the distal forearm (bowing of forearm bones), knee, & costochondral junction.
- **Delayed fontanel closure,** craniotabes (soft skull bones), growth delays, delayed dentition, **genu varum (lateral bowing of the femur & tibia),** parietal & frontal bossing, widening of the wrist.

DIAGNOSIS
- Depends on the cause but classic labs reveal **decreased calcium, phosphate, & 25-hydroxyvitamin D levels** (calcipenic). **Increased alkaline phosphatase** & parathyroid hormone (PTH) in calcipenic.
- Radiographs: widening of the epiphyseal plate, **costochondral junction enlargement of the chest (rachitic rosary), and long bones appear to have a less distinct ("fuzzy") cortex.**

MANAGEMENT
- **Vitamin D supplementation** first-line — **vitamin D2 (Ergocalciferol)** or D3 (Cholecalciferol).
- **Exclusively breastfed infants should receive 400 international units of vitamin D per day.**
- Vitamin D supplementation given to infants who consume < 32 ounces (1 liter) of formula per day.

VITAMIN A

- Vitamin A Function: vision, immune function, embryo development, hematopoiesis, skin, and cellular health (epithelial cell differentiation).
- Sources: found in the kidney, liver, egg yolk, butter, and green leafy vegetables.

VITAMIN A EXCESS

- Acute toxicity: blurred vision, nausea, vomiting, vertigo, **Idiopathic intracranial hypertension.**
- Chronic toxicity: **teratogenicity**, alopecia, ataxia, visual changes skin disorders, hepatotoxicity.

VITAMIN A DEFICIENCY

DEFICIENCY RISK FACTORS

- Patients with liver disease, alcoholics, fat-free diets (Vitamin A is a fat-soluble vitamin), fat malabsorption (eg, Cystic Fibrosis, Crohn ileitis, short bowel syndrome, bariatric surgery).

CLINICAL MANIFESTATIONS

- **Visual changes: especially night blindness, xerophthalmia (dry eyes),** retinopathy. **Bitot's spots: white spots on the conjunctiva due to squamous metaplasia of the corneal epithelium**.
- **Impaired immunity** (poor wound healing, frequent infections). Poor bone growth, loss of taste.
- Dry skin: follicular hyperkeratosis and dryness.
- **Squamous metaplasia** — conjunctival, respiratory epithelium, urinary tract.

DIAGNOSIS

- Clinical. Decreased serum retinol levels below the normal range of 30–65 mg/dL.

MANAGEMENT

- Vitamin A 30,000 IU orally daily for 1 week.

VITAMIN B DEFICIENCY

RIBOFLAVIN (B2) DEFICIENCY

- May occur in patients who are malnourished, Anorexia nervosa, Malabsorption syndrome, malignancy, short bowel syndrome.

CLINICAL MANIFESTATIONS

Oral, ocular, genital syndrome.

- Oral: pharyngitis (sore throat), stomatitis, hyperemia & edema of the pharyngeal mucous membranes, lesions of mouth, **magenta colored tongue**, glossitis, angular cheilitis.
- Ocular: photophobia, corneal lesions.
- Genital: scrotal dermatitis.
- Other findings: Normocytic normochromic anemia, and Seborrheic dermatitis.

MANAGEMENT

- Administration of Riboflavin 5–15 mg/day until clinical findings resolve is usually adequate.
- Prevention: The United States recommended dietary allowance (RDA) for Riboflavin is 0.5-0.9 mg/day in children, 1.3 mg/day for adults.

PYRIDOXINE (B6) DEFICIENCY

ETIOLOGIES

- Chronic alcoholism, **Isoniazid,** Penicillamine, Levodopa + Carbidopa, oral contraceptives, Hydralazine.

CLINICAL MANIFESTATIONS

- **Neurologic: peripheral neuropathy** (classic but rare), seizures, headache, mood changes.
- Stomatitis, cheilosis, glossitis, flaky skin, seborrheic dermatitis, **anemia**.

THIAMINE (B1) DEFICIENCY

ETIOLOGIES
- **Chronic alcohol use disorder (most common cause in the US),** weight loss surgery, Malabsorption.

CLINICAL MANIFESTATIONS
- Thiamine deficiency in the diet causes two main presentations: [1] Beriberi (infantile and adult) & [2] Wernicke-Korsakoff syndrome.
- **[1] "Dry" Beriberi: nervous system changes: symmetric peripheral neuropathy with sensory & motor neuron impairment, predominantly involving the distal extremities** — paresthesias, impaired coordination, impaired reflexes, anorexia, muscle cramps, & wasting (legs > arms).
- **[2] "Wet" Beriberi: high-output Heart failure, Dilated cardiomyopathy,** tachycardia.
- Infantile Beriberi — often clinically manifests in infants 2-3 months of age in infants who are breastfed by mothers with a thiamine-deficient diet. May include a fulminant cardiac syndrome with cardiomegaly, tachycardia, a loud piercing cry, cyanosis, dyspnea, vomiting and pulmonary hypertension. Older infants may have neurologic symptoms resembling Aseptic meningitis.

Wernicke-Korsakoff syndrome: 2 different syndromes that are different stages of the same disease.
- **[3] Wernicke encephalopathy: acute syndrome characterized by the triad of (1) ataxia (difficulty walking & balance), (2) global confusion** (eg, disorientation, inattentiveness, indifference), and **(3) ophthalmoplegia** (eg, paralysis or abnormalities of the ocular muscles – nystagmus, conjugate gaze palsies, lateral rectus palsy); Considered a neurologic emergency requiring emergency treatment to prevent neurological morbidity & death. **Most common in chronic alcohol use disorder.**
- **[4] Korsakoff dementia: memory loss (especially short-term) & confabulation.** Chronic condition as a consequence of Wernicke's encephalopathy and **usually irreversible.**

MANAGEMENT
Beriberi:
- **IV Thiamine administration if the patient is critically ill, followed by oral Thiamine** [eg, 5-30 mg/dose IV, 3 times daily for several days), followed by oral Thiamine, 5 to 30 mg/day].
- **Some clinicians prefer to replace Thiamine before glucose** (delay giving dextrose until Thiamine supplementation has been initiated) to avoid precipitating Wernicke encephalopathy (WE) in individuals with alcohol use disorder, prolonged starvation, or other high risk for developing WE.

NIACIN [NICOTINIC ACID (VITAMIN B3)] DEFICIENCY
- Sources of B3 (Niacin/Nicotinic acid): meats, grains, legumes.

ETIOLOGIES
- **US: Alcohol use disorder.** Anorexia nervosa, malabsorption, bariatric surgery. Isoniazid therapy.

Resource poor countries:
- **Often due to diets high in untreated corn or sorghum (lacks niacin & tryptophan), diets which lack tryptophan, alcoholism, anorexia, or malabsorption.** Isoniazid therapy.

Other:
- Carcinoid syndrome: increased tryptophan metabolism due to the production of serotonin.
- Hartnup disease: decreased tryptophan absorption in the kidneys & small intestine.

CLINICAL MANIFESTATIONS
Pellagra (3 Ds): dermatitis, diarrhea, & dementia.
- **Dermatitis: photosensitive hyperpigmented dermatitis (pigmentation and scaling similar to sunburn, especially on sun-exposed areas).** Casal's necklace: ring of dermatitis around the neck.
- **Diarrhea:** due to malabsoprtion & proctitis. Bright red glossitis.
- **Dementia:** irritability, anxiety, insomnia, disorientation, delusions, dementia, & encephalopathy.

MANAGEMENT:
- Oral supplementation with 100-200 mg of Nicotinamide or Nicotinic acid 3 times daily for 5 days.

B12 (COBALAMIN) DEFICIENCY

- <u>Sources of B12:</u> **natural sources mainly animal in origin** (eg, fish, meats, eggs, dairy products).
- <u>Absorption:</u> **B12 is released by the acidity of the stomach and combines with intrinsic factor** (produced by the parietal cells) in an acidic environment, **later absorbed mainly via distal ileum.**
- <u>Function of B12:</u> Vitamin B12 is essential for neurologic function, red blood cell production, and DNA synthesis; it is a cofactor for 3 major reactions: conversion of methylmalonic acid to succinyl coenzyme A; conversion of homocysteine to methionine; & conversion of 5-MTH to tetrahydrofolate.
- Substantial hepatic B12 stores may delay manifestations for 5-10 years after the onset of deficiency.

ETIOLOGIES

Decreased B12 absorption:

- **Decreased intrinsic factor: Pernicious anemia most common cause of B12 deficiency** (lack of intrinsic factor due to parietal cell antibodies, leading to gastric atrophy), gastric bypass, post gastrectomy, gastritis, achlorhydria, tropical sprue, Gastrinoma (Zollinger-Ellison syndrome).
- **Ileal disease: Crohn disease** (affects the terminal ileum), Ileal resection, Fish tapeworm (rare).
- <u>Medications:</u> **H2 blockers & Proton pump inhibitors** (decrease acid), decreased nucleic acid synthesis (**Metformin**, Zidovudine, Hydroxyurea), anticonvulsants. **Chronic alcohol use.**

<u>Decreased intake:</u> **Vegans** (due to lack of consumption of meat and meat products).

CLINICAL MANIFESTATIONS

- **Anemia symptoms similar to Folate deficiency but associated with spinal cord involvement.**
- <u>Hematologic:</u> fatigue, exercise intolerance, pallor. <u>Epithelial:</u> glossitis, diarrhea, malabsorption.
- **Neuropsychiatric symptoms: symmetric paresthesias & numbness most common initial symptom** (especially involving the legs). Later, **lateral and <u>posterior spinal cord demyelination & degeneration</u>** — **gait ataxia, weakness, vibratory, sensory, & proprioception deficits,** including difficulty with balance. May develop dementia, psychosis, or seizures. On examination, **decreased deep tendon reflexes** (hypotonia) or ⊕ Babinski may be seen.

DIAGNOSIS

- **CBC with peripheral smear: increased MCV (macrocytic anemia) + megaloblastic anemia (macro-ovalocytes & hypersegmented neutrophils with >5 lobes).** Mild pancytopenia may be seen [leukopenia, reticulocytes, and/or thrombocytopenia (B12 deficiency affects all cell lines)].
- Increased serum LDH & indirect bilirubin due to intramedullary destruction of developing abnormal erythroid cells.
- **Decreased serum B12 levels:** <200 pg/mL; symptomatic patients are often <100 pg/mL.
- **Increased homocysteine nonspecific (can be seen in both B12 and Folate deficiencies).**
- **Increased methylmalonic acid [MMA] distinguishes B12 from Folate deficiency,** (FD is associated with increased homocysteine & normal MMA). ↑MMA in B12 deficiency occurs because B12 is a cofactor in conversion of methylmalonyl-CoA to succinyl-CoA.

MANAGEMENT

B12 replacement

- <u>Routes of administration:</u> oral, sublingual, nasal and intramuscular/deep subcutaneous injection.

Symptomatic anemia or neurological findings:

- **Start with Intramuscular (IM) Cyanocobalamin** injection weekly until the deficiency is corrected & then once monthly. Patients can be switched to oral therapy after resolution of symptoms. **Patients with Pernicious anemia need lifelong monthly IM therapy (or high-dose oral therapy).**
- With adequate treatment, a brisk reticulocytosis occurs in 5–7 days, and the hematologic picture normalizes in 2 months.
- Hypokalemia may complicate the first several days of therapy, particularly if the anemia is severe (due to placement of potassium into the newly formed cells).

<u>Dietary deficiency:</u> Oral B12 replacement.

INGUINAL HERNIAS

INDIRECT HERNIA
- Type of inguinal hernia with bowel protrusion at the internal inguinal ring.
- The origin of the sac is **LATERAL** to the inferior epigastric artery.
- **Indirect hernia is the most common type of hernia in both sexes** (although more common in men), **young children, and young adults.**

PATHOPHYSIOLOGY
- **Often congenital due to a <u>persistent patent processus vaginalis</u>.** An increase in abdominal pressure may force the intestines through the internal ring into the inguinal canal & may follow the testicle & spermatic cord tract into the scrotum in men; may tract to the labia majora in women.

CLINICAL MANIFESTATIONS
- <u>Asymptomatic:</u> swelling or fullness at the hernia site. Enlarges with increased intrabdominal pressure and/or standing. **May develop scrotal swelling.**
- <u>**Incarcerated:**</u> **painful, enlargement of an irreducible hernia** (unable to return the hernia contents back into the abdominal cavity). Nausea & vomiting if bowel obstruction present.
- <u>**Strangulated:**</u> **ischemic incarcerated hernias with systemic toxicity** (irreducible hernia with compromised blood supply). Severe painful bowel movement (may refrain defecation).

DIAGNOSIS
- Clinical. Groin ultrasound often the initial imaging of choice of an occult uncomplicated inguinal hernia. CT or MRI are alternatives.

MANAGEMENT
- Inguinal hernias often require surgical repair. Strangulated hernias are surgical emergencies.

DIRECT INGUINAL HERNIAS
- Type of inguinal hernia with bowel protrusion where the origin of the sac is **MEDIAL to the inferior epigastric artery within Hesselbach's triangle.** When you send a **D**irect **M**essage (DM – Direct is Medial). Directly behind the superficial inguinal ring due to a defect of the transversalis fascia.
- <u>**Hesselbach's triangle:**</u> "RIP" — **R**ectus Abdominis: medial border. **I**nferior epigastric vessels: lateral border. **P**oupart's (inguinal) ligament: inferior border.
- <u>Pathophysiology:</u> occurs as a result of weakness in the floor of the inguinal canal through weakened fascia in the abdominal wall (defect of the transversalis fascia).
- Most commonly found on the right side; more common in middle aged to older men.

CLINICAL MANIFESTATIONS
- <u>Asymptomatic:</u> swelling or fullness at the hernia site. Enlarges with increased intrabdominal pressure and/or standing.
- <u>**Incarcerated:**</u> **painful, enlargement of an irreducible hernia** (unable to return the hernia contents back into the abdominal cavity). Nausea & vomiting if bowel obstruction present
- <u>**Strangulated:**</u> **ischemic incarcerated hernias** with **systemic toxicity** (irreducible hernia with compromised blood supply). Severe painful bowel movement (may refrain defecation).

DIAGNOSIS
- Clinical. Groin ultrasound often the initial imaging of choice of an occult uncomplicated inguinal hernia. CT or MRI are alternatives.

MANAGEMENT
- Inguinal hernias often require surgical repair. Strangulated hernias are surgical emergencies.

FEMORAL HERNIAS

- Protrusion of the contents of the abdominal cavity through the femoral canal (below the inguinal ligament).
- **Most commonly seen in women.** They occur later in life compared to inguinal hernias.
- **Because the femoral ring is smaller in women, Femoral hernias often become incarcerated or strangulated** compared to inguinal hernias.
- **Most commonly located in the upper thigh,** medial to the femoral vein.

UMBILICAL HERNIAS

- Hernia through the umbilical fibromuscular ring. Congenital (failure of umbilical ring closure).
- Usually due to loosening of the tissue around the ring in adults.

MANAGEMENT

- Observation: usually resolves by 2 years of age.
- **Surgical repair may be indicated if still persistent in <u>children 5 years of age or older</u>** to avoid incarceration or strangulation.

INCISIONAL (VENTRAL) HERNIAS

- Herniation through weakness in the abdominal wall.
- Incisional hernias most commonly occur with vertical incisions and in obese patients due to breakdown of the fascial closure from prior surgery.

OBTURATOR HERNIAS

- Rare hernia through the pelvic floor in which abdominal/pelvic contents protrude through the obturator foramen.
- Most common in women (especially multiparous) or women with significant weight loss.

LATERAL VENTRAL (SPIGELIAN) HERNIAS

- Defect through the spigelian fascia, bulge often **lateral to the rectus abdominus.** Rare.
- High strangulation risk. Most common on the right side.

CHAPTER 4 – MUSCULOSKELETAL SYSTEM

ANTIPHOSPHOLIPID SYNDROME (APS)

- **Idiopathic disorder characterized by <u>recurrent venous or arterial thromboses</u> or small-vessel thrombosis due to antibodies against negatively charged phospholipids.**
- Can occur as a primary disease or in the setting of other diseases, such as other autoimmune disorders, eg, **Systemic lupus erythematosus (~35%).** More common in women.

PATHOPHYSIOLOGY
- The autoantibodies react against platelet membranes or prothrombin-platelet membrane complex, activating endothelial cells, platelets, and complement-mediated thrombosis.
- <u>Triggers:</u> smoking, prolonged immobilization, estrogen (eg, oral contraceptive use, pregnancy, postpartum period, hormone replacement therapy), malignancy, hyperlipidemia, and Hypertension.

CLINICAL MANIFESTATIONS
- **<u>Increased risk of venous & arterial thromboses:</u> <u>venous</u>: recurrent DVT (most common) PE, or atypical sites; <u>arterial</u>: atherosclerosis, TIA, cerebrovascular accidents, recurrent fetal loss.**
- <u>Pregnancy complications</u> including spontaneous abortions ≥10 weeks' gestational age, preterm birth, or complications due to eclampsia, pre-eclampsia, or placental insufficiency; or ≥3 spontaneous abortions <10 weeks' gestational age.
- Livedo reticularis, skin ulcers, valvular heart disease, neurologic symptoms (eg, stroke, TIA, cognitive defects, mental status changes), thrombocytopenia, mental status changes, microangiopathic nephropathy, and cardiac valvular thickening &/or vegetations.

<u>Physical examination:</u>
- Cutaneous findings include livedo reticularis — reticular (lacy) or mottled violaceous rash.

DIAGNOSIS
<u>Antiphospholipid antibody testing:</u>
- **<u>Anticardiolipin antibodies:</u> IgG and IgM** by enzyme-linked immunosorbent assay (ELISA). Associated with **false-positive testing for Syphilis — positive RPR or VDRL** with a negative confirmatory FTA-ABS because the screening tests (RPR and VDRL) contain cardiolipin.
- **Anti-Beta-2 glycoprotein 1 autoantibodies** IgG & IgM.
- **<u>Lupus anticoagulant:</u> <u>increased partial thromboplastin time (PTT)</u> but associated with thrombosis.** Despite its name, lupus anticoagulant positivity is associated with hypercoagulability.

<u>Other testing:</u>
- <u>Coagulation studies:</u> Normal or slightly prolonged prothrombin time (PT), normal bleeding time. **Prolonged PTT due to the presence of lupus anticoagulant.** Thrombocytopenia may be seen but does not decrease the risk of thrombosis.
- **<u>Mixing studies:</u> <u>failure to correct PTT after mixing</u>** the patient's blood with normal plasma due to the **presence of an inhibitor** (unlike clotting deficiency disorders where mixing study corrects PTT).
- **<u>Prolonged Russell viper venom test:</u> most specific for lupus anticoagulant.** In the presence of a lupus anticoagulant, the RVVT is prolonged and does not correct with mixing studies but does with the addition of excess phospholipid. Official diagnosis requires 2 positive results with samples taken at least 12 weeks apart.
- <u>CBC:</u> thrombocytopenia is common (usually <100,000) but does not reduce the risk of thrombosis.

MANAGEMENT
- **<u>Asymptomatic patients</u> do not need to be treated (pregnant and nonpregnant patients).**
- **<u>Nonpregnant patients:</u> <u>Lifelong Warfarin therapy</u> remains the cornerstone for long-term treatment APS with thromboses (Target INR 2-3).** In patients who experience recurrent arterial or venous thrombosis despite therapeutic range INR, options can include (1) higher intensity Warfarin (INR 3–4) or (2) switching to Low molecular weight Heparin (eg, Enoxaparin).
- DOACs are not recommended as they are less effective than Warfarin in managing APS.
- **<u>Pregnancy (or history of fetal loss):</u> Low molecular weight Heparin (eg, Enoxaparin) plus low-dose Aspirin** to prevent fetal loss during pregnancy and can be given up to 8-12 weeks postpartum.

SYSTEMIC LUPUS ERYTHEMATOSUS (SLE)

- **Idiopathic, chronic systemic, multi-organ autoimmune inflammatory disorder characterized by autoantibodies to nuclear antigens that can affect virtually any organ.**
- **Primarily a Type III hypersensitivity reaction** due to antigen-antibody immune complexes.

RISK FACTORS
- **Increased estrogen: most common in females of reproductive age** (onset 20-40s), oral contraceptive use, hormone replacement therapy.
- Increased in Black, Hispanic, & Native American women.
- Genetic: high frequency in DR2 and DR3 haplotypes, other autoimmune disorders, ⊕ family history.
- Environmental: eg, **sunlight exposure,** infections, medications.

PATHOPHYSIOLOGY
- Interaction between immune dysfunction as well as genetic and environmental factors.
- **Type III hypersensitivity reaction** (antigen-antibody immune complexes) – autoantibodies precipitate immune complexes in multiple organs, including the kidneys, skin, brain.
- Polyclonal activation of B cells with the production of autoantibodies against DNA. Complement factors and cytokines also play a key role.

CLINICAL MANIFESTATIONS
- **Constitutional symptoms: fatigue (most common),** fever, chills, night sweats, malaise, weight loss.
- **Triad: [1] joint pain + [2] fever + [3] malar "butterfly" photosensitive rash is classic for SLE.**
- **Mucocutaneous:** 4 types of rashes — [1] photosensitive rash over areas exposed to sunlight; [2] **Malar rash: raised or flat erythematous "butterfly rash" on cheeks/nose and spares nasolabial folds after sun exposure most common;** [3] **discoid lesions: erythematous raised plaques with keratotic scale and follicular plugging that tend to scar,** and [4] **oral &/or nasal ulcers,** which are usually painless. Alopecia is usually nonscarring (may scar with Discoid lupus).
- **Musculoskeletal:** Joint symptoms (eg, arthralgias) with or without active synovitis (>90%) are often the earliest manifestations. Myalgias are common. Arthritis is often migratory, polyarticular, and symmetrical. Usually does not cause joint erosion and is rarely deforming. Osteoporosis.
- **Hematologic:** anemia, leukopenia, thrombocytopenia, autoimmune hemolytic anemia, immune thrombocytopenia, and thrombotic thrombocytopenic purpura.
- **Discoid lupus: annular, erythematous patches on the face & scalp that heal with scarring.**
- **Serositis: pleuritis with or without pleural effusions, pericarditis with or without pericardial effusion (most common cardiac manifestation of SLE),** myocarditis.
- **Neurologic:** stroke, seizures, headaches, psychiatric or behavioral changes, cognitive impairment, delirium, psychosis, peripheral and cranial neuropathies, transverse myelitis, meningitis.
- **Kidney involvement:** 50% — associated with significant cause of morbidity & mortality. Hematuria, proteinuria, Nephrotic syndrome, Glomerulonephritis (eg, lupus nephritis), hypertension.
- Pulmonary: Pleuritis (with or without effusion). Pneumonitis, interstitial lung disease, pulmonary hypertension.
- Cardiovascular: may involve the pericardium, myocardium, valves, conduction system, and coronary arteries (increased risk of Coronary artery disease). Heart failure may result from myocarditis and hypertension. Cardiac arrhythmias. Verrucous (Libman-Sacks) endocarditis.
- Ocular: keratoconjunctivitis sicca, retinal vasculopathy (cotton wool spots, episcleritis, scleritis and optic neuropathy).
- Raynaud phenomenon: intermittent acral pallor followed by cyanosis and erythroderma.
- Vasculitis: cutaneous (eg, palpable purpura, petechiae, papulonodular lesions, livedo reticularis).
- Thromboembolic disease: arterial thrombotic event (ATE) or venous thrombotic event (VTE).
- **Glomerulonephritis, central nervous system disease, and complications of antiphospholipid antibodies are major sources of disease morbidity.**

DIAGNOSIS
- **Anti-nuclear antibodies (ANA):** initial screening test of choice for SLE — **most sensitive** (nearly 100%) **but not specific** (seen in many other autoimmune disorders as well as asymptomatic individuals). If the ANA is ⊕, test for specific antibodies (eg, anti-dsDNA, anti-Sm, Ro/SSA, La/SSB).
- **Anti-Smith: most specific for SLE** (more than anti-dsDNA) but not sensitive (present in only 30%).
- **Anti-double-stranded DNA (dsDNA): highly specific for SLE** but not sensitive (seen in only 70%). **During flares, dsDNA antibodies rise & complement decreases (C3, C4, CH50); dsDNA used in monitoring response to treatment** (response = decreased dsDNA & increased compliment).
- **Antiphospholipid antibodies: increased risk of arterial & venous thrombi** (eg, atherosclerosis & DVTs) — Anticardiolipin antibody, Lupus anticoagulant, & Anti–beta2 glycoprotein 1.
- Pancytopenia: anemia of chronic disease (more common), hemolytic anemia, leukopenia, lymphopenia & thrombocytopenia.
- **Decreased complement levels (eg, C3, C4, CH50) during disease flares**; often return toward normal in remission.
- Increased Erythrocyte sedimentation rate (ESR) and/or C-reactive protein (CRP) levels.
- Urinalysis: proteinuria or hematuria may indicate renal disease. Urine protein-to-creatinine ratio.
- Other autoantibodies: SSA/Ro, SSB/La, ribonucleoprotein (RNP). Neonatal lupus can cause heart block in babies of women with SLE expressing anti-Ro/SSA and anti-La/SSB.

MANAGEMENT
- All patients with lupus should receive education, counseling, and support; smoking cessation ideal.
- **Photoprotection:** UVA/UVB sunscreen while outdoors; avoidance of prolonged sun exposure.

Mild lupus: (skin, joint, &/or mucosal involvement).
- **Hydroxychloroquine with or without NSAIDs,** and/or short-term use of low-dose glucocorticoids.
- Milder skin lesions often respond to the topical administration of corticosteroids.
- Minor joint symptoms may often be alleviated by NSAIDs alone.

Moderate (significant but non-organ threatening disease):
- **Antimalarials (Hydroxychloroquine or Chloroquine) plus short-term glucocorticoid therapy helpful in reducing skin & joint manifestations. Hydroxychloroquine is the cornerstone of SLE management** because it reduces the incidence of disease flares and prolongs survival in SLE. **Adverse effects of Hydroxychloroquine: retinal toxicity**; neuropathy and myopathy are rare.

Severe [life or organ-threatening (eg, CNS, cardiac, or renal involvement)]:
- Indications for systemic glucocorticoids include Glomerulonephritis, hemolytic anemia, myocarditis, alveolar hemorrhage, central nervous system involvement, and severe thrombocytopenia.
- **High-dose oral glucocorticoids or intermittent IV "pulses" of Methylprednisolone** with other immunosuppressive agents (eg, Cyclophosphamide, Mycophenolate, Rituximab).
- Immunosuppressive agents (Cyclophosphamide, Mycophenolate mofetil, Azathioprine, Methotrexate, or Tacrolimus) are used for long-term control of disease.
- **Belimumab:** monoclonal antibody that inhibits B-lymphocyte stimulator binding to B cells, which inhibits B-cell survival. It was designed for SLE & is usually reserved for active antibody positive SLE cutaneous or musculoskeletal disease unresponsive to other therapies (eg, glucocorticoids or other immunosuppressive agents). Adverse effects: nausea, diarrhea, & respiratory tract infection.

Lupus nephritis:
- Induction phase & maintenance phase. **Induction phase: Mycophenolate mofetil** (1000 mg or 1500 mg orally twice daily) **or Cyclophosphamide** are first-line induction treatments for Lupus nephritis & are **generally given with corticosteroids to achieve disease control.** Belimumab (FDA approved drug for Lupus nephritis), can improve renal response when added to Cyclophosphamide or Mycophenolate mofetil. **Maintenance phase: Mycophenolate mofetil or Azathioprine.**
- When higher doses of Cyclophosphamide are required, gonadotropin-releasing hormone analogs can be given to protect a woman against the risk of premature ovarian failure.
- Rituximab is usually reserved for life-threatening or organ-threatening manifestations that have failed conventional therapies.

American College of Rheumatology has 11 classification criteria for lupus. If a patient meets at least four criteria, lupus can be diagnosed with 95% specificity and 85% sensitivity.

DIAGNOSTIC CRITERIA for SYSTEMIC LUPUS ERYTHEMATOSUS
At least 4 of the 11 needed

ANA SMITH was stranded on an island & developed a RASH when the RAIN made way for the sun

- **R**ash: Malar, Discoid, Oral ulcers, **Photosensitivity** (each count as 1)
- **A**rthritis
- **S**erositis: pericarditis, pleuritis, peritonitis
- **H**ematologic: hemolytic anemia, leukopenia, leukocytosis, thrombocytopenia

@pance_prep_pearls

- **R**enal disease: glomerulonephritis, proteinuria
- **A**nti-nuclear antibody (ANA)
- **I**mmunologic disorders: anti-double stranded DNA, anti-Smith, false-positive tests for syphilis (RPR, VDRL) with a negative FTA.
- **N**eurologic: seizures or psychosis in absence of any other causes.

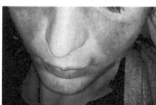 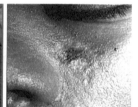

Malar (butterfly) rash   Discoid lupus

DRUG-INDUCED LUPUS (DIL)

- Autoimmune disorder similar to SLE caused by the use of certain drugs. Equal in males & females.
- **Procainamide (most common), Hydralazine, Isoniazid, Quinidine** (all high yield on exams).
- Methyldopa, Chlorpromazine, Pyrazinamide, D-penicillamine, Carbamazepine, Phenytoin, Minoxidil.
- **Minocycline**, particularly among young women being treated for Acne.

CLINICAL MANIFESTATIONS
- SLE-type symptoms: rash, fever, arthralgias, arthritis, myalgias, & serositis (pleuritis, pericarditis). Pleuritis is common especially with Procainamide not as much with Quinidine.
- Cutaneous manifestations less than with idiopathic SLE.
- Unlike SLE, DIL is <u>NOT</u> usually associated with alopecia, hematologic, kidney injury, CNS symptoms, or major organ-threatening complications.

DIAGNOSIS
- **Anti-histone antibodies are hallmark (>95%), especially in patients on Procainamide, Hydralazine, Quinidine, & Chlorpromazine. Positive Antinuclear antibodies (ANA).**
- Anti-Ro/SSA antibodies: >80% with drug-induced subacute cutaneous lupus erythematosus (SCLE).
- Hypocomplementemia & anti-double-stranded DNA antibodies are <u>not</u> usually seen.

MANAGEMENT
- **Discontinuation of the offending agent** is associated with resolution of the clinical manifestations of the disease usually within several weeks but sometimes up to several months after the offending drug has been discontinued. The ANAs often persist for a greater duration than the symptoms and physical findings, and in most patients, autoantibodies persist indefinitely.
- NSAIDs may be used for arthralgias & serositis. Topical corticosteroids for cutaneous symptoms.

SJÖGREN SYNDROME

- **Systemic autoimmune disease primarily affecting the <u>exocrine glands</u> (eg, salivary & lacrimal glands), primarily characterized primarily by <u>dryness of the mouth & eyes</u>.**
- <u>Primary:</u> occurs alone as a solitary process.
- <u>Secondary:</u> associated with other autoimmune disorders (eg, Hashimoto, SLE, Rheumatoid arthritis).
- Sjögren syndrome most common in females (90%), 40-60 years. Associated with HLA-DR52.
- Sjögren syndrome is one of the three most common systemic autoimmune diseases.

<u>PATHOPHYSIOLOGY</u>
- Inflammatory destruction of the exocrine glands characterized by focal lymphocytic infiltration (aggregation of lymphocytes, primarily CD4+ T-cells and memory cells) of the exocrine glands.

<u>CLINICAL MANIFESTATIONS</u>
- **<u>Dry mucous membranes</u>: dry mouth (xerostomia, from decreased saliva production), dry eyes** (keratoconjunctivitis sicca from **decreased tear production), vaginal dryness** (may present as **dyspareunia** from decreased vaginal secretions).
- <u>Constitutional:</u> generalized pain, fever, fatigue, weakness, sleep disturbances, anxiety, depression.
- <u>Extraglandular:</u> arthralgias, nonerosive arthritis, GI symptoms, Raynaud phenomenon, peripheral neuropathy. <u>ENT:</u> nasal dryness, chronic cough, sensorineural hearing loss; pericarditis; fever.
- <u>Complications:</u> **Increased risk of Non-Hodgkin lymphoma,** pneumonitis, interstitial nephritis.
Physical examination:
- <u>Ocular examination:</u> ocular dryness (xerophthalmia), conjunctivitis, corneal ulcers.
- <u>Oral examination:</u> decreased salivary pool, dry mucous membranes, soreness, ulceration. Dental caries, periodontal disease. **Bilateral parotid gland enlargement** (may be tender).

<u>DIAGNOSIS</u>
- **<u>Screening labs:</u> ⊕ Antinuclear antibodies (ANA), especially Anti SSA/Ro (most specific), Anti SSB/La are best initial tests.** Anti SSA/Ro, Anti SSB/La can cross the placenta and cause neonatal heart block in women with Sjögren syndrome. Rheumatoid factor may be positive.
- **<u>Ocular tests:</u> <u>Positive Schirmer test:</u> decreased tear production** (wetting of <5 mm of the filter paper placed in the lower eyelid for 5 minutes). **<u>Rose Bengal stain:</u>** abnormal corneal epithelium.
- **<u>Minor salivary gland (lip) biopsy</u> (or parotid gland biopsy) criterion standard to confirm the diagnosis.** Findings include gland fibrosis, lymphocytic infiltration, glandular & ductal atrophy.
- <u>Other labs:</u> positive Rheumatoid factor (RF), anemia, leukopenia, ↑ESR, hypergammaglobulinemia.
- <u>Oral tests:</u> Salivary flow rate, sialochemistry, sialography, or scintigraphy (all are seldom used).

<u>MANAGEMENT</u>
- **<u>Lifestyle:</u> increase mucosal secretions — artificial tears to prevent corneal ulcers, increase fluid intake,** sugar-free gum, artificial saliva, and fluoride treatments. Vitamin D supplementation because Vitamin D deficiency may increase the risk of neuropathy & lymphoma. Cyclosporine ophthalmic.
- **<u>Cholinergic drugs</u> (muscarinic agonists) Pilocarpine or Cevimeline** lead to increased secretions in patients with dry eyes and dry mouth. Anticholinergics and decongestants avoided if possible.

PILOCARPINE & CEVIMELINE

- <u>Mechanism of action:</u> **Cholinergic (muscarinic) drug that increases lacrimation and salivation.**
- <u>Indications:</u> **Sjögren syndrome (improves dry mouth and dry eyes).** Topical used for Acute angle-closure glaucoma (causes pupillary constriction, opening the angle).
Cholinergic (muscarinic) adverse effects:
- **Diaphoresis, flushing, sweating, bradycardia, diarrhea, nausea, vomiting, incontinence, blurred vision, and bronchoconstriction.** Cevimeline has less effect on cardiac and lung tissues.
- Think SLUDD-C (**S**alivation, **L**acrimation, **U**rination, **D**efecation, **D**igestion, **C**onstriction of pupil).

DERMATOMYOSITIS (DM)

- Idiopathic autoimmune disorder leading to **dermatologic manifestations + muscle inflammation,** primarily involving the proximal limbs, neck, and pharynx.
- May affect the heart, lungs & GI tract. **Associated with cancer in 25% of cases** — eg, lung, ovarian, breast, colorectal, cervical, bladder, esophageal, pancreatic, and renal cancer.

PATHOPHYSIOLOGY
- Inflammatory myopathy due to **CD4+ lymphocyte infiltration of the perimysium (perivascular involvement).**

CLINICAL MANIFESTATIONS
- **Progressive symmetric proximal muscle weakness (shoulders, hips)** — may have difficulty combing hair, raising arms, rising from a chair, and climbing stairs due to weakness (similar to PM).
- Distal muscle weakness, if present, tends to be milder than proximal muscle weakness and usually does not cause significant functional impairment. Muscle pain and tenderness are uncommon.
- Systemic symptoms: dysphagia, polyarthralgia, low-grade fever, fatigue, weight loss.

PHYSICAL EXAMINATION
- **Decreased muscle strength** — especially the proximal muscles, often symmetrical (due to muscle inflammation). Muscle atrophy may be present.

Skin findings in Dermatomyositis:

Gottron papules and the heliotrope eruption are pathognomonic features of Dermatomyositis.
- **Gottron papules: raised violaceous scaly patches on** extensors surfaces of fingers, elbows, & knees.
- **Heliotrope rash: edema & blue or purple discoloration of the upper eyelids.**
- Malar rash that involves the nasolabial folds (unlike SLE), Photosensitive poikiloderma: shawl sign (erythema of the shoulder, upper chest and back) or V sign (erythema of the neck & upper chest). Holster sign: changes on the lateral aspect of the thigh.
- Nailfold changes, scalp involvement, and calcinosis cutis.

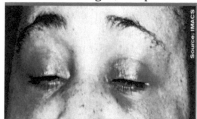
Heliotrope rash: eyelids.

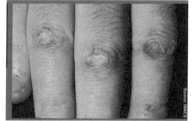
Gottron papules

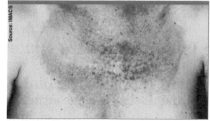
Poikiloderma

DIAGNOSIS
- **Elevated muscle enzymes best initial test** — **creatine kinase (CK), aldolase,** aspartate aminotransferase (AST), and alanine aminotransferase (ALT), lactate dehydrogenase (LDH).
- **Autoantibodies: Anti Jo-1 [myositis-specific antibody associated with interstitial lung fibrosis and "mechanic hands"** (hyperkeratotic palms with dirty appearance)] seen in both PM and DM. **Anti-Mi-2 more associated with DM.**
- Positive ANA. Increased ESR & CRP, Rheumatoid factor. Normocytic normochromic anemia.
- Abnormal electromyography.
- **Muscle biopsy: definitive diagnosis** (most accurate) — **CD4+ lymphocyte infiltration of the perimysium (perivascular involvement).**

MANAGEMENT
- **High-dose glucocorticoids are the cornerstone of initial therapy for Dermatomyositis and PM.**
- Sun protection for all patients.
- **Hydroxychloroquine useful for skin lesions** with no benefit to muscle disease.
- Steroid-sparing agents: either Azathioprine or Methotrexate (see Polymyositis).

POLYMYOSITIS (PM)

- Idiopathic autoimmune disorders leading to **muscle inflammation,** primarily involving the proximal limbs, neck, and pharynx. May affect the heart, lungs, & GI tract. Most common in women 30-50y.
- Inflammatory myopathy due to <u>**CD8+ lymphocyte infiltration of the endomysium.**</u>

CLINICAL MANIFESTATIONS

- **Progressive symmetric <u>proximal skeletal muscle weakness</u> (shoulders, hips)** evolving over weeks to months — may have difficulty combing hair, raising arms, rising from a chair, carrying bags, and climbing stairs due to weakness. In more severe cases, weakness of the neck flexors (head drop), pharyngeal weakness (dysphagia), and diaphragmatic weakness (respiratory compromise).
- <u>Systemic symptoms:</u> dysphagia, polyarthralgia, inflammatory arthritis (joint pain and swelling).
- <u>Constitutional symptoms:</u> low-grade fever, fatigue, weight loss. Muscle pain & tenderness uncommon.

Physical examination:
- **<u>Decreased muscle strength</u> — especially the <u>proximal</u> girdle muscles** (eg, proximal arm muscles, especially the deltoids & neck flexors, with biceps and triceps often involved; hip flexors are the most commonly affected leg muscles but hamstrings & quadricep weakness also common), often symmetrical due to muscle inflammation. Muscle atrophy may be present.

DIAGNOSIS

- **<u>Elevated muscle enzymes</u> best initial tests — creatine kinase (CK), aldolase,** aspartate aminotransferase (AST), and alanine aminotransferase (ALT), lactate dehydrogenase (LDH).
- <u>Autoantibodies:</u>
  - **<u>Anti Jo-1</u> myositis-specific antibody often associated with interstitial lung fibrosis and "mechanic hands" (hyperkeratotic palms with a dirty appearance)** seen in both PM and DM.
  - **<u>Anti-signal recognition protein</u> more associated with PM.** Antinuclear antibodies (ANA).
- Increased ESR, CRP, positive Rheumatoid factor. Abnormal electromyography.
- **<u>Muscle biopsy</u>: definitive diagnosis (most accurate) — <u>endomysial inflammation (CD8+).</u>***

MANAGEMENT

- **High-dose glucocorticoids are the cornerstone of initial therapy for DM and Polymyositis (PM).** Glucocorticoid therapy improves strength and preserves muscle function (eg, Prednisone 1 mg/kg per day, to a maximum daily dose of 80 mg). Pulse Methylprednisolone (1,000 mg per day for 3 days) may be used at the initiation of therapy for severely ill patients.
- **Steroid-sparing agents: either Azathioprine or Methotrexate** are (1) generally initiated with glucocorticoid treatment to reduce the cumulative dose of Prednisone to reduce glucocorticoid-induced morbidity or (2) first-line agents in patients in whom glucocorticoids are contraindicated. Azathioprine preferred if contraindications to Methotrexate (eg, interstitial lung disease, underlying liver disease, or individuals unwilling to abstain from alcohol) due to Methotrexate adverse effects.
- <u>Azathioprine adverse effects</u>: flu-like reaction (eg, fever GI symptoms), bone marrow suppression, pancreatitis, and liver toxicity. Long-term adverse effects may include increased risk of malignancy.
- <u>Methotrexate adverse effects</u>: stomatitis, GI symptoms, & leukopenia, (reduced with Folic acid or Leucovorin). Hepatotoxicity & pulmonary toxicity (eg, Pneumonitis).
- <u>Intravenous immune globulin</u> added to glucocorticoids may be used in selected patients with severe life-threatening weakness or patients with severe dysphagia at risk for aspiration.

EXAM TIP: Polymyalgia rheumatica (PMR) vs. Polymyositis (PM)
- Both can have hip and shoulder pain, difficulty rising from chair and combing their hair.
- **Polymyositis: <u>decreased muscle strength</u> on physical examination,** symmetrical proximal muscle weakness reproducible on physical exam (decreased muscle strength), **elevated muscle enzymes (creatinine kinase & aldolase),** abnormal EMG.
- **Polymyalgia rheumatica <u>normal muscle strength</u>** (no objective weakness on examination) with decreased range of motion of the joints & **normal muscle enzymes.**

POLYMYALGIA RHEUMATICA (PMR)

- **Idiopathic inflammation of the joints, bursae, and tendons** (eg, shoulder & hip girdle).
- **Closely associated with Giant cell arteritis (GCA);** can occur alone or as part of GCA.
- **Most common >50 years of age,** women, Caucasians (>90%).

CLINICAL MANIFESTATIONS
- **Pain & stiffness** in the proximal joints — **shoulder & hip girdles, neck, torso, & lower back. Worse with inactivity & after immobilization, resulting in nocturnal bilateral aching, pain, and stiffness and morning predominance, with morning stiffness >45 minutes,** often >2 weeks. The shoulders and arms are more commonly involved (70–95%) than the hips and thighs (50–70%). May have difficulty combing hair & rising from a chair.
- Constitutional symptoms: fatigue, malaise, anorexia, weight loss, low-grade fever.
- **Absence of cranial manifestations** (headache, visual changes) distinguish PMR from GCA.

PHYSICAL EXAMINATION
- **Decreased active and passive range of motion of the shoulders, hip, and neck.**
- **Absent of cranial symptoms.** Headache, jaw claudication, or vision changes suggest coexisting GCA.
- **Normal muscle strength** no muscle inflammation or objective weakness.
- Swelling, erythema, or warmth are usually absent.

DIAGNOSIS
- **Primarily a clinical diagnosis. Increased CRP & ESR.** Normocytic normochromic anemia.
- Normal muscle enzymes (eg, creatine kinase & aldolase) distinguishes PMR from Polymyositis.

MANAGEMENT
- **Low-dose corticosteroids initial treatment of choice** (eg, 10-25 mg/day), associated with rapid response. After ~4 weeks, on the initial dose, Prednisone is gradually tapered over 9–12 months.
- Methotrexate alternative if corticosteroids are contraindicated. IL-6R blockade with Tocilizumab.

FIBROMYALGIA

- A disorder characterized by abnormal pain perception of unknown etiology.
- **Most common in women 20-55 years.** Increased incidence with history of autoimmunity.

PATHOPHYSIOLOGY
- Patients with Fibromyalgia have altered pain processing compared to normal individuals — eg, increased subjective sensitivity to pain, enhanced CNS pain processing, increased substance P.

CLINICAL MANIFESTATIONS
- **Pain: chronic, widespread multisite musculoskeletal pain & stiffness.**
- **Nonrestful sleep & cognitive disturbances** (fibro fog), headache, neurologic symptoms (eg, numbness).
- **Extreme fatigue:** persistent, moderate-severe mental or physical fatigue worse with mild exertion.
- **Psychiatric disturbances:** 30-50% have Anxiety and/or Depression at the time of diagnosis.

DIAGNOSIS
- Primarily a clinical diagnosis. Associated with normal laboratory tests. Sleep studies show no REM cycle.
- **Tenderness in at least 11 out of 18 trigger points + chronic pain ≥3 months.** Normal labs.

MANAGEMENT
- **Conservative measures:** multidisciplinary approach: patient education, sleep hygiene, **low-impact aerobic exercise (swimming & water aerobics,** walking, & biking), cognitive behavioral therapy.
- Medical: **Low-dose Tricyclic antidepressants (eg, Amitriptyline) first-line medical agent in patients not responsive to conservative measures. Prominent fatigue: SNRI (eg, Duloxetine) or Milnacipran. Pregabalin** especially helpful for sleep disturbances (Gabapentin alternative).

SYSTEMIC SCLEROSIS (SCLERODERMA)

Systemic autoimmune connective tissue disorder characterized by:
- **[1] <u>fibrosis of the skin</u>**, muscles, soft tissues, & internal organs (eg, lung, heart, kidney, & GI tract).
- **[2] <u>vascular dysfunction</u>** eg, Raynaud phenomenon and Pulmonary arterial hypertension.

PATHOPHYSIOLOGY
- <u>Sclerosis:</u> excessive deposition of collagen & other elements of the extracellular matrix in skin & internal organs, fibroproliferation of microvasculature causing a noninflammatory vasculopathy, and chronic inflammation resulting in fibrosis.
- Most common in women 30–50 years of age. Older age, males, & African Americans have ↑mortality.

2 MAIN TYPES
- **[1] <u>Limited:</u> 80% — characterized by tight, shiny, thickened skin confined only to the face, neck, as well as <u>distal to the elbows & knees.</u>** Spares the trunk. Pulmonary hypertension with advanced disease. **C**alcinosis cutis, **R**aynaud's phenomenon: red-white-blue vasospastic changes of the digits, **E**sophageal motility disorder, **S**clerodactyly (claw hand), **T**elangiectasias (CREST features). Less severe multisystemic internal organ involvement compared to Diffuse scleroderma.

- **[2] <u>Diffuse:</u> (20%) — tight, shiny, thickened skin involving the <u>trunk & proximal extremities.</u> Associated with greater internal organ involvement** (eg, restrictive lung disease due pulmonary fibrosis, myocardial fibrosis, renal involvement). May have some of the "CREST" features (eg, RP).

DIAGNOSIS
- **<u>Anti-centromere antibodies:</u> associated with & specific for Limited Scleroderma.**
- **<u>Anti-SCL-70 antibodies (anti-topoisomerase) I:</u> associated with diffuse Scleroderma & multiple organ involvement.** Poorer prognosis than limited.
- <u>ANA:</u> nonspecific but sensitive — positive in >90% in patients with Scleroderma.

MANAGEMENT: Treatment is organ specific:
- <u>Skin (without visceral involvement):</u> Methotrexate or Mycophenolate for progressive skin sclerosis.
- <u>GERD:</u> Proton pump inhibitors (PPIs).
- <u>Hypertensive renal disease:</u> ACE inhibitors, especially if ⊕ RNA polymerase III autoantibodies.
- <u>Raynaud:</u> vasodilators — calcium channel blockers. Prostacyclin (prostaglandin).
- <u>Severe:</u> DMARDs: Methotrexate or Mycophenolate. Cyclophosphamide reserved for refractory cases.
- <u>Pulmonary fibrosis:</u> Mycophenolate preferred (greater efficacy & safety) over Cyclophosphamide.
- <u>Pulmonary hypertension:</u> Bosentan, Sildenafil, Prostacyclin analogues.

BEHÇET'S SYNDROME

- Multisystemic autoimmune disorder characterized by **<u>recurrent, painful oral & genital ulcers</u>** (aphthous), **erythema nodosum**, eye (**uveitis,** conjunctivitis), arthritis, & CNS involvement (may mimic Multiple sclerosis). Initial presentation usually 20-40 years.
- **Increased incidence in Asian or Middle Eastern or Mediterranean persons.**

DIAGNOSIS
- **Primarily a clinical diagnosis.** Increased ESR, CRP, and leukocytes.
- **<u>Pathergy</u> = sterile skin papules or pustules from minor trauma (eg, needle stick)** – less common in patients from N. America or N. Europe.
- <u>Biopsy</u> for definitive diagnosis (leukocytoclastic vasculitis or lymphocytic vasculitis).

MANAGEMENT
- **<u>Corticosteroids</u> during flares.** Other options include Colchicine, Cyclophosphamide, Azathioprine.

TAKAYASU ARTERITIS

- Chronic <u>large-vessel granulomatous vasculitis</u> **that affects the aorta & its primary branches (aortic arch & pulmonary arteries)** — causes vascular stenoses &/or dilation.
- <u>Risk factors:</u> **young women — women (80-90%), age of onset 10-40 years; Asian descent.**

CLINICAL MANIFESTATIONS
- <u>Constitutional:</u> (early symptoms) — weight loss, low-grade fever, fatigue, myalgia, arthralgia.
- **Vessel ischemia:** coronary arteries, carotid arteries (TIA, stroke), renal artery (hypertensive crisis), **Extremity claudication: Upper extremity claudication** (exertional arm fatigue & pain due to subclavian artery involvement) develops more often than lower extremity. Aneurysm rupture.
- <u>Cardiac involvement:</u> Volume overload (eg, aortic insufficiency), pressure overload (eg, Hypertension due to aortic narrowing or renal artery stenosis), Myocardial ischemia (eg, coronary arteritis causing angina), and myocarditis may lead to LV dysfunction.

Physical examination:
- <u>Vascular:</u> **Bruits** (carotid, subclavian, or abdominal), **diminished/absent pulses, asymmetric blood pressure measurements between arms (>10 mmHg), Hypertension,** Peripheral arterial disease.

DIAGNOSIS
- **Angiography [MRA (preferred) or CTA] necessary to confirm diagnosis** and extent of the disease.
- <u>Nonspecific:</u> may have increased ESR, CRP, normochromic, normocytic anemia, leukocytosis.
- **Definitive diagnosis requires vascular imaging (eg, MRI/MRA, CTA) showing narrowing or occlusion of the aorta and/or its primary branches** or biopsy (seldomly used).

MANAGEMENT
- **Moderate to high-dose corticosteroids mainstay (with or without an immunosuppressant).**
- **Immunosuppressant: Methotrexate or Azathioprine;** Mycophenolate, Leflunomide. Biologic agents.
- Revascularization if thrombosis or occlusion (eg, coronary artery) and thoracic aortic aneurysms.

KAWASAKI SYNDROME (MUCOCUTANEOUS LYMPH NODE SYNDROME)

- Medium & small vessel necrotizing vasculitis which may include the **coronary arteries;** self-limited.
- Thought due to a respiratory agent or viral pathogen with a propensity towards vascular tissue.

Risk factors:
- **Children 3 months–5 years, boys, & Asian descent, especially Japanese** (highest risk).

DIAGNOSIS
Warm + CREAM = high-grade fever (over 39°-40°C) **at least 5 DAYS + 4 of the following 5:**
- **Conjunctivitis: bilateral nonexudative conjunctivitis** (begins shortly after the onset of fever).
- **Rash: polymorphous rash** (eg, erythematous or morbilliform or macular).
- **Extremity changes: edema, erythema, or desquamation of palms & soles** (acute phase), periungual desquamation 2-3 weeks after fever onset; Beau's lines (transverse nail grooves), arthritis.
- **Adenopathy (cervical)** >1.5 cm, usually unilateral, involving the **anterior cervical nodes.**
- **Mucositis: strawberry tongue;** lip swelling or fissures or cracking, pharyngeal erythema (no ulcers).
- <u>Labs:</u> nonspecific — elevated WBC and platelet counts, transaminases, and acute-phase reactants (eg, ESR & CRP), as well as anemia and sterile pyuria, are suggestive of KD.
- <u>Complications:</u> **coronary vessel arteritis: coronary artery aneurysm,** myocardial infarction, pericarditis, myocarditis. **Echocardiogram & ECG are recommended to look for complications.**

MANAGEMENT
- **IV Immunoglobulin + Aspirin:** IVIG reduces coronary complications. A single dose of IVIG given ideally in the first 10 days of the illness. IVIG still beneficial if >10 days + ↑ESR, CRP, persistent fever, or presence of coronary artery aneurysms. Aspirin (anti-inflammatory & anti-platelet activity).
- If increased risk of IVIG resistance, glucocorticoids may be added to initial IVIG therapy.

POLYARTERITIS NODOSA (PAN)

- **Systemic vasculitis primarily of medium-sized arteries & muscular arterioles (necrotizing).**
- Most commonly affects the vessels of the skin, peripheral nerves, GI tract, & kidneys.
- PAN differs from other systemic vasculitis with [1] confinement to arteries only, [2] **sparing of the lung**, [3] absence of granulomatous inflammation, & [4] lack of any association with a known autoantibody.

PATHOPHYSIOLOGY
- Type III hypersensitivity reaction leads to ischemia & microaneurysms of the affected vessels.
- Most common in men 40-60 years of age. **Increased association with chronic Hepatitis B & C.**

CLINICAL MANIFESTATIONS
- Constitutional symptoms: fever, chills, arthralgia, arthritis, myalgias, malaise, weight loss, weakness.
- Derm: lower extremity nodules, papules, & ulcers; **livedo reticularis, (starburst),** purpura, Raynaud.
- **Renal: Renin-mediated Hypertension** (due to renal ischemia), proteinuria, &/or hematuria, **no** RBC casts. Because PAN spares small blood vessels (capillaries), PAN is **not** associated with glomerulonephritis, although it can cause renovascular hypertension & renal infarctions.
- **GI: postprandial abdominal pain** (intestinal angina), weight loss, nausea, vomiting, bowel infarction.
- **Neurologic: Mononeuritis multiplex. Multiple peripheral neuropathies** — peroneal nerve (foot drop) most common, sural, ulnar nerve, & radial, etc. CNS involvement includes stroke.

DIAGNOSIS
- Labs: increased ESR, proteinuria. Autoantibody tests are usually negative.
- **Classic PAN is ANCA negative.** In a minority of cases, P-ANCA is positive (<20%).
- **Renal or Mesenteric angiography: microaneurysms with abrupt cut-off of small arteries (beading).** The diagnosis requires either a tissue biopsy or an angiogram showing microaneurysms.
- **Biopsy:** (eg, skin) definitive — **necrotizing medium-vessel vasculitis & _no granulomas_.**

MANAGEMENT
- **Glucocorticoids mainstay of treatment.** Azathioprine or Methotrexate may be added if needed.
- Severe or refractory: Cyclophosphamide or biologic agents may be added to Glucocorticoids.
- **ACEIs or ARBs for Hypertension.** Treatment for HBV and possibly plasmapheresis if HBV-positive.

EOSINOPHILIC GRANULOMATOSIS WITH POLYANGIITIS [EGPA (CHURG-STRAUSS)]

- **Systemic small- & medium-sized granulomatous necrotizing vasculitis.**
- Can be a rare adverse effect of Montelukast and Zafirlukast.

CLINICAL MANIFESTATIONS
- **Triad: [1] Asthma + [2] peripheral eosinophilia (>10%) + [3] chronic rhinosinusitis.**
- Prodromal phase: **Asthma (>90%), atopic disease, allergic rhinitis, & nasal polyposis.** Adult-onset Asthma with no previous history of atopy or less commonly previously controlled Asthma becomes difficult to treat. Lung is the most common organ involved, followed by the skin.
- Eosinophilic phase: peripheral blood eosinophilia & organ infiltration (lung, skin, GI) — subcutaneous nodules, palpable purpura, ulcers, pulmonary opacities, abdominal pain, GI bleed, colitis.
- Vasculitic phase: constitutional symptoms (eg, fever, weight loss, malaise), **vasculitic neuropathy** (eg, Mononeuritis multiplex), Congestive heart failure is the most common cardiac manifestation.

DIAGNOSIS
- Labs: **eosinophilia & ⊕ P-ANCA (myeloperoxidase) hallmark.** ↑ESR, CRP, IgE, ⊕ rheumatoid factor.
- Biopsy: most accurate test — granulomatous necrotizing vasculitis without immune deposits.

MANAGEMENT
- **Nonsevere: Glucocorticoids mainstay of treatment** with or without Mepolizumab.
- **Severe: Glucocorticoids** with either Cyclophosphamide or Rituximab. Azathioprine for maintenance.

GRANULOMATOSIS WITH POLYANGIITIS [(GPA) WEGENER'S GRANULOMATOSIS]

- **Small vessel vasculitis (granulomatous inflammation) & necrosis** affecting the nose, lungs, & kidney.
- Silica exposure & α_1-antitrypsin deficiency increases risk of developing GPA.

CLINICAL MANIFESTATIONS

Triad: [1] upper respiratory tract + [2] lower respiratory tract + [3] Glomerulonephritis:

- **Upper respiratory tract & nose: nasal (90%)** — congestion, **saddle nose deformity, rhinorrhea with brown or bloody crusts,** nasal perforation, **rhinosinusitis. Otitis media,** mastoiditis, stridor.
- **Lower respiratory tract: lung involvement** — cough, dyspnea, hemoptysis, wheezing; pulmonary infiltrates, nodules, or cavitation on imaging (usually does not improve with antibiotics).
- **Glomerulonephritis: may be rapidly progressive (crescentic glomerulonephritis seen on biopsy).** Hematuria, **RBC casts,** proteinuria, rising serum creatinine.
- Other: **Cutaneous involvement** include purpura (especially the lower extremities). **Neurologic involvement** may include multiple mononeuropathy (Mononeuritis multiplex), sensory neuropathy, cranial nerve abnormalities, central nervous system mass lesions, external ophthalmoplegia, and sensorineural hearing loss. Polyarthralgias and arthritis.

DIAGNOSIS

- Chest radiograph: nonspecific changes (eg, nodules, cavitation) that resemble malignancy or infection.
- ⊕ **C-ANCA [anti-proteinase 3 (PR3)]: best initial lab test.** Cytoplasmic anti-nuclear cytoplasmic antibody positivity is hallmark (but not seen in all cases).
- Biopsy: definitive (lung preferred over sinus or kidney biopsy) — large **necrotizing granulomas.**

MANAGEMENT

- **Organ- or life-threatening:** Glucocorticoids PLUS either Rituximab or Cyclophosphamide.
- Non-organ- & non-life-threatening GPA not involving the kidney: initial therapy with Glucocorticoids combined with Methotrexate, rather than Cyclophosphamide or Rituximab.

MICROSCOPIC POLYANGIITIS (MPA)

- MPA is a [1] small & medium-vessel vasculitis **(predominantly small-sized artery vasculitis** but affects capillaries, arterioles, or venules [2] necrotizing vasculitis **with few or no immune deposits,** & [3] **tropism for the kidneys and lungs,** in addition to other organs.
- **MPA presents similar to GPA, except MPA is rarely associated with significant lung disease, has less ENT involvement (no destructive sinusitis,** less nasopharyngeal symptoms), ⊕ **P-ANCA,** & **not associated with granulomatous inflammation** (as in GPA & EGPA); MPA affects the capillaries & venules (capillary involvement not seen with PAN & PAN only affects arteries & arterioles).

CLINICAL MANIFESTATIONS

- 5 most common manifestations of MPA are glomerulonephritis (~80%), weight loss (>70%), mononeuritis multiplex (60%), fever (55%), and cutaneous vasculitis (>60%).
- Constitutional: **fever, weight loss,** migratory arthralgias or arthritis, malaise, fatigue.
- **Lung:** cough, dyspnea, **hemoptysis (alveolar hemorrhage** due to pulmonary capillitis in~12%).
- **Cutaneous involvement palpable purpura** (lower extremities), skin ulcers, papules.
- **Neurologic: Mononeuritis multiplex** (can cause sensory &/or motor symptoms).
- **Renal: acute glomerulonephritis — often rapidly progressive (crescentic).**

DIAGNOSIS

- ⊕ **P-ANCA [anti-neutrophil myeloperoxidase (MPO)] hallmark** — 55-75% of cases.
- Chest radiographs: nonspecific abnormalities. May show alveolar hemorrhage.
- Biopsy: criterion standard diagnosis — **non-granulomatous inflammation** (may be necrotic).

MANAGEMENT

- **Organ- or life-threatening:** Glucocorticoids PLUS either Rituximab or Cyclophosphamide.
- Non-organ- & non-life-threatening GPA not involving the kidney: initial therapy with Glucocorticoids combined with Methotrexate (rather than Cyclophosphamide or Rituximab).

	INCIDENCE	PATHOPHYSIOLOGY	CLINICAL	DIAGNOSIS	MANAGEMENT
Large vessels					
GIANT CELL (TEMPORAL) ARTERITIS	• **Older women** • **>50 years of age**	• **Cranial artery vasculitis** eg, temporal artery	• **Headache** • **Jaw claudication** • **Visual loss**	• ↑ESR, CRP • Clinical diagnosis • Temporal artery bx.	• **Corticosteroids (high dose)** • Tocilizumab

TAKAYASU ARTERITIS	• Young women <40y
	• Asians
		• **Aorta & primary branches**
		  • **aortic arch**
		  • **pulmonary arteries**
			• Vessel aneurysm (TIA, CVA, MI)
			• Extremity claudication
			• ↓pulses, hypertension
				Angiography
				• **(CTA or MRA)**
					• **Corticosteroids** (high dose)

Medium vessels — Affects arterioles					
KAWASAKI DISEASE	• **Children <5 years** • Asians	• Necrotizing vasculitis	• **"warm + CREAM"** • Coronary aneurysms	• Clinical diagnosis • ↑ESR, CRP	• **IVIG + Aspirin**
POLYARTERITIS NODOSA	• Males, >40 years • **Hepatitis B** associated	• Necrotizing vasculitis • Capillaries not involved	• CNS, GI, Derm, Renal • **Renovascular HTN** • **Lungs not involved**	• Angiogram negative • **ANCA negative** • **No granulomas**	• **Corticosteroids** • Methotrexate or Azathioprine
Small vessels: affects arterioles, venules, capillaries					
GRANULOMATOUS EOSINOPHILIC GPA	• Males, >40 years	• Necrotizing granulomatous	• <u>Triad:</u> **Asthma, Allergic rhinitis, Eosinophilia**	• ↑ eosinophils • ⊕ <u>**P-ANCA**</u>	• Corticosteroids • Cyclophosphamide • Mepolizumab
GRANULOMATOSIS WITH POLYANGIITIS (GPA) (WEGENERS)	• Men = women • Peaks 30-40 years	• Necrotizing granulomatous	<u>Triad:</u> • **Upper resp. tract** • **Lower resp. tract** • **Glomerulonephritis**	• ↑ESR, CRP • ⊕ <u>**C-ANCA**</u>	• **Corticosteroids PLUS Cyclophosphamide or Rituximab** • Steroids + MTX
NONGRANULOMATOUS MICROSCOPIC POLYANGIITIS (MPA)	• Males, >50 years	• Capillaries, arteries, veins	• Lung symptoms • Glomerulonephritis	• ⊕ <u>**P-ANCA**</u>	• **Corticosteroids PLUS Cyclophosphamide or Rituximab**
HENOCH-SCHONLEIN PURPURA (HSP)	• **Children 3-15 years**	• **IgA deposition vasculitis** • **Often postviral**	• <u>H</u>ematuria • <u>S</u>ynovial (arthritis) • <u>P</u>alpable purpura • <u>A</u>bdominal pain	• ↑IgA • Normal coags • Normal platelets • <u>UA:</u> RBCs, proteinuria	• <u>Supportive:</u> often self-limited.

IMMUNOGLOBULIN A (IgA) VASCULITIS [HENOCH-SCHÖNLEIN-PURPURA]

- Acute systemic IgA-mediated small-vessel vasculitis leading to **nonthrombocytopenic purpura**.
- **>90% occur in children**, especially 3-15 years of age; 10% in adults. More common in males.
- **Often occurs after infection** (eg, URI, GABHS, Parvovirus B-19).

PATHOPHYSIOLOGY
- The purpura is caused by inflammation the capillaries & venules of the superficial dermis as a result of IgA deposition in the affected organs, <u>not</u> due to thrombocytopenia or coagulopathy.

CLINICAL MANIFESTATIONS
4 cardinal symptoms: **HSP** affects Ig**A**:
- **H**ematuria (macroscopic or microscopic); Azotemia (↑BUN/Creatinine), proteinuria.
- **S**ynovial (**arthritis or arthralgia**) — hips, knees, & ankles most common; ±wrists, elbows, & hands.
- **P**alpable purpura, especially on the lower extremities and buttocks. Localized skin edema.
- **A**bdominal pain typically colicky & may worsen after eating ("intestinal angina"). GI bleeding.

DIAGNOSIS
- **Usually a clinical diagnosis** (biopsy usually not needed in most).
- Labs: **Usually normal PT, aPTT, & platelets** — the purpura is due to vasculitis, not due to thrombocytopenia or coagulopathy. 60% have an elevated serum IgA.
- Urine microscopy: normal or may show hematuria with or without RBC casts; mild or no proteinuria.
- Kidney biopsy: definitive diagnosis — **mesangial IgA deposits & leukocytoclastic vasculitis**.

MANAGEMENT
- **Supportive treatment mainstay** — oral hydration, bed rest, symptomatic relief of joint and abdominal pain (NSAIDs if no active GI bleeding, hematuria, or renal disease). Usually self-limited.
- Severe symptoms or progressive renal insufficiency may require hospitalization & glucocorticoids.

ANTIGLOMERULAR BASEMENT MEMBRANE (ANTI-GBM) ANTIBODY DISEASE [GOODPASTURE SYNDROME]

- <u>Type II hypersensitivity reaction:</u> IgG autoantibodies against type IV collagen of the [1] alveoli in the lungs & [2] glomerular basement membrane of the kidney.

CLINICAL MANIFESTATIONS
Symptoms limited to the lung & the kidney (Pulmonary-renal syndrome):
- **Lung:** hemoptysis (alveolar hemorrhage), dyspnea, dry cough, chest pain.
- **Kidney:** hematuria, oliguria, unexplained edema, elevated blood pressures.
- Systemic symptoms of vasculitides are usually absent or mild (fever weight loss, arthralgias, etc.)

DIAGNOSIS
- **Glomerulonephritis:** ↑BUN/creatinine, <u>UA</u>: **hematuria, dysmorphic RBCs, RBC casts,** proteinuria.
- ⊕ **anti-glomerular basement membrane (GBM) antibodies** — **best initial test after UA.**
- May have anemia (Iron deficiency anemia is common).
- Chest radiographs are usually abnormal but nonspecific (eg, diffuse bilateral alveolar infiltrates).
- **Biopsy of glomerulus or alveoli: definitive (criterion standard):**
  - **Linear IgG deposits** on immunofluorescence (anti-GBM antibodies & complement deposits).
  - **Kidney: Crescentic (rapidly progressive) glomerulonephritis.** Focal or segmental necrosis.

MANAGEMENT
- **Glucocorticoids PLUS Cyclophosphamide + Plasmapheresis first-line therapy.**

Think **G**ood**P**asture = ❶ **G**lomerulonephritis (rapidly progressing) + ❷ **P**ulmonary hemorrhage (hemoptysis) & Treatment also "GP".

SERONEGATIVE SPONDYLOARTHROPATHIES

- Joint diseases affecting the vertebral column, associated with **rheumatoid factor & ANA negativity.**

RISK FACTORS
- Most common in **young males, <40 years of age** at initial presentation, <u>**HLA-B27 positivity.**</u>
- **Characterized by axial skeleton involvement (vertebral column, sacroiliitis), uveitis, dactylitis, & enthesitis** (inflammation at the site of attachment of a tendon or ligament to the bone). Common sites of enthesitis includes the Achilles tendon, plantar fascia, pelvic bone, & epicondyles.

<u>DISEASES:</u> **PEAR** — **P**soriatic arthritis, **E**nteropathic arthritis (associated with Crohn or Ulcerative colitis), **A**nkylosing spondylitis, **R**eactive arthritis.

PSORIATIC ARTHRITIS (PsA)

- Chronic inflammatory arthritis in patients with Psoriasis affecting the skin, joints, and axial spine.
- 15-20% of patients with Psoriasis develop Psoriatic arthritis.
- 80% will have Psoriasis preceding the arthritis by months to years.

CLINICAL MANIFESTATIONS
- **Arthritis:** Asymmetric inflammatory oligoarthritis (<5 small and/or large joints). Distal arthritis may be asymmetric, symmetric, or clinically indistinguishable from Rheumatoid arthritis (RA) but **unlike RA, PsA often involves the DIP joint & often asymmetric.** May involve more joints.
- **Dactylitis** uniform swelling of the fingers or toes **(sausage digits).** Axial involvement.
- **Sacroiliitis & spondylitis:** lower back pain, neck, buttocks, hip pain, or thigh pain, worse after rest.
- **Enthesitis:** Achilles tendon, plantar fasciitis, medial & lateral epicondyles.
- <u>Ocular:</u> uveitis & conjunctivitis.
- **Psoriasis: erythematous plaques with thick silvery-white scales, nail pitting, and nail oil spots.**

DIAGNOSIS
- <u>Radiographs:</u> **best initial test — "pencil in a cup" deformities** (description of the appearance of the periarticular bony erosions & bone resorption). The bony erosions look like the thin end of one bone is being inserted into a thicker bone, similar to a pencil in a cup.

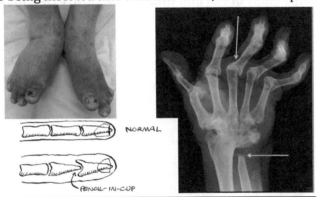

<u>Dactylitis:</u> **sausage-shaped digits**

<u>Radiographs:</u> **pencil in cup deformities**

- <u>Labs:</u> "usually negative" Rheumatoid factor and Antinuclear antibody (ANA) in most patients.

MANAGEMENT
- **Nonaxial (eg, Dactylitis, Enthesitis, Arthritis): NSAIDs initial management if mild oligoarticular disease (<5 joints) with no joint damage; TNF-inhibitor or nonbiologic DMARD (eg, Methotrexate) if no response to NSAIDs. TNF inhibitors preferred in severe arthritis** (eg, **Adalimumab, Golimumab, Etanercept;** alternatives include Infliximab or Certolizumab).
- **Mild axial disease: NSAIDs first-line therapy** (eg, Naproxen, Indomethacin, Celecoxib).
- **Moderate-severe axial disease: TNF-inhibitor (eg, Etanercept, Infliximab, Adalimumab);** IL-17 inhibitor (eg, Secukinumab or Ixekizumab); JAK inhibitor (Tofacitinib, Upadacitinib).

ENTEROPATHIC ARTHRITIS: associated with IBD: **Crohn, Ulcerative Colitis.**

ANKYLOSING SPONDYLITIS & NONRADIOGRAPHIC AXIAL SPONDYLOARTHRITIS

- Chronic inflammatory arthropathy of the axial skeleton — spine & sacroiliac joints with progressive stiffening of the spine (ankylosis = stiffness of joints due to fusion of the joints).

RISK FACTORS
- **Young males 15-30 years of age, HLA-B27 positivity.**

CLINICAL MANIFESTATIONS
- **Low back pain & neck pain:** insidious onset of back pain, stiffness, & decreased range of motion that is worse at night & in the morning, not improved with rest, & <u>improves</u> with exercise & activity. "Inflammatory" back pain (1) has insidious onset, (2) age of onset <40 years, (3) improves with exercise & activity, (4) not improved with rest, & (5) pain at night (with improvement upon arising). Progressive kyphosis & limitation of back motion over time, with limited chest expansion. Limited spine flexibility (positive Schober test).
- **Sacroiliitis & arthritis:** transient acute large joint arthritis — most commonly the ankles, hips, knees, shoulders, and the sternoclavicular joints.
- **Enthesopathy:** pain, stiffness, and tenderness of insertions, usually without much swelling at the Achilles tendon at its insertion or calcaneal attachment to the plantar fascia, (heel pain).
- **Dactylitis uniform swelling of the fingers & toes (sausage digits).**
- Extraarticular: **Anterior uveitis most common extraarticular manifestation of Ankylosing spondylitis** (eye pain, photophobia) in 25-35%. Inflammatory bowel disease (IBD), cardiac (eg, AV cardiac blocks, aortic regurgitation), Pulmonary fibrosis (decreased chest expansion).

DIAGNOSIS
- Labs: Increased ESR. **HLA-B27 positivity.** Negative serologies [eg, Rheumatoid factor (RF) & ANA].
- Radiographs:
  - **Radiograph of the SI joint often initial test ordered.** Findings include **sacroiliitis** — erosions, sclerosis, joint space widening or narrowing, and eventually, bony ankylosis (fusion).
  - **Bamboo spine = straightening of the spine (loss of normal lumbar curvature) + squaring & fusion of the vertebrae by bridging syndesmophytes is a classic but late finding.**

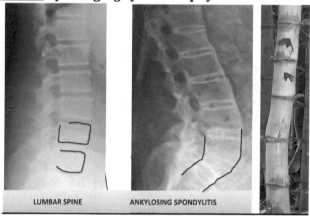

LUMBAR SPINE   ANKYLOSING SPONDYLITIS

- MRI: most accurate test.

MANAGEMENT
- **NSAIDs first line and may slow radiographic progression of spinal disease** (eg, Naproxen, Ibuprofen); exercise program, & physical therapy. If inadequate response, switch to a second NSAID.
- **Anti-TNF drugs used if no response to at least 2 NSAIDs consecutively** (eg, Etanercept, Adalimumab, Infliximab, Golimumab, Certolizumab).
- **IL-17 inhibitors** Secukinumab & Ixekizumab are alternatives to a TNF inhibitor as initial biologic.

REACTIVE ARTHRITIS

- Inflammatory arthritis due to cross reactive antibodies in response to an infection or inflammation in another part of the body (coexisting or recent antecedent extraarticular infection).
- **Seen 1-4 weeks after a gastrointestinal or genitourinary infection** [eg, *Chlamydia trachomatis* **(most common)**, *Salmonella, Shigella, Campylobacter, Yersinia, C. difficile*]. *C. pneumoniae.*
- ⊕ **HLA-B27** 50-80% of patients. Most common in young adults 20-40 years & males.

PATHOPHYSIOLOGY
- Although triggered by infection, organisms are generally not recovered or cultured from the affected joints — the arthritis is "reactive and aseptic" not "septic".

CLINICAL MANIFESTATIONS
- **Triad:** [1] **arthritis** + [2] **ocular (conjunctivitis, uveitis)** + [3] **genital (urethritis,** cervicitis, balanitis).
- Arthritis **asymmetric sterile mono- or oligoarthritis commonly involving the lower extremities (eg, knees, ankles),** associated with **enthesitis** — eg, swelling, warmth, & tenderness to the Achilles tendon or plantar fascia, **dactylitis:** fusiform swelling of the finger or toe, **inflammatory low back pain** — insidious in onset, worse after rest, improved with activity & exercise. Sacroiliitis.
- **Keratoderma blennorrhagicum — hyperkeratotic lesions on the palms & soles.**
- **Mucocutaneous: Circinate balanitis** — painless erythematous lesions with small, shallow ulcers on the glans penis & urethral meatus. **Painless oral mucosal ulcers.** Psoriasis-like nail changes — eg, onycholysis, subungual keratosis, or nail pits.

DIAGNOSIS
- **Arthrocentesis to rule out Septic arthritis** — findings of Reactive arthritis are similar to other inflammatory arthritides — increased WBC count but <50,000, predominantly neutrophils, & negative cultures & gram stain (no evidence of Septic arthritis — no organism recovered).
- Nonspecific: increased ESR. May show positive stool cultures or ⊕ Chlamydia NAAT. ⊕ **HLA-B27.**

MANAGEMENT
- **NSAIDs first-line treatment of Reactive arthritis** — eg, Naproxen, Diclofenac, Indomethacin.
- **Second-line: Intraarticular glucocorticoid injection.** If no response, switch to low-moderate dose of systemic glucocorticoids. If no response, nonbiological DMARD (Sulfasalazine; Methotrexate).
- Antibiotics do not reverse Reactive arthritis once the joint pain has begun but may be indicated to treat the underlying cause (eg, active ongoing *Chlamydia trachomatis*).

TUMOR MARKER	MAIN ASSOCIATIONS
ALPHA FETOPROTEIN	• **Hepatocellular carcinoma** • **Nonseminomatous germ cell testicular cancer** • Decreased in Down syndrome "AFP is down in Down syndrome"
Beta-hCG	• **Nonseminomatous germ cell testicular cancer** • **Choriocarcinoma,** Teratomas • **Trophoblastic tumors** (eg, Hydatidiform molar pregnancy)
CA-125	• **Ovarian cancer**
CA 19-9	• **Pancreatic cancer** • GI – colorectal, esophageal, & hepatocellular cancer.
CALCITONIN	• **Medullary thyroid cancer**
CEA	• **Colorectal cancer** • Medullary thyroid, pancreatic, gastric, lung, & breast cancers
PROSTATE SPECIFIC ANTIGEN	• **Prostate cancer** • Can also be elevated in BPH & Prostatitis

ARTHRITIS SYNDROMES

GOUT

- **Uric acid (monosodium urate crystal) deposition in the soft tissues, joints, & bones.**
- **90% occur in middle-aged to elderly men.** Increased incidence in postmenopausal women.

ETIOLOGIES
- **Renal uric acid underexcretion (90%)** — worsened with renal insufficiency, Thiazides, Aspirin;
- Uric acid overproduction (10%) — increased cell turnover (eg, cancer, chemotherapy, hemolysis).

TRIGGERS
- Attacks associated with **purine-rich foods** (alcohol, liver, seafood, yeasts) causing rapid changes in uric acid concentrations. Trauma, surgery, starvation, fatty food, initiation of urate lowering meds.
- Medications: **Thiazide & loop diuretics, ACEI, Pyrazinamide, Ethambutol, Aspirin,** & ARBs (**notable exception is Losartan**, which decreases uric acid levels).

CLINICAL MANIFESTATIONS
Acute gouty arthritis:
- **Usually begins as an intermittent, acute mono- or oligoarthritis, especially of the first metatarsophalangeal joint. Flares are most frequent overnight and in the early morning** (between midnight and 8 am). Flares begin suddenly and typically peak with maximal intensity within 12-24 hours with resolution, even without treatment, in 2 weeks.
- **First MTP joint of the great toe most common (podagra)** & lower extremity (knees, feet, & ankles).
- Systemic features may include fever, chills, general malaise, and fatigue (their presence does not distinguish Cellulitis or Septic arthritis from Gout or Pseudogout).

Physical examination:
- **Signs of inflammation: severe joint pain, erythema, warmth, swelling, & exquisite tenderness, with limited range of motion,** often extending beyond the confines of involved joint.
- **Tophi may be seen in longstanding disease.** Tophi are subcutaneous depositions of urate that form nodules, typically occurring in the joints, ears, finger pads, tendons, and bursae.

DIAGNOSIS
- **Arthrocentesis diagnostic test of choice — negatively birefringent, needle-shaped crystals.** Increased WBC count (but usually < 50,000), predominantly neutrophils.
- **Radiographs: punched out erosions with sclerotic & overhanging margins (mouse or rat bite lesions).** Tophi may be seen in longstanding disease.

ACUTE MANAGEMENT (ATTACKS)
- **NSAIDs initial treatment of choice** (eg, Indomethacin, Naproxen, Ibuprofen, Celecoxib). NSAIDs should be avoided in patients with active or recent Peptic ulcer disease, patients with kidney disease, or active cardiovascular disease. Avoid Aspirin. **Intraarticular glucocorticoids** alternative.
- **Glucocorticoids also first-line or reserved if refractory to NSAIDs or if NSAIDs are contraindicated (eg, renal disease).** Can be injected into a single joint or given as oral therapy.
- **Colchicine usually reserved if unable to use NSAIDs or Corticosteroids. Adverse effects include diarrhea and bone marrow suppression (neutropenia).** Avoided in patients with kidney disease.
- Refractory cases: Interleukin 1 (IL-1) inhibitor (eg, Anakinra) may be used for refractory cases.

CHRONIC MANAGEMENT (PROPHYLAXIS)
- Lifestyle: decrease alcohol consumption (especially beer), weight loss, decrease high-purine intake (eg, meats, seafood). Colchicine is the only drug that can be used for both acute flares & prophylaxis.
- **Allopurinol (first line) & Febuxostat are xanthine oxidase inhibitors that decrease uric acid production.** Not started during acute attacks. Allopurinol safe in renal insufficiency.
- Uricosurics: Probenecid & Sulfinpyrazone. Contraindicated in renal failure & urate overproducers.

ACUTE GOUT MANAGEMENT

NSAIDs (eg, Naproxen, Indomethacin, Ibuprofen)

- Mechanism: anti-inflammatory agents that reduce inflammatory mediators in the gouty joint & inhibit neutrophil phagocytosis of uric acid crystals. NSAIDs are superior to Colchicine.
- Indications: **initial management of choice for acute Gout, especially in patients <60 years of age without significant cardiovascular, renal, or active GI disease. Avoid Aspirin.**
- Contraindications: **renal insufficiency, active duodenal or gastric ulcer,** cardiovascular disease.

Glucocorticoids (eg, oral Prednisone, intraarticular Triamcinolone)

- Mechanism: glucocorticoids reduce the synthesis of inflammatory mediators in the gouty joint.
- Indications: **An NSAID or a glucocorticoid is preferred for the treatment of acute Gouty arthritis. Glucocorticoids can also be used for acute Gout refractory to NSAIDS or if NSAIDs are contraindicated (eg, severe renal disease) or in older patients.** Intraarticular or oral versions.
- Adverse effects: mood changes, hyperglycemia, increased blood pressure, and fluid retention.
- Cautions: caution in patients with glucose intolerance, Heart failure, or poorly controlled Hypertension.

Colchicine

- Mechanism: anti-inflammatory that impairs neutrophil chemotaxis & other anti-inflammatory effects.
- Indications: **patients who cannot use either NSAIDs or Corticosteroids.** Colchicine is the only medication that can be used in the management of both an acute flare & chronic Gout (prophylaxis).
- Adverse reaction: **GI irritation most common. Myelosuppression. Dose adjusted or avoided in patients with impaired kidney or liver function** (may be safe if in some with mild renal disease).

CHRONIC GOUT MANAGEMENT

Medications used in the chronic management of Gout are NOT initiated during an acute attack.

Allopurinol, Febuxostat

- Mechanism: **xanthine oxidase inhibition leads to decrease uric acid production.** Febuxostat is a nonpurine inhibitor of xanthine oxidase that is more selective than Allopurinol.
- Indications: **Allopurinol first-line prophylaxis for Gout** (not used for acute attacks). Prevents urate nephropathy from Tumor lysis syndrome. Allopurinol safe in patients with renal insufficiency.
- Allopurinol adverse reactions: **GI upset, hypersensitivity** (eg, rash, Stevens-Johnson syndrome, allergic interstitial nephritis), hemolysis. Rarely, peripheral neuritis, vasculitis, or bone marrow dysfunction, including aplastic anemia.
- Contraindication of Allopurinol: Renal insufficiency. Febuxostat can be used safely in renal insufficiency.
- Adverse effects of Febuxostat: liver function abnormalities, headache, and gastrointestinal upset. It carries a black box warning for increased risk of cardiovascular death and all-cause mortality.

Colchicine

- Mechanism: anti-inflammatory (eg, impairs neutrophil chemotaxis).
- Indications: **patients who cannot use either NSAIDs or Corticosteroids.** Safe in mild renal injury. The only medication that can be used in both an acute flare & chronic Gout (prophylaxis).

Uricosuric drugs

Probenecid, Sulfinpyrazone
- Mechanism: **increase urinary uric acid excretion** (uricosurics). Used in uric acid underexcreters.
- Indications: second-line urate-lowering prophylaxis for Gout alone or with Allopurinol.
- Adverse effects: uric acid calculi, GI intolerance, Gout flares, and prolonged Penicillin levels.
- Contraindications: renal insufficiency, prior history of uric acid renal calculi.

Pegloticase

- Mechanism: **dissolves uric acid — recombinant uricase** (catalyzes metabolism of uric acid to allantoin, which is more water soluble & inactive). **Not used with urate-lowering therapy.**
- Indications: approved only for the treatment of refractory chronic gout; not used in acute flares.
- Adverse effects: increased risk of new gout flare, muscle pain and cramps. Contraindicated if G6PDD.

CALCIUM PYROPHOSPHATE DIHYDRATE DEPOSITION DISEASE (CPPD)

- **Calcium pyrophosphate dihydrate deposition in the joints & soft tissue, leading to inflammation & bone destruction.** Most common in older patients >60 years.
- **Risk factors:** Hemochromatosis, Hyperparathyroidism, & Hypomagnesemia.
- Joints involved: **knee most common, followed by wrist. Elbow & MCP joints also common.**

CLINICAL MANIFESTATIONS

- **[1] Asymptomatic: (majority)** — incidental finding of chondrocalcinosis on radiographs.
- **[2] Acute CPP crystal arthritis (Pseudogout):** clinically indistinguishable from Gout — **sudden severe joint pain, erythema, warmth, swelling, & tenderness, with limited range of motion.** Up to 50% may have a low-grade fever.
- [3] Chronic CPP: mimics RA [pseudo-RA] — inflammation, joint pain, and morning stiffness.
- [4] Pyrophosphate arthropathy: resembles Osteoarthritis [pseudo-OA] — asymmetrical bony enlargement, tenderness, effusions, crepitus, and decreased range of motion.

DIAGNOSIS OF PSEUDOGOUT

- **Arthrocentesis: diagnostic test of choice — positively birefringent, rhomboid-shaped calcium pyrophosphate crystals** & increased WBC count 2,000 – 50,000, primarily neutrophils.
- **Radiographs: chondrocalcinosis (linear calcification of the cartilage)** supports the diagnosis.

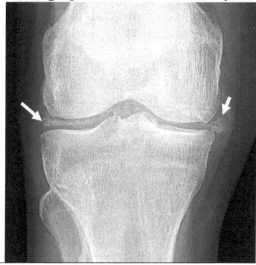

Evidence of tricompartmental marginal osteophytes of the knee.

Chondrocalcinosis: an associated calcification of the patellar hyaline articular cartilage as well as both knee menisci (arrows).

Photo credit:
Case courtesy of Fakhry Mahmoud Ebouda, Radiopaedia.org, rID: 33384

PSEUDOGOUT MANAGEMENT

- Symptomatic relief (eg, ice application, resting the affected area, and analgesic medications) and anti-inflammatory therapy for most patients.

1 or 2 joints amenable to joint aspiration:
- **Corticosteroids: joint aspiration and intraarticular corticosteroids if 1 or 2 joints.**

≥3 joints:
- **Systemic treatment of acute inflammation involving ≥3 joints, often with Nonsteroidal anti-inflammatory drugs (NSAIDs) or if NSAIDs are contraindicated, systemic glucocorticoids or Colchicine.**
- **NSAIDs: first-line option if >2 joints.** Contraindications include renal insufficiency, active PUD, GI bleed, cardiovascular (eg, Heart failure, uncontrolled Hypertension), or anticoagulant use.
- Oral corticosteroids is an option if >2 joints.
- **Colchicine:** first-line option that can be used in acute & chronic CPP disease (can be used as prophylaxis between acute attacks).
- Refractory cases: Interleukin 1 (IL-1) inhibitor (eg, Anakinra) may be used for refractory cases.

PROPHYLAXIS

- Colchicine can be used in patients with ≥3 attacks of Pseudogout annually.

	GOUT	PSEUDOGOUT
PREVALENCE	• 17-20 per 1,000 individuals. • **Mostly adult men** Postmenopausal women.	• <1 per 1,000 individuals. • **Female predominance, elderly**
CRYSTAL CHEMISTRY	**Monosodium urate**	**Calcium pyrophosphate dihydrate**
SYNOVIAL FLUID CRYSTALS	<u>NEGATIVELY BIREFRINGENT; NEEDLE-SHAPED.</u>	<u>WEAKLY POSITIVE; RHOMBOID-SHAPED.</u>
MOST FREQUENTLY AFFECTED JOINTS	• **First MTP joint MC (Podagra)** 50% initially; 90% eventually. • **80% monoarticular typically lower extremities** (ankle, knees, foot)	• Knees, wrists, MCP joints, elbows, MTP.
RADIOGRAPH FINDINGS	• **"MOUSE BITE" (PUNCHED OUT) EROSIONS** Tophi Needle-shaped crystals Podagra Sclerosis with overhanging margins	• **CHONDROCALCINOSIS** - calcification of the cartilage
THERAPEUTIC OPTIONS	**ACUTE ATTACKS** • **NSAIDs 1st line** • Corticosteroids • Colchicine **CHRONIC MANAGEMENT** • **Uric acid-lowering agents** **Allopurinol**, Febuxostat, Probenecid • Colchicine	**ACUTE ATTACKS** • **Intraarticular steroids 1st line.** • NSAIDs, Colchicine, oral steroids **CHRONIC MANAGEMENT** • NSAIDs • ± Colchicine

Note that the **medications used in the chronic management of Gout are NOT initiated during an acute attack** (because it may precipitate an attack). Colchicine can be used for acute & chronic.
Any acute increase OR decrease in serum uric acid levels can cause an acute attack.
Note that measuring serum uric acid levels are generally not helpful to determine if the attack is due to gout.

ARTHOCENTESIS ANALYSIS OF FLUID			
	WBCs (/μL)	MICROSCOPIC	CULTURES
NORMAL	200		
INFLAMMATORY ARTHRITIS			
• GOUT	<50, 000 (mostly PMN)	• Needle shaped crystals; negatively birefringent • Uric acid crystals	Negative
• PSEUDOGOUT	<50, 000 (mostly PMN)	• Rhomboid-shaped crystals; positively birefringent • Calcium Pyrophosphate crystals	Negative
• REACTIVE ARTHRITIS & OTHER INFLAMMATORY ARTHRITIS	<50, 000 (mostly PMN) PMN = Polymorphonuclear neutrophils		Negative
SEPTIC ARTHRITIS	≥50,000 (>90% PMNs)	Bacteria, Cloudy	Positive

ANTIBODIES/AUTO ANTIBODIES	CLASSIC DISEASE ASSOCIATION
ACETYLCHOLINE RECEPTOR	Myasthenia Gravis
β-2 GLYCOPROTEIN 1	Antiphospholipid Antibody Syndrome (SLE)
CARDIOLIPIN	Antiphospholipid Antibody Syndrome (SLE)
CENTROMERE	CREST syndrome (Limited Systemic Sclerosis)
CYCLIC CITRULLINATED PEPTIDE (PROTEIN) – CCP	Specific for Rheumatoid Arthritis. Rheumatoid Factor used for screening but is not specific.
DOUBLE-STRANDED DNA	Systemic Lupus Erythematosus (*specific*, not sensitive)
ENDOMYSIAL	Celiac disease
GLOMERULAR BASEMENT MEMBRANE	Anti-GBM disease (Goodpasture's syndrome)
HISTONE	Drug-induced Lupus
JO-1	Polymyositis, Dermatomyositis
LA (SS-B)	Sjögren syndrome
LUPUS ANTICOAGULANT	Antiphospholipid Antibody Syndrome (SLE)
Mi-2	Dermatomyositis
MITOCHONDRIAL	Primary Biliary Cirrhosis
MUSK (Muscle specific receptor tyrosine kinase)	Myasthenia Gravis - may be positive in AChR-negative patients with MG.
P-ANCA	Microscopic Polyangiitis (MPA), Churg Strauss Ulcerative Colitis, Primary Sclerosing Cholangitis
RHEUMATOID FACTOR	Rheumatoid Arthritis
RIBONUCLEOPROTEIN (RNP)	Mixed Connective Tissue disease, SLE
RO (SS-A)	Sjögren syndrome, Systemic Lupus Erythematosus
SACCHAROMYCES CEREVISIAE	Crohn disease
SCL-70 (TOPOISOMERASE)	Diffuse Systemic Sclerosis (Scleroderma)
SIGNAL RECOGNITION PROTEIN (SRP)	Polymyositis
SMITH	Systemic Lupus Erythematosus (*specific,* not sensitive)
SMOOTH MUSCLE	Autoimmune hepatitis
THYROGLOBULIN	Hashimoto's thyroiditis, Autoimmune thyroiditis
THYROID PEROXIDASE (TPO)	Hashimoto's thyroiditis, Autoimmune thyroiditis
TOPOISOMERASE (SCL-70)	Diffuse Systemic Sclerosis (Scleroderma)
TRANSGLUTAMINASE (IgA)	Celiac disease, Dermatitis Herpetiformis
TSH (THYROTROPIN) RECEPTOR/ THYROID STIMULATING IGs	Graves' disease
VOLTAGE-GATED CALCIUM CHANNEL	Lambert-Eaton Myasthenic Syndrome (LEMS)

JUVENILE IDIOPATHIC ARTHRITIS (JIA)

- **Heterogenous autoimmune mono or polyarthritis in children <16 years of age for >6 weeks.**

3 types:

[1] Oligo (pauci) articular JIA:
- **<5 joints involved.** Most commonly affects medium to large joints (eg, knees, ankles, and wrists).
- **Iridocyclitis (Anterior uveitis) especially if ANA positive.** Temporomandibular joint affected.
- **Systemic manifestations** (eg, fever, rash, constitutional symptoms) **are characteristically absent.**

[2] Polyarticular JIA:
- **≥5 small joints** (usually symmetric).
- **Most similar to adult RA** (including morning stiffness). **Worse prognosis if Rheumatoid factor positive.**
- **Iridocyclitis (anterior uveitis) more common with positive ANA** & RF-negative; rare in RF-positive).

[3] Systemic JIA (Still's disease):
- **Daily or diurnal high fever,** daily arthritis.
- **Salmon-colored pink migratory rash on the trunk & extremities** that classically appears in conjunction with the fever & fades as the temperature normalizes.
- **No iridocyclitis but classically associated with systemic symptoms [hepatomegaly, splenomegaly, generalized lymphadenopathy, or serositis** (eg, Pericarditis, Pleural effusion)].

DIAGNOSIS
- **Primarily a clinical diagnosis.**
- Increased ESR & CRP. ⊕ANA in oligoarticular & RF-negative in polyarticular.
- Systemic (Still's) usually associated with increased ferritin and negative RF & ANA.

MANAGEMENT
- **NSAIDs first-line therapy.** Glucocorticoids if no response to biologic DMARD. Physical therapy.
- Second line or severe disease: Anakinra (intereukin-1 receptor inhibitor), Methotrexate, Leflunomide.
- **ANA positivity associated with increased risk of Iridocyclitis,** so routine eye exam every 3 months is recommended.

OLIGO (PAUCI) ARTICULAR JIA 50%	POLYARTICULAR JIA 35%	SYSTEMIC JIA (STILL'S DISEASE) 15-20%
• Children 1-3y; rare >10 years	• 2-5 years; 10-14y	**Clinical features:**
	Clinical features:	• **Arthritis** (destructive)
Clinical features:	• **Arthritis: 5 or more joints; symmetric & destructive joint (most similar to RA).**	• **Fever: daily spike or diurnal**
• **Arthritis (1-4 joints) weightbearing (eg, knees, ankles, wrist, TMJ); asymmetric & nondestructive.**	• Mild systemic symptoms	• **Rash: salmon-pink colored often on trunk or extremities (migratory, worse with fever)**
• **No systemic symptoms (no fever)**		
		• **Hepatosplenomegaly,** lymphadenopathy, **serositis**
• **Uveitis (iridocyclitis) 20% (especially if ANA+, RF+)** perform routine eye exams	• **Uveitis (iridocyclitis) 10-20%.** **Perform routine eye exams.**	• Heart, lung, or liver involved
Labs	**Labs**	**Labs**
• **Positive ANA**	• **Positive ANA**	• **Negative ANA & RF***
• RF negative (pos if severe)	• **RF positive 10-15%** (worse)	• **Increased ESR,** leukocytosis
• Normal ESR	• ESR mild to mod increased	• **High ferritin***
Management:	**Management:**	**Management:**
• NSAIDs	NSAIDs	• NSAIDs
• Corticosteroids	Corticosteroids	• IL-1 or IL-6 inhibitors
• Methotrexate	Methotrexate	• Corticosteroids
• TNF inhibitors	TNF inhibitors	• Methotrexate

SEPTIC ARTHRITIS

- Infection in joint cavity (synovium) & synovial fluid by microorganisms; most commonly bacterial.
- Septic arthritis is a medical emergency because it can lead to rapid destruction of the joint.
- **Knee most common joint involved in older children and adults** (>50%); hips, wrists, & ankles.
- **Hip joint most common in younger children. Sternoclavicular joint seen in IV drug users.**

PATHOPHYSIOLOGY
- Occurs through either [1] **hematogenous infection** (~75%) & [2] contiguous spread of organisms — percutaneous inoculation, penetrating trauma, arthroscopic surgery, or orthopedic fixation devices.

RISK FACTORS
- **Preexisting joint disease** (eg, Rheumatoid arthritis, Gout, Osteoarthritis). Prosthetic joint/surgery.
- Extremes of age, chronic diseases, immunosuppression (medications, HIV, IVDU, Diabetes mellitus).

NOTABLE ORGANISMS
- **Staphylococcal species:** *S. aureus* **most common organism in all age groups** (>50%) including IV drug users (especially MRSA). *Staphylococcus epidermidis* (coagulase-negative) seen with increased incidence with recent prosthetic joint placement or steroid injections into the joints.
- **Streptococcal species: second most common cause.** Group A *Streptococcus*. Group B *Streptococcus*: neonates, infants <3 months, and older adults. *Streptococcus pneumoniae*.
- *Neisseria gonorrhoeae:* **sexually active young adults. Disseminated gonococcal infection may present with the triad of extensor tenosynovitis, migratory arthralgias without purulent arthritis, & dermatitis [vesicular pustules with erythematous halos (especially the distal extremities)].**
- Pseudomonas: increased incidence in immunocompromised (eg, IV drug use, older adults, neonates) or with trauma. Mycobacteria & fungi (eg, Candida) less common causes.

CLINICAL MANIFESTATIONS
- **Acute monoarthritis: swollen warm, painful, and tender joint, with decreased ROM** (tenderness with micromotion). Gonococcal septic arthritis may also be polyarticular.
- Constitutional symptoms: **fever,** chills, night sweats, diaphoresis, myalgias, malaise.
- Findings may include warmth, effusion, erythema, and guarding against range of motion testing.

DIAGNOSIS
- **Arthrocentesis: best initial and most accurate test — WBC ≥50,000, primarily neutrophils** (Septic arthritis can be present at lower counts). Prosthetic joint: WBC >1,100 considered positive. Aspirate also examined for crystals, gram stain, & culture. Positive gram stain often seen.
- **Increased ESR & CRP** nonspecific markers of inflammation. Although WBC, ESR, & CRP are usually monitored to assess response to treatment, **CRP is more useful**.
- Other tests: Blood cultures positive in 50%. Radiographs may show soft tissue swelling. MRI/CT.

MANAGEMENT
- **Treatment is multimodal, including [1] prompt IV antimicrobial therapy & [2] effective joint drainage, with debridement as needed.**
- Joint drainage: arthrotomy (open surgical drainage), needle aspiration, or arthroscopic drainage.

GRAM STAIN	ANTIBIOTIC REGIMEN
NO ORGANISM SEEN (EMPIRIC)	**Vancomycin + Ceftriaxone** (or other 3rd or 4th generation Cephalosporin). (± anti-Pseudomonal agent if Pseudomonas is suspected).
GRAM POSITIVE COCCI	**Vancomycin 1st-line.** MSSA suspected: Nafcillin, Oxacillin, or Cefazolin.
GRAM NEGATIVE COCCI	**Ceftriaxone,** Cefotaxime, Ceftazidime or Cefepime; Fluoroquinolone. **Gonococcal: Ceftriaxone 1g IV every 24h** + Azithromycin 1g x 1 dose PO.
GRAM NEGATIVE RODS	**Pseudomonas coverage: Ceftazidime or Cefepime or Gentamicin** Dual therapy (eg, neutropenia, sepsis, severe burns, bacteremia). Ciprofloxacin can be substituted if Penicillin allergic.

OSTEOARTHRITIS (OA) [DEGENERATIVE JOINT DISEASE]

- Chronic disease characterized by (1) loss of articular cartilage, (2) joint degeneration, (3) minimal or absent inflammation, and (4) hypertrophy of bone at the articular margins.

RISK FACTORS

- Nonmodifiable: **increasing age (most common ≥45years) most important overall risk factor for OA (mostly a disease of aging).** Female gender & family history.
- **Obesity important modifiable risk especially at weightbearing joints, trauma;** heavy labor.
- Most common in **weight-bearing joints** (eg, knees, hips, spine, wrists). Arthroscopic meniscal surgery.

CLINICAL MANIFESTATIONS

- **Triad of [1] usage-related joint pain, [2] joint stiffness, & [3] restriction of movement.** The joint pain is worse with activity (usually worse in the late afternoon & evening) and relieved with rest.
- **Evening joint stiffness — worsens throughout the day** & with weather changes. **If morning stiffness is present, it is of brief duration, lasting ≤30 minutes** (compared to RA >60 minutes).

Physical examination:
- **Joint hard, cool, & bony; decreased ROM, crepitus, audible grating sound.** No inflammatory signs.
- **Heberden node** (DIP enlargement) & **Bouchard nodes** (PIP enlargement). DIP involvement > PIP or MCP.

DIAGNOSIS

- **Radiographs:** [1] **asymmetric** joint-space narrowing, [2] **marginal osteophytes** (bone spurs), &/or [3] thickened **subchondral bone sclerosis** (density) or bony cysts are classic findings.
- Labs: lack of inflammatory markers — normal ESR, CRP, ANA, and Rheumatoid factor (RF) usually.

MANAGEMENT

- **Nonpharmacologic interventions are the mainstay of OA management and should be tried first, followed by or in concert with medications to relieve pain when necessary.** Nonpharmacologic therapies including weight management, regular exercise, braces, and foot orthoses for patients suitable to these interventions. Assistive devices (eg, cane, walker) can reduce the load on joints.

NSAIDs (topical or oral):
- **Topical NSAIDs (eg, Diclofenac) if one or few joints are affected (especially knee and/or hand OA) due to their similar efficacy compared with oral NSAIDs and their better safety profile.**
- **Oral NSAIDs may be used if inadequate symptom relief with topical NSAIDs, symptomatic OA in multiple joints, and/or patients with hip OA.** NSAIDs may be used if no contraindications exist (eg, renal disease, Heart failure, Peptic ulcer disease, GI bleeds). Oral NSAIDs are associated with increased adverse effects in the elderly (eg, GI bleeding, Peptic ulcers, renal injury, cardiovascular). Patients with increased risk of NSAID-induced GI toxicity may use it with PPIs or use Celecoxib.

Other options:
- Duloxetine in some patients with multiple joint involvement in whom NSAIDs are contraindicated.
- Topical Capsaicin if one or a few joints & other meds do not work (± cause local burning or irritation).
- Intraarticular corticosteroids provide temporary relief (usually ~4 weeks). No long-term benefit.
- Joint replacement if function is significantly compromised.

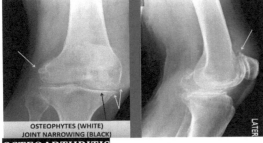

OSTEOARTHRITIS
- **Asymmetric joint narrowing**
- Marginal **osteophytes**
- **Subchondral bone sclerosis,** bone cysts.

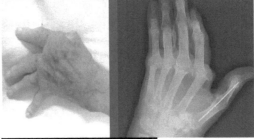

RHEUMATOID ARTHRITIS
- **Symmetric joint narrowing**
- **Osteopenia, bone & joint erosions.**
- Ulnar deviation in severe cases

RHEUMATOID ARTHRITIS (RA)

- Chronic systemic autoimmune inflammatory disease characterized by (1) symmetric polyarthritis, (2) bone erosion & cartilage destruction & (3) joint structure loss.

PATHOPHYSIOLOGY
- Hyperplastic synovial tissue (pannus) formation leads to T-cell mediated joint destruction.
- Risk factors: women, Women 30–40 years; Men 50–60 years, smoking, HLA-DRB 1 & 4.

CLINICAL MANIFESTATIONS
- Systemic (constitutional) symptoms: fatigue, fever, weight loss, anorexia.
- Joint pain, stiffness, & swelling: insidious onset. Worse in the morning, with morning stiffness >1 hour after initiating movement, improves later in the day. Decreased ROM.
- Small joints most commonly affected: wrist, MCP, PIP, MTP; ankle, knees. Usually spares the DIP.
- Extra-articular disease: subcutaneous nodules, interstitial lung disease, pleural effusion, pericarditis, splenomegaly, scleritis, and vasculitis.
- Felty syndrome: RA + splenomegaly + neutropenia
- Caplan syndrome: RA + Pneumoconiosis + pulmonary nodules
- Cervical spine subluxation: especially C1-C2 subluxation (atlantoaxial instability).

PHYSICAL EXAMINATION
- Symmetric inflamed joints — tender, soft "boggy" effusion; warmth or erythema. Ulnar deviation of the hand, swan neck & boutonniere deformities, rheumatoid nodules over bony prominences.

DIAGNOSIS
- Labs: Rheumatoid factor best initial test (⊕ in 60-80%), ⊕ Anti-cyclic citrullinated peptide antibodies (Anti-CCP) most specific (ordered after RF); Increased ESR & CRP. Anemia.
- Radiographs: [1] symmetric joint narrowing, [2] osteopenia, [3] bone & joint erosions. Severe disease is associated with joint subluxation. Plain radiographs are often normal in early disease.

MANAGEMENT
- Prompt initiation of DMARD to slow disease progression (eg, Methotrexate or Leflunomide) + simultaneous symptom relief with an anti-inflammatory (eg, NSAIDs or glucocorticoids).
- Methotrexate or Leflunomide preferred initial DMARD for high disease activity & advanced disease.
- Other DMARDs: TNF inhibitor, IL-6 inhibitor (eg, Tocilizumab), Janus kinase inhibitors, Tofacitinib.

DISTINGUISHING BETWEEN RHEUMATOID ARTHRITIS (RA) AND OSTEOARTHRITIS (OA)

FEATURES	RHEUMATOID ARTHRITIS (RA)	OSTEOARTHRITIS (OA)
Primary joints affected	Wrists, MCP, PIP (DIP usually spared)	DIP, thumb (CMC)
Heberden's nodes	Absent	Frequently present
Joint Characteristics	Soft (spongy, boggy), tender, warm	Bony, hard, and cool
Stiffness	• Worse after resting • Morning stiffness, often >1 hour • MORNING STIFFNESS >60 minutes	• Worse after effort • Evening stiffness. • If morning stiffness present, it is usually ≤30 minutes
Radiograph findings	• Osteopenia • SYMMETRIC joint narrowing	• Osteophytes • ASYMMETRIC joint narrowing • Subchondral sclerosis
Laboratory findings	Positive: RF, anti-CCP Ab, ESR, CRP	Negative: RF, anti-CCP Ab, ESR, CRP

NONBIOLOGIC DMARDS
METHOTREXATE
- Mechanism: folic antagonist.
- Indications: **initial DMARD in most patients with RA.** Can be used in combination with biologic DMARDs. Methotrexate and Leflunomide good for severe disease or high disease activity.
- Adverse effects: **liver, lung, marrow: hepatitis, interstitial pneumonitis, & bone marrow suppression.** Contraindicated in liver disease, alcohol use disorder, HBV, HCV, renal impairment.
- Contraindications: chronic hepatitis, pregnancy, & in any patient with significant kidney dysfunction.

LEFLUNOMIDE
- **T-cell inhibitor that is an alternative to Methotrexate with similar efficacy.**
- Adverse effects: diarrhea, rash, reversible alopecia, weight loss, hepatic injury, and teratogenicity.

HYDROXYCHLOROQUINE
- Indications: reserved for very mild disease or if the diagnosis is uncertain. Can also be used in combination with Methotrexate & Sulfasalazine. Safe in pregnancy.
- Adverse effects: **retinal toxicity (eye exams required every 12 months while on therapy),** ototoxicity.

SULFASALAZINE
- Indications: usually reserved for patients unable to take Methotrexate or Leflunomide.
- Adverse effects: **hemolysis (especially if G6PD deficient),** rash, hepatitis, & marrow suppression. CBC should be monitored every 2–4 weeks for the first 3 months, then every 3 months.

BIOLOGIC DMARDS
All patients on biologic DMARDs should have a PPD to rule out Tuberculosis before initiating therapy.
TNF (TUMOR NECROSIS FACTOR) INHIBITORS
Etanercept, Infliximab, Adalimumab, Golimumab, Certolizumab
- Adverse effects: reactivation of Tuberculosis & other chronic infections, such as Hepatitis B and C (screen for latent TB before using). Avoided in patients with Multiple sclerosis.

ANAKINRA
- Mechanism of action: **interleukin-1 receptor antagonist.**
- Indications: often used when treatment with other DMARDs are not effective. Increased activity when used with Methotrexate.

RITUXIMAB
- Mechanism of action: **anti-CD20 B cell-depleting monoclonal antibody.**
- Indications: used with Methotrexate in patients not responding to TNF-inhibitors.
- Adverse effects: reactivation of chronic infections, such as Tuberculosis, HBV, HCV. Infusion reaction.

ABATACEPT
- Mechanism of action: **T-cell inhibitor** used if no response to combination TNFi & Methotrexate.
- Adverse effects: reactivation of chronic infections, such as Tuberculosis, HBV, HCV.

ANTI-INFLAMMATORY MEDICATIONS FOR SYMPTOM CONTROL
NSAIDS
- Mechanism: analgesic & anti-inflammatory. **First-line for symptom control** but does not affect disease course so DMARD must also be initiated to slow down progression.
- Adverse effects: GI (gastritis, peptic ulcer disease), renal insufficiency, cardiovascular, ↑bleeding.

CORTICOSTEROIDS
- Mechanism of action: suppresses inflammation. Low-dose oral, IV, or intraarticular routes.
- Adverse effects: hyperglycemia, cataracts, weight gain, fluid retention, immunosuppression, hypertension, osteopenia (prevented with Calcium + Vitamin D).

ACUTE OSTEOMYELITIS

- Infection of the bone. Most commonly seen in children.
- **Femur & tibia most common bones affected in children.**
- **Vertebrae most common bones affected in adults, especially with IV drug use.**

RISK FACTORS
- Sickle cell disease, Diabetes mellitus, immunocompromised, preexisting joint disease, catheters.

SOURCES
- **[1] Acute hematogenous spread: most common route in children.**
- [2] Direct Inoculation: infection close to bone, post traumatic (eg, open fractures, puncture wounds), surgical (eg, insertion of a prosthetic joint).
- [3] Contiguous spread with vascular insufficiency: eg, DM, Peripheral vascular disease.

NOTABLE ORGANISMS
- *Staphylococcus aureus*: **most common organism overall.** Group A *Streptococcus* (S. pyogenes).
- *Staphylococcus epidermidis* **(coagulase-negative)** — increased incidence after recent **prosthetic joint placement,** neonates, & children with indwelling catheters (eg, chronic hemodialysis).
- *Salmonella* **pathognomonic for** Sickle cell disease.
- *Group B streptococcus* — **increased incidence in neonates.**
- *Pseudomonas aeruginosa* — **calcaneal Osteomyelitis associated with puncture wounds through tennis shoes.**
- *Pasteurella multocida* should be covered in treatment of Osteomyelitis due to **dog or cate bites.**

CLINICAL MANIFESTATIONS
- Nonspecific constitutional symptoms: eg, **fever,** chills, malaise.
- **Signs of bone inflammation: bone pain, warmth, swelling, tenderness.**
- **Limitation of function:** restricted use of the extremity, decreased ROM, limp, refusal to bear weight.

DIAGNOSIS
- Labs: **increased ESR & CRP (CRP more useful).** WBC may be increased. Blood cultures ⊕ in 50%.
- **Radiographs: usually the initial imaging test ordered.** However, evidence of bone infection may not be evident for up to 2 weeks after symptom onset (frequently falsely negative).
     Early: soft tissue swelling & **periosteal reaction.** Later: lucent areas of cortical destruction.
- **MRI: most sensitive test in early disease.** CT scan often used for surgical planning.
- Radionuclide bone or Gallium scan: sensitive in early disease; may also detect multiple infection sites.
- **Bone Aspiration (biopsy): criterion standard (definitive).**

AGE	COMMON ORGANISMS	EMPIRIC THERAPY
MANAGEMENT OF ACUTE OSTEOMYELITIS: Antibiotics 3-6 weeks (at least 2 weeks via IV). May need debridement.		
Birth to 3 months	**Group B Streptococcus** Gram negative organisms	• **3rd or 4th generation Cephalosporin** [eg, **Cefotaxime** (preferred if <3 months), **Ceftriaxone,** or **Ceftazidime**] **PLUS** anti-staphylococcal agent - **Vancomycin (preferred),** Nafcillin, or Oxacillin.
>3 months - adults	**Empiric management**	
>3 months – adults	**Methicillin Sensitive (MSSA)** *S. aureus*	• **Nafcillin, Oxacillin, Cefazolin,** Ceftriaxone. (Clindamycin or Vancomycin if PCN allergic)
	Methicillin Resistant (MRSA)	• **Vancomycin.** Alternative: Daptomycin.
Sickle cell	**Salmonella,** S. Aureus	• **3rd generation Cephalosporin OR** • **Fluoroquinolone (Ciprofloxacin** or Levofloxacin).
Puncture wound	**Pseudomonas**	• Ceftazidime of Cefepime. • Ciprofloxacin can be used in adults.

CHRONIC OSTEOMYELITIS

- Chronic infection of the bone (months to years).
- Etiologies: *Staphylococcus aureus, Staphylococcus epidermidis* (eg, prosthetic joint infections);
  Gram negative: *Pseudomonas* (IV drug abuse), Serratia, *E. coli*. May be polymicrobial.

Sources:
- **Direct inoculation:** infection close to bone s/p trauma, surgery, insertion of a prosthetic joint.
- **Contiguous spread with vascular insufficiency:** eg, Diabetes mellitus, Peripheral vascular disease.
- Acute hematogenous spread: Not a common cause in adults. Vertebral osteomyelitis is the most common cause of hematogenous Osteomyelitis in adults. Hematogenous spread in children.

CLINICAL MANIFESTATIONS
- Sinus tract drainage and nonspecific symptoms are hallmark.
- The involved limb may be edematous, warm, swollen, tender, with decreased ROM (due to pain).

DIAGNOSIS
- Radiographs: soft tissue swelling, periosteal reaction, osteopenia, bone destruction. **Sequestrum** segments of necrotic bone that has become separated from normal bone; **Involucrum** = new periosteal bone formation that surrounds necrotic bone (sequestrum).
- MRI or CT scan: more sensitive than radiographs.
- Bone biopsy: essential to identify pathogens and obtain sensitivities.

MANAGEMENT
- **Surgical debridement + cultures initial treatment of choice for chronic Osteomyelitis.** Unlike acute Osteomyelitis, empiric antibiotics are generally not recommended.
- Antibiotic treatment is based on culture and sensitivity in chronic Osteomyelitis.

ACUTE COMPARTMENT SYNDROME

- **Muscle & nerve ischemia (decreased tissue perfusion)** when the closed muscle compartment pressure > perfusion pressure due to limited space, compromising circulation and function.

ETIOLOGIES
- **Trauma: most common after fracture of the long bones (75%), especially involving the lower extremities (tibial fractures most common); In children, supracondylar fractures** of the humerus and both ulnar and radial forearm fractures are associated with ACS. Crush injuries, constriction (eg, tight casts, splints, & circumferential burns).

CLINICAL MANIFESTATIONS
- **Pain out of proportion to injury most specific.** Pain & paresthesia are the earliest symptoms.

Physical examination:
- **Pain with passive stretching of the affected muscles is the most sensitive earliest exam finding.**
- **Tense swollen compartment** with a firm or "wood-like" feel.
- Pulselessness, pallor, decreased sensation, & paresis (late findings); Capillary refill usually preserved.

DIAGNOSIS
- **Increased intracompartmental pressure** >30 mmHg or Delta (Δ) pressure <20-30 mmHg indicates the need for fasciotomy. Δ pressure = Diastolic BP – measured compartment pressure.
- Increased muscle enzymes: creatinine kinase & myoglobin.

MANAGEMENT
- **Prompt decompression: emergent Fasciotomy to decompress the compartmental pressure (surgical consultation for decompression).**
- While awaiting decompression: place the limb at the level of the heart without elevation prior to decompression. Supportive management — removal of constrictive dressings, IV fluids, oxygen.

OSTEOPOROSIS

- **Loss of bone density (both mineral & matrix) over time due to imbalance of increased bone resorption > formation of new bone (decreased)**. Osteopenia is a precursor to Osteoporosis.

PRIMARY
- Type I: **Postmenopausal and in men (most common type)** & Type II: **senile** (>75 years).
- Risk factors: **Caucasians** > Asians > African Americans; low BMI **(thin body habitus)**, corticosteroid use, smoking, chronic kidney disease, alcohol, low calcium & vitamin D intake, physical inactivity.

SECONDARY
- Due to chronic disease or medications — hypogonadism, high cortisol states (eg, **Glucocorticoid use, Cushing's syndrome)**, Hyperthyroid states, Diabetes mellitus, low estrogen, malignancy, **Heparin, Phenytoin, Lithium, Levothyroxine, Proton pump inhibitors**, SSRIs, Warfarin, alcohol use, smoking.

CLINICAL MANIFESTATIONS
- Usually asymptomatic until a fracture occurs.
- **Bone fractures:** may develop pathologic fractures, back pain or deformity. **Pathologic fractures — spine (vertebrae) most common**, hip, wrist (eg, distal radius) and pelvis.
- **Spine compression** — lumbar & thoracic. **Loss of vertebral height** (shortening of stature), kyphosis ("hunchback" bowing forward curvature of spine with forward thrust of head). **Back pain.**

DIAGNOSIS

DEXA scan (bone densitometry) best diagnostic test:
  Normal = T-score ≥-1.0. T score compares bone density with the bone density of a young woman. **Osteoporosis: bone density T-score -2.5 or less; Osteopenia: T-score between -1.0 and -2.5.**

Ancillary
- Normal serum calcium, phosphate, PTH, & alkaline phosphatase. Slight elevations of alkaline phosphatase may occur after acute fractures. Decreased Vitamin D; screen for thyroid, celiac disease.

MANAGEMENT
- **Lifestyle modification:** **Vitamin D** (eg, Ergocalciferol 800mg/IU) + **calcium supplementation initial therapy** (1,500 mg/IU), phosphorus intake, weightbearing exercise (eg, weightlifting, high impact, resistance training, jogging, jumping, walking), smoking cessation, fall prevention. Periodic height & bone mass measurements.
- **Bisphosphonates: first-line medical management & prevention of Osteoporosis,** including FRAX-determined 10-year hip fracture risk >3%. They inhibit osteoclast-mediated bone resorption & turnover. Taken with water on an empty stomach an hour before food & other medications & must sit upright for 30-60 minutes. Not recommended for patients with renal impairment. **Adverse effects: rare, atypical fractures or jaw osteonecrosis possible with prolonged use.**
- Denosumab: RANKL inhibitor that is an option for initial therapy in certain patients with high risk for fracture intolerant or unresponsive to other therapies. Superior to Bisphosphonates at increasing BMD at femur & femoral neck, (similar efficacy at spine BMD). May cause Hypocalcemia & infection.
- Teriparatide: anabolic recombinant human PTH analog that is an option in men or postmenopausal women with **severe** Osteoporosis (T-score -3.5 or less even in the absence of fractures, or T-score of -2.5 or less plus a fragility fracture). Monitor serum calcium, uric acid & renal function (may cause Hypercalcemia). **Not used for >18 months due to increased risk of Osteosarcoma.**
- Romosozumab: anabolic agent. Only used for 12 months because bone-making activity wanes after 1 year.
- Raloxifene: SERM (selective estrogen receptor modifier) that inhibits bone resorption and reduces the risk of vertebral fractures in postmenopausal women. It has an additional benefit of Breast cancer prophylaxis. May also be used to prevent Osteoporosis. Adverse effects include increased DVT risk.
- Calcitonin (nasal) usually used as last-line therapy because of its relatively weak effect on bone density, poor antifracture effects, and increased risk of cancer. Reduces pain from fracture.

Screening:
- **DEXA scan in patients 65 years or older** (or anyone with the risk = that of a 65y Caucasian female).

PAGET DISEASE OF THE BONE (OSTEITIS DEFORMANS)

- **Abnormal bone remodeling** in aging bone (increased osteoclastic bone resorption & disordered osteoblastic bone formation), **leading to focal areas of larger, weaker bone formation.**
- Risk factors: persons of **Western European descent.** 40% autosomal dominant, >40 years. Males.

CLINICAL MANIFESTATIONS
- **Most are asymptomatic (>70%).** Found incidentally on radiographs or because of an incidentally **high alkaline phosphatase** on routine lab testing. May cause high-output Heart failure.
- **Bone pain: most common symptom. Pelvis, spine**, skull, & long bones are most commonly affected.
- Bowing deformities of the long bones, compression fractures, radiculopathy (nerve compression).
- **Skull enlargement: deafness** (bony compression of CN VIII), headache. **Osteosarcoma is rare.**

DIAGNOSIS
- Labs: **isolated markedly elevated alkaline phosphatase.** Normal calcium, phosphate, and parathyroid hormone levels in most. ↑urinary pyridinoline & N-telopeptide, ↑serum C-telopeptide.
- **Plain radiograph: initial test.** Radionuclide bone scan if positive radiograph to assess disease extent.
  Lytic phase: "blade of grass or flame shaped" lucency. Mixed phase (lucency + sclerosis).
  Sclerotic phase: **increased trabecular markings and thickened cortex.**
  Skull radiographs: cotton wool appearance — poorly defined fluffy sclerotic patches as a result of thickened, disorganized trabeculae, which leads to sclerosis in previously lucent bone.

MANAGEMENT
- **Asymptomatic patients do not usually require treatment unless moderate disease is present.**
- **Bisphosphonates first-line (eg, Zoledronate).** Vitamin D & calcium supplementation to prevent hypocalcemia during bisphosphonate treatment. Normalization of alkaline phosphatase levels indicates response to treatment. NSAIDs for pain.
- **Calcitonin in patients unable to take Bisphosphonates.**

BISPHOSPHONATES
- Newer nitrogen-containing bisphosphonates — IV: Zoledronate, Pamidronate. **Zoledronate has greater efficacy than the other agents in severe Paget disease of the bone.**
- Oral: Alendronate, Risedronate. Etidronate is a non-nitrogen bisphosphonate that is rarely used.

INDICATIONS
- **First-line medical management of Paget disease of the bone & Osteoporosis.**

MECHANISM OF ACTION
- **Inhibits osteoclast activity, decreasing bone resorption & turnover.**
- Alendronate & Risedronate inhibit both osteoclast & osteoblast activity.

CONSIDERATIONS
- Taken with 8 ounces of plain water as well as 1-2 hours before meals (minimum 30 minutes), Aspirin, Ca, Mg, Al & antacids. Poor oral absorption.
- **Calcium & vitamin D supplementation recommended.**

ADVERSE EFFECTS
- **Esophagitis (especially Alendronate) so must stay upright for at least 30 minutes.**
- Musculoskeletal pain, nephrotoxicity, thrombocytopenia, GI symptoms & Flu-like symptoms during initial treatment in naïve patients (IV forms).
- **Rare but notable adverse effects are atypical femur fractures & osteonecrosis of the jaw.**

CONTRAINDICATIONS FOR ORAL BISPHOSPHONATES
- Esophageal disorders, certain bypass procedures. Chronic kidney disease is a CI for both oral & IV.
- Alendronate contraindicated if esophageal stricture, dysphagia, or hiatal hernia.

RHABDOMYOLYSIS

- Potentially life-threatening acute breakdown & necrosis of skeletal muscle.

ETIOLOGIES
- **Traumatic or muscle compression: crush injuries to muscles**, prolonged immobilization. Snake bites.
- Nontraumatic exertional: **strenuous physical activity**, seizures, hypothermia, hyperthermia, psychomotor agitation (eg, Neuroleptic malignant syndrome), hyperthyroid states.
- Nontraumatic nonexertional: illicit drug use (eg, alcohol, cocaine, amphetamines, heroin), infections (viral most common causes in children, especially Influenza), electrolyte disorders (eg, hypokalemia, hypophosphatemia).
- Medications: eg, **Statin therapy** (except Rosuvastatin & Pravastatin), especially in combination with other medications, such as Macrolides or Fibrates. Colchicine.

PATHOPHYSIOLOGY
- Myolysis leads to leakage of muscle intracellular components (eg, potassium, creatine kinase, myoglobin, phosphates, organic acids) into the bloodstream, leading to complications.
- **Nonprotein heme pigment released from myoglobin during muscle breakdown is extremely nephrotoxic to the renal tubular cells, leading to heme-induced Acute kidney injury (AKI).**

CLINICAL MANIFESTATIONS
- **Classic triad: [1] muscle pain (myalgia) + [2] muscle weakness or swelling + [3] dark urine (red or brown urine)** due to myoglobinuria. Many patients are asymptomatic with only dark urine.
- Muscle pain: when present, is usually most prominent in proximal muscle groups (eg, shoulders, thighs) and in the lower back and calves. Muscle stiffness and cramping may occur.
- If severe, tachycardia, fever, malaise, abdominal pain, nausea, or vomiting may occur.
- Physical examination: muscle weakness, tenderness, and swelling may be seen. Hypovolemia.

Complications:
- **Early complications include severe Hyperkalemia** with subsequent cardiac arrhythmia & arrest.
- **Acute kidney injury (Acute tubular necrosis)** 10-40%. Disseminated intravascular coagulation.

DIAGNOSTIC WORKUP
- **ECG: most important initial test to look for signs of life-threatening Hyperkalemia.**

Workup for Rhabdomyolysis:
- **Urine dipstick & UA: first lab tests ordered — dipstick positive for heme (blood) but microscopic examination of urine is negative for significant amount of blood** (usually <5 RBCs/hpf), indicating myoglobin spillage into the urine. ↑urine myoglobin most specific urine test (not always positive). ATN (epithelial cell or muddy brown casts, protein, red blood cells).
- Increased muscle enzymes: **increased creatinine kinase most specific serum marker** (usually ≥5 times the upper limit of normal, and usually >5,000 IU/L), often declines within 3-5 days of cessation of muscle injury. Other elevated muscle enzymes include **LDH, ALT, AST, & myoglobin.**
- Electrolytes: **hyperkalemia, hyperuricemia, hypocalcemia, & increased creatinine classic. Hyperphosphatemia** (more common) or Hypophosphatemia. Metabolic acidosis.

MANAGEMENT
- **IV fluids: early and aggressive fluid resuscitation (eg, 0.9% normal saline) mainstay of treatment to prevent or treat AKI** (target urine output 0.5–1.0 mL/kg/h). Diuresis diminishes renal toxicity of heme pigments. **Treat the underlying cause & fluid resuscitation mainstay.**
- ECG changes of Hyperkalemia: Calcium gluconate stabilize cardiac membranes + Insulin with glucose because insulin shifts potassium intracellularly.
- Sodium bicarbonate may be added in some patients with severe disease as long as Hypocalcemia is not present, the arterial pH is < 7.5, and serum bicarbonate <30 mEq/L. Alkalinization of the urine may diminish the renal toxicity of heme pigments. Osmotic diuretics (eg, Mannitol) rarely used.
- Hypocalcemia is usually not treated unless it is causing severe cardiac arrhythmias.

DISORDERS OF THE BACK & SPINE

HERNIATED DISC (NUCLEUS PULPOSUS)

- **Most common at L5-S1** (because it is the junction between the mobile & non-mobile spine); L4-L5.

ETIOLOGIES
- Chronic: **structural most common cause — disc degeneration leading to intervertebral disc herniation or degenerative spondylolysis.** Increased strain on the annulus fibrosus, resulting in tears and fissures, facilitating the nucleus pulposus herniation.
- Acute: axial overloading applies a large biomechanical force on a healthy disc, resulting in extrusion and bulging of disc material through a failing annulus fibrosus.
- Infection, trauma, inflammation, neoplasm, and vascular disease.

PATHOPHYSIOLOGY
- The annulus fibrosus is thinner on the posterolateral aspect and lacks support from the posterior longitudinal ligament, making it more prone to herniations. Due to the proximity of the nerve root, a posterolateral herniation is more likely to result in nerve root compression.

CLINICAL MANIFESTATIONS
Radicular back pain:
- **Usually unilateral, may radiate down the leg with paresthesias or numbness in a dermatomal pattern.** Pain may increase with coughing, straining, bending, prolonged sitting, flexion, & Valsalva.

PHYSICAL EXAMINATION
- **Positive straight leg raise test:** pain is elicited by lower limb flexion at an angle <45°.
- **Positive crossover test:** pain in the involved limb at 40° of hip flexion of the uninvolved limb.

Sensory, weakness, and reflex findings:

	L4	L5	S1
Sensory **"ALP"**	• ANTERIOR thigh pain into the knee and medial aspect of leg. • Sensory loss to the medial ankle.	• LATERAL thigh/leg, hip groin paresthesias & pain. • **Dorsum of the foot:** especially between 1st & 2nd toes.	• POSTERIOR leg/calf, gluteus into the foot. • **Plantar surface of the foot.**
Weakness	• ANKLE DORSIFLEXION	• BIG TOE EXTENSION **(big toe dorsiflexion).** • **Walking on heels more difficult** than on toes.	• PLANTAR FLEXION • **Walking on toes more difficult** than on heels.
Reflex Diminished	• LOSS OF KNEE JERK. • Weak knee extension – quads).	Reflexes usually normal. ± loss of ankle jerk.	• LOSS OF ANKLE JERK. (ACHILLES TENDON)

DIAGNOSIS
- Clinical. Imaging only necessary if progressive or severe weakness or if high-risk clinical features.
- Radiographs: normal or loss of disc height, loss of lordosis due to spasm, or degenerative changes.
- **MRI: diagnostic test of choice** that is usually reserved for suspected herniation, persistent pain, or refractory pain, or risk for a condition associated with neurological impairment.

MANAGEMENT
- **Conservative: preferred initial management — analgesics (eg, NSAIDs or Acetaminophen) + continuation of ordinary activities within the limits permitted by pain.** If bed rest is advised, it should be brief (1-2 days). Physical therapy. Muscle relaxers or oral steroid taper in select patients.
- Epidural corticosteroid injection: second line if refractory to first-line therapy. Usually performed after MRI confirmation of disc disease.
- Operative: laminectomy & discectomy if persistent disabling pain >6 weeks not responding to nonoperative options or evidence of cauda equina syndrome.

CAUDA EQUINA SYNDROME AND CONUS MEDULLARIS SYNDROME

- Constellation of symptoms as a result of compression of the nerve roots in the lumbosacral region.
- <u>Lower motor neuron lesion:</u> It is not a true spinal cord syndrome because the cauda equina are peripheral nerve roots (eg, lumbar, sacral, and coccygeal nerve roots) arising from L1-L5 levels.
- **Conus medullaris syndrome: compressive damage to the spinal cord from T12-L2.**
- **CES & CMS are considered neurosurgical emergencies and may have overlapping symptoms.**

<u>ETIOLOGIES</u>
- **Massive lumbar disc herniation most common** (45%).
- Spinal stenosis, from trauma, tumors, epidural abscess, epidural hematoma, & vertebral fractures.

<u>CLINICAL MANIFESTATIONS</u>
<u>Back pain</u> plus any one of the following:
- <u>Radiculopathy:</u> **bilateral leg radiation of pain** and weakness in multiple root distributions (L3-S1) [progressive motor and/or sensory deficits in the lower extremities]. May be unilateral.
<u>Involvement of S2-S4 spinal nerve roots:</u>
- **Saddle anesthesia — decreased sensation to the buttocks, perineum**, and inner surfaces of the thigh. Erectile dysfunction in men.
- **New onset of urinary or bowel dysfunction: eg, urinary or fecal retention or incontinence.**
- **Decreased anal sphincter tone** on physical examination (decreased anal wink test).

<u>DIAGNOSIS</u>
- **<u>MRI:</u> Urgent MRI of the lumbar spine initial imaging of choice.**
- <u>CT myelography</u> if unable to perform MRI (eg, pacemaker).

<u>MANAGEMENT</u>
<u>Neurosurgical or orthopedic consultation:</u>
- **Emergent decompression** (eg, laminectomy) to preserve sphincter function & ambulation.
- Corticosteroids to reduce inflammation.

VERTEBRAL COMPRESSION FRACTURE

- Most traumatic lumbar vertebral body fractures result from injuries producing anterior wedging or compression; often occur at midthoracic (T7-T8) spine & thoracolumbar junction (T12-L1).
- "Burst" fractures in children from jumping/fall from height [vertebral body & posterior elements].
- **Pathologic lumbar compression fractures** may occur in the **elderly** (eg, osteoporosis), **malignancy** (eg, Multiple myeloma, Prostate cancer), or systemic illness. **Pathologic fractures may occur with coughing, sneezing, sudden bending, lifting, or a fall.**

<u>CLINICAL MANIFESTATIONS</u>
- **Localized back pain with focal midline tenderness at the level of fracture.** Sitting, spine extension, Valsalva maneuver, & movement often aggravate the pain; may have muscle spasms.
- Nerve root deficits may be present in the presence of retropulsed bone fragments in the spinal canal.

<u>DIAGNOSIS</u>
- **<u>Radiographs:</u> localized vertebral compression**, loss of vertebral height, or kyphosis may be seen.
- MRI or CT usually not necessary but may provide additional information. Imaging indicated if neurologic deficits are present.

<u>MANAGEMENT</u>
Orthopedic & neurosurgery consult to determine appropriate workup & management.
- <u>Conservative:</u> observation, analgesics (pain control), gradual return to activity, bracing (for some).
- <u>Surgical:</u> kyphoplasty may be used if symptoms are severe or persistent.

LUMBAR SPINAL STENOSIS [(Pseudo claudication) (Neurogenic)]

- **Narrowing of the intraspinal (central) vertebral canal,** lateral recess and/or neural foramina with impingement of the nerve roots.

ETIOLOGIES
- **Degenerative arthritis or Spondylolysis most common — especially >60 years of age.**
- Post-surgical, congenital, traumatic, inflammatory.

CLINICAL MANIFESTATIONS
- **Back pain, numbness, & paresthesias** that may radiate to buttocks, legs, & thighs bilaterally. Because extension of the lumbar spine causes bulging of the disc into the canal, the **symptoms are:**
  - <u>worsened with extension:</u> prolonged standing, walking upright, walking downhill, lying prone.
  - <u>relieved with flexion:</u> **sitting, bending forward, leaning over a shopping cart, walking uphill, cycling** (unlike claudication), lying flexed. Lumbar flexion increases the canal volume.
- Relieved by sitting and not worsened with Valsalva (unlike Herniated disc).
- Unlike vascular claudication, symptoms are often provoked by standing without walking.

DIAGNOSIS
- <u>**MRI:** test of choice.</u> MRI or CT with myelography help to better define bony anatomy and visualize soft tissues and neural structures.
- <u>Radiographs:</u> nonspecific degenerative changes.

MANAGEMENT
- <u>**Conservative:**</u> **pain control (eg, NSAIDs, Acetaminophen), exercise, physical therapy (eg, cycling, swimming).**
- Lumbar corticosteroid injections (epidural or foraminal) may reduce need for surgical intervention.
- <u>Surgical management</u> for severe or refractory cases (eg, decompression laminectomy).

LUMBOSACRAL SPRAIN OR STRAIN

- Acute strain or tear of the paraspinal muscles, especially after twisting or lifting injuries.
- Most common cause of lower back pain.

CLINICAL MANIFESTATIONS
- <u>**Back pain & muscle spasms**</u> **that are activity-related, does not radiate to the legs, and is not associated with neurological symptoms.**
- May develop stiffness & difficulty bending.

PHYSICAL EXAMINATION
- <u>**Paraspinal muscle tenderness**</u> **& spasms** may be seen, **no neurological changes.** Decreased ROM.

DIAGNOSIS
- Clinical. Radiographs are not needed unless symptoms are persistent, or alarm symptoms are present.

MANAGEMENT
- **Analgesics (eg, NSAIDs) & resumption of ordinary activity or activity modification is the preferred management of Lumbar sprain or strain.**
- If not tolerable, BRIEF bed rest (no more than 1-2 days) may be indicated if moderate pain.
- Muscle relaxers may help with spasm in some cases.

SPINAL CORD COMPRESSION

- External compression of the spinal cord (eg, due to **malignancy or infection).**
- A neurologic emergency.

CLINICAL MANIFESTATIONS
- **Sudden onset of focal neurologic deficits** (eg, at a sensory level)
- Hyperreflexia below the level of compression.

DIAGNOSIS: MRI imaging of choice

MANAGEMENT
- Systemic glucocorticoids for acute neurologic symptoms, management of the underlying cause.
- Surgical decompression if not responsive to initial management.

SPINAL EPIDURAL ABSCESS

- **Pus-filled collection often associated with Osteomyelitis & Discitis.** The abscess can expand, compressing the brain or the spinal cord. Posterior most common type.
- Two-thirds of epidural infections result from hematogenous spread of bacteria from the skin (furunculosis, surgical wound, IV drug use), soft tissue (pharyngeal or dental abscesses; sinusitis), or deep viscera (bacterial endocarditis).

Microbiology:
- ***Staphylococcus aureus* most common** (60%), gram-negatives (eg, *E. coli*), *Streptococci,* coagulase-negative *Staphylococci. Mycobacterium tuberculosis* in the developing world.

RISK FACTORS
- >50y, **IV drug abuse, immunodeficiency** (eg, Diabetes mellitus, HIV, immunosuppressive medications, such as corticosteroids, alcoholism, malignancy), recent spinal procedure, epidural catheter placement, and infections of the skin or other tissues.

CLINICAL MANIFESTATIONS
Classic triad for Epidural abscess is [1] fever + [2] spinal pain + [3] progressive neurologic deficits.
- **Back pain: usually midline, focal (localized), & severe over the abscess** (most common symptom), often aggravated by movement. **Tenderness to percussion or palpation over the area.**
- **Radiculopathy** pain that radiates along the nerve root.
- **Myelopathy (neurologic deficits) & cord compression** — progressive motor, sensory, bowel, or bladder dysfunction. Paralysis & other signs of myelopathy are associated with increased risk of irreversibility. Reflexes may be hypoactive, absent, brisk, or spastic.

DIAGNOSIS
- **MRI with gadolinium: imaging modality of choice** — will reveal a ring-enhancing lesion. CT scan may be used if MRI is contraindicated. Radiographs are usually normal.
- Inflammatory markers: increased ESR, CRP. May have an elevated WBC count.

MANAGEMENT
Primary goals are elimination or reduction of the inflammatory mass & treatment of the organism.
- **Surgical consultation for drainage (eg, aspiration) & antibiotics:** eg, decompression **laminectomy & drainage** usually indicated if neurologic deficits, large abscess, or spinal instability.
- **Antibiotics: Vancomycin PLUS either Cefotaxime or Ceftriaxone.** Cefepime or Ceftazidime if *Pseudomonas aeruginosa* is suspected.
- IV Corticosteroids may be used in some cases to control the acute neurologic deficits.
- Conservative (nonsurgical): systemic antibiotics alone (as above) may be used in selected patients (eg, no neurologic deficits, patient not a surgical candidate due to medical comorbidities).

VERTEBRAL OSTEOMYELITIS

- **Hematogenous seeding of one or more vertebral bodies from a distant focus.**
- Routes of infection: Vertebral osteomyelitis occurs by 3 main mechanisms: **hematogenous spread from a distant site or focus of infection (most common)**, direct inoculation from trauma or spinal surgery, and contiguous spread from adjacent soft tissue infection
- The primary source of infection is usually the skin or urinary tract. Other common sources of bacteremia are IV drug use, endocarditis, poor dentition, lung abscess, IV catheters, or postoperative wound sites. Vertebral osteomyelitis and discitis may occur together or independent of each other.

MICROBIOLOGY

- ***Staphylococcus aureus* most common bacteria in Vertebral osteomyelitis (>50%).**
- Coagulase-negative staphylococci and *Propionibacterium acnes* after spinal surgery, enteric gram-negative bacilli, *Candida, Pseudomonas aeruginosa, Mycobacterium tuberculosis* (Pott's disease).

CLINICAL MANIFESTATIONS

- **Back or neck pain,** with or without fever, gradually increasing over weeks to months.

Physical examination:

- **Local point tenderness** to percussion over the involved vertebra or posterior spinous process.

DIAGNOSIS

- **MRI most sensitive for early detection of Osteomyelitis. MRI and CT are sensitive and specific.** The intervertebral disc can also be affected by infection (discitis) and rarely by tumor. Extension of the infection posteriorly from the vertebral body can produce a spinal epidural abscess.
- Laboratory evaluation: Elevated erythrocyte sedimentation rate (ESR) or C-reactive protein (CRP).
- Blood cultures: positive in 50-70% of patients.

MANAGEMENT

When possible, antimicrobial therapy should be withheld until a microbiologic diagnosis is confirmed.

- **Most cases of vertebral Osteomyelitis respond to antimicrobial therapy** (minimum of 6 weeks).
- **Methicillin-susceptible *Staphylococcus*: Nafcillin or Oxacillin or Cefazolin.**
- **MRSA: Vancomycin.** Daptomycin alternative (eg, Vancomycin allergy).
- **Gram-negative bacilli: Third-generation Cephalosporin** (eg, Ceftriaxone or Ceftazidime or Cefotaxime). Fourth generation Cephalosporin (eg, Cefepime). Fluoroquinolones.

Surgery

- Surgery is necessary in a minority of patients with vertebral osteomyelitis; Indications include focal neurologic deficits, epidural or paravertebral abscess, and/or cord compression.

RED FLAGS OF BACK PAIN

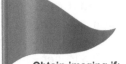

1. Tumor: **night pain, weight loss, not relieved with rest, >50 years**
2. Bone or disc infection: **fever, chills, sweats, immunodeficiency, recent spinal instrumentation**
3. Fracture: **Focal bony tenderness**
4. Cauda equina: **bilateral radiation, saddle anesthesia, urinary/bowel retention**
5. Spondyloarthropathy: **morning stiffness in an adult**
6. Spinal epidural hematoma: **coagulopathy**
7. **Extremes of age**

Obtain imaging if:
- Fever
- Trauma

- history of cancer
- neurologic deficits
- weight loss
- extremes of age
- focal bony tenderness
- coagulopathy.

SCOLIOSIS

- **Lateral curvature of the spine** that is usually accompanied by rotation.
- May be associated with **kyphosis** (humpback) **or lordosis** (sway back).
- Most common in girls & positive family history.
- **Adolescent idiopathic: Cobb angle ≥10 degrees**, age of onset at least 10 years of age, & no underlying etiology (eg, neuromuscular, congenital). Most common type.

SCREENING
- **Adams forward bend test most sensitive physical finding.** Asymmetry (thoracic or lumbar prominence on one side) is seen with Scoliosis. Forward bending sitting test.
- **Scoliometer: measurement of the angle of trunk rotation (ATR) if asymmetry is noted on Adams test.** Scoliometer is considered positive for Scoliosis if a ≥7-degree curve is measured.
- Assessment includes leg length, waistline asymmetry, midline skin defects, cafe-au-lait spots, foot deformities, and abdominal reflex asymmetry.

CONFIRMATORY
- **Radiographs** — **Cobb's angle ≥10 degrees** measured on AP & lateral films.
- MRI: not part of the initial evaluation without red flags or abnormal curve types but indicated if rapid curve progression, left thoracic curve, abnormal reflexes, excessive kyphosis, or foot abnormalities.

MANAGEMENT
Based on skeletal maturity of the patient, severity of the deformity, & curve progression:
- **Observation: Cobb angle 11-24° & Risser grade 0 to 2 at time of presentation.** Regular follow up to monitor progression every 6-9 months (11-19°) or every 4-6 months if 20-24°. Bracing may be recommended if the Cobb angle increases ≥5° over a 3- to 6-month period.
- **Bracing may be needed to stop progression if Cobb angle 25-39°**, in patients with a flexible deformity & still skeletally immature: (1) if the Cobb angle increases ≥5° over a 3- to 6-month period or (2) some patients with Cobb angle of 30–39°.
- Bracing is contraindicated if skeletally mature, little growth remaining, Cobb angle ≥50° or <20°.
- **Surgical correction: alternative to bracing if >40° & Risser grade 0 to 2 (skeletally immature).**

THORACIC OUTLET SYNDROME (TOS)

- **Idiopathic compression of brachial plexus [(nTOS) most common], subclavian vein (vTOS), or subclavian artery (aTOS)** as they exit the narrowed space between shoulder girdle & first rib and behind the clavicle. **TOS are due to rib anomalies, muscular anomalies, or a result of injury.**

CLINICAL MANIFESTATIONS
- Nerve compression: **ulnar neuropathy,** arm pain, weakness, or paresthesia to the forearm or arm.
- Vascular compression: **swelling and/or discoloration of the arm, especially with abduction of the arm (erythema, edema, or cyanosis of affected arm).** Thromboembolism to the hand or arm. Features of arm/hand ischemia include pain, paresthesia, pallor, and coolness.
- Venous compression leads to upper extremity swelling and cyanosis with or without deep venous thrombosis. Due to swelling, some patients may complain of hand paresthesias.
- Physical examination: ⊕ **Adson sign** — **loss of radial pulse with head rotated to affected side.**

DIAGNOSIS
- Cervical spine radiographs or chest radiographs to assess the anatomy. MRI may be helpful.
- Arterial or venous duplex ultrasounds may be used for aTOS or vTOS, respectively.

MANAGEMENT
- Controversial. **Physical therapy first line**, avoid strenuous activity. Orthopedic consult, surgery.
- Thrombolysis for DVT due to vTOS; Embolectomy for aTOS.

SPONDYLOLYSIS

- **Pars interarticularis defect** due to failure of fusion or stress fracture. **90% occur at L5-S1.**

MECHANISM OF INJURY
- Often from repetitive hyperextension trauma (eg, football players, gymnasts, weightlifters).
- Often the first step to Spondylolisthesis (forward slipping of a vertebra on another).

CLINICAL MANIFESTATIONS
- **Most cases are asymptomatic** (~90%). May develop hamstring tightness. Radicular symptoms rare.
- **Low back pain especially with activity.** Most common form of back pain in children & adolescents.

DIAGNOSIS
- **Lateral radiographs:** lateral view — radiolucent defect in pars.
- **Oblique radiographs:** the normal appearance of the lumbar spine has been described to resemble a **scotty dog**. If spondylolysis is present, the pars interarticularis (neck of the scotty dog) will have a defect or break (looks like a collar around the neck). CT scan. Bone scan.

MANAGEMENT
- Low-grade or asymptomatic: observation with no activity limitations if asymptomatic & low grade.
- Symptomatic: physical therapy, spinal stabilization, & activity restriction in some patients.
- Spinal bracing may be helpful for acute pars stress reaction or if failed physical therapy.

SPONDYLOLISTHESIS

- **Forward anterior displacement/slipping (subluxation) of a vertebra on another due to a bilateral fracture or defect of the pars interarticularis.**
- May also place stress on the adjacent intervertebral disc, resulting in degenerative disc disease.
- Mechanism: **usually a complication of Spondylolysis** (lytic spondylolysis).

CLINICAL MANIFESTATIONS
- Most cases are asymptomatic. **Lower back pain most common symptom if symptomatic.**
- **Nerve compression: sciatica (L5 radiculopathy) resulting in weakness of ankle dorsiflexion and extension of the great toe as well as diminish the Achilles tendon reflex.** L4 radiculopathy may present with weakness at the quadriceps and a decreased patellar tendon reflex.
- Bowel or bladder dysfunction and neurologic deficits if severe.

DIAGNOSIS
- **Radiographs: forward slipping of a vertebra.** Lateral views used to measure slip angle and grade. Flexion & extension views can help to evaluate stability.
- **MRI:** indicated if neurologic symptoms are present to assess for stenosis or complications.

MANAGEMENT
- Mild: **treated like Spondylolysis: conservative — NSAIDs, physical therapy, activity modification if symptomatic, stretching, and in some, lumbosacral orthosis.**
- Severe cases that do not respond to initial nonsurgical management may need surgical intervention.

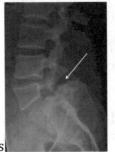 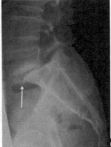

Spondylolysis   Spondylolisthesis

HIP & PELVIS INJURIES

DEVELOPMENTAL DYSPLASIA OF THE HIP

- Abnormality in the shape and/or stability of the shape of the femoral head and acetabulum due to abnormal development of the proximal femur and the acetabulum.
- Examination of the hip is performed during newborn assessment soon after birth and at every well-check visit until about 9 months of age and/or the child is ambulating independently.

RISK FACTORS
- **Breech presentation at delivery,** first-born children, females, positive family history.

PHYSICAL EXAMINATION
Assess for hip instability, asymmetry, &/or limited abduction:

Hip dislocation assessment using the Barlow & Ortolani maneuvers.
- **Barlow maneuver:** gentle adduction without downward pressure to **feel for dislocatability,** resulting in a "click", "clunk" or "jerk".
- **Ortolani maneuver:** abduction and elevation to **feel for reducibility,** resulting in a "click", "clunk" or "jerk".
- Other findings may include asymmetry (eg, skin folds, femur length, or gait) and restricted hip abduction.
- In infants >3 months, the dislocation may become relatively fixed and the Galeazzi test can be used instead.

ORTOLANI MANEUVER:
Reduces the hip

BARLOW MANEUVER:
Dislocates the hip

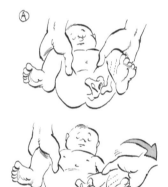
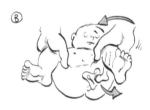
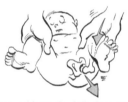

Examiner grasps the medial aspect of the knee & abducts the hips while applying anterior force to the femur, resulting in *reduction of the hip joint* (may feel a clunk).

Examiner adducts the fully flexed hip while applying posterior force to the femur, *resulting in dislocation of the hip.*

DIAGNOSIS
- Clinical with confirmation with imaging. **Infants with a positive Ortolani maneuver should be referred to an orthopedic surgeon.** If positive Barlow maneuver, serial follow-up examinations by the primary care provider or an orthopedic surgeon.
- **Ultrasound: often used in children <4 months of age.** Ultrasound at 4–6 weeks (adjusted for prematurity) if risk factors: breech at >34 weeks, FH of DDH, Hx of clinical instability on examination.
- **AP radiographs** in older children **(>4-6 months of age).**

MANAGEMENT
- **≤ 6 months of age: Pavlik harness abduction splint first-line management.**
- 6 months-2 years: reduction under anesthesia (closed or open); may need an arthrogram.
- Monitoring with routine hip radiographs until the child is skeletally mature may be needed.

PELVIC FRACTURES

- <u>MECHANISM OF INJURY</u>: **high-impact injuries** (eg, MVA). Low-impact injuries.
- **Intraabdominal bleeding up to 40% of cases**, but there also may be intrathoracic, retroperitoneal, or compartmental bleeding, especially with Acetabular fractures.
- **Soft tissue injuries:** lacerations of the perineum (rectum or vagina). May have **perineal ecchymosis.**
- **Neurologic injuries** may involve the L5 or S1 nerve roots. Sacral fractures may lead to S2-S5 sacral nerve root injury, which may result in bowel or bladder incontinence and sexual dysfunction.

DIAGNOSIS
- <u>Imaging:</u> radiographs. CT or MRI may be indicated if radiographs are negative or to get more details.
- <u>Labs:</u> CBC to monitor any blood loss, blood type and screen.

MANAGEMENT
- **Nonsurgical: weight bearing as tolerated, with early mobilization is often encouraged** in the management of some pelvic ring injuries (eg, APC Type I and LC Type I fractures). **Minimally displaced pelvic fractures & most pubic rami factures can often be treated non-operatively.**
- **For bleeding, a pelvic binder & IV fluid resuscitation is often used initially** with vessel embolization in refractory cases. **ORIF for more severe fractures.**

Mechanical stabilization:
- External compression device such as a **pelvic binder or sheet centered over the greater trochanter can help to stabilize the pelvic ring as well as help restrict internal bleeding from the venous plexus in APC type pelvic ring injuries** but should be avoided in lateral compression type pelvic ring injuries with an internal rotation component.
- **Skeletal traction is the appropriate stabilization for a vertical shear pelvic ring injury.** If appropriate, the patient can be taken for skeletal external fixation of the pelvis, which will provide the best stability in hemodynamically unstable patients, and generally can be performed in conjunction with an emergent laparotomy.

HIP DISLOCATIONS

MECHANISM OF INJURY
Trauma most common cause (eg, **MVA**, fall from height). Orthopedic emergency.
- **Posterior: most common type (90%).** Mechanism of injury: hip flexion, adduction, internal rotation, or axial loading on an adducted femur.
- <u>Anterior:</u> mechanism — axial loading with hyperabduction, extension, & externally rotated femur.
- <u>Associated conditions:</u> fractures of the hip & pelvis, knee injuries (eg, meniscus), sciatic nerve damage.

PHYSICAL EXAMINATION
- **Posterior** (90%) — **hip pain with the <u>leg shortened, internally rotated & adducted</u>** with the hip/knee slightly flexed.
- <u>Anterior</u> (10%) — hip pain with the leg shortened, externally rotated, & abducted.

RADIOGRAPHS
- <u>Posterior:</u> the femoral head appears smaller than the contralateral side and femur appears adducted.
- <u>Anterior:</u> the femoral head appears larger and the femur appears abducted.

MANAGEMENT
- **Conservative (nonoperative): closed reduction under conscious sedation.** Not performed if there is an associated ipsilateral femoral neck fracture.
- <u>Operative (surgical):</u> Open reduction.

<u>COMPLICATIONS:</u> **Avascular necrosis** up to 13% (reduced with early closed reduction <6 hours). **Sciatic nerve injury,** DVT, bleeding. Femoral nerve injury (anterior dislocations).

HIP FRACTURES

- Most common in osteoporotic women. Common in the elderly & patients with decreased bone mass.
- Mechanism of injury: Minor or indirect trauma in the elderly, high-impact injuries in younger patients. May be pathological (eg, malignancy or Bisphosphonate use).

3 MAIN TYPES

- Femoral neck fractures: proximal (cephalad) to the trochanters. **Fractures of the femoral head and neck are associated with a higher incidence of avascular necrosis.**
- Intertrochanteric: between the greater and lesser trochanters.
- Subtrochanteric: distal (below) the trochanters
- Intertrochanteric & subtrochanteric are extracapsular. Femoral head & neck fractures are intracapsular.

CLINICAL MANIFESTATIONS

- **Hip, thigh, or groin pain** may be referred to medial side of the thigh & knee. Inability to bear weight.
- Physical examination: **The affected leg is classically shortened, abducted, & externally rotated.** Pain with palpation in the groin or greater trochanter, axial loading of the hip.

DIAGNOSIS

- **Radiographs: traction-internal rotation AP hip is best initial test for defining fracture type.** Cross-table lateral, full-length femur views.
- MRI: gold standard imaging test — helpful to rule out occult fracture.
- CT: helpful in determining displacement & degree of comminution in some patients.
- Bone scan: helpful to rule out occult fracture.
- Duplex Scanning: may be needed to rule out DVT if delayed presentation to hospital after hip fracture.

MANAGEMENT

- **Operative: ORIF (open reduction & internal fixation) or Arthroplasty** (total hip replacement or hemiarthroplasty) **are surgical options.** Hip prosthesis may be used for femoral neck fractures.
- **Nonoperative management is generally reserved for debilitated patients (eg, non-ambulatory), and high surgical risk patients, but may be reasonable in patients with stable, impacted fractures.**
- Stable trochanteric fractures: pinning — intramedullary nails and sliding hip screws may be used.

COMPLICATIONS

- **Infection and thromboembolism are potentially life-threatening complications associated with Hip fractures for which prophylaxis should be given.** Avascular necrosis, Nonunion.
- **Bleeding: a large volume of blood can be lost into the thigh and hemodynamic status should be closely monitored.**

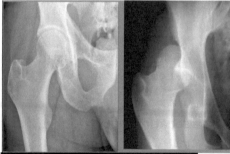

POSTERIOR HIP DISLOCATION

- **Hip pain with the leg shortened, internally rotated, & adducted** with hip/knee slightly flexed.

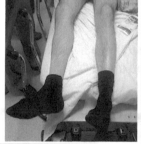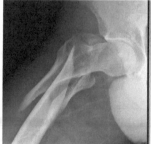

HIP FRACTURE

- Hip, thigh, or groin pain with the affected **leg shortened, abducted, & externally rotated**

LEGG-CALVÉ-PERTHES DISEASE (LCP)

- **Idiopathic avascular necrosis** (Osteonecrosis) of the capital femoral epiphysis of the femoral head in children due to ischemia of capital femoral epiphysis.

RISK FACTORS
- **Children 3-12 years (peak incidence 5-7 years),** 3-4 times **more common in boys** (4:1), low birth weight, skeletal immaturity, coagulopathies and thrombophilias (eg, Factor V Leiden), Whites and Asians most commonly affected. Low incidence in Blacks.

CLINICAL MANIFESTATIONS
- **LCP typically presents as acute or insidious onset of hip pain and/or limp (limp is usually painless), worsened continued activity,** especially at the end of the day.
- Pain, if present, is mild and intermittent and may radiate to the hip, thigh, knee, or groin.

Physical examination:
- Restricted range of motion: **decreased abduction & internal rotation.** May have atrophy of the thigh muscles (from pain leading to disuse). Patients may lag in bone age & height or leg length discrepancy. Antalgic Gait (acute): Short-stance phase secondary to pain in weight-bearing leg. Trendelenburg gait (chronic): Downward pelvic tilt away from affected hip during swing phase.

RADIOGRAPHS
- **Early:** Initial radiographs are often normal; **increased density and smaller appearance of the femoral epiphysis,** widening of the cartilage space (epiphyseal cartilage hypertrophy).
- **Advanced: deformity, positive crescent sign** — curved subchondral radiolucent line due to subchondral microfractures on the proximal femoral head with collapse of the bone); flattening of the femoral head, fragmentation, healing (sclerosis).
- Bone scan may show decreased perfusion to the femoral head.
- MRI may show marrow changes suggestive of Legg-Calvé-Perthes.

MANAGEMENT
- **Observation: activity restriction (nonweight bearing initially) with pediatric orthopedist follow up is initial treatment in most cases** (usually self-limiting with revascularization within 2 years). The orthopedist may advocate for protected weight bearing during early stages until reossification is complete. **Physical therapy or brace/cast.** NSAIDs for pain management.
- **Surgical: Pelvic osteotomy may be indicated in some children >8 years of age, more advanced disease (eg, lateral pillar B and B/C).**

LEGG-CALVÉ-PERTHES DISEASE
- Idiopathic avascular necrosis of the femoral head in children due to ischemia of the femoral epiphysis.

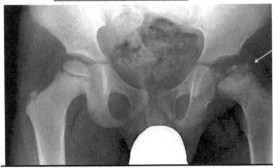

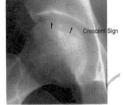

Crescent Sign

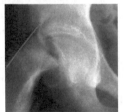

LEGG-CALVE-PERTHES (LCP)
- **Children 3-12 years (peak incidence 5-7 years)**
- Children to be shorter in stature
- **Whites highest risk**

- Radiographs: Normal, crescent sign deformity, or destruction of the femoral epiphysis.

Management:
- Initial: nonweight bearing and ortho follow-up
- Femoral osteotomy for some patients.

SLIPPED CAPITAL FEMORAL EPIPHYSIS (SCFE)
- **Children 8-16y** (mean age 12y in females; 13.5 in m
- **Children to be obese**
- **Blacks highest risk**

- Radiographs: **Displacement of the femoral neck**

Management:
- ORIF with (internal fixation with screw)

SLIPPED CAPITAL FEMORAL EPIPHYSIS (SCFE)

- Displacement of the femoral head (epiphysis) posterior and inferior from the femoral neck through the growth plate (type I Salter-Harris fracture).

RISK FACTORS
- **Children 8-16y [mean age 12y in females & 13.5y in males], obese, Blacks, males during adolescent growth spurt** (due to weakness of the growth plate & hormonal changes at puberty).
- If seen in children before puberty, suspect hormonal or systemic disorders (eg, **Hypothyroidism,** Hypopituitarism).

CLINICAL MANIFESTATIONS
- <u>Pain & altered gait</u>: **Ipsilateral nonradiating dull, achy hip, groin, thigh, or knee pain with a painful limp worse with physical activity.** May develop inability to walk after minor trauma.
- <u>Physical examination</u>: **externally rotated leg** on the affected side — **limited internal rotation,** abduction, and flexion on ROM of the hip. Altered gait.

DIAGNOSIS
- <u>Plain radiographs</u>: **posterior displacement of femoral epiphysis, similar to ice cream slipping off a cone.** Best seen on frog-leg lateral pelvis or cross table lateral hip view.

MANAGEMENT
- **[1]** <u>**Strict nonweight bearing**</u> (eg, crutches, wheelchair, and bed rest) **to prevent further slippage, followed by [2]** <u>**operative stabilization**</u> **(eg, internal fixation with a single cannulated screw fixation),** usually involving pinning in situ (eg, without attempt at reduction).

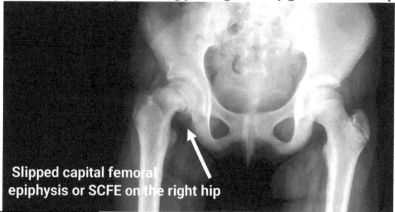

Slipped capital femoral epiphysis or SCFE on the right hip

POPLITEAL (BAKER'S) CYST

- Popliteal synovial fluid (effusion) is displaced with subsequent cyst formation.
- <u>Mechanism</u>: degenerative or inflammatory joint disease.

CLINICAL MANIFESTATIONS
- Most are small, asymptomatic, & only noted incidentally on imaging.
- <u>Symptomatic</u>: posterior knee pain and stiffness, mass or fullness behind the knee in the popliteal fossa more prominent in knee extension and becomes smaller when the knee is flexed to 45° (Foucher sign). Difficulty fully flexing the knee, or knee effusion.
- **Ruptured cysts may present with pseudothrombophlebitis syndrome, mimicking a DVT (tenderness, warmth, and erythema of the calf with a positive Homan's sign).**

DIAGNOSIS: Doppler often performed to rule out DVT (also helpful to identify the cyst).

MANAGEMENT
- **Conservative: initial management of choice (eg, ice, assisted weight bearing, NSAIDs), arthrocentesis of the knee, & intraarticular injection with glucocorticoids (eg, Triamcinolone).**
- Surgical excision often reserved for refractory cases.

MCL (Medial) & LCL (lateral) COLLATERAL LIGAMENT INJURIES

- **Medial collateral ligament:** resists valgus force on the knee (lateral trauma). **MCL injury most common.**
- Lateral collateral ligament: resists varus force on the knee (medial trauma).

CLINICAL MANIFESTATIONS
- Localized knee pain, swelling, ecchymosis, stiffness.
- **Lateral collateral ligament (LCL): pain & laxity with varus stress testing.**
- **Medial collateral ligament (MCL): pain & laxity with valgus stress testing.**

MANAGEMENT
- **Grades I (sprains) & II (incomplete tears): conservative: pain control, functional rehabilitation (physical therapy)** to restore range of motion & muscle strength, RICE, NSAIDs, knee immobilizer.
- Grades III (complete tears): long leg braces to provide stability; may require surgical repair.
- Surgery may be indicated for injuries refractory to exhaustive conservative treatment, those with gross knee instability, associated intra-articular injury, or multiple ligamentous injuries.

ANTERIOR CRUCIATE LIGAMENT (ACL) INJURIES

- **ACL is the most common knee ligamental injury;** may be associated with meniscal tears.
- 70% of injuries are sports related. More common in female athletes.

Mechanism of injury:
- **[1] Noncontact pivoting injury — running or jumping athlete who suddenly decelerates & changes direction (eg, cutting) or pivots or lands in a way that involves rotation or lateral bending** (eg, valgus stress) of the knee.
- [2] Less common: blow to lateral aspect of the knee [valgus (lateral) stress, lateral bending of knee].

CLINICAL MANIFESTATIONS
- **Audible "pop" in the knee & acute swelling, followed by knee effusion (hemarthrosis).**
- **May develop knee buckling (instability or "giving out"),** often with inability to bear weight.

PHYSICAL EXAMINATION
- **Lachman test: most sensitive** — the knee is placed at 15° in supine position. Forward anterior translational movement >2 mm when the tibia is pulled forward is positive for ACL injury.
- **Pivot shift (Losee) test** while maintaining internal rotation, valgus force is applied to knee while it is slowly flexed. Positive if the tibia's position on the femur is reduced or there is anterior subluxation with extension. Quadricep avoidance gait: does not actively extend the knee.
- **Anterior drawer test:** similar to Lachman but at 90° — least reliable (spasms may stabilize the knee).

DIAGNOSIS
- Plain radiographs: usually the initial test to rule out fracture but not used to diagnose an ACL injury.
  - ± **Segond fracture: avulsion of the lateral tibial condyle** with varus stress to the knee. If present, ligamental injuries are most likely present. **Segond fracture is pathognomonic for ACL tear.**
- **MRI: best test to assess ACL tears** — highly sensitive and specific for ACL injuries.

MANAGEMENT
Controversial (depends on activity level of the patient). Therapy vs. surgical.
- **Immediate: acutely, placed in a knee immobilizer, given crutches, & made non-weight bearing.**
- Conservative: rest, NSAIDs, ICE, compression, physical therapy, ACL brace.
- Surgical reconstruction: significant knee instability with desired activities, young active patients <40y, those with high demand jobs or athletes. May be performed with allograft.

Unhappy (O'Donoghue's) triad: injury to ❶ ACL + ❷ medial collateral ligament + ❸ medial meniscus.

POSTERIOR CRUCIATE LIGAMENT (PCL) INJURIES

- The posterior cruciate ligament (PCL) is the largest and strongest of the intraarticular ligaments of the knee. The PCL resists excessive posterior translation of the tibia at the knee joint.

MECHANISM OF INJURY
- **High-energy mechanisms** of PCL injury typically involve **an anterior force or posteriorly directed sheer force applied to a flexed knee [eg, a direct blow to the anterior tibia with the knee flexed, such as knee striking a dashboard during a motor vehicle collision (MVC) with dashboard injuries]**. Often in association with damage to other knee & ligamental structures.
- Sporting activities are the second most common cause of PCL injury — direct blow injury or fall on a flexed knee. Usually associated with other ligamentous injuries & neurovascular injuries.

CLINICAL MANIFESTATIONS
- **Posterior knee pain, anterior bruising** (especially to the anteromedial aspect of proximal tibia). Large knee effusion.

Physical examination:
- **Posterior drawer test — posterior translational movement of the tibia is a positive test**.
- **Posterior sag sign** (obvious set-off at the anterior tibia), quadriceps active test. May have gross knee instability so assessment of ACL, MCL, and lateral collateral ligament (LCL) should be assessed.

DIAGNOSIS
- Plain radiographs of the knee: part of the initial diagnostic imaging. **MRI most sensitive imaging.**

MANAGEMENT
- **Conservative: rest, ice, compression, and elevation (RICE) therapy, NSAIDs & knee immobilization if isolated PCL injury.** Progressive physical therapy for isolated PCL injuries with maintaining the knee in full extension for ~2 weeks initially to reduce posterior lag.
- Surgical intervention may be indicated if acute injury or if associated with multiple injuries.

MENISCAL TEARS

MECHANISM OF INJURY
- Degenerative tear more common in individuals >40 years with minimal or no trauma.
- **Acute: axial loading & rotation** (eg, squatting, twisting, compression, or trauma with femur rotation on the tibia) **while the foot is planted. Medial tears 3 times more common** than lateral tears.

CLINICAL MANIFESTATIONS
- **Popping, clicking, catching, locking** (inability to fully extend the knee), **knee "giving out," during ambulation** or climbing or descending stairs, **effusion after activities over 24 hours or later.**

PHYSICAL EXAMINATION
- **Positive McMurray sign: pop or click (catching on the joint line) when the knee is flexed and then externally rotated and extended.** McMurray and joint line tenderness specific tests.
- **Positive Thessaly test**: Pain or a locking or catching sensation with knee rotation (most sensitive).
- **Joint line tenderness & pain with deep squatting; joint effusion, & swelling.**
- Apley compression test: prone-flexion compression.

DIAGNOSIS
- Plain radiographs for initial imaging.
- **MRI most sensitive test to assess for and characterize meniscal injuries.**

MANAGEMENT
- **Conservative: rest, ice, NSAIDs, compression, & elevation**; orthopedic follow up, physical therapy.
- Surgical: arthroscopic repair or partial meniscectomy — may be indicated if severe symptoms or persistent symptoms despite conservative management, or if occupational or sports-related profession require it.

PATELLAR FRACTURE

- <u>Mechanism of injury</u>: **[1] direct blow most common (eg, fall on a flexed knee)** or **[2] indirect force** applied through a contracting quadriceps. Most common in young patients.

CLINICAL MANIFESTATIONS
- Pain, swelling, &/or deformity to the anterior patellar area. A palpable defect may be noted.
- Limited knee extension with pain; inability to extend the leg against gravity.

DIAGNOSIS
- <u>Radiographs:</u> **sunrise view**; cross table lateral views allow better visualization of the patella.

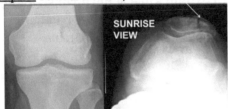 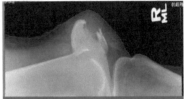

MANAGEMENT
- **<u>Nondisplaced</u>: Initial treatment includes immobilization of the knee in extension with a knee immobilizer.** <u>Definitive treatment</u>: continued immobilization with a walking cylinder cast from the groin to the ankle (ending just proximal to the malleoli), with the knee in extension, for 4-6 weeks.
- <u>Displaced</u>: surgery (ORIF) if fragments are displaced >3 mm or if the articular step-off is >2 mm.

OSGOOD-SCHLATTER DISEASE (TIBIAL TUBEROSITY AVULSION)

- **<u>Apophysitis of the tibial tuberosity</u>** (inflammation of the patellar tendon at the insertion of the tibial tubercle) **due to overuse (repetitive stress microtrauma) or small avulsions from repetitive knee extension & quadriceps contraction.**
- The apophysis is a muscle-tendon-bone attachment that is subject to injury from repetitive stress or an acute avulsion injury.

RISK FACTORS
- **Most common in males, 10-15 years, during growth spurts, athletes.**

CLINICAL MANIFESTATIONS
- **<u>Activity-related anterior knee pain & swelling</u>** eg, running, jumping, kneeling, cutting, squatting, climbing stairs, walking uphill; relieved with rest.
- **Bony prominence, swelling, enlargement, & <u>tenderness over the anterior tibial tubercle</u>.**

DIAGNOSIS
- **Clinical diagnosis (enlarged tibial tubercle).** Imaging usually not necessary in classic presentations.
- <u>Radiographs:</u> elevation, heterotopic ossification, &/or bone fragmentation of the tibial tuberosity.

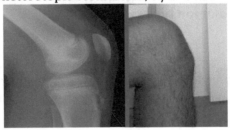

MANAGEMENT
- **<u>Conservative:</u> mainstay of treatment** — RICE (rest, ice, elevation), NSAIDs, quadriceps stretching, continued sports participation, physical therapy. Most symptoms resolve within 12–24 months or with physeal closure.
- Surgery rare (only in refractory cases). If done, usually performed after growth plate has closed.

PATELLAR & QUADRICEPS TENDON RUPTURES

MECHANISM OF INJURY
- **Forceful quadriceps contraction** (eg, fall on a flexed knee, walking up or down stairs).
- Quads > patellar. Quads rupture usually occurs >40 years; Patellar rupture usually occurs <40 years.

RISK FACTORS
- **Males >40y, history of systemic disease** (eg, DM, Gout, obesity, renal disease).

CLINICAL MANIFESTATIONS
- Sharp proximal knee pain with ambulation, **inability to extend knee & perform straight leg raise**.
- **Quadriceps tendon rupture: palpable defect above** the knee and low riding patella.
- **Patellar tendon rupture: palpable defect below** the knee and high riding patella.

DIAGNOSIS
Plain radiographs:
- **Quadriceps tendon rupture: patella baja** (low-riding patella).
- **Patellar tendon rupture: patella alta** (high-riding patella).

NORMAL KNEE	PATELLAR TENDON RUPTURE	QUADRICEPS TENDON RUPTURE
Lateral View	"Patella Alta" Lateral View	"Patella Baja" - Lateral View

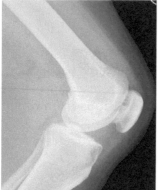 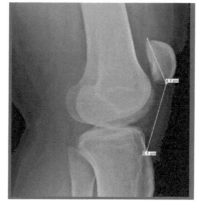 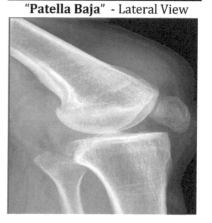

MANAGEMENT
- **[1] Non-operative: Knee immobilization in brace with partial tears with intact knee extensor mechanism. Non or partial weight bearing.**
- **[2] Operative: Surgical fixation in complete tears or non-intact extensor mechanism.** Surgical repair usually performed within 7-10 days to reduce the risk of tendon or muscle retraction.

PATELLAR DISLOCATION

- <u>MECHANISM OF INJURY</u>: **valgus stress** after twisting injury, direct blow.
- **Lateral patellar dislocation most common type.**
- **Most common in females.**

DIAGNOSIS
- **Apprehension sign:** patient exhibits anxiety/forcefully contracts the quadriceps when the examiner pushes laterally. Only performed if patellar is already reduced. Radiographs.

MANAGEMENT
- **Closed reduction — push anteromedially on the patella while gently extending the leg.**
  Post reduction films. **After reduction and complete evaluation, the knee should be placed in a patellar-stabilizing brace or in a knee immobilizer** with crutches to assist with ambulation until a brace may be obtained. Physical therapy (quads strengthening).

KNEE (TIBIAL-FEMORAL) DISLOCATIONS

- **Severe limb-threatening emergency. Anterior most common**; posterior (highest incidence of popliteal artery injury); lateral, rotational, or medial. Fractures present in 60% of dislocations.

MECHANISM OF INJURY
- **Anterior dislocation: High velocity trauma with <u>hyperextension of the knee</u>, often associated with multiple trauma. 50% spontaneously reduce before arriving to ED (so believe patients).**
- Posterior dislocation: direct blow to the anterior tibia with the knee flexed. May show a "dimple" sign.

MANAGEMENT
- **<u>Immediate orthopedic consult for prompt reduction</u>** via longitudinal traction with vascular status check. If intact, place a splint with 15-20° flexion. Most will need emergent surgical intervention.

COMPLICATIONS
- <u>**Vascular:** popliteal artery injury</u> **in 1/3 of patients — in patients with no hard findings of vascular injury but the ABI/API is <0.9, immediate vascular surgical consultation, perfusion surveillance, and further vascular imaging is performed**, either duplex ultrasonography, or CT angiography, or conventional angiography (criterion standard). Serial exams if ABI >0.9.
- **<u>Neurologic</u>: <u>peroneal injury</u> most common.** Tibial nerve injury less common.

FEMORAL CONDYLE FRACTURES

MECHANISM OF INJURY
- **Axial loading** eg, fall from height; direct blow to the femur.

CLINICAL MANIFESTATIONS
- Pain, swelling, deformity, rotation, shortening, or inability to bear weight.

Complications:
- **Peroneal nerve injury: foot drop or decreased sensation in the posterior first web space of foot.**
- **Popliteal artery injury.**

MANAGEMENT: immediate orthopedic consult. ORIF. Usually heals poorly.

TIBIAL PLATEAU FRACTURES

- <u>Location:</u> **lateral plateau most common fracture type** > bicondylar > medial.

MECHANISM OF INJURY
- Axial loading, rotation, direct trauma to the knee (most commonly seen in children in MVAs).

CLINICAL MANIFESTATIONS
- Pain, swelling, hemarthrosis, limitation of motion. If displaced, **check for peroneal nerve injury — foot drop or decreased sensation in the posterior first web space of foot.**

DIAGNOSIS
- <u>Radiographs:</u> may be hard to see. <u>CT scan</u> may be done for further definition & pre-surgical planning.

MANAGEMENT
- <u>Conservative:</u> non-weight bearing with crutches initially; hinged knee brace + partial weight bearing & passive ROM + orthopedic follow up may be an option if nondisplaced.
- <u>Surgical:</u> if displaced or severe. ORIF in acute setting vs. delayed fixation after soft tissue swelling subsides.

COMPLICATIONS
- **Often associated with soft tissue injuries** — meniscal & ligamental tears (ACL and MCL injuries with lateral plateau fractures; PCL and LCL with medial plateau fractures), Compartment syndrome.
- Post degenerative arthritis (>50%), loss of joint congruity.

PATELLOFEMORAL SYNDROME (CHONDROMALACIA)

- Idiopathic softening or fissuring of the patellar articular cartilage from overuse.

RISK FACTORS
- **Most commonly in seen in runners ("runner's knee) or cyclists.** More common in women.

CLINICAL MANIFESTATIONS
- **Anterior knee pain behind or around the patella** worsened with loaded knee hyperflexion & **bending** (eg, prolonged sitting, jumping, kneeling, squatting, climbing up or down hills or stairs).
Physical examination:
- **Pain with squatting most sensitive sign.**
- Compression of the patella during knee extension will produce symptoms or a **positive apprehension sign** (anticipated pain).
- Provoked pain with quadriceps contraction: isometric contraction of the quadriceps with the knee flexed — **The combination of [1] pain with quadriceps contraction and [2] pain with squatting or lunging (most sensitive sign) are highly suggestive of Patellofemoral syndrome.**
- **Atrophy or weakness of the quadriceps or hip abductors is common;** rotational or varus/valgus malalignment.

MANAGEMENT
Conservative:
- **Ice, rest, NSAIDs, & rehabilitation (physical therapy) initial management of choice** (strengthening the vastus medialis obliquus of the quadriceps); weight loss if indicated.
- Short-term: NSAIDs, icing, and activity modification; Long-term: physical therapy.
- **Knee orthotics:** Elastic knee sleeve for patellar stabilization.

ILIOTIBIAL BAND (ITB) FRICTION SYNDROME

- Inflammation of the iliotibial band bursa due to lack of flexibility of the ITB bursa.

PATHOPHYSIOLOGY
- Excessive friction between the iliotibial band & the lateral femoral condyle.

RISK FACTORS
- **Most commonly affects runners & cyclists.**

CLINICAL MANIFESTATIONS
- **Lateral knee pain (activity related)**, especially where the ITB courses over the lateral femoral epicondyle. The pain is classically sharp or burning & **worse with changes in terrain (eg, climbing stairs or running downhill);** usually relieved with rest.

PHYSICAL EXAMINATION
- **Tenderness over the lateral condyle** (not on the joint line). Pain reproduced with single leg squat.
- **Positive Noble compression test:** positive if pain over the distal ITB especially at 30 degrees of knee flexion with pressure applied to the ITB.
- **Positive Ober test to assess for ITB tightness — pain or resistance (tightness) to adduction of the leg parallel to the table in neutral position.** Also tests the tensor fascia lata.

MANAGEMENT
- **Conservative: initial management of choice — eg, NSAIDs, ice, avoid overuse, physical therapy, & stretching of the iliotibial band,** quadriceps, and gluteal muscles. Running on flat terrain, changing the gait pattern, lowering the seat height, & adjusting the pedals in cyclists helpful.
- Steroid injections (seldom); surgical intervention rarely may be indicated if chronic or refractory.

ACHILLES TENDON RUPTURE

Rupture usually occurs 4-6 cm above the calcaneal insertion in the hypovascular region.

MECHANISMS OF INJURY
- Mechanical overload from eccentric contraction of gastrocsoleus complex.
- **Sudden forced plantar flexion**
- **Sudden violent dorsiflexion with a plantar flexed foot** (often sports-related).

RISK FACTORS
- 75% occur as a sports-related injury; episodic athletes "weekend warriors". Common 30-50 years.
- **Fluoroquinolone use.**
- Corticosteroids: **eg, Corticosteroid injections.**
- **Diabetes mellitus**

CLINICAL MANIFESTATIONS
- **Sudden severe calf or heel pain after push-off movement, "pop", sudden, sharp calf pain.**
- Inability to bear weight. Weakness and difficulty walking.

PHYSICAL EXAMINATION:
- **Positive Thompson test: positive if weak or absent plantar flexion when the gastrocnemius (calf) is squeezed.** Palpable gap. Difficulty walking on the tip toes.

DIAGNOSIS
- **Clinical diagnosis (positive Thompson test).** Diagnostic imaging usually not needed
- Standard ankle radiographs: may be performed to rule out ankle fracture.
- **MRI: best test if equivocal physical examination or pre-surgical for chronic ruptures.**

MANAGEMENT
[1] Immediate management:
- **Ice, analgesics** (Acetaminophen and/or NSAIDs); rest (eg, non-weightbearing with crutches).
- **Immobilization with the ankle in some plantar flexion (eg, short-leg splint in resting Equinus position)**, and referral to an orthopedic surgeon to determine operative vs. nonoperative treatment.
- Further treatment may be nonoperative or operative depending on patient age, patient activity demands, and chronicity of injury.

[2] Nonoperative management:
- **Serial functional bracing or casting initially in mild resting plantar flexion (resting equinus)** with subsequent splinting employing **gradual dorsiflexion towards neutral + functional rehab.**
- If a cast is used, it should remain for at least 6-12 weeks.
- **Equivalent plantar flexion strength, ROM, and rates compared to operative treatment.** May have similar re-rupture rates.
- **Nonoperative management has fewer short-term complications compared to operative.**

[3] Operative management:
Open vs. percutaneous Achilles tendon repair
- **Allows for early range of motion.** Indicated in acute (<6 weeks) rupture.
- **Increased short-term complications rates with operative repair: wound healing complications, such as infection, (5-10%), especially in smokers.**
- Traditionally, surgical treatment was favored due to the low rates of re-rupture. **However, a growing body of evidence suggests that surgery does not lead to better long-term functional outcomes than nonoperative management and is associated with higher rates of some short-term complications (eg, infection),** although re-rupture rates are similar or lower.

ANKLE SPRAINS

- **Lateral sprain:** 85% of ankle sprains involve the <u>lateral ligament complex</u>: **Anterior talofibular (ATFL) most common injured ligament in ankle sprains,** Calcaneofibular (CFL), or Posterior talofibular ligament (rare). **ATFL is the main stabilizer during <u>inversion and plantarflexion</u>.**

Eversion:
- **A syndesmotic injury or "high ankle" sprain often involves the anterior *tibio*fibular ligament** in the anterolateral aspect of the ankle, superior to the anterior *talo*fibular ligament. The mechanism of injury often involves the foot being turned out or externally rotated and everted.
- **<u>Medial sprain:</u> deltoid ligament sprains are usually due to <u>eversion injuries</u>.**

<u>CLINICAL MANIFESTATIONS</u>
- Patient often report "turning the ankle" during a fall or after landing on an irregular surface, followed by a "pop" followed or localized swelling, pain, inability to bear weight. May be ecchymotic.
- <u>Inversion:</u> The anterior, inferior aspect below the lateral malleolus is most often the point of maximal tenderness in anterior talofibular and calcaneofibular ligament injuries
- <u>Eversion ("High"):</u> severe and persistent pain, reduced ROM, difficulty with weight bearing. Point of maximal tenderness over anterior tibiofibular ligament (higher than the ATFL). Palpate the proximal fibula to rule out proximal syndesmotic ligament injury and Maisonneuve fracture.

	Ligament disruption	Ecchymosis & swelling	Pain with weight bearing
Grade I	**None** (mild stretching or microscopic tears)	Mild swelling and tenderness No joint instability	**Able to bear weight and ambulate.**
Grade II	**Incomplete tear**	Moderate pain, swelling, tenderness, & ecchymosis. Mild to moderate joint instability; some loss of range and function.	**Typically, painful with weightbearing.**
Grade III	**Complete tear of the ligament**	Severe pain, swelling, tenderness, ecchymosis.	Significant joint instability, loss of range and function. **Inability bear weight or ambulate.**

<u>DIAGNOSIS</u>
- **Anterior drawer test assesses ATFL integrity. Talar tilt test assesses CFL stability.**

OTTAWA ANKLE RULES	
ANKLE FILMS	**FOOT FILMS**
Pain along the **lateral malleolus**	**Bone tenderness at the navicular bone** (midfoot).
Pain along the **medial malleolus**	**Bone tenderness at the base of the 5th metatarsal.**
Inability to walk ≥4 steps at the time of injury & in the ED.	

<u>MANAGEMENT</u>
Grade 1:
- <u>Mild</u> — **RICE (rest, ice, compression, elevation), NSAIDs, no immobilization, soft compression (elastic) wrap or sleeve.**
- **<u>Modified activity:</u> weight bearing as tolerated** or crutches as needed.

Grade 2:
- **RICE, NSAIDs. May need ankle support (eg, elastic wrap + air cast, ankle brace, or similar splint)** for up to a few weeks. Ankle support in patients with mild or moderate sprains should not interfere with early rehabilitation.

Grade 3 (severe):
- **<u>Brief period of immobilization</u> in some patients** (eg, below-knee cast). Prolonged immobilization will weaken the ligaments and is not recommended for either athletes or non-athletes who have sustained an Ankle sprain. **As soon as acute inflammation has resolved, early mobilization with a stabilizing orthosis, and active range of motion while bearing weight is preferred.**
- May need surgical reconstruction in severe cases.

HIGH ANKLE SPRAINS & SYNDESMOTIC INJURIES

- High Ankle Sprain & Syndesmosis Injuries are traumatic injuries that affect the distal tibiofibular ligaments and most commonly occur due to sudden external rotation of the ankle.
- The distal tibiofibular syndesmosis includes the anterior-inferior tibiofibular ligaments (AITFL), posterior-inferior tibiofibular ligament (PITFL), interosseous membrane, interosseous ligament (IOL), and the inferior transverse ligament (ITL).

DIAGNOSIS

- Diagnosis is suspected clinically with tenderness over the syndesmosis aggravated with squeezing of the tibia and fibula together at the midcalf.
- Plain stress radiographs of the ankle are required to diagnosis complete syndesmosis injuries with tibiofibular diastasis.

MANAGEMENT

- Nonoperative for syndesmotic sprains without diastasis or ankle instability.
- Operative management is indicated for patients with diastasis of the tibiofibular joint or injuries with associated fractures.

MAISONNEUVE FRACTURE

- **Spiral fracture of the proximal third of the fibula associated with a distal medial malleolar fracture or rupture of the deep deltoid ligament**.
- The proximal fibular fracture is a result of tearing of the distal talofibular syndesmosis and the interosseous membrane.
- Proximal films performed in distal fractures to rule out proximal fracture (Maisonneuve fracture).

PROXIMAL   **DISTAL**

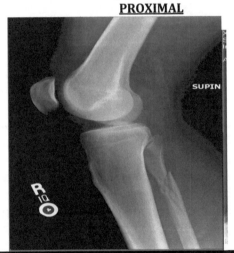   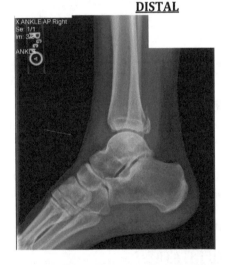

WEBER ANKLE FRACTURE CLASSIFICATION

Way to classify ankle fractures on the basis of the lateral malleolus (fibular bone).

NORMAL	WEBER A	WEBER B	WEBER C
	• Fibular fx BELOW syndesmosis	• Fibular fx AT LEVEL of syndesmosis	• Fibular fx ABOVE Mortise
	• Tibiofibular syndesmosis intact	• Tibiofibular syndesmosis intact or mild tear (talofibular joint not widened).	• Tibiofibular syndesmosis torn c widening of talofibular joint
	• Deltoid ligament intact	• Deltoid ligament intact or may be torn	• Deltoid ligament damage or
	• Usually stable	• Can be Stable or Unstable	• Medial malleolar fx
	• ± medial malleolar fracture		• Unstable – requires ORIF

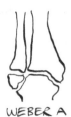

LEVEL OF FIBULAR FRACTURE RELATIVE TO THE SYNDESMOSIS

A- BELOW THE SYNDESMOSIS

B- LEVEL OF SYNDESMOSIS

C- ABOVE LEVEL OF SYNDESMOSIS

WEBER A   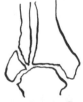 WEBER B   WEBER C

TIBIAL PLAFOND (PILON) FRACTURE

- **Fracture of the distal tibia from impact with the talus (high-energy rotational or axial load)**, interrupting the ankle joint space eg, high-impact trauma. The fracture extends into the ankle joint.

CLINICAL MANIFESTATIONS
- Severe pain, swelling, deformity.

MANAGEMENT
- **Surgical management: ORIF.** In a majority most cases, an external fixator is placed to primarily stabilize the fractures and allow for soft tissues healing. Subsequently, definitive reconstruction using internal fixation can be performed with the goals of restoring fibula length and stability along with the tibial articular surface.
- Complications may include associated fibula or talus fractures, compartment syndrome, or open injuries.

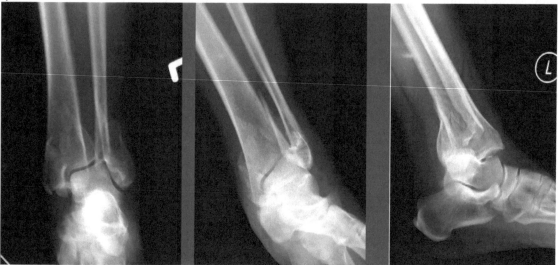

STRESS (MARCH) FRACTURE

- **Fracture due to overuse or high-impact activities (eg, athletes, military personnel)**, often after abrupt increase in activity, exercise, or repetitive microstress.
- **Most common bones involved are the metatarsals (distal second metatarsal, third, and fourth metatarsals most common metatarsals)**, tibia, fibula, navicular bones.
- Risk factors: females, repetitive activities, decreased physical fitness, inadequate vitamin D and calcium intake, eating disorders, increased age, decreased bone density, and low body mass index.

CLINICAL MANIFESTATIONS
- **Insidious onset of localized aching pain, swelling & tenderness that increases with activity.**
- **Localized bone tenderness** at the fracture site.
- May develop pain with weight bearing as it progresses.

DIAGNOSIS
- Radiographs: 50% of radiographs will be negative initially (especially in the first 2 weeks), so mainly a clinical diagnosis. Radiographs may be positive for a healing fracture (periosteal callous).
- MRI or Bone scan usually only performed if radiographs are negative in high-risk areas (eg, proximal fourth or fifth metatarsal, navicular, talus, or patella) or if symptoms persist.

MANAGEMENT
- **Conservative — rest, avoidance of high-impact activities, ice, splint or post-op shoe, analgesia.**
- Orthopedic surgery may be needed for high-risk fractures (eg, fifth metatarsal).

PLANTAR FASCIITIS

- **Heel pain due to inflammation of the plantar fascia aponeurosis at its origin on the calcaneus.**

PATHOPHYSIOLOGY
- The deep plantar fascia (plantar aponeurosis) is a thin layer of connective tissue that supports the arch of the foot and provides shock absorption.
- **Chronic overuse stress** (repetitive trauma and strain) leads to recurrent inflammation & microscopic tears of the plantar fascia at its origin on the calcaneus [especially in patients with pes planus (flat feet), high arches, or heel spurs]. May cause calcaneal apophysitis.
- Epidemiology: Most common in females, 40-60 years of age, older, & obese patients.

CLINICAL MANIFESTATIONS
- **Heel pain** in the plantar region of the foot (inferior and medial heel, sole of the foot), often sharp, usually worse **after** period of rest when initiating walking (eg, **first few steps out of bed in the morning or standing after rest**) — patients may prefer to walk on toes initially. **The pain then decreases after further ambulation, massage, & stretching** but worsens towards the end of the day with prolonged weight bearing with a return of the pain at night and during sleep.

Physical exam:
- **Local point tenderness** to palpation of the plantar fascia and plantar medial calcaneal **tuberosity** at the site of the plantar fascial insertion on the heel bone (underside of the heel).
- **Pain can also be reproduced with passive dorsiflexion of the foot and toes** (stretching of the plantar fascia). Tight Achilles heel cord (limited ankle dorsiflexion), pes planus, pes cavus.

DIAGNOSIS
- **Mainly a clinical diagnosis — [1] plantar heel pain + [2] local point plantar fascia tenderness.**
- Radiographs are not necessary for the diagnosis — may show a flat foot deformity or a heel spur.

MANAGEMENT
- **Conservative:** NSAIDs are considered first line treatment, along with relative rest, ice, and shoe inserts with heel/arch support (orthotics), massage, physical therapy (plantar fascia & Achilles tendon stretching exercises), & activity modification. Most resolve within 12 months.
- **Foot orthotics:** cushioned heel inserts, prefabricated shoe inserts, arch taping, night splints, and walking casts. Avoidance of flat shoes (eg, slippers) & barefoot walking.
- Corticosteroid injections: reserved for pain refractory to NSAIDs because may lead to fat pad atrophy or planta fascia rupture.
- Surgery in severe cases or refractory to conservative and corticosteroid injections.

TARSAL TUNNEL SYNDROME

- **Posterior tibial nerve compressive neuropathy as the nerve travels through the tarsal tunnel.**
- Compression may be a result of overuse, restrictive footwear, or edematous states.

CLINICAL MANIFESTATIONS
- **Compression symptoms:** alternating poorly localized (ill-defined) pain & numbness at the medial malleolus, plantar aspect of the foot, heel, & sole. The pain increases throughout the day, is worse at night, with dorsiflexion, does not improve with rest. Pronation of the foot may cause pain and paresthesias in the medial aspect of the ankle, heel, and foot.
- **Positive Tinel sign:** tapping at the tarsal tunnel (posterior medial malleolus) reproduces symptoms.

DIAGNOSIS
- [1] Clinical + [2] Tinel sign at the tarsal tunnel; [3] Electromyography confirms the diagnosis.

MANAGEMENT
- **Conservative initial therapy of choice — rest, NSAIDs, properly fitted shoes, & orthotics.**
- Corticosteroid injection if refractory to initial treatment. Surgical: tunnel release in severe cases.

HALLUX VALGUS (BUNION)

- **Hallux valgus deformity at the <u>first metatarsophalangeal joint</u>** with **<u>lateral deviation</u> of the hallux (great toe).** It causes the toenail to face medially (eversion).
- **History of wearing poorly fitted, tight, or pointed shoes most common**, pes planus (flat feet), rheumatoid arthritis, women.

CLINICAL MANIFESTATIONS
- Pain over the great toe at the MTP joint with a lateral deformity.

MANAGEMENT
- **Conservative:** footwear modification (eg, comfortable, wide toe box, low-heeled shoes). Analgesics.
- Orthotics: if persistent discomfort despite footwear modification.
- Surgical referral if severe or refractory (no response to conservative treatment for at least 3 months).

HAMMER TOE

- **<u>Deformity of PIP joint</u>: flexion of PIP joint & hyperextension of MTP & DIP joint.**
- Seen if 2nd, 3rd, or 4th toe is longer than the first, people who wear tight fitting shoes, OA, RA.
- Clinical manifestations: **PIP pain** (due to contact with shoe). PIP deformity.

NEUROPATHIC OSTEOARTHROPATHY (CHARCOT JOINT)

MECHANISM OF INJURY
- **Loss of sensation resulting in joint damage & destruction as a result of peripheral neuropathy** from Diabetes mellitus, peripheral vascular disease, or other diseases.

PATHOPHYSIOLOGY
- **Joint denervation:** Decreased sensation & proprioception, autonomic dysfunction, & repetitive microtrauma with daily activity leads to bone resorption & weakening. This is followed by a hypertrophic repair phase, where the damaged joint is replaced with abnormal bone and cartilage.
- **Most commonly affects the midfoot & ankle.** Neuropathic arthritis of the knee can be seen with Diabetes mellitus & rarely with Tabes dorsalis (a form of tertiary Syphilis).

CLINICAL MANIFESTATIONS
- Acute: unilateral nontender, swollen, warm & erythematous joint, with edema over the foot/ankle.
- Chronic: **joint or foot deformity, alteration of the shape of the foot, ulcer, wound or skin changes.**

DIAGNOSIS
- Radiographs: **obliteration of the joint space**, fragmentation of bone, increased bone density (bony sclerosis), joint subluxation, & **disorganization of the joint**. Osteolysis that mimics Osteomyelitis.
- MRI or Bone scintigraphy followed by indium scintigraphy may be needed in some cases to rule out Osteomyelitis.
- Labs: usually associated with normal WBC & inflammatory markers but may have an elevated ESR.

MANAGEMENT
- Conservative: **offloading the foot is the most important intervention with mechanical devices** (eg, carried non-removable, total contact cast walker, prosthetic walker, crutches, or a wheelchair), **avoidance of weightbearing on the affected joint should be advised until resolution of edema and erythema occurs, accommodative footwear and orthoses, Physical therapy.**
- Surgical correction rarely performed and is best avoided in most patients but may be done in selected patients (select patients with severe deformity). Arthrodesis, with or without orthobiologics.

INTERDIGITAL (MORTON) NEUROMA

- **Compressive neuropathy of the forefoot interdigital nerve (digital branch of the medial plantar nerve)** against the distal end of the transverse metatarsal ligament during dorsiflexion of the toes.
- **Most commonly occurs in the third web space (between the third and fourth metatarsals)** because it is narrower compared to other spaces.

PATHOPHYSIOLOGY
- Repetitive microtrauma leading to degeneration, proliferation, & thickening of the interdigital nerve.

RISK FACTORS
- **Most common in women 25-50 years, especially if they wear tight-fitting shoes, high heels** (overpronation and hyperextension) **or have flat feet.**

CLINICAL MANIFESTATIONS
- **Lancinating, shooting, or burning forefoot pain** (ball of the foot) most commonly in the <u>third intermetatarsal space</u> **(between the third and fourth metatarsal heads)** that may radiate into the toes, worse with walking, tight-fitted, narrow toe box, or high-heeled shoes; relieved with resting or removing shoes. Pain may be described as stabbing or tingling with electric sensations.
- **Numbness or paresthesia of the toes or plantar aspect of the web space** may occur.
- With prolonged walking, the pain can radiate to the hindfoot, leg, or toes; cause cramps, or feel like walking on a stone or marble.

Physical examination:
- **Reproduction of symptoms** (eg, pain in the forefoot) **by compressing together the metatarsal heads of the second and third or the third and fourth toes.**
- May have a palpable, painful mass near the tarsal heads.
- **Mulder's sign (click): compression of the forefoot (squeezing the metatarsal joints) in the mediolateral direction while palpating the affected space often results in a significant crunching or clicking feeling.** <u>Sullivan sign</u>: the affected toes may also appear to spread apart.

DIAGNOSIS:
- **Clinical diagnosis** based on history and physical examination.
- <u>Radiographs:</u> plain weightbearing radiographs should be taken to rule out bony masses, dislocation, or subluxation.
- <u>Ultrasound</u> is an inexpensive method for neuroma detection — noncompressible dumbbell shaped soft tissue lesion with hypoechogenicity within the intermetatarsal space
- <u>MRI</u> may be obtained based on the clinical scenario, especially to rule out other pathologies. The classic finding is a dumbbell shaped soft tissue lesion >5 mm within the intermetatarsal space.

NONOPERATIVE MANAGEMENT
- **Conservative: initial management of choice to relieve pressure on the nerve — wide laced shoe with a wide toe box and low heel; soft metatarsal support or pad** (placement of inserts just proximal to the metatarsal head). **Avoiding tight shoes or high heels.** Metatarsal pads, orthotics.
- **Single glucocorticoid injection** and local anesthetic under ultrasound guidance with a **dorsal approach may be used if refractory to initial management** (eg, Triamcinolone + Lidocaine). The effect is usually not long-lasting. <u>Adverse effects</u> include atrophy of the subcutaneous fat and plantar fat pad, discoloration of skin and disruption of the joint capsule adjacent to the injected site.
- Anti-inflammatory medications, tricyclic antidepressants such as Amitriptyline, and anti-seizure medications such as Gabapentin can be used to reduce the severity of related nerve symptoms.

SURGICAL RESECTION
- Surgical removal of the neuroma and nerve may be necessary in patients who failed 9 to 12 months of nonoperative therapy. Dorsal approached preferred over plantar approach.
- <u>Complications</u> include permanent numbness or residual stump neuroma (may be more painful than the original neuroma).

JONES FRACTURE

- **Acute transverse fracture through the <u>proximal diaphysis</u> of the fifth metatarsal at the <u>metaphyseal–diaphyseal junction</u> or intermetatarsal zone (Zone 2).**
- Acute proximal diaphyseal fractures extend **into or towards** the intermetatarsal joint (4th-5th metatarsal articulation) within 1.5 cm of the metatarsal tuberosity.

MECHANISM OF INJURY
- [1] Ankle inversion or [2] adduction when then heel is off the ground while the forefoot is plantar flexed.
- <u>Complications:</u> **15-50% <u>risk of nonunion or malunion</u>** because of the vascular watershed area.

CLINICAL MANIFESTATIONS
- **Pain over the fifth metatarsal area & lateral border** of the midfoot, especially with weight bearing.

<u>Physical examination:</u>
- Tenderness to palpation along the bone at the fracture site. Difficulty with weight bearing.
- Edema and/or ecchymosis at the fracture site (lateral aspect of the foot).

DIAGNOSIS
- <u>Radiographs:</u> **acute proximal diaphyseal fractures with the medial fracture line extending into or towards the intermetatarsal joint** (articulation between the bases of the fourth and fifth metatarsals). **With acute fractures, the fracture line is sharp, and the surrounding bone appears normal.** With stress fractures (Zone 3), surrounding bone will appear abnormal.

MANAGEMENT
- **<u>Immediate management</u>: immobilization in a posterior splint, strict non-weight bearing (crutches are required), analgesics, and orthopedic follow-up in 3-5 days.** Icing (while keeping the splint dry); elevation of the injured foot above the heart level to minimize swelling.
- **<u>Nonoperative (conservative) management</u>: Non-weight bearing short leg cast for 4-6 weeks,** followed by 4-6 weeks in walking boot or hard-sole shoe, until both clinical and radiographic evidence of fracture union. Usually placed 3-5 days postinjury, after swelling has begun to subside.
- **<u>Operative management:</u> Jones fractures frequently requires surgical management — eg, intramedullary screw fixation (surgical standard of treatment)** or open reduction internal fixation with plate and screws. **Surgery reduces the risk of non-union.** 30-50% will re-fracture.

PSEUDO-JONES FRACTURE

- **<u>Proximal tuberosity base or styloid avulsion fracture of the fifth metatarsal</u>** due to plantar flexion with inversion (**Zone 1**). Much more common and less serious than a true Jones fracture.
- Pain to the lateral border of the forefoot. May have difficulty with weight bearing.

MANAGEMENT
- **<u>Nondisplaced:</u> Stiff-soled shoe or weight-bearing immobilization (short-leg walking cast or boot)** for up to 6-8 weeks. It may extend into the articular surface (cubometatarsal joint).
- <u>Displaced:</u> ORIF (surgical fixation) if >30% of articular surface or with an articular step off of 2 mm.

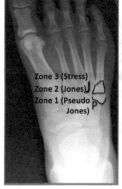
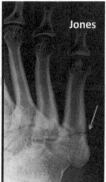
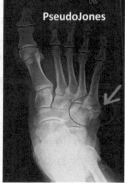
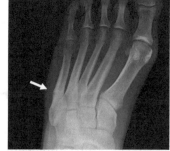

Stress fracture (Zone 3): proximal diaphyseal fracture. Case courtesy of Andrew Dixon, Radiopaedia.org, rID: 36631

LISFRANC INJURY

- <u>Lisfranc joint:</u> bases of the first 3 metatarsal heads & their respective cuneiforms.
- <u>Lisfranc Injury:</u> injury where **one or more of the metatarsal bones are displaced from the tarsus.**

PATHOPHYSIOLOGY
Tarsometatarsal (TMT) joint complex injury:
- **Tarsometatarsal fracture-dislocation:** disruption between the articulation of the medial cuneiform & the base of the second metatarsal, leading to ligamentous injury (dislocation) and or fracture.
- <u>Mechanism of injury</u> **severe foot plantar flexion**: Varied but includes rotational (midfoot) & **severe axial load placed on a plantar-flexed foot** that then forcibly rotates, bends, or is compressed.

CLINICAL MANIFESTATIONS
- **Pain at the dorsum midfoot: pain, bruising, &/or swelling at the tarsal-metatarsal joints.**
- Severe pain and inability to bear weight or standing on their toes.

Physical examination:
- **Plantar ecchymosis (hematoma) is highly suggestive a TMT joint complex injury if present.**
- **Pain with forefoot rotation against a stabilized hindfoot (calcaneus).**
- <u>Instability</u> (dorsal subluxation with dorsal force to the forefoot). Tenderness over the TMT joint.

RADIOGRAPHS
- Most common variant is one metatarsal away from the other ones.
- **Fleck sign — fracture at the base of the second metatarsal pathognomonic for disruption of the tarsometatarsal ligaments.** May be associated with multiple fractures of the metatarsals.

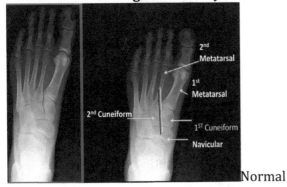
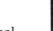
Normal
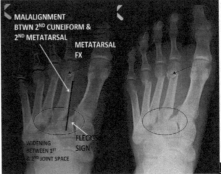
Lisfranc

MANAGEMENT
Immediate management:
- **Initial treatment includes PRICE-M — protection with short-leg splint or boot, rest (non-weightbearing, ice, compression with elastic wrap, elevation** of the extremity above the level of the heart, and medication (analgesia).
- **Posttraumatic arthritis most common complication of Lisfranc injuries.**

Operative management:
- **ORIF (open reduction internal fixation) followed by non-weight bearing cast for 6-8 weeks for Lisfranc injuries with any evidence of instability or bony fracture.** At that time, re-evaluation is performed, and a walking boot or cast can be considered as clinical presentation indicates. This cast or boot is then usually worn for another 6 weeks.

Nonoperative management:
- <u>Indications:</u> **Nonoperative management only reserved for anatomically stable and non-displaced injuries — non-weight bearing and placed in a cast or boot.** Repeat evaluation and radiographs should be performed after 2 weeks to rule out any diastasis that may need surgical management. After at least 6 weeks, if the patient is completely nontender and radiographs are again negative, weightbearing and a rehabilitation program may be begun. If there is any tenderness but still no displacement, then the patient should be in a boot or cast again for at least another 4 weeks before starting rehabilitation. Any diastasis or displacement requires surgical fixation.

PEDIATRIC FRACTURES

GREENSTICK FRACTURES

- **Incomplete fracture** break on one side of the cortex (cortical disruption) & periosteal tearing on the convex side of the fracture (intact periosteum on the concave side) similar to a broken branch of a young tree **"bowing"**. Usually heals without long-term complications since it is incomplete.
- Management: **Immobilization followed by casting** — all greenstick fractures should be treated in a well-molded long arm splint or cast. Fractures with >15° of angulation in girls ≤8y & boys ≤10y and younger or fractures >10° in older children also require closed reduction.

TORUS (BUCKLE) FRACTURES

- **Incomplete fracture with "wrinkling or bump" due to trabecular decompression of the metaphyseal-diaphyseal junction** (where the dense bone meets the more porous bone) due to axial loading.
- Management: **Torus fractures are considered stable & are treated via application of a removable splint for 3 weeks**. Follow-up radiographs are usually not necessary, as the fractures are stable and heal well with a splint.

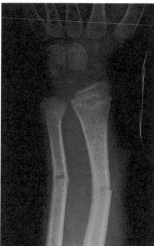
GREENSTICK FRACTURE

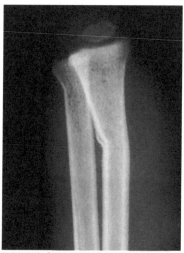
TORUS (BUCKLE) FRACTURE

SALTER- HARRIS CLASSIFICATION OF FRACTURES

- **Growth (Epiphyseal) Plate Fractures. "SALTR" useful mnemonic IN RELATION TO PLATE**

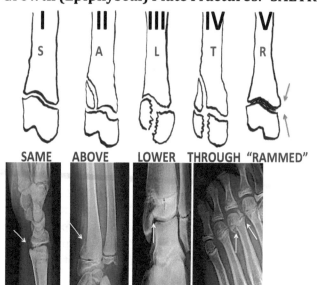

I — S — SAME
II — A — ABOVE
III — L — LOWER
IV — T — THROUGH
V — R — "RAMMED"

Type I: isolated growth plate fracture (may look normal). Best outcome.

Type II: growth plate fracture + **fracture of the metaphysis (good prognosis). MC of all Salter-Harris Fractures.**

Type III: growth plate fracture + **fracture of the epiphysis.** (good prognosis).

Type IV: fracture **extending across the metaphysis, growth plate & epiphysis (needs reduction).**

Type V: Growth plate compression injury (may arrest growth). **Worst type!**

MALIGNANT BONE TUMORS

OSTEOSARCOMA

- Malignant tumor with production of osteoid (new bone) or immature bone by the malignant cells.
- **Most common primary bone malignancy in children and young adults.**
- **90% occur in the metaphysis of the long bones (distal femur most common)**, proximal tibia, & proximal humerus. **Most common METS to the lungs** (most common cause of death).
- Bimodal: **Most common in adolescents** (80% occur <20y); **second peak 50-60y especially if history of Paget disease of the bone or radiation therapy. Retinoblastoma is a risk factor.**

CLINICAL MANIFESTATIONS
- **Localized bone pain** (may occur after injury); **worse at night. Joint swelling** (no systemic symptoms).
- Physical exam: **palpable soft tissue mass (may be tender to palpation).**

DIAGNOSIS
- Radiographs: **"hair on end" or "sunburst" appearance due to tumor spicules of calcified bone radiating in right angles is classic** (not specific). Other findings: mixed sclerotic & lytic lesions. Codman's triangle: ossification of raised periosteum (can also be seen in Ewing sarcoma). MRI.

Hair On End

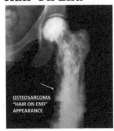

Codman's Triangle

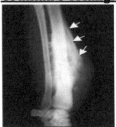

- **Biopsy: definitive diagnosis** - malignant osteoid within the tumor & malignant sarcomatous stroma.
- Labs: **increased alkaline phosphatase** (due to increased osteoblastic activity) — ALP the biochemical marker most closely associated with Osteosarcoma that is useful for diagnosis, prognosis, treatment response, and recurrence detection. Increased LDH.
- CT scan: may be used to evaluate the thorax for metastatic disease to the lungs.
- Radionuclide bone scan to detect bony metastasis or presence of multiple lesions.

MANAGEMENT
- **Neovascular: Preoperative chemotherapy followed by limb-sparing surgery, followed by postoperative chemotherapy.** Doxorubicin, Ifosfamide, Cisplatin, Methotrexate with Leucovorin.
- Not neovascular: limb-sparing resection.

CHONDROSARCOMA

- **Cancer of the cartilage** [produces chondroid (cartilage) matrix]. Most common in adults 40-75 years.
- Location: proximal femur, pelvic bones, and proximal humerus most common sites.

CLINICAL MANIFESTATIONS
- **Localized pain and swelling** (signs of inflammation), especially at night. Pathologic fractures.

DIAGNOSIS
- Radiographs: lobular mineralized mottled or punctate appearance of the chondroid matrix with **punctate, popcorn, or ring & arc appearance to calcification**.
- CT or MRI provide more details. Histology: increased malignant cartilage matrix production.

MANAGEMENT
- Surgical resection: **wide surgical excision for nonmetastatic Chondrosarcoma mainstay.**
- Chemotherapy may be used in select cases of advanced disease (most are resistant to chemotherapy).

EWING SARCOMA

- **Second most common primary bone malignancy in adolescents and young adults (after Osteosarcoma)** — peak incidence of 10-15 years of age.
- Due to translocation between chromosomes 11 & 22. The tumors originate from unique mesenchymal progenitor cells.
- Most common in Caucasian males.

LOCATION:
- **50% found in the diaphysis of the long bones** — **proximal femur most common; pelvis,** axial skeleton, tibia, & fibula are common sites.
- Metastases: bone, bone marrow, & lung are common sites for metastasis. Lung METS is a common cause of death.

CLINICAL MANIFESTATIONS
- **Localized bone pain & swelling** over the site of involvement for a few weeks to months' duration. The pain may be intermittent and worse at night or with exercise.
- Systemic symptoms (eg, fever, fatigue, malaise, weight loss, leukocytosis) especially if metastatic.

PHYSICAL EXAM
- May have a palpable soft tissue mass, local tenderness, or joint swelling.

DIAGNOSIS
- **Radiographs: multilayered periosteal reaction with an "onion skin/peel" appearance,** destructive lytic lesions that become confluent over time with a **"moth-eaten" appearance**. Codman's triangle: ossification of raised periosteum (can also be seen in Osteosarcoma).
- Labs: increased ESR, leukocytosis. **LDH carries prognostic significance.**
- Bone scan, MRI, and CT scan of the chest are required for initial staging to look for metastasis.
- Histology: sheets of monotonous small round blue cells. May have pseudo-rosettes (circle of cells with central necrosis). The presence of p30/32, the product of the *mic-2* gene is a cell-surface marker for Ewing's sarcoma

MANAGEMENT
- **Systemic chemotherapy mainstay of therapy, followed by limb-sparing resection when possible.** Interval-compressed therapy with alternating cycles of Vincristine, Doxorubicin, Cyclophosphamide (VDC) and Ifosfamide-Etoposide (VDC/IE). Dactinomycin.
- Radiation therapy when complete excision is not possible. Topotecan or Irinotecan + alkylating agent.

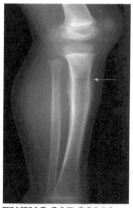

EWING SARCOMA
"Onion" peel appearance
(periosteal reaction)

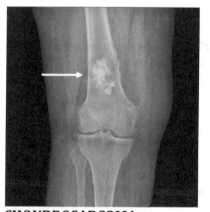

CHONDROSARCOMA
Punctate or ring & arc appearance calcification
Case courtesy of Domenico Nicoletti, Radiopaedia.org, rID: 30655

BENIGN BONE TUMORS

OSTEOCHONDROMA

- Cartilage-capped bony overgrowth arising on the external surface of a bone & areas of tendon insertion (eg, proximal tibia, femur, & proximal humerus). Does not cause bone destruction.
- **Most common benign bone tumor.** 10% may become secondary Chondrosarcomas.
- **Most commonly seen in between 10-20 years of age & in males.**
- Begins in childhood & grows until skeletal maturity.

CLINICAL MANIFESTATIONS
- Most asymptomatic. **Painless, palpable mass.** May develop symptoms of neurovascular compression.

DIAGNOSIS
- <u>Radiographs:</u> **often pedunculated (narrow stalk) that <u>grows away from the growth plate</u> &** involves the medullary tissue. CT or MRI. <u>Biopsy:</u> definitive.

MANAGEMENT
- **Observation if asymptomatic.**
- <u>Marginal resection</u> including cartilage cap if it becomes painful or if located in the pelvis (pelvis most common site of malignant transformation). Usually delayed until skeletal maturity.

OSTEOID OSTEOMA

- **Benign bone tumor characterized by a <u>small radiolucent nidus</u>** (usually <1 to 1.5 cm in diameter).
- Most commonly presents in the second decade. More common in males.
- <u>Locations:</u> proximal femur most common, tibia, the remainder of the femur, and spine.
- <u>Pathophysiology:</u> **the nidus produces high levels of prostaglandins.**

CLINICAL MANIFESTATIONS
- **Progressively increasing <u>pain that is worse at night</u> and unrelated to activity. The <u>pain is relieved within 20-25 minutes of administration of NSAIDs</u>** (prostaglandin inhibition).
- May develop a limp, localized tenderness over the region, and limitation of range of motion.

DIAGNOSIS
- **<u>Radiograph:</u> small round lucency (nidus) with a dense sclerotic margin.** CT or MRI more sensitive.

MANAGEMENT
- **<u>Conservative</u>: NSAIDs with serial examinations or radiographs every 6 months.**
  Untreated Osteoid osteoma often spontaneously resolves over several years.
- Surgical resection for symptomatic lesions not responsive to conservative treatment.

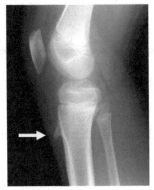

OSTEOCHONDROMA
Pedunculated stalk that **grows away from the growth plate.**

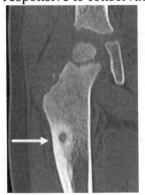

OSTEID OSTEOMA
Small round lucency (nidus) with a sclerotic margin
Case courtesy of Micheál Anthony Breen, Radiopaedia.org, rID: 25971

UPPER EXTREMITY NERVE INJURIES

AXILLARY NERVE INJURIES

The axillary nerve is derived from the posterior cord of the brachial plexus.

Sensory deficits:
- Decreased <u>deltoid pinprick sensation</u> over the lateral shoulder.

Motor deficits:
- **Weakened shoulder abduction:** the axillary nerve innervates the teres minor & deltoid.

Associated conditions:
- **Proximal** humerus fracture
- Shoulder dislocations. Sleep in a prone position with the arms raised above the head.

RADIAL NERVE INJURIES

Sensory deficits:
- **Posterior first webspace (dorsoradial side of the hand);** may extend up the posterior forearm.

Motor deficits:
- **Radial nerve palsy: leads to weakness of wrist extensors resulting in a <u>wrist drop</u>** because the radial nerve is responsible for wrist extension. Forearm pain & weakness of finger dorsiflexion with posterior interosseus neuropathy.
- **Radial nerve palsy (Saturday night palsy): Radial nerve compression from prolonged direct pressure** on the medial arm or axilla by an object or surface or use of crutches.
  Management: splinting the wrist, physical therapy, and pain management. Remember the radial nerve is formed from nerve roots C5 through T1.

Associated conditions:
- Elbow dislocations, Monteggia Fracture, Supracondylar fracture, Humeral shaft fracture.

ULNAR NERVE INJURIES

Sensory deficits:
- 5th finger and ulnar side of the 4th finger.

Motor deficits:
- **Adductor pollicis of the thumb is innervated by the ulnar nerve** (may have **thumb adduction deficits** if damaged): **Froment's sign** (when pinching a piece of paper between the thumb & index finger against resistance, the thumb IP joint will flex if the adductor pollicis is weak), Jeanne's sign, problem with index finger abduction (scissors motion). Weakness in wrist and finger flexion.
- Claw hand if severe: atrophy of the hand intrinsic muscles and clawing of the fourth and the fifth digits.

Associated conditions:
- Elbow dislocations, Olecranon Fractures, Cubital Tunnel syndrome, elbow flexion at night.

MEDIAN NERVE INJURIES

Sensory deficits:
- **1st 3 fingers & radial side of 4th finger** (eg, sensation at the volar tip of the index finger).

Motor deficits:
- Normally, thenar eminence muscles allow for thumb abduction "**Thumbs Up**". Damage leads to **loss of thumb abduction. "OK" sign (pincer function of the thumb and index finger) or oppose thumb & fifth finger. Weakness &/or atrophy of the thenar eminence.**

Associated conditions:
- **Carpal Tunnel syndrome,** Supracondylar Fracture, Colles Fracture,
- **Pronator syndrome: proximal forearm pain** (but no pain at night).
- Elbow dislocations & injury to the anterior interosseous nerve that branches at the elbow.

BRACHIAL PLEXUS INJURIES

- The brachial plexus begins at the neck and crosses the upper chest to the armpit. Anatomically, the brachial plexus stems from the C4-T1 cervical roots and ultimately from the lateral, posterior, and medial cords. At the lateral border of the pectoralis minor, these cords ultimately form the 5 major peripheral nerves of the arm (musculocutaneous, axillary, radial, median, and ulnar nerves).

MECHANISMS OF INJURY
- **Often occurs when the arm is forcibly pulled or stretched**, fall onto the shoulder; penetrating, compression, or closed traction injuries. **High speed motor vehicle or motorcycle crashes.**

CLINICAL MANIFESTATIONS

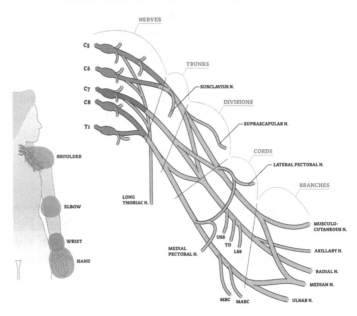

BRACHIAL PLEXUS

- **Upper extremity paresthesias & shoulder weakness (neck & shoulder girdle & upper arm),** with pain-free ROM of the cervical spine. Cervical radiculopathy.
- Weakness, reflex, & sensory deficits.
- **Adduction & internal rotation of the shoulder indicate weakness of the deltoid & infraspinatus muscles (C5); elbow extension is due to weakness of the biceps (C6), and flexion of the digits and wrists is due to weakness of extensors (C7).**
- <u>Mucocutaneous nerve injury:</u> **numbness to the lateral forearm.**
- Paresthesias &/or motor loss in may be transient (eg, neuropraxia) or permanent.

MANAGEMENT
- Depends on the extent of the injuries. Orthopedist referral.
- Electromyography/nerve conduction velocity (EMG/NCV) can help localize the lesion and aid in prognosis. Can show changes as early as 3 weeks after injury.

LONG THORACIC NERVE INJURIES

MECHANISM OF INJURY
- Traction, blunt trauma, or iatrogenic surgical injury may cause injury to the long thoracic nerve.

CLINICAL MANIFESTATIONS
- <u>Winging of the scapula</u> **due to palsy of the serratus anterior** (the scapula moves medial and the medial border wings away from the thorax). Iatrogenic surgical injury is more commonly associated with spinal accessory nerve injury, and this results in lateral winging of the scapula (scapula moves lateral and the medial border wings away from the thorax).
- May be painless, but often, medial scapula pain is present.

MANAGEMENT
- **Treatment after traction and blunt trauma is usually conservative initially, with rehabilitation during return of function.** EMG/NCV can help localize the lesion and aid in prognosis.
- When paralysis is permanent, pectoralis transfer facilitates treatment of long thoracic nerve palsy, and levator scapulae transfer facilitates treatment of spinal accessory nerve palsy.

SHOULDER INJURIES

ANTERIOR GLENOHUMERAL DISLOCATION

- <u>Mechanism of injury:</u> **most common after a blow to an abducted, externally rotated, and extended upper extremity;** fall on an outstretched hand (FOOSH), or posterior humeral force.
- **Anterior glenohumeral dislocation is the most common type of shoulder dislocation.**

PHYSICAL EXAMINATION
- **Arm held in slight abduction & external rotation** (elbow pointing outward). Prominent acromion.
- Humeral head is often palpable inferiorly with loss of the deltoid contour or **"squared off shoulder".**

DIAGNOSIS
- <u>Shoulder radiographs:</u> initial test of choice. **Axillary & scapular "Y" views most helpful to distinguish anterior vs. posterior dislocations** — humeral head <u>displaced inferior & medially</u>. <u>Hill-Sachs lesion:</u> **humeral head groove fracture.** <u>Bankart lesion:</u> **glenoid rim fracture.**
- <u>CT or MRI:</u> gives more details about any associated soft tissue injuries.

MANAGEMENT
- **Reduction & immobilization**: **[1] Shoulder reduction with [2] pre & post assessment of the Axillary nerve (deltoid pinprick sensation), followed by [3] immobilization by sling & swath (Velpeau sling).** Follow up with orthopedist in 1 week (or 1-2 days if complicated). For patients <40 years, physical therapy should begin after 3 weeks (after 1 week if >40 years).
- <u>Complications</u> include **injuries to the axillary nerve (most common),** axillary artery, brachial plexus, suprascapular nerve & radial nerve. Neurovascular examination done pre & post reduction.

POSTERIOR GLENOHUMERAL SHOULDER DISLOCATION

- <u>Mechanisms of injury:</u> **forced adduction, internal rotation — seizures, electrocution, or trauma (direct blow to anterior shoulder with posterior directed force).** Less common than anterior shoulder dislocations.

PHYSICAL EXAMINATION
- **Arm is usually adducted & internally rotated.** Inability to externally rotate the arm.
- The anterior shoulder appears flat with a prominent humeral head & coracoid process.

DIAGNOSIS
- <u>Shoulder radiographs:</u> **initial test of choice. Scapular "Y" & Axillary lateral views best to distinguish anterior vs. posterior.** AP films may show the **"light bulb" sign** (the appearance of the humeral head looks like a light bulb or ice cream cone). CT or MRI to assess for complications.

MANAGEMENT
- **Reduction & immobilization with close follow-up.** Neurovascular compromise is uncommon.
- Glenolabral and capsular injuries may lead to posterior shoulder instability. Reverse Hill-Sachs.

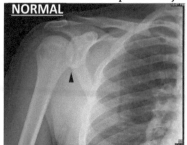

NORMAL AP: humeral head articulates with glenoid (arrowhead). Appears overlapped.

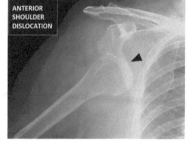

ANTERIOR DISLOCATION: Humeral head **anterior & inferior to** glenoid

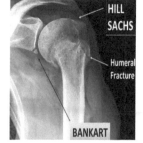

HILL-SACHS: Humeral head groove
BANKART: fracture of glenoid rim

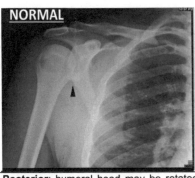
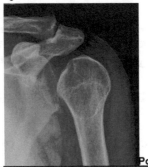
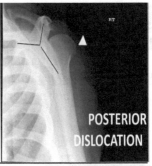

Posterior: humeral head may be rotated (**ice cream on cone/light bulb appearance**) and isn't centered on the glenoid. **Humeral head posterior to the glenoid and inferior to the acromion.** May look normal on AP view or may show increased distance from the glenoid rim (normally there is overlap between glenoid rim & the humeral head).

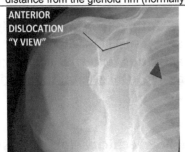
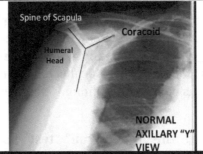
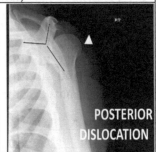

ACROMIOCLAVICULAR JOINT DISLOCATION (SHOULDER SEPARATION)

- <u>Mechanism of injury:</u> Direct blow to an adducted shoulder.
- <u>Physiology:</u> the acromioclavicular ligament provides horizontal stability. The coracoclavicular ligament provides vertical stability.

CLINICAL MANIFESTATIONS
- Pain with lifting arm, unable to lift the arm at the shoulder. Decreased range of motion (ROM).
- There may be a deformity (step-off) at the AC joint. Prominent distal clavicle may be seen.

DIAGNOSIS
- Radiographs taken without weights or with weights to reveal mild separations.
- Both shoulders may be visualized to compare the separation.

MANAGEMENT
- **Nonoperative: in most Type I, type II, & most type III.** Conservative management includes ice, brief sling immobilization, & rest. Early rehabilitation + ROM exercises for ROM preservation (7-14 days).
- <u>Surgical:</u> Type IV and above with <2 cm clavicular displacement, Type V, Type VI, and some patients with Type III (eg, athletes, cosmetic concerns).

SHOULDER SEPARATION

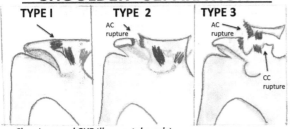

- Class I: *normal CXR (ligamental sprain)*
- Class II: *slight widening (Acromioclavicular ligament ruptured)*
  Coracoclavicular ligament sprained
- Class III: *significant widening: rupture of both AC & CC ligaments*
- Class IV: AC & CC rupture + displacement of clavicle into/through trapezius
- Class V: Class IV + disruption of the clavicular attachments

GRADE 2 SHOULDER SEPARATION
- **Acromioclavicular (AC) ligament RUPTURED**
- **Coracoclavicular (CC) ligament sprained**

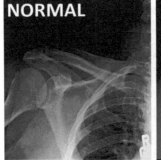
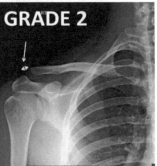

ROTATOR CUFF INJURIES

- **SITS** supraspinatus **(abduction)**, infraspinatus (external rotation), teres minor (external rotation), subscapularis (internal rotation). **Supraspinatus is the most commonly injured muscle/tendon.**
- Mechanism of injury: chronic erosion, trauma. Impingement of the supraspinatus tendon. Common in athletes or laborers performing **repetitive overhead movements**, older age, smokers.

TENDONITIS
- Inflammation often associated with subacromial bursitis; **Most common in adolescents & <40 years.**

ROTATOR CUFF TEAR
- **Most common cause of shoulder pain >40 years of age.** Trauma, degeneration, or chronic overuse.

CLINICAL MANIFESTATIONS
- **Anterolateral shoulder (deltoid) pain: with overhead activity & lifting arm; worse at night (persistent night pain), with inability to sleep on the affected side** (especially with tears).
- **Decreased range of motion (ROM), especially with overhead activities, external or internal rotation or >90° abduction** (combing hair, reaching for wallet). **Passive ROM greater than active.**
- Weakness, atrophy, & continuous pain more commonly seen with tears.

PHYSICAL EXAMINATION
- **Supraspinatus strength test: the "open can" test has 90% specificity for assessing supraspinatus.** Resisted shoulder abduction at 90° with slight forward flexion to ~45°.
- Impingement tests: positive Hawkins test, Drop arm test, and Neer test.
   - ⊕ **Hawkins test** elbow/shoulder flexed at 90°: **sharp anterior shoulder pain with internal rotation.**
   - ⊕ **Drop arm test:** pain with inability to lift arm above shoulder level, or hold it, or severe pain when slowly lowering the arm after the shoulder is abducted to 90°. ⊕ Jobe test.
   - ⊕ **Neer test:** arm fully pronated (thumbs down) with pain during forward flexion while the shoulder is held down to prevent shrugging.
- Supraspinatus: pain with abduction against resistance. Subscapularis: IR weakness at 0° abduction.
- Infraspinatus: ER weakness at 0° abduction; Teres minor: ER weakness at 90° abduction and 90° ER.
- **Subacromial lidocaine test:** may help to distinguish tendinopathy from tears. **Normal strength with pain relief = tendinopathy. Persistent weakness classically seen with large tears.**
- **MRI: most accurate test to diagnose Rotator cuff tears.** Ultrasound: can be helpful.

MANAGEMENT OF TEARS
- **Conservative: NSAIDs for pain management, ice, rest; physical therapy for rehabilitation, range of motion, and muscle strengthening exercises.**
- Intraarticular corticosteroids usually reserved for patients who fail NSAID management of pain.
- Surgery: patients who fail conservative management within 6 months or patients with complete tears.

MANAGEMENT OF TENDINITIS
- **Physical therapy: shoulder pendulum/wall climbing exercises.**
- Activity modification, physical therapy, oral Nonsteroidal anti-inflammatory drugs (NSAIDs), & ice.

ROTATOR CUFF INJURIES
PHYSICAL EXAMINATION

Impingement of subscapular nerve/supraspinatus between acromial process & humeral head:
- ⊕*Hawkins test**: Elbow/shoulder flexed @90° c̄ sharp anterior *shoulder pain on passive internal rotation* of humerus

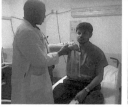
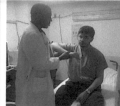

ROTATOR CUFF INJURIES
PHYSICAL EXAMINATION

Impingement of subscapular nerve/supraspinatus between acromial process & humeral head:
- ⊕*Neer test: arm fully pronated (thumb's down) c̄ pain during forward flexion* (shoulder is held down to prevent shrugging)

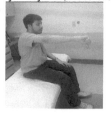
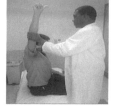

PROXIMAL HUMERUS & HUMERAL HEAD FRACTURES

- <u>Mechanism of injury:</u> Fall on an outstretched hand (FOOSH), direct blow, high-energy trauma.
- Common site for pathologic fractures in metastatic breast cancer & Osteoporosis. Surgical neck MC.
- <u>Physical examination:</u> arm held in adducted position. **Decreased ROM, pain, swelling, & ecchymosis.**

DIAGNOSIS
- Shoulder radiographs usually the initial test. Neer classification used for determining type.
- <u>CT scan:</u> may be used to further evaluate (eg, preoperative planning). MRI

MANAGEMENT
- **Conservative management: 80% of proximal humeral fractures are impacted or nondisplaced & can be treated conservatively — application of a sling and swath (Velpeau sling)** ±closed reduction for most nondisplaced or minimally displaced fractures. Early mobilization & ROM, with progressive rehabilitation after 2 weeks with pendulum exercises to prevent Frozen shoulder.
- <u>Surgical fixation vs. arthroplasty</u> — often reserved for complex fractures (eg, significantly displaced).

Complications
- **Nerve injury: axillary (most common) and suprascapular nerve injury (second most common).** Radial nerve injuries may occur with significant displacement of mid to distal shaft fractures. Median and ulnar nerve injuries are uncommon. Brachial plexus injury.
- <u>Vascular injury:</u> axillary artery most common (5-6%). Fractures at the anatomic neck may disrupt the blood supply, leading to osteonecrosis (avascular necrosis) of the humeral head.

HUMERAL SHAFT (DIAPHYSIS) FRACTURE

MECHANISM OF INJURY
- Fall on an outstretched hand (FOOSH), direct trauma (direct blow that produces a bending force).

CLINICAL MANIFESTATIONS
- Severe arm pain in the mid-arm; the pain may be referred to the elbow or shoulder.

<u>Physical examination:</u>
- Local pain, swelling, ecchymosis, crepitus, tenderness, decreased ROM. **Rule out radial nerve injury.**
- **Radial nerve injury most common nerve injured by midshaft humerus fractures — weakness of wrist, finger, and thumb extension,** weakness of elbow supination, and **wrist drop.** Sensory loss may be present on the dorsum of the hand and is easily tested at the **dorsal web space between the thumb and index finger.** Median nerve and ulnar injuries are uncommon.

MANAGEMENT
- **The majority of both proximal and midshaft humerus fractures are nondisplaced and can be treated conservatively (nonsurgical)** — ice, immobilization, analgesia, and referral.
- **Nonoperative: coaptation (sugar-tong) splint or sling & swathe** & prompt orthopedic follow up.
- <u>Operative:</u> ORIF for open fractures, vascular, or neuronal injuries with pain and weakness.

PROXIMAL HUMERUS FRACTURE
arm usually held in adducted position.
Check deltoid sensation, brachial plexus injury*
± crepitus/ecchymosis

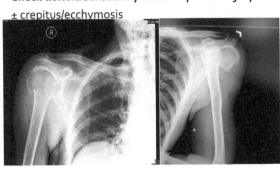

HUMERAL SHAFT FRACTURE
- **MOI:** FOOSH, direct trauma.
- *R/o radial nerve injury (may develop a wrist drop)**

NORMAL PATH OF RADIAL NERVE

AXILLARY NERVE

RADIAL NERVE

ULNAR NERVE

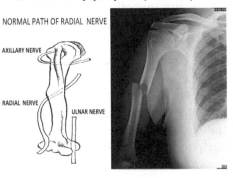

ADHESIVE CAPSULITIS (FROZEN SHOULDER)

- **<u>Shoulder stiffness</u> due to inflammation.** Most common age 40–60 years and in women.
- **<u>Associations</u>: Diabetes mellitus, Hypothyroidism,** or other systemic disorders.
- May occur following shoulder bursitis, tendinitis, fractures, surgery, or without an antecedent event.

CLINICAL MANIFESTATIONS
- **<u>Shoulder pain/stiffness</u> decreased range of motion [ROM], especially with external rotation.**
  Pain initially, then diminishes. Pain is usually worse at night. Stiff-pain cycle is common.
- Associated with a gradual return of range of motion (may last 18-24 months).

Physical Examination:
- **<u>BOTH decreased active AND passive ROM</u> (especially with external rotation). All ranges of motion of the shoulder are diminished only on the affected side.**

MANAGEMENT
- **Usually, a self-limited disease with spontaneous recovery within 18-30 months.**
- **Treatment is mainly symptomatic relief and improving ROM — prolonged physical & occupational therapy (gentle ROM exercise),** NSAIDs, massage therapy, hydrodilatation.
- Anti-inflammatories, intraarticular steroid injection & heat may be helpful. Surgery if refractory.

CLAVICLE FRACTURES

- **Most commonly fractured bone in children, adolescents, & newborns during birth.**

MECHANISM OF INJURY
- Mid-high energy direct impact to the area or fall on an outstretched hand (FOOSH).
- If no history of trauma, think malignancy, Rickets, or child abuse (especially in children <2 years of age).

PHYSICAL EXAMINATION
- **Pain with ROM, swelling, deformity, crepitus, & tenderness overlying the clavicle.** May have tenting of the skin (impending open fracture). May hold arm against chest to protect against motion.

CLASSIFICATION
- **<u>Group I</u> (midshaft) middle 1/3 of the clavicle is the most common type of clavicular fracture.**
- **<u>Group II</u>: lateral (distal) third.** Treatment is immobilization or surgery, depending on severity.
- **<u>Group III</u>: proximal (medial) third often due to high-mechanism injuries & intrathoracic trauma.**

Normal 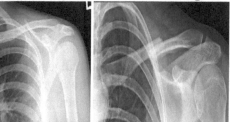 **Clavicular fracture**

MANAGEMENT
- **<u>Mid 1/3:</u> <u>Nonoperative:</u> sling immobilization in most adults with early ROM. Sling or figure-of-eight splint in children, with early ROM.** <u>Operative:</u> indicated for open fractures, displaced fractures with skin tenting, subclavian artery of vein injuries, severe displacement, or shortening.
- **<u>Proximal 1/3:</u> Emergent orthopedic consult (may cause compromise of mediastinal structures).**
- Clinical union is usually achieved by 6-12 weeks in adults and 3-6 weeks in children.

Complications:
- Pneumothorax, hemothorax, coracoclavicular ligament disruption (distal), & brachial plexus injuries.
- <u>Brachial plexus injury</u> can occur at the time of presentation or during the healing and callus formation of the clavicle. Excessive callus formation can lead to compression of the brachial plexus, resulting in peripheral neuropathy.

SUPRACONDYLAR HUMERUS FRACTURES

- <u>Mechanism:</u> fall on outstretched hand (FOOSH) with hyperextended elbow. Extension type (90-98%).
- Most common elbow fracture in children, especially in children 5-10 years of age (peak 5-7 years).
- <u>Clinical manifestations:</u> pain, swelling, tenderness, and decreased ROM at the elbow.

DIAGNOSIS
- **<u>Nondisplaced:</u> [1] <u>displaced anterior fat pad sign</u> &/or [2] <u>posterior fat pad sign</u> (hemarthrosis) is suggestive of fracture** (may be the only initial evidence of a fracture).
- **<u>Displaced:</u> abnormal anterior humeral line** may be seen on the lateral radiographs.

COMPLICATIONS
- <u>Neuropraxia:</u> 11.3% incidence. **<u>Anterior interosseous nerve</u> injury is the most common nerve injury in displaced extension type fractures** [may affect the flexor pollicis longus: sole motor deficits: inability to flex either the thumb IP joint or the index finger DIP joint, difficulty pinching between the thumb & index finger (**thumb & index finger form a flat & triangular shape instead of normal round "OK" sign**)]. **Radial nerve injury (second most common).** Median or ulnar nerve.
- **<u>Volkmann ischemic contracture:</u> due to Median nerve & brachial artery injury** (claw-like deformity from ischemia with flexion/contracture of wrist).
- **<u>Compartment syndrome:</u> most common cause of forearm Compartment syndrome in children.**

MANAGEMENT
<u>Nondisplaced (Garland Type I) or minimally displaced (<2 mm) fractures:</u>
- **Usually treated with a short period of rest & a sling or posterior splint with the elbow at 90° of flexion to support the extremity.** Orthopedic follow-up within 7 days.

<u>Type II and III:</u>
- **<u>Urgent orthopedic consultation in the ED</u> and closed reduction & percutaneous pinning or ORIF:** indicated for type II and III supracondylar fractures, flexion type, and median column collapse.

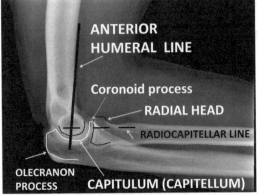

NORMAL LATERAL VIEW: the radial head dissects the capitellum. A line drawn from the anterior humerus should also dissect the capitellum.

SUPRACONDYLAR FRACTURE

DIAGNOSIS
- *Abnormal anterior humeral line* on lateral view

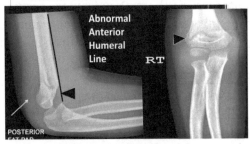

SUPRACONDYLAR FRACTURE: abnormal anterior humeral line (does not dissect the capitellum). Posterior fat pad sign. Fracture (arrowhead).

SUPRACONDYLAR FRACTURE

DIAGNOSIS
- ⊕ Anterior or Posterior fat pad sign (hemarthrosis)

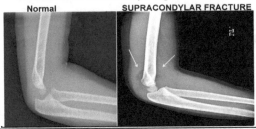

SUPRACONDYLAR FRACTURE:
The anterior humeral line may be normal & the only clue is an abnormal anterior or ⊕ posterior fat pad (joint effusion) [white arrows].
Posterior fat pads are always abnormal.
Anterior fat pads may be seen as a normal variant if they are small and almost parallel to the humerus.
Anterior/posterior fad pad = supracondylar fracture in children (= radial head fracture in adults).

RADIAL NECK AND HEAD FRACTURES

- Mechanism: fall on outstretched hand (FOOSH) or direct elbow trauma. Usually intraarticular.
- Physical examination: lateral (radial) elbow pain, **inability to fully extend the elbow.**

DIAGNOSIS
- Notoriously difficult to see. The neck is fractured more commonly than the head.
- **Radiographs: Positive posterior fat pad or displaced anterior fat pad sign (both due to hemarthrosis) may be the only radiologic evidence of occult fractures.**

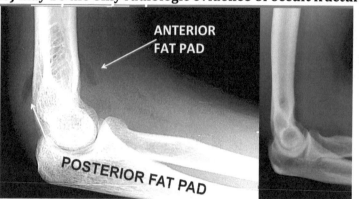
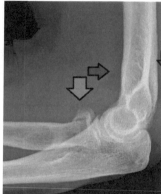

Photo credit: James Heilman, MD, *Wikimedia commons*

MANAGEMENT
- **Nondisplaced: immobilization (eg, sling or long arm splint 90°) with early ROM.** Reduction is often necessary when angulation is >35° or displacement is >60%.
- Displaced or complicated: surgical (eg, ORIF).

SUPPURATIVE FLEXOR TENOSYNOVITIS

- Infection of the flexor tendon & the synovial sheath of the finger; may also involve the wrist.
- ***Staphylococcus aureus* most common (including MRSA).** *Staphylococcus epidermidis*, group A *Streptococcus*; Others: *Pseudomonas aeruginosa* or mixed flora. *Eikenella* (human bites).
- Mechanism: often due to penetrating trauma or contiguous spread from adjacent tissues.
- Risk factors: Diabetes mellitus, IV drug use, immunocompromised patients.

CLINICAL MANIFESTATIONS
- Pain & swelling especially to the palmar aspect of the affected finger.
4 Kanavel's signs: FLEXor tenosynovitis
- **Finger held in flexion.**
- **Length of tendon sheath is tender** (tenderness along the tendon sheath).
- **Enlarged finger** (fusiform swelling of the finger).
- **Xtension of the finger causes pain (pain with passive extension).**

DIAGNOSIS
- Radiographs & MRI are often obtained but definitive diagnosis is made via aspiration &/or biopsy.

MANAGEMENT
- **Urgent incision & drainage with irrigation of the tendon sheath, debridement, & IV antibiotics.**
Empiric antibiotics:
- **Mechanism unknown or trauma: Vancomycin + a third-generation Cephalosporin (eg, Ceftriaxone).** Known water exposure: Vancomycin + antipseudomonal antibiotic (Ceftazidime).
- **Dog or cat bite: Ampicillin-sulbactam (IV) preferred or Amoxicillin-clavulanate (PO).** Alternatives include antibiotics vs. *Pasteurella multocida* (eg, Doxycycline, TMP-SMX, Penicillin V, Ciprofloxacin, Levofloxacin) PLUS anaerobic coverage (either Clindamycin or Metronidazole).

OLECRANON FRACTURES

- <u>Mechanism of injury:</u> direct blow (fall on a flexed elbow); triceps contraction while elbow is flexed.

CLINICAL MANIFESTATIONS
- **Pain, swelling, inability to fully extend the elbow (loss of triceps extensor mechanism),** bony defect.

COMPLICATIONS
- **Ulnar neuropathy,** posttraumatic arthritis, anterior interosseous nerve injury, & loss of extension strength. May occur in association with fractures of the radial head or neck.

MANAGEMENT
- <u>**Nondisplaced or minimally displaced with intact extensor mechanism:** reduction & posterior long arm splint (45°-90° flexion or with slight extension),</u> ortho follow up in 3 days, short period of immobilization, followed by early range of motion. Surgical management if loss of extensor mechanism.
- <u>Unstable:</u> surgical intervention (eg, tension band wiring, plate & screw fixation, intramedullary nails).

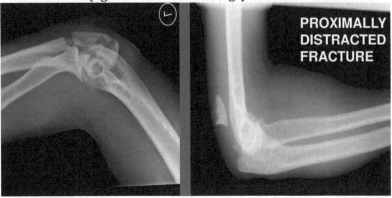

PROXIMALLY DISTRACTED FRACTURE

OLECRANON BURSITIS

- The olecranon bursa fills with fluid or blood; may become inflamed or infected.

ETIOLOGIES
- <u>Direct trauma:</u> eg, repetitive microtrauma, pressure, or contact to the elbow. Gout, inflammation.
- <u>Infectious (septic bursitis)</u> can occur after penetrating injury or break in the skin. *Staphylococcus aureus* is the most common organism of Septic bursitis.

CLINICAL MANIFESTATIONS
- **"Goose egg" boggy swelling to the posterior olecranon process area.**
- <u>Repetitive trauma or chronic:</u> usually painless or minimally tender. Often associated with full passive range of motion, decreased active ROM, or mild discomfort with full flexion.
- <u>Inflammatory or infectious:</u> **may have erythema, warmth, tenderness with painful, limited ROM.** Evaluate for skin breaks or overlying Cellulitis if suspected Septic bursitis.

DIAGNOSIS
- **Clinical diagnosis in most patients** — boggy swelling to the posterior olecranon process area.
- **Aspiration of the bursa** usually reserved for suspected Septic bursitis or if Gout is the suspected cause. WBC count <500/mm³ usually indicates noninfectious, non-crystalline bursitis. WBC count >2,000 cells/mm³ is often septic.

MANAGEMENT
- <u>**Olecranon bursitis:** conservative — avoid further trauma, joint protection (eg, padding to the area), NSAIDs (if painful or inflammatory), ice or heat application, ACE wrap for compression.</u> If the bursa persists or recurs, aspiration of the fluid with an 18-gauge needle may be performed.
- <u>Septic bursitis:</u> drainage of infected bursal fluid and antibiotic therapy (eg, oral Dicloxacillin or Clindamycin).

ULNAR SHAFT (NIGHTSTICK) FRACTURE

- <u>Mechanism:</u> direct blow to the forearm on the ulnar side. May present with localized pain & swelling.
- <u>Nightstick fracture:</u> fracture of the middle portion of the ulnar shaft without any associated fractures.

MANAGEMENT
- **<u>Nondisplaced distal third</u>: short arm cast.**
- **<u>Nondisplaced mid-proximal third (Nightstick)</u>: long arm posterior splint with the elbow at 90° and the wrist at neutral and slight extension for 7-10 days, which may be followed by cast or functional brace for 4-6 more weeks.** Closed reduction may be attempted when fracture angulation >10° or displacement >50%.
- <u>Displaced >50%:</u> open reduction & internal fixation.

MONTEGGIA FRACTURE

- **[1] Fracture to the proximal 1/3 of the ulnar shaft + [2] radial head dislocation.**
- <u>Mechanism of injury:</u> direct blow to the forearm or after a fall an outstretched hand (FOOSH).

CLINICAL MANIFESTATIONS
- Elbow pain and swelling, thumb paresthesias. Evaluate radial and posterior interosseus nerves.
- **<u>Radial nerve injury</u>** (17%) due to the radial head dislocation (may develop a **wrist drop**).

MANAGEMENT:
- **<u>Immediate immobilization:</u>** double-sugar-tong splint & immediate orthopedic surgery referral.
- **<u>Surgical</u>: most are unstable fractures requiring open reduction & internal fixation (ORIF).**

GALEAZZI FRACTURE

- **[1] Mid-distal radial shaft fracture with [2] dislocation of the distal radioulnar joint (DRUJ).**
- <u>Mechanism:</u> FOOSH (fall on an outstretched hand) or direct blow.

CLINICAL MANIFESTATIONS
- Fracture & deformity on the radial side of the wrist. Additionally, the ulnar head will appear prominent at the wrist (because it is dorsally displaced).

MANAGEMENT
- <u>Adults:</u> **ORIF (it is an unstable fracture).** Long arm or double sugar tong splint initial immobilization.

COMPLICATIONS
- <u>Anterior interosseous nerve injury:</u> loss of pinch between the thumb and index finger.
- Compartment syndrome.

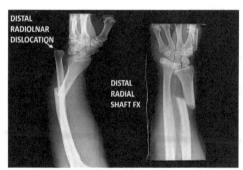

GALEAZZI FRACTURE

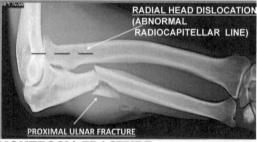

MONTEGGIA FRACTURE

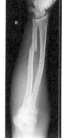

Ulnar shaft fracture

MU GR: **M**onteggia: proximal **U**lnar shaft fracture + radial head dislocation. **G**aleazzi: distal **R**adial fracture + dislocation of the distal radioulnar joint.

Case courtesy of Henry Knipe, Radiopaedia.org, rID: 33936

RADIAL HEAD SUBLUXATION (NURSEMAID'S ELBOW)

- **Radial head is wedged into the stretched annular ligament.**
- **Most common in children 1-4 years of age (<5 years of age).** Rare >5 years of age.

MECHANISM
- **Lifting, swinging, or pulling the arm** (longitudinal traction) while the forearm is pronated & extended.
- Physical examination: **arm slightly flexed, passive pronation, & child refuses to use the arm** (usually no swelling). Tenderness to palpation of the radial head (lateral elbow).

DIAGNOSIS: Clinical diagnosis. Radiographs are normal & usually unnecessary prior to reduction.

MANAGEMENT
- **Closed reduction: via (1) hyperpronation or (2) supination/flexion method (Hyperpronation method is associated with a higher rate of successful RHS reduction).** Following successful reduction (click may be heard or felt), there is pain relief. Reduction is confirmed after observation of the child and noting the child moving the affected arm (usually within 5 to 10 minutes).
- **If the initial reduction is not successful** (eg, the patient is not moving the arm after a period of observation of up to 20 minutes), **reevaluate for subtle signs of fracture. If no signs of fracture are present (no swelling, bony tenderness, or deformity), then reduction can be repeated up to two times.** If the arm remains immobile after 2-3 reduction attempts, obtain plain radiographs to rule out possible fracture.

LATERAL EPICONDYLITIS (TENNIS ELBOW)

- Inflammation of the tendon insertion of the **extensor carpi radialis brevis muscle** due to **repetitive pronation of the forearm & excessive wrist extension against resistance** [eg, backhand stroke in racket sports (eg, tennis, squash, badminton)], supination against resistance.

CLINICAL MANIFESTATIONS
- **Lateral elbow pain especially with gripping** (eg, shaking hands, opening doors), forearm pronation & **pain worse with wrist extension against resistance**. Pain exacerbated by passive wrist flexion.
- May radiate down the forearm & dorsum or wrist; worsen when lifting objects with the forearm prone.

MANAGEMENT
- **Conservative: activity modification, RICE, NSAIDs, physiotherapy, counterbalance braces, friction massage;** Intraarticular corticosteroid injections may provide short-term benefit (6 weeks).
- Surgery if refractory to conservative management (eg, at least 6-12 months) prior to consideration.

MEDIAL EPICONDYLITIS (GOLFER ELBOW)

- Not as common as lateral epicondylitis. Common 40-60 years of age.
- Mechanism: Inflammation of the **pronator teres-flexor carpi radialis** muscles due to repetitive overuse & stress at the tendon insertion of flexor forearm muscle (wrist flexion & pronation).
- Most common in golfers, throwing baseballs, & individuals who do household chores.

CLINICAL MANIFESTATIONS
- **Medial epicondyle tenderness that is worse with pulling activities.**
- Physical examination: **pain reproduced by performing wrist flexion against resistance** with the elbow fully extended. Pain exacerbated by passive wrist extension.

MANAGEMENT
- Similar to Lateral epicondylitis but more difficult to treat — activity modification, RICE, NSAIDs, physiotherapy, counterbalance brace; Intraarticular steroid injections (short-term benefit).
- Surgery if refractory to conservative management (eg, at least 6-12 months) prior to consideration.

ELBOW DISLOCATION

- <u>Mechanism:</u> fall on outstretched hand (FOOSH) with hyperextension (high energy) & axial loading.
- **<u>Posterior</u> most common type (often with lateral displacement).** Most common in males (70%).

PHYSICAL EXAMINATION
- **Flexed elbow, marked olecranon prominence,** & inability to extend elbow.
- Often associated with radial head or coronoid process fracture.
- Must rule out brachial artery; median, ulnar, or radial nerve injuries. **<u>Ulnar neuropathy</u> occurs in 10% of all dislocations** and may be associated with medial epicondyle entrapment.

RADIOGRAPHS

NORMAL

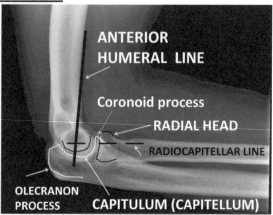

ANTERIOR HUMERAL LINE

Coronoid process

RADIAL HEAD

RADIOCAPITELLAR LINE

OLECRANON PROCESS CAPITULUM (CAPITELLUM)

POSTERIOR ELBOW DISLOCATION

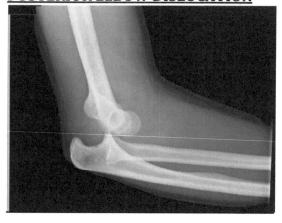

MANAGEMENT
- **<u>Stable:</u> EMERGENT reduction, immobilize with long arm posterior splint at 45°-90° of flexion,** postreduction films to confirm reduction, orthopedic follow up within 1 week, and early range of motion (ideally within 5-10 days) to prevent elbow stiffness.
- <u>Unstable:</u> open reduction internal fixation (ORIF).

COMPLICATIONS
- **Loss of 5°-10° terminal extension is the most common sequelae** (often expected).
- **<u>Elbow joint stiffness</u> most common complication**; contractures if the splint is left on >3 weeks.
- Compartment syndrome.

CUBITAL TUNNEL SYNDROME (ULNAR NEUROPATHY AT THE ELBOW)

- **Ulnar nerve compression at the cubital tunnel** between the medial epicondyle & the olecranon.

CLINICAL MANIFESTATIONS
- **Paresthesias, tingling, numbness, & pain along ulnar nerve distribution (ulnar half of the fourth finger, entire fifth finger,** & ulnar dorsal hand), **worse with elbow flexion.** Nocturnal awakening.

PHYSICAL EXAMINATION
- ⊕ **<u>Tinel's sign at elbow</u>.** Weakness & atrophy of ulnar-innervated hypothenar & lumbrical muscles.
- ⊕ **<u>Froment sign</u>:** ulnar nerve evaluation via adductor pollicis: holds paper & compensates for **<u>thumb adductor weakness</u>** with flexion of IP joint of the thumb — weak pinch.
- Decreased sensation to the fifth and the ulnar side of the fourth finger. Elbow or forearm weakness.
- **<u>Clinical diagnosis</u>** but can be confirmed by electrodiagnostic testing with or without neuroimaging.

MANAGEMENT
- **Nighttime elbow extension splinting, NSAIDs, activity modification, use of elbow pads.**
- Intraarticular steroids (chronic). <u>Refractory:</u> Surgery to decompress the nerve in the cubital tunnel.

WRIST INJURIES

SCAPHOID (NAVICULAR) FRACTURE

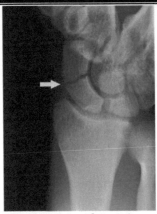

65% occur at the waist
25% proximal third
10% distal third

- **Most commonly fractured carpal bone.** 65% occur at the waist.
- Mechanism: fall on outstretched hand (FOOSH) on extended wrist.

CLINICAL MANIFESTATIONS
- **Pain along dorsal radial surface of the wrist with <u>anatomical snuffbox tenderness</u>.** Swelling, limited range of motion, or rarely, ecchymosis.
- Scaphoid tubercle tenderness, pain with axial loading.

DIAGNOSIS
- **<u>Radiographs:</u> the fracture may not be evident for up to 2 weeks. If snuffbox tenderness is present, treat as fracture because of the <u>high incidence of avascular necrosis or nonunion</u> since the blood supply to the scaphoid is distal to proximal.**
- **If negative initially, options include [1] <u>repeat radiograph films</u> in 7-14 days, OR [2] <u>MRI or CT of the wrist</u>: more sensitive, OR [3] <u>Radionuclide bone scan</u> in 3-5 days.**

MANAGEMENT
- **<u>Nondisplaced fracture or snuffbox tenderness:</u> Thumb spica splint or cast** until ortho follow-up or evidence of union seen on radiographs.
- Displaced >1 mm: percutaneous pin placement or ORIF if significant.

SCAPHOLUNATE DISSOCIATION (SCAPHOLUNATE LIGAMENT INJURY)

- **Widened space >3 mm between the scaphoid & lunate bones.**
- Mechanism: fall on outstretched hand (FOOSH).

CLINICAL MANIFESTATIONS
- Pain on the dorsal radial side of the wrist with minimal swelling.
- Pain is increased with dorsiflexion; click with wrist movement.

MANAGEMENT
- **<u>Initial management:</u> radial gutter splint.**
- Surgical repair of the scapholunate ligament usually required to prevent SLAC of the wrist (**often unstable**).

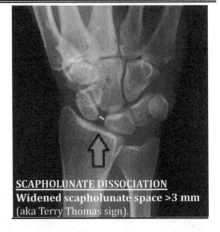

SCAPHOLUNATE DISSOCIATION
Widened scapholunate space >3 mm
(aka Terry Thomas sign).

OSTEOGENESIS IMPERFECTA (BRITTLE BONE DISEASE)

- **Autosomal dominant disease leading to <u>defects in the gene that encodes for type I collagen</u>.**
- Associated with fetal or perinatal death & intrauterine growth retardation in its most severe form.

CLINICAL MANIFESTATIONS
- **<u>Severe premature osteoporosis</u> — multiple recurrent spontaneous fractures with minimal or no trauma in childhood leading to limb deformities & shortening.** Short stature, Scoliosis.
- **Presenile deafness.** Easy bruisability, increased laxity of the joints & skin, basilar skull deformities.

PHYSICAL EXAMINATION: **blue-tinted sclerae hallmark. Brown teeth.**

DIAGNOSIS: Clinical and radiologic findings. Confirmed with DNA or protein testing.

MANAGEMENT: Combination of Bisphosphonates, physical therapy, & surgical interventions.

COLLES' FRACTURE

- Distal radius fracture with dorsal angulation. **Ulnar styloid (Chauffer) fracture also seen in 60%.**
- Mechanism: **fall on outstretched hand (FOOSH) with wrist extension.**
- Clinical manifestations: wrist pain worse with passive motion, swelling, ecchymosis, pain on ROM.
- Physical examination: **dinner fork deformity appearance to the wrist (dorsal displacement).**

DIAGNOSIS
- Radiographs: lateral view shows **dorsally displaced or angulated extraarticular fracture of the distal radius.** Lateral view needed to distinguish Colles' vs Smith's.
- **Barton's fractures intra-articular dorsal or volar rim fractures of the distal radius,** often with fracture-dislocation of radiocarpal joint.

MANAGEMENT
- **Stable: closed reduction followed by Sugar tong splint or cast is the initial management.**
- Surgery: ORIF if comminuted or unstable (>20° angulation, intraarticular, >1 cm shortening).

COMPLICATIONS
- **Extensor pollicis longus tendon rupture most common complication.**
- Malunion, nonunion, joint stiffness, **median nerve compression** (most common neurological complication), residual radius shortening, Complex regional pain syndrome, Carpal tunnel syndrome.

SMITH'S (REVERSE COLLES') FRACTURE

- Extra-articular distal radius fracture with ventral angulation of the distal fragment.
- Mechanism: **fall on outstretched hand (FOOSH) with the wrist flexed.**
- Clinical manifestations: wrist pain worse with passive motion.
- Physical examination: **garden spade deformity appearance of wrist (volar/palmar displacement).**

DIAGNOSIS
- Radiographs: lateral view shows **ventrally/volarly displaced or angulated** extraarticular **fracture of the distal radius.** Lateral view needed to distinguish Colles vs Smith.

MANAGEMENT
- Stable: **closed reduction followed by Sugar tong splint or cast is the initial management.**
- ORIF if comminuted or unstable.

COLLES' FRACTURE
DORSAL angulation.

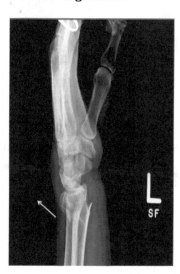

SMITH'S FRACTURE
VENTRAL angulation.

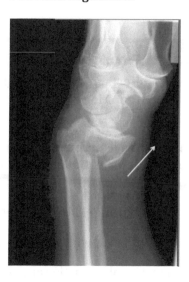

BARTON'S FRACTURE
Intra-articular distal radius fracture with **carpal displacement.**

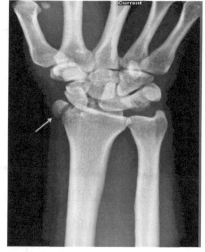

LUNATE DISLOCATION

- **The lunate does not articulate with both the capitate and the radius.**
- Mechanism: high energy injuries causing forceful dorsiflexion while the wrist is extended & ulnarly deviated and impact on the outstretched hand (eg, fall from height, motor vehicle collision).

CLINICAL MANIFESTATION
- Acute wrist swelling & pain. Often associated with other injuries (eg, fractures, median neuropathy).

DIAGNOSIS
- AP view: **lunate appears triangular in shape ("piece-of-pie" sign).**
- Lateral view: **volar displacement & tilt of the lunate towards the palm ("spilled teacup" sign).**

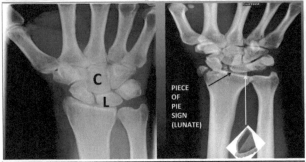 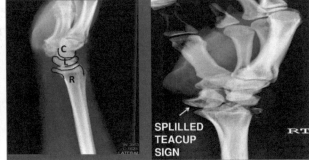

| Normal | Lunate dislocation | Normal | Lunate dislocation |

"Piece of pie sign" seen on the AP view.   **" Spilled teacup" sign"** seen on the lateral view.

MANAGEMENT
- **Emergent closed reduction & splint followed by ORIF** (open reduction internal fixation). Lunate & perilunate dislocations are considered orthopedic emergencies.
- Referral to a hand surgeon is important to reduce the long-term risk of avascular necrosis.

PERILUNATE VS LUNATE DISLOCATION

PERILUNATE: the lunate does not articulate with the capitate but still articulates with the radius.

LUNATE: the lunate doesn't articulate with the capitate OR radius "spilled teacup" sign on the lateral view.

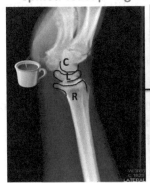 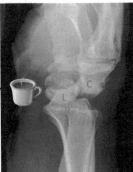 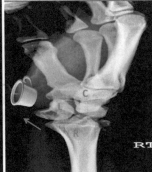 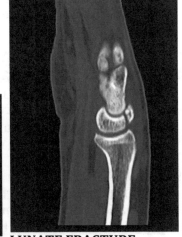

NORMAL LATERAL   **PERILUNATE**   **LUNATE**

LUNATE FRACTURE
Case courtesy of Henry Knipe,
Radiopaedia.org, rID: 70427

LUNATE FRACTURE

- **Most serious carpal fracture** since the lunate occupies two-thirds of the radial articular surface. Radiographs are often negative.
- Complications: **avascular necrosis of the lunate bone (Kienböck's disease).**

MANAGEMENT
- Immobilization with orthopedic follow up.

COMPLEX REGIONAL PAIN SYNDROME (CRPS)

- Formerly known as reflex sympathetic dystrophy (RSD).
- **Autonomic dysfunction following bone or soft tissue injuries** (eg, wrist fracture or post-surgery). 30% have no history of injury.
- EPIDEMIOLOGY: Most commonly affects the upper extremities, women & >30 years.

CLINICAL MANIFESTATIONS
Characterized by 4 main symptoms after an initiating event:
- **[1] Sensory: pain, hyperalgesia often out of proportion to the initial injury,** pain with light touch.
- **[2] Motor/trophic changes**: decreased range of motion & motor dysfunction with trophic changes **(increased hair & nail growth initially followed by decreased growth).**
- **[3] Sudomotor/edema swelling or sweating changes.**
- **[4] Vasomotor: temperature & skin color asymmetry with autonomic dysfunction.**

DIAGNOSIS:
- **Mainly a clinical diagnosis.**
- Radiographs: may show patchy osteoporosis. Bone scintigraphy: increased uptake/activity.

Diagnostic criteria:
- An initiating event, or immobilization
- Persistent pain, allodynia, or hyperalgesia out of proportion to the initiating event
- Symptoms of edema, changes in skin blood flow, or abnormal sudomotor activity
- No other obvious diagnosis that could explain the symptoms.

MANAGEMENT
- **Initial management: NSAIDs, physical therapy, & occupational therapy** (multidisciplinary).
- **Cognitive behavioral therapy** is a necessary component in the management.
- Anesthetic blocks, antidepressants — eg, **Duloxetine, Tricyclic antidepressants** (eg, **Amitriptyline or Nortriptyline**), anticonvulsants (eg, **Gabapentin**), Transdermal Lidocaine, Transcutaneous electric nerve stimulation, etc. Bisphosphonates short-term if abnormal uptake on Bone scan.

DE QUERVAIN (TENDINOPATHY) TENOSYNOVITIS

- **Stenosing inflammation of the tendons (entrapment tendinitis) of the abductor pollicis longus (APL) & extensor pollicis brevis (EPB)** as they pass through first dorsal compartment of the wrist.
- Mechanism: excessive thumb use with repetitive action (thumb abduction & extension). Seen in golfers, clerical workers, **women postpartum** (from lifting the newborn), **diabetics**, posttraumatic.

CLINICAL MANIFESTATIONS
- **[1] Atraumatic radial wrist pain: pain along the radial aspect of the wrist & base of the thumb radiating to the forearm, especially with thumb extension or gripping.**
- **[2] Radial styloid pain & tenderness** at the radial side of the distal wrist (first dorsal compartment).
- Swelling & thickness over the tendon sheath may be present.

DIAGNOSIS
Clinical diagnosis: [1] atraumatic radial wrist pain, [2] radial styloid pain, [3] ⊕ Finkelstein test.
- **⊕ Finkelstein test: pain over the first dorsal compartment over the radial styloid with ulnar deviation while the thumb is flexed in the palm or pain with thumb extension.**

MANAGEMENT
- **Thumb spica splint** (forearm-based with free IP joint), **NSAIDs, & physical therapy.**
- Glucocorticoid injection into the tendon sheath may be used if initial treatment is unsuccessful.
- Surgical release (decompression) usually reserved for cases refractory to nonoperative management.

MALLET (BASEBALL) FINGER

- **<u>Avulsion of the extensor tendon</u>** of the finger near the DIP joint.

MECHANISM OF INJURY
- High velocity injury to the end of the digit with **sudden blow to the tip of the finger causing <u>forced hyperflexion of the DIP joint of an extended finger</u>** (eg, when a ball hits the end of the finger).

CLINICAL MANIFESTATIONS
- **Pain at the DIP joint with <u>inability to actively extend the injured DIP joint</u>**. The DIP joint is held in flexion due to unopposed action of the flexor digitorum profundus. Passive extension often intact.
- Pain, swelling, and tenderness may be present over the DIP joint. May be associated with a fracture.

DIAGNOSIS
- <u>Radiographs</u>: **normal or avulsion fracture of the distal phalanx at the tendon insertion site.**

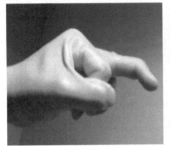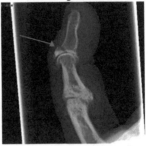

MANAGEMENT
- **<u>Nonoperative</u>: uninterrupted (full-time) hyperextension volar splint of DIP joint for 6-8 weeks.** The proximal interphalangeal (PIP) & metacarpophalangeal (MCP) joints should be allowed to move freely. **Complications of untreated Mallet fingers include a Swan neck deformity.**
- <u>Operative</u>: Closed reduction & surgical percutaneous pinning if displaced Mallet finger with subluxation. ORIF or tendon reconstruction if the above cannot be done.

GANGLION CYST OF THE WRIST & HAND

- **Fluid-filled swelling overlying a joint or tendon sheath**, especially on the dorsal side of the wrist (but can be volar). When appearing on the hand, they are often found on the volar surface.
- **Ganglion cysts are the most common soft tissue tumor of the hand** (mucin-filled cystic lesions).

CLINICAL MANIFESTATIONS
- **Can be asymptomatic or produce wrist, joint, or local pain with direct pressure or during certain wrist motions.** May increase in size or become painful with time.
- May cause nerve compression if large.
- **They are well circumscribed, smooth, rounded, rubbery mass that may feel fluid filled.** If they are large enough, then they can be **transilluminated with a small penlight.**

DIAGNOSIS
- The diagnosis can be made clinically. The diagnosis can also be confirmed with an MRI, CT scan, or Ultrasound if the physical examination is inconclusive. May be calcified on radiographs.

MANAGEMENT
- **<u>Asymptomatic lesions</u> observed and reassurance that >50% resolve on their own, especially if they are small and have been present for <1 year.** Avoiding weight-bearing with wrist extension may help to reduce the pain associated with dorsal wrist ganglia.
- **<u>Bothersome symptoms</u>: Aspiration can be performed** in the clinic, but patient should be informed recurrence rates after aspiration are 50–70%. Injection with steroid has no added benefit and has been shown to have an increased incidence of skin depigmentation and subcutaneous fat atrophy.
- <u>Surgical excision</u> of the ganglion cyst can be performed for symptomatic ganglia that do not respond to conservative treatment.

BOUTONNIERE & SWAN NECK DEFORMITIES

- <u>Mechanism:</u> sharp force against the tip of a partially extended digit ⇨ hyperflexion at the PIP joint with hyperextension at the DIP. Disruption of extensor tendon at the base of the middle phalanx.

<u>MANAGEMENT:</u>
- Splint PIP in extension x 4-6weeks with hand surgeon follow up.

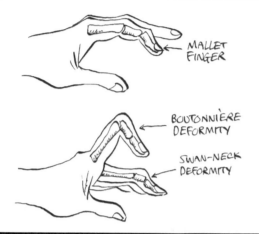

MALLET FINGER
Finger flexed at the DIP joint
  unable to extend at the DIP joint

BOUTONNIERE DEFORMITY
Finger flexed @ PIP joint &
  hyperextended @ DIP joint

SWAN NECK DEFORMITY
Finger hyperextended @ PIP joint &
  flexed @ DIP joint

FLEXOR TENDON INJURY OF THE DIP JOINT (JERSEY FINGER)

- <u>**Acute rupture of the flexor digitorum profundus (FDP) tendon**</u> at its insertion at the distal phalanx. The tendon may retract to the proximal interphalangeal (PIP) joint or all the way to the palm.

<u>MECHANISM OF INJURY</u>
- **Rupture of the FDP is caused by a sudden, <u>forceful hyperextension of the distal interphalangeal (DIP) joint.</u>**

<u>CLINICAL PRESENTATION</u>
- Pain and swelling at the palmar DIP joint or along the distal volar aspect of the involved finger.
- **Inability to actively flex the DIP joint** (weak incomplete flexion may indicate a partial tear).

<u>MANAGEMENT</u>
- <u>**Surgical referral: Definitive treatment is surgical in all cases,**</u> and some injuries require surgical repair within 7 to 10 days, so urgent hand surgeon referral is recommended for all cases.

TRIGGER FINGER (STENOSING FLEXOR TENOSYNOVITIS)

- <u>**Painless locking and snapping of a finger during flexion**</u> due to a mismatch in the size of the flexor tendons and the surrounding retinacular pulley system, as the first annular (A1) pulley. The flexor tendon catches when it attempts to glide through a relatively stenotic sheath.
- **Patients initially describe painless snapping, catching, or locking of one or more fingers during flexion of the affected digit (inability to smoothly flex the finger).** This often progresses to painful episodes in which the patient has difficulty spontaneously extending the affected digits.

<u>MANAGEMENT</u>
- <u>**Initial management (acute symptoms):**</u> **conservative therapy for 4-6 weeks — activity modification or splinting as well as a concurrent trial of nonsteroidal antiinflammatory drugs (NSAIDs).**
- <u>**Persistent symptoms:**</u> **local glucocorticoid injection** (eg, Methylprednisolone or Triamcinolone) rather than surgical therapy. May be repeated in 6 weeks if <50% symptom improvement.
- <u>Surgical therapy</u> for persistent pain and locking persist despite conservative therapy and at least 1 or 2 local glucocorticoid injections (eg, US-guided percutaneous & open surgical A1 ligament release).

ULNAR COLLATERAL LIGAMENT INJURY [GAMEKEEPER'S (SKIER'S) THUMB]

- **Sprain or tear of the <u>ulnar collateral ligament (UCL) of the thumb</u> ⇨ instability of MCP joint.**
- <u>Skier's thumb:</u> acute condition (eg, after fall); <u>Gamekeeper's:</u> chronic hyperabduction injury.
- <u>Mechanism of injury:</u> **Forced hyperabduction (radial deviation) & hyperextension of the metacarpophalangeal (MCP) joint** (eg, downhill skier falling and their thumb is thrust forcibly against a planted ski pole). Normally, the UCL functions to resist against valgus forces.

CLINICAL MANIFESTATIONS
- **<u>Thumb far away from the other digits</u> (especially with valgus stress** — pulling thumb away from the hand), MCP tenderness, weakness in pinch strength. Tenderness over the ulnar border of thumb.
- **± Fracture at the base of the proximal phalanx** (if UCL ruptures, it may pull off piece of bone).

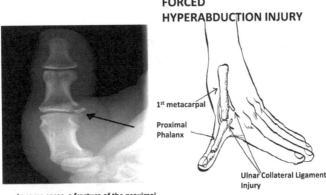

FORCED
HYPERABDUCTION INJURY

1st metacarpal

Proximal
Phalanx

Ulnar Collateral Ligament
Injury

In some cases, a fracture of the proximal
phalanx on the ulnar side may be seen.

MANAGEMENT
- **<u>Initial management:</u> Thumb spica splint including the MCP joint, often for up to 6 weeks + RICE therapy** (rest, ice, compression, and elevation). **Follow-up with orthopedic hand surgeon.**
- Most complete ulnar collateral ligament tears need urgent surgery. Generally, early surgical intervention is required for complete tears to prevent a displaced UCL tear (eg, Stener lesion).

FIFTH (OR FOURTH) METACARPAL NECK [BOXER (BRAWLER) FRACTURE]

- **Fracture through the fifth metacarpal neck (may involve the fourth finger).**
- <u>Mechanism:</u> direct trauma to a closed fist against a hard surface (eg, punching a wall or solid object).

CLINICAL MANIFESTATIONS
- Pain along the dorsum of the fifth metacarpal of the hand with swelling, ecchymosis. May have loss of the prominence of the knuckle if angulated.
- May have rotational deformity.

DIAGNOSIS: Radiographs to measure angulation.

MANAGEMENT
- <u>Initial:</u> **Ulnar gutter splint** with joints in at least 60° flexion. **Closed reduction required prior to splinting of any fracture >25°-30° angulation.**
- <u>Open reduction internal fixation</u> if fifth finger remains >40° degrees angulated (>30° for the ring finger).
- **Always check for bite wounds. If present, copious irrigation, wound debridement treat with the appropriate antibiotics [eg, Ampicillin-sulbactam (IV) Amoxicillin-clavulanate (oral)].**

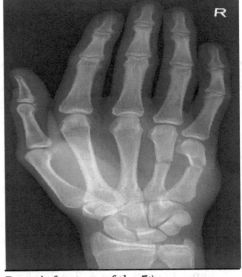

R

Boxer's fracture of the 5th.
4th metacarpal fracture also seen here.

THUMB METACARPAL FRACTURE [BENNETT FRACTURE–DISLOCATION & ROLANDO FRACTURE]

- **Metacarpal fractures involving the base of the thumb into the carpometacarpal (CMC) joint.**
- **Bennett fracture: <u>non-comminuted</u> partial intra-articular fracture** into the CMC joint.
- **Rolando fracture: <u>comminuted</u> complete intra-articular fracture** into the CMC joint.

MECHANISM ON INJURY
- Axial force applied to a partially flexed thumb, often with forced thumb abduction.

CLINICAL MANIFESTATIONS
- Pain, dorsal swelling at thumb base, ecchymosis, and tenderness to the CMC joint (base of thumb).
- Pain & decreased motion at the metacarpophalangeal (MCP) and carpometacarpal (CMC) joints.

DIAGNOSIS
Radiographs:
- **Bennett fracture: small fragment of first metacarpal base articulating with the trapezium.**
- **Rolando fracture: T or Y sign** — splitting of the first metacarpal base into dorsal and volar fragments.

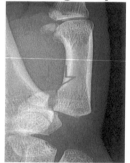 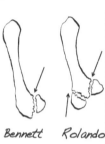 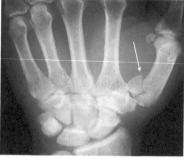

Bennett   Rolando

MANAGEMENT
- **Immediate management: <u>Thumb spica splint</u> for temporary stabilization. Intra-articular fractures require orthopedic referral and generally require surgical fixation.**
- <u>Bennett:</u> immobilization. Closed reduction & percutaneous pinning, ORIF if large fragment and joint displacement.
- <u>Rolando:</u> unstable often needing ORIF, external fixation, or closed reduction & percutaneous pinning.

Other thumb fractures:
- 80% of thumb fractures involve the metacarpal base: the most common pattern is extraarticular epibasal fracture and may be treated in many cases with Thumb spica immobilization.

PRONATOR TERES SYNDROME

- **<u>Proximal forearm median nerve compression & entrapment</u>** in the antecubital fossa where the nerve traverses between the 2 muscular heads of the pronator teres muscle.

CLINICAL MANIFESTATIONS
- **<u>Median neuropathy:</u> paresthesia or pain of the lateral palmar aspect of the first 3 (& radial half of the fourth) digits similar to Carpal tunnel syndrome (CTS) but with <u>pain more prominent over the proximal volar forearm</u>** than in the hands or fingers (with CTS).
- **Sensory changes over the palmar cutaneous branch (palm of hand & thenar eminence)** unlike CTS.
- **Symptoms are usually NOT worse at night** (compared to Carpal tunnel syndrome).
- **Tenderness over the proximal median nerve aggravated by repetitive pronation of the forearm against resistance.** ⊕ Tinel's sign at the proximal volar forearm (rather than at the wrist in CTS).
- Nerve conduction studies with EMG can establish both diagnoses and rule out other neuropathies.

MANAGEMENT
- **<u>Initial management:</u> reduction in the symptom-inducing activity, splinting, & NSAIDs for pain.**
- <u>Glucocorticoid injections</u> (eg, Methylprednisolone) if no relief with NSAIDs.
- <u>Surgical decompression</u> in cases refractory cases after 3-6 months or if motor loss is significant.

CARPAL TUNNEL SYNDROME

- **Median nerve entrapment & compression** as is passes through the carpal tunnel at the wrist.
- Increased incidence: women, **Diabetes Mellitus, pregnancy,** Hypothyroidism, Rheumatoid arthritis, occupations with repetitive extension & flexion of the wrists (eg, typing).

CLINICAL MANIFESTATIONS

- **Median neuropathy: paresthesias (numbness & tingling) or pain of the palmar (volar) aspect of the first 3 (& radial half of the fourth) digits <u>worsening at night</u> or with gripping** (may have to shake the hand or massage it to relieve the symptoms). Clumsiness & weakness uncommon.
- **Sensory deficits of the median-innervated fingers, but Thenar eminence sensation is spared** (unlike in PTS). Thenar muscle wasting and atrophy may be seen in advanced cases.

DIAGNOSIS

- Workup may include electromyography & nerve conduction velocity studies.
- ⊕ **Durkan test (carpal tunnel compression test)** symptom reproduction with pressing thumbs over the carpal tunnel and holding pressure for 30 seconds (**most sensitive test to diagnose CTS**).
- ⊕ **Phalen test if flexion of both wrists for 30-60 seconds reproduces the symptoms.**
- ⊕ **Tinel test if percussion of the median nerve produces symptoms** (less sensitive than Phalen).

MANAGEMENT

- **Conservative: nocturnal volar splint in neutral position initial management,** NSAIDs, avoiding repetitive wrist movements. Corticosteroid injection if patient refuses splinting at night.
- **Corticosteroid injection** into the carpal tunnel adjunctive if no response to initial management.
- **Carpal tunnel surgery in refractory or severe cases (eg, denervation, axonal loss, thenar atrophy).**

DIFFERENTIAL DIAGNOSIS:

PRONATOR TERES SYNDROME Median nerve compression in the proximal forearm. May develop paresthesias in the same distribution as CTS. However, unlike CTS, **Pronator teres syndrome (PTS) is associated more with proximal forearm pain than wrist/hand pain, reduced thenar eminence sensation, Tinel sign at the forearm, & not associated with pain at night.**

DUPUYTREN CONTRACTURE

- **Progressive fibrosis and thickening of the palmar and digital fascia of the hand leading to contracture deformities** as a result of fascial nodules or longitudinal bands (cords) in the palm.

RISK FACTORS

- **Men >40y, Northern Europeans, <u>Diabetes mellitus</u>,** Chronic alcohol use, Cirrhosis, smoking.

CLINICAL MANIFESTATIONS

- **Visible or palpable painless nodules (may be pitted) first, then cords, & contractures over the distal palmar crease or palmar side of the proximal phalanx [ring finger (most common) & little finger]** along the course of the flexor tendons. Loss of motion of the affected fingers.

Physical examination:

- May have finger thickening, bands, or puckering in the palmar fascia. Pit and grooves may be present.
- The nodules may be tender; the cords & contractures are usually painless.
- **Fixed flexion deformity at the MCP joint with limited extension of the MCP or PIP joint.**

MANAGEMENT

- **Conservative management: observation if painless stable disease and no impairment in function.** Physical and occupational therapy, including passive stretching.
- **Intralesional corticosteroid injections.** Flexion contractures: Intralesional *Clostridium histolyticum* collagenase injection. High recurrence rate after injections (50%). Needle aponeurotomy.
- Surgical correction (fasciotomy or fasciectomy) in advanced or refractory cases, or impaired function.

PHOTO CREDITS

CHAPTER 5 – ENT (EARS, NOSE, & THROAT DISORDERS)

SCLERITIS

- **Inflammation of the sclera, the outer covering of the eye (potentially vision threatening).** May also involve the cornea, adjacent episclera, & uveal tract. Average age at onset is 48 years.
- <u>**Scleritis is often associated with systemic disease**</u>, such as systemic rheumatologic and inflammatory disorders — **Rheumatoid arthritis, Granulomatosis with polyangiitis, infection.**

CLINICAL MANIFESTATIONS

- <u>Anterior scleritis</u> — <u>**intense eye pain**</u> **(deep, constant boring pain radiating to head, periorbital area & neck;** worse at night/early morning hours), <u>**local tenderness**</u> **to touch, pain worse with eye movements, <u>edema & deep purple-blue (violaceous hue) redness of the sclera</u>** (diffuse or local) that is purpuric or deeper in color compared to Conjunctivitis or Episcleritis. **Photophobia &/or vision loss.**
- <u>Posterior scleritis</u> nonvisible portion of the sclera — the eye appears "white" (no redness) & uninflamed on external exam, rather than violaceous or red. Variable amounts of pain (often severe) & often difficult to localize. Diplopia and pain upon eye movement is common. Reduced vision.

Physical examination:

- **Slit-lamp exam: scleral edema & profound dilatation of the deep episcleral vascular plexus.**
- **No vessel blanching with the installation of 2.5% topical Phenylephrine.** Episcleral redness improving with instillation of Phenylephrine drops suggests Episcleritis vs. Scleritis.

MANAGEMENT OF NONINFECTIOUS SCLERITIS

- **<u>Diffuse or nodular Scleritis</u>: systemic NSAIDs (eg, Indomethacin) initial treatment of choice. Topical corticosteroids (eg, Prednisolone acetate 1.0%) may be added to systemic NSAIDs.**
- **<u>Necrotizing or posterior Scleritis</u>: High-dose Glucocorticoids (eg, Prednisone) with or without an immunosuppressive agent [eg, Rituximab (preferred) or Cyclophosphamide].**
- Patients with suspected Scleritis should be **referred for ophthalmologist evaluation** within a few days.

EPISCLERITIS

- **Localized inflammation of vessels lining the episclera (between the sclera & the conjunctiva).**
- ~70% occur in women. Most common in young & middle-aged adults (mean age 45 years).

ETIOLOGIES

- <u>Thought to be an autoimmune process</u> — most commonly idiopathic (most have no underlying systemic disease) but may be seen with connective tissue diseases.
- <u>Autoimmune associations</u>: eg, RA, IBD, ANCA vasculitis, SLE, Seronegative spondyloarthropathies.

CLINICAL MANIFESTATIONS

- **<u>Nonpainful localized eye redness without vision loss</u>: abrupt onset of unilateral <u>sectoral redness</u> (local erythema confined to 1 quadrant with overlying conjunctival vessel injection),** irritation, & possible watery discharge. May be nodular. **Pain & vision loss are uncommon.**
- **Mild if any ocular discomfort** (achiness associated with nodular variant). Normal visual acuity.
- <u>Physical examination</u>: sclera may appear blotchy with **areas of bright redness over episcleral vessels.**

MANAGEMENT
Asymptomatic:

- **Treatment generally not needed because it is self-limiting & non-sight threatening** — symptoms and findings typically resolve spontaneously over several weeks. Ophthalmology follow-up.

Symptomatic:

- **[1] <u>Topical lubricants</u> & artificial tear preparations that do not contain preservatives** (eg, Bion tears, Refresh plus).
- **[2] <u>Topical NSAID</u>** (eg, Diclofenac ophthalmic drops 2-4 times daily) if significant discomfort or refractory to topical lubricants. Topical corticosteroids may be used if refractory to topical NSAIDs
- **[3]** <u>Topical corticosteroid</u>: Fluorometholone 0.1%, Loteprednol etabonate 0.5%, Prednisolone acetate 1%.
- **[4]** <u>Oral NSAIDs</u> eg, Ibuprofen, Naproxen, Indomethacin. Oral Corticosteroids.

BACTERIAL CONJUNCTIVITIS

- **Most commonly due to *Staphylococcus aureus* in adults**, *Streptococcus pneumoniae, H. influenzae* (most common in children), *Moraxella catarrhalis. N. gonorrhoeae, Chlamydia trachomatis.*
- Transmitted by direct contact with infected substance and autoinoculation.

CLINICAL MANIFESTATIONS
Purulent or mucopurulent ocular discharge, conjunctival erythema, ocular irritation, & tearing:
- **Mucopurulent or purulent discharge usually thick, globular, and often painless;** may be yellow, white, or green. Purulent discharge at the lid margins and in the corners of the eye which may reappear within minutes of wiping the lids. **Lack of itching**; often no prior history of conjunctivitis.
- Lid-crusting: adherence of the eyelid "stuck shut" and eyelid matting in the morning — nonspecific, (can also be seen with Viral and Allergic conjunctivitis).
- **Conjunctival erythema** diffuse redness or injection, involving the bulbar (globe) conjunctiva 360° as well as the palpebral (tarsal) conjunctiva (the mucus membrane on the inner surface of the lids). No ciliary injection (limbal flush).
- **Vision is usually normal or not significantly changed** (reduced only slightly if affected).

DIAGNOSIS
- **Usually clinical.** Fluorescein staining to look for Keratitis or Corneal abrasions.
- Limited role for testing — culture & gram stain of the discharge not necessary for diagnosis in most.

MANAGEMENT
- Bacterial conjunctivitis is frequently self-limited, lasting 10-14 days if left untreated, but antibiotic treatment shortens course of symptoms if given before day 6. Frequent handwashing important.
Topical antibiotics:
- **Noncontact lens wearers: Erythromycin ophthalmic ointment or Trimethoprim-Polymyxin B drops first-line agents.** Ointment preferred over drops in children; Ointments can blur vision for 20 minutes. Fluoroquinolones (eg, Moxifloxacin, Ofloxacin) or Sulfacetamide are alternatives.
- **Contact lens wearer: cover for *Pseudomonas aeruginosa* (eg, topical Ciprofloxacin, Ofloxacin, Moxifloxacin).** Patients should discontinue contact lens use until the eye is white and there is no ocular discharge after 24 hours after the completion of antibiotic therapy. Topical aminoglycosides (eg, Tobramycin or Gentamicin) are alternatives.

GONOCOCCAL CONJUNCTIVITIS

Hyperacute bacterial conjunctivitis due to *N. gonorrhoeae* after exposure to genital secretions.
- **Profuse (copious) purulent discharge amount often striking.** May reaccumulate after wiping.
- Rapid progression of eye redness, irritation, and tenderness of the globe to palpation. Eyelid edema.
- **Marked chemosis** (conjunctival edema), **eyelid swelling, & tender preauricular adenopathy common.**

DIAGNOSTIC TESTING
- Conjunctival scrapings should be sent for immediate Giemsa and Gram stains to identify **gram-negative diplococci (*N. gonorrhoeae*).** Polymerase chain reaction (PCR).

MANAGEMENT OF GONOCOCCAL CONJUNCTIVITIS:
- **Emergent ophthalmologist evaluation,** topical & systemic antibiotics (may lead to perforation).
Systemic antibiotics:
- **Single 1 gram IM dose of Ceftriaxone and presumptive treatment for Chlamydia coinfection** [eg, Doxycycline 100 mg orally twice daily for 7 days OR Azithromycin (1 gm oral), single dose].
- **Severe: IV Ceftriaxone** 1 gram intravenously every 12-24 hours until resolution.
Topical antibiotics:
- **A topical Fluoroquinolone, saline irrigation to promote resolution, and daily assessment are also recommended** because of the increased risk of corneal involvement and perforation.

VIRAL CONJUNCTIVITIS

- Viral inflammation of the conjunctiva. **Adenovirus is the most common cause (90%).** HSV.

TRANSMISSION
- Highly contagious; spread from direct contact with patients and their secretions or contaminated surfaces. **Swimming pool most common source during outbreaks.** Most common in children.

CLINICAL MANIFESTATIONS
- **Watery or mucoserous discharge** with scant, stringy quality; tearing & itching.
- Foreign body, sandy, burning, or gritty sensation; ocular erythema. No significant visual changes.
- **Often starts unilateral and progresses to bilateral involvement within 24-48 hours.**
- Viral symptoms (fever, pharyngitis, coryza, nasal congestion) may precede or accompany symptoms.
- Lid-crusting: adherence of the eyelid "stuck shut" and eyelid matting in the morning (nonspecific, can be seen with Viral and Allergic conjunctivitis). Cobblestone mucosa seen in Viral and allergic.

PHYSICAL EXAMINATION
- Copious (profuse) watery tearing; may have mucoid discharge.
- **Ipsilateral enlarged & tender preauricular lymphadenopathy.**
- The tarsal conjunctiva may have a follicular or "bumpy" appearance with lid eversion of the palpebral conjunctiva. Chemosis (conjunctival edema). **Visual acuity is usually at or near baseline vision.**
- Slit examination: punctate staining may be seen.

MANAGEMENT
- **Supportive mainstay of treatment (self-limited) — symptomatic relief with warm or cool compresses, artificial tears, antihistamines for itching & redness (eg, Olopatadine), Topical antihistamines with decongestants (eg, Pheniramine-Naphazoline).** No specific treatment except for HSV infection. Symptoms may worsen for 3-5 days after onset & persist for 2-3 weeks.
- Frequent hand and linen hygiene to minimize spread of infection.

ALLERGIC CONJUNCTIVITIS

- Inflammation of the conjunctiva in response to contact with an allergen, triggering a type I (IgE) reaction, causing local mast cell degranulation and release of histamine.

CLINICAL MANIFESTATIONS
- **Conjunctival erythema (bilateral eye redness) & clear, watery, mucoserous, or scant stringy discharge, with no significant visual changes** (vision at or near the patient's baseline vision).
- **Allergic symptoms: marked ocular pruritus (hallmark & cardinal symptom)** distinguishes allergic from viral. Nasal congestion, sneezing. Ocular grittiness, burning, or irritation.
- May have history of or complain of other allergic symptoms (eg, nasal congestion, sneezing, wheezing) or an atopic history (eg, Hay fever).

Physical examination:
- Similar to Viral conjunctivitis: **Cobblestone mucosa** [bumpy follicular appearance to the inner upper eyelid & tarsal conjunctiva (seen in both viral and allergic)], erythema, **watery or mucoid stringy discharge, chemosis (conjunctival edema). Eyelid edema.** No significant visual deficits.
- Lid-crusting: adherence of the eyelid "stuck shut" in the morning (nonspecific). Gritty sensation.

MANAGEMENT
Supportive mainstay of treatment (self-limited) — symptomatic relief with:
- **Topical Antihistamines (H$_1$ blockers): Olopatadine (antihistamine/mast cell stabilizer), Pheniramine-Naphazoline (antihistamine & decongestant),** Emedastine (antihistamine).
- Cromolyn (mast cell stabilizer). Topical NSAIDs (eg, Ketorolac).
- Systemic antihistamines (eg, Loratadine) if Allergic eye symptoms + associated nonocular symptoms.

KERATITIS (CORNEAL ULCER/INFLAMMATION)

BACTERIAL KERATITIS
- **Cornea ulceration** & or inflammation. **May rapidly progress & be sight-threatening** because of the risk of corneal clouding, scarring, and perforation.

MICROBIOLOGY:
- Include *S. aureus, Streptococci.* ***Pseudomonas aeruginosa*** **increased in contact lens wearers.**

RISK FACTORS
- **Improper contact lens wear greatest risk factor for Bacterial keratitis.**
- Dry ocular surfaces (eg, inability to fully close eyes with Bell palsy).
- Topical corticosteroid use and immunosuppression.

CLINICAL MANIFESTATIONS
- **Ocular pain, photophobia, eye redness, vision changes, watery or mucopurulent ocular discharge,** tearing, foreign body sensation, and difficulty keeping the affected eye open.

PHYSICAL EXAM
- **Conjunctival erythema, ciliary injection (limbal flush), hazy cornea [corneal opacification, infiltration, & ulceration (often a round white spot)].** The tarsal conjunctiva usually spared.
- Hypopyon (layer of white cells due to pus in the anterior chamber) may be seen in severe cases.
- Slit lamp: **increased fluorescein uptake** (deeper than an abrasion due to disruption of the corneal epithelium), a cloudy corneal opacity or stromal infiltrate (typically a round white spot), & inflammatory cellular reaction in the anterior chamber. Hypopyon may be seen in severe cases.

MANAGEMENT
- **Fluoroquinolone topical (eg, Moxifloxacin, Gatifloxacin, Ciprofloxacin, Ofloxacin) ideally after obtaining corneal scraping & cultures if possible + same-day ophthalmology follow-up.**
- **Do not patch the eye.** Contact lens should not be worn during an active eye infection.
- Use of topical corticosteroids controversial, so usually left to the discretion of an ophthalmologist.

HERPES (HSV) KERATITIS
- Corneal infection and inflammation usually due to **reactivation of Herpes simplex virus in the trigeminal ganglion.** HSV keratitis is a major cause of blindness in the US. HSV-1 most common.

CLINICAL MANIFESTATIONS
- Acute onset of unilateral **ocular pain, photophobia, eye redness,** watery discharge, **blurred vision.**
Physical examination:
- Conjunctival erythema, **limbic injection (ciliary flush),** hazy cornea. Preauricular lymphadenopathy.

DIAGNOSIS
- **Dendritic (branching) corneal ulceration with fluorescein staining hallmark of HSV keratitis.**

MANAGEMENT
- **Antivirals: either [1] topical: Acyclovir 3% ophthalmic ointment (preferred topical), Ganciclovir 0.15% gel, Trifluridine 1%; OR [2] oral Acyclovir or Valacyclovir.** Famciclovir.
- Corneal transplantation may be needed in severe cases.

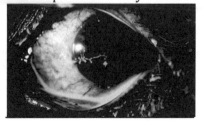

Dendritic (branching) lesion of HSV keratitis
Photo credit: Shutterstock (used with permission)

PHOTOKERATITIS [ULTRAVIOLET (UV), ACTINIC] KERATITIS

- **Radiation burn resulting in severe eye pain that begins 6 to 12 hours after exposure to UV light** [eg, high intensity sun exposure (while skiing), sun lamps, tanning booths, exposure to welding arc].
- The surface layer of the corneal epithelium is desquamated, exposing subepithelial nerve endings; the surface regenerates with resolution of symptoms in 24 to 72 hours.

CLINICAL MANIFESTATIONS
- **Patients usually present about <u>6–12 hours post-exposure</u> complaining of agonizing eye pain, foreign body sensation, blepharospasm, tearing, and severe photophobia.**
- <u>Physical examination</u>: generalized eye injection and edema. Facial and lid erythema.
- **<u>Fluorescein staining superficial punctate epithelial surface irregularities</u> that usually cover the entire surface of the cornea.** If the patient's eyelid was partially closed during the exposure, a well-demarcated line may distinguish normal from damaged corneal epithelium.

MANAGEMENT
- **<u>Supportive management</u>: with topical lubricant antibiotic ointment (eg, Erythromycin, Bacitracin, Polymyxin-Bacitracin) and oral analgesics (eg, NSAIDs, mild oral opioids).** Topical anesthetics should **not** be dispensed or prescribed, although they may be used during the initial examination. Patients should **not** be treated with cycloplegics or eye patching.
- **<u>Prevention</u>: Protective eyewear should be worn for occupational or recreational exposure.**

UVEITIS (IRITIS)

- **<u>Anterior uveitis:</u> inflammation of iris (iritis) or ciliary body (cyclitis) — most common type.**
- <u>Intermediate uveitis</u>: inflammation in the vitreous humor.
- **<u>Posterior uveitis:</u> inflammation of the choroid or retina.**

ETIOLOGIES
- **<u>Systemic inflammatory & autoimmune diseases</u>:** eg, HLA-B27 spondyloarthropathies, Sarcoidosis, Inflammatory bowel disease, Juvenile idiopathic arthritis, Behçet's disease.
- <u>Infectious</u>: Toxoplasmosis, Syphilis, Tuberculosis, fungal, viral (eg, HSV, CMV), parasitic. Immunodeficiency. Trauma. 30% have no underlying identifiable etiology.

CLINICAL MANIFESTATIONS
- **<u>Anterior uveitis:</u> sudden onset of usually unilateral severe ocular pain, photophobia, eye redness, tearing, blurred or decreased vision.**
- **<u>Posterior & intermediate:</u> blurred or decreased vision, floaters,** photopsia. **May not be painful.**

PHYSICAL EXAMINATION
- **Conjunctival erythema, <u>ciliary injection (limbal flush)</u>, consensual photophobia.**
- **<u>Constricted pupil</u> (miosis).** <u>Hypopyon</u> layered collection of leukocytes in the anterior chamber.
- **<u>Slit lamp</u>: inflammatory "cells & flare" — [1] cells [WBCs (lymphocytes neutrophils)] in the anterior chamber & [2] flare (haziness due to proteins in the aqueous humor).** <u>Intermediate & posterior Uveitis</u>: cells in the vitreous (vitreous haze), subretinal & retinal exudates, macular edema, & optic nerve swelling.

MANAGEMENT IF NOT DUE TO INFECTION
- **<u>Anterior uveitis</u>: topical glucocorticoids (eg, Prednisolone) + relief of spasms of the ciliary body with mydriatics [Scopolamine or topical cycloplegics (eg, Cyclopentolate, Homatropine)] + ophthalmology follow-up;** Cycloplegics reduce pain & prevent formation of posterior synechiae. Oral glucocorticoids if resistant to topical therapy. <u>Immunosuppressives</u>: Methotrexate, Azathioprine, or Mycophenolate are alternatives or may be used in chronic cases.
- **<u>Posterior uveitis</u>: systemic (oral) glucocorticoids or intravitreal glucocorticoids.**
- <u>Infectious uveitis</u>: treat as appropriate (viral, bacterial, etc.).

OPHTHALMIA NEONATORUM (NEONATAL CONJUNCTIVITIS)

Neonatal conjunctival infection contracted by newborns during delivery.

Day 1:
- **Chemical conjunctivitis** due to silver nitrate. Artificial tears may be helpful once it occurs.

2-5 days after birth:
- **Gonococcal (*N. gonorrhoeae*) most likely cause.** Presents with purulent conjunctivitis with **profuse exudate and swelling of the eyelids**. Increased risk for corneal rupture.
- Diagnosis: Nucleic acid amplification testing (NAAT), gram stain of exudate, & culture of exudate.
- Management: **single dose of IM or IV Ceftriaxone** [25-50 mg/kg (maximum dose 250 mg)].
- **Prophylaxis: Topical Erythromycin used prophylactically to prevent infection.**

5-7 days after birth (may occur up to 23 days after birth):
- *Chlamydia trachomatis* **most common.** Mild swelling, watery or mucopurulent discharge.
- Complication: 5-30% of neonates also develop Pneumonia (staccato cough, nasal congestion).
- Management: **Oral Azithromycin or Erythromycin.**

PREVENTION (PROPHYLAXIS):
- Gonococcal conjunctivitis: **Erythromycin ointment 0.5% is the standard neonatal prophylaxis against Gonococcal conjunctivitis given immediately after birth.** Other options include topical Tetracycline 1.0%, Silver nitrate, or Povidone-iodine 2.5%.
- Neonatal ocular prophylaxis is **NOT** effective in preventing neonatal Chlamydial conjunctivitis. **Maternal screening & treatment of Chlamydial infection** is the best method for prevention.

OCULAR FOREIGN BODY & CORNEAL ABRASION

CLINICAL MANIFESTATIONS
- **Pain (excruciating eye pain), foreign body sensation, photophobia, blurring of vision, tearing, erythema, blepharospasms (hard to open the eye due to photophobia).**

DIAGNOSIS
- Check visual acuity first — visual acuity is usually normal or blurring of vision.
- **Fluorescein staining: corneal abrasion ("ice rink"/linear abrasions) & epithelial defect with increased fluorescein uptake but no infiltrate or corneal opacity seen.** Because the foreign body may be underneath the eyelid, evert the eyelid to look for any retained foreign bodies.
- **Pain often relieved with instillation of ophthalmic anesthetic drops (eg, Proparacaine or Tetracaine).**

MANAGEMENT
24-hour ophthalmology follow-up + Antibiotic drops for both corneal abrasions & foreign bodies:
- **Non-contact lens wearers: Erythromycin ointment,** Polymyxin-Trimethoprim, Sulfacetamide.
- **Contact lens wearers: antipseudomonal coverage (eg, topical Ciprofloxacin or Ofloxacin).** Topical Tobramycin or Gentamicin are alternatives.
- Foreign body removal: remove with sterile irrigation or moistened sterile cotton swab (needle via slit lamp if experienced). Topical NSAIDs (eg, Ketorolac, Diclofenac) or oral NSAIDs for pain.
- Corneal abrasions: **patching is not indicated for small abrasions or in contact lens wearers.** May patch the eye in some large abrasions (>5 mm) but do not patch longer than 24 hours. Do not send home with topical anesthetics (may delay healing and cause corneal toxicity) or steroids.
- Rust ring: remove rust ring at 24 hours usually with rotating burr by an ophthalmologist.

CONTRAINDICATIONS
- **Do not patch if *Pseudomonas aeruginosa* infection is suspected.**
- Antibiotics containing Corticosteroids are **NOT** used as they can prolong healing and increase susceptibility to superinfection.

OCULAR CHEMICAL BURNS

- Ophthalmologic emergency that may result in permanent vision loss.
- **Alkali injuries: worse than acids — cause liquefactive necrosis,** denature proteins & collagen, cause thrombosis of vessels. Household agents (lye, ammonia) and building material contain alkali.
- **Acid injuries: coagulative necrosis,** with denaturing of protein forming a coagulum that acts as a barrier to further tissue penetration. Penetrates slower and less deep than alkali burns.

CLINICAL PRESENTATION

- Ocular pain, decreased vision, blepharospasm (inability to open the eyelids), photophobia, erythema.

MANAGEMENT

- **Immediate continuous irrigation achieved** with 2-3L **Lactated ringers or Normal saline following a topical anesthetic until a neutral pH (7.0–7.4).** LR ideal because it is closer to a normal pH & is less irritating. Any particulate is removed. Unless there is a strong suspicion for Globe rupture, do not delay irrigation. Often irrigated for at least 30 minutes. Once the pH is normal, the eye can safely be examined.
- **Topical antibiotic:** Polymyxin-Trimethoprim, Erythromycin ointment, or Moxifloxacin. Artificial tears.
- Obtain ophthalmologic consultation. Tetanus prophylaxis if needed.

HYPHEMA

- **Grossly visible layering of blood in the anterior chamber of the eye (gross fluid level).**
- ETIOLOGIES: most common as a result of trauma **(eg, blunt or penetrating injury to the eye).**

DIAGNOSIS

- The primary evaluation is to rule out life or visual-threatening injuries (eg, Globe rupture, orbital Compartment syndrome). Patients may have decreased visual acuity.
- CT scan of the eye without contrast if Globe rupture is suspected. Check intraocular pressure.

MANAGEMENT

- Placement of an eye shield, bed rest, & dim lighting. Ophthalmology consultation.
- **Elevation of the head to 30-45°** reduces permanent staining of the cornea, aids in the clearance of blood & maintains arterial flow to the eye. Avoid antiplatelets and anticoagulants.
- Once Globe rupture has been ruled out, topical Tetracaine for pain control may be used. Topical glucocorticoids reduce the risk of bleeding.

Indications for admission:

- Large Hyphemas occupying ≥50% of the anterior chamber, patients with bleeding or clotting disorders, increased intraocular pressure or patients with sickle hemoglobinopathy.

HYPOPYON

- **White blood cells layered out in the anterior chamber.** A type of anterior uveitis.

ETIOLOGIES

- **HLA-B27-associated Uveitis most common in the US.**
- **Infectious keratitis or Endophthalmitis:** bacterial or fungal infection within the eye, including involvement of the vitreous and/or aqueous humors.
- Behçet disease (not common).

DIAGNOSIS

- Anterior chamber or vitreous tap for PCR and culture may be needed in some to rule out infection, including exogenous or endogenous endophthalmitis, Herpes simplex virus, & Syphilis.

MANAGEMENT

- Same day evaluation by an ophthalmologist to look for Keratitis vs. Endophthalmitis.
- Treat the underlying cause.

ECTROPION

- **Eyelid & lashes are turned outward (everted)** due to relaxation of the orbicularis oculi muscle.
- Risk factors: most commonly seen in the elderly (tends to be bilateral) but can be congenital, infectious, or part of a cranial nerve 7 palsy.
- Clinical manifestations: irritation, ocular dryness, tearing, sagging of the eyelid, increased sensitivity.

MANAGEMENT
- Lubricating eye drops & moisture shields for symptom relief.
- Surgical correction if needed.

ENTROPION

- **Eyelid & lashes are turned inward (inverted).** Most commonly seen in the elderly.
- Pathophysiology: may be caused by spasms of the orbicularis oculi muscle.

CLINICAL MANIFESTATIONS
- Eyelashes may cause corneal abrasion or ulcerations, erythema, tearing, or increased sensitivity.

MANAGEMENT
- Lubricating eye drops & moisture shields for symptom relief. Surgical correction if needed.

BLEPHARITIS

Inflammation of the eyelid margins associated with eye irritation.
- **Posterior: Meibomian gland dysfunction** (inner portion of the eyelid). **Most common type.**
- Anterior: inflammation of the eyelid skin & base of the eyelashes. 2 types: **[1] Infectious** (*Staphylococcus aureus* or *Staphylococcus epidermidis*), viruses; or **[2] Seborrheic.**
- RISK FACTORS: Down syndrome, Atopic dermatitis, Rosacea, Seborrheic dermatitis.

CLINICAL MANIFESTATIONS
- **Eyelid: burning, erythema, crusting, scaling, & red rimming of the eyelid** (pink or erythematous eyelid edges), **gritty sensation, & flaking on the lashes or lid margins.** ± Entropion or Ectropion.

MANAGEMENT
- **Eyelid hygiene mainstay of treatment** — warm wet compresses applied for 5-10 minutes, eyelid scrubbing, gentle eyelid massage, and lid washing with baby shampoo, & artificial tears.
- **Severe or refractory: patients who do not respond to supportive measures should be managed by an ophthalmologist. Topical antibiotics for flares** [ointment (eg, Bacitracin, Erythromycin) or Azithromycin solution]; Chronic blepharitis should undergo lid biopsy to exclude carcinoma.
- Oral antibiotics: eg, Doxycycline, Tetracycline, Azithromycin. Topical steroids, topical Cyclosporine.

DACRYOCYSTITIS

- **Infection of the lacrimal sac often due to obstruction of the nasolacrimal duct.**
- Etiologies: *Streptococcus pneumoniae, Staphylococci, S. pyogenes, H. influenzae, Pseudomonas.*

CLINICAL MANIFESTATIONS
- Acute: **unilateral tearing and signs of infection — pain, tenderness, edema, erythema, & warmth to the inferior medial canthal (nasal) side/lower lid area. May have purulent discharge.**
- Chronic: mucupurulent drainage from the puncta without other signs of infection, tearing, matting of the eyelashes.

MANAGEMENT
- **Acute: warm compresses + systemic antibiotics:** Mild: oral Clindamycin, Cefuroxime, Cefazolin. IV Vancomycin + Ceftriaxone if severe.
- **Chronic or severe acute: Dacryocystorhinostomy.** Topical antibiotics may be used prior to surgery.

DACRYOADENITIS

- **Inflammation of the <u>lacrimal gland</u>.**

CHRONIC DACRYOADENITIS:

- **<u>Chronic Dacryoadenitis</u> inflammation >1 month caused by <u>noninfectious inflammatory</u> <u>disorders</u>** — eg, Sjögren syndrome, Sarcoidosis, Thyroid eye disease. More common than acute.
- Chronic Dacryoadenitis is often seen in older patients and is often a result of a tumor or associated **inflammatory disorders** — eg, Graves', Sjögren syndrome, Sarcoidosis, SLE, IgG4-related diseases.
- <u>Infectious causes</u> are uncommon but include Syphilis, Tuberculosis, Leprosy, and Trachoma.

ACUTE DACRYOADENITIS:

- **<u>Acute Dacryoadenitis</u> is <u>usually infectious</u>** — Bacterial (eg, *S. aureus* **most common bacterial cause**), streptococci, *Neisseria gonorrhoeae*, *Chlamydia trachomatis*, and *Brucella melitensis*); viral (eg, Epstein-Barr virus, mumps virus, coxsackievirus, cytomegalovirus, and varicella-zoster virus).
- Acute Dacryoadenitis most commonly affects children and young adults with systemic infections.

CLINICAL MANIFESTATIONS

- **Soft tissue swelling or fullness, erythema, and tenderness, especially localized in the region of the lateral (outer one-third) upper lid.** Ptosis of the eyelid and diplopia may be seen.
- Infectious causes may be associated with systemic symptoms (eg, malaise, fever, myalgias).
- **<u>Bacterial Dacryoadenitis</u>: intense severe eye discomfort, tenderness, and erythema.**
- <u>Viral Dacryoadenitis</u> causes less intense discomfort and erythema than bacterial dacryoadenitis.

DIAGNOSIS

- Often laboratory workup for inflammatory etiologies reveals little; however, biopsy of the gland may be needed, especially to differentiate Dacryoadenitis from a neoplastic process.

MANAGEMENT

- **<u>Chronic dacryoadenitis</u> involves management of the underlying systemic disorder causing it.**
- **<u>Bacterial Dacryoadenitis</u>: oral or parenteral antibiotics against *S. aureus*. <u>Mild infections</u>: oral first-generation Cephalosporin (eg, Cephalexin), Trimethoprim-sulfamethoxazole, Amoxicillin-clavulanate, or Linezolid. <u>Severe</u>: IV Nafcillin IV Ampicillin-sulbactam; IV Vancomycin if MRSA is suspected.** Patients should return to the ED if symptoms suggestive of Orbital cellulitis occur (eg, pain with eye movement, decreased ocular motility, or proptosis).
- <u>Viral Dacryoadenitis</u> (eg, Mumps or Epstein-Barr virus) — supportive management (eg, warm compresses, analgesia) are recommended. Resolution occurs spontaneously.

DACRYOSTENOSIS

- **Congenital or acquired nasolacrimal duct narrowing or obstruction** seen in 6% of all newborns.

CLINICAL MANIFESTATIONS

- **<u>Excessive eye watering</u> (epiphora), eyelash matting, & tears appearing thicker & yellowish in color.** Overflow of tears when exposed to "stress" (eg, wind, cold, or during times of nasal obstruction).
- **<u>Lack of accompanying signs or symptoms of infection</u>** (eg, fever, irritability, or conjunctivitis). Evaporation of the aqueous layer of poorly draining tears, results in a residual yellow mucus layer that may resemble Conjunctivitis. **Palpation of the lacrimal sac may cause reflux of tears.**

DIAGNOSIS

- **<u>Lack of normal Fluorescein clearance</u>:** Fluorescein applied to the eye and left for 5 minutes will accumulate, whereas it normally would be cleared by the lacrimal system. **Clinical diagnosis.**

MANAGEMENT

- **<u>Conservative management</u> usually resolves symptoms (no antibiotics needed). "<u>Crigler (lacrimal sac) massage</u>": instruction on gentle massage in a downward motion to the nasolacrimal duct 3-4 times a day to promote drainage. <u>Lacrimal probing</u> if it persists >6-10 months.**
- If still present >12 months of age, ophthalmology referral is indicated for possible dilation of the duct.

HORDEOLUM (STYE)

- **Localized abscess of the eyelid margin.** Rapid development common, often within 1-2 days.
- Etiologies: ***Staphylococcus aureus* most common cause (>90%).**
- Increased risk with Seborrheic dermatitis & Rosacea.

TYPES:
- External: infection of an eyelash follicle or external sebaceous glands near the lid margin with production of pus in the gland of Moll or gland of Zeis.
- Internal: inflammation or infection of a Meibomian gland. They are found deep from the palpebral margin under the eyelid.

CLINICAL MANIFESTATIONS
- **Focal abscess: localized erythematous, painful, warm, tender nodule or pustule on the eyelid on the conjunctival surface.** May also be located at or near the eyelash follicle.

MANAGEMENT
- **Warm moist compresses mainstay of treatment 5-10 minutes for 4 times a day, followed by eyelid massage after compresses to promote drainage.** Most eventually point & drain spontaneously and do not require specific intervention.
- **May add topical antibiotic ointment** (eg, Erythromycin, Bacitracin) **if actively draining in some.**
- Incision & drainage may be needed if there is no spontaneous drainage after 48 hours.

CHALAZION

- **Painless indurated granulomatous inflammation of the internal Meibomian sebaceous gland** away from the eyelid margin.
- Pathophysiology: obstruction of the Zeis or Meibomian glands due to thickened secretions.

CLINICAL MANIFESTATIONS
- **Painless, localized, hard, rubbery, & non-tender eyelid swelling (nodule) on the conjunctival surface of the eyelid above the eyelashes.** May cause mild erythema of the affected eyelid.
- **Chalazions are often larger, firmer, slower growing, & less painful than Hordeola.**

MANAGEMENT
- **Conservative: eyelid hygiene & warm compresses** 5-10 minutes 4 times daily. Small Chalazia will often resolve without intervention in days to weeks. Antibiotics are not usually indicated.
- **Refractory: ophthalmologist referral** for glucocorticoid injection or incision + curettage if no resolution by 1-2 months. Persistent or recurrent lesions are often biopsied to rule out malignancy.

PINGUECULA

- Slow growing thickening of the bulbar conjunctiva that remains confined to the conjunctiva.
- Pinguecula consists of fat, protein, & calcium.

RISK FACTORS
- Often develop when the eye is irritated (eg, outdoor, sandy, dry, windy, or sunny conditions; trauma).

CLINICAL MANIFESTATIONS
- **Grey, white yellow slightly elevated nodule (mass) most common on bulbar conjunctiva** on the nasal side of the sclera near the limbal conjunctiva — **does not grow onto the cornea (stays confined to the nasal or temporal conjunctiva).** Does not affect visual acuity.

MANAGEMENT
- **No treatment is needed in most.** Patients should safeguard their eyes from UV light, wind, and dust. Patients should use sunglasses & wide-brimmed hats to avoid sunlight exposure during the day.
- May be resected if chronically inflamed or for cosmetic reasons.

PTERYGIUM

- Slow-growing thickening of the bulbar conjunctiva tissue that may extend onto the corneal surface.

RISK FACTORS
- **Outdoor exposure: associated with ultraviolet light exposure in sunny climates (tropics), sand, wind, & dust exposure. The use of hats and sunglasses reduce the incidence.**

CLINICAL MANIFESTATIONS
- **Elevated, superficial fleshy, triangular-shaped <u>growing</u> fibrovascular mass** that usually starts **medially (nasal side of the eye)** & extends laterally.
- Local symptoms: may cause irritation, erythema, or foreign body sensation.
- May impair vision with corneal extension or if it causes astigmatism via its effect on the visual axis.

MANAGEMENT
- **Supportive management: Topical lubricants (artificial tears) may help irritation & erythema.**
- **Surgical removal only needed if the growth affects vision** (if it advances over the cornea or causes astigmatism) or significant cosmetic impact. However recurrent Pterygium after initial removal can be more symptomatic & problematic to remove than the primary Pterygium.

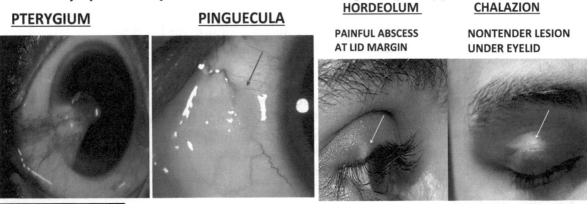

PTERYGIUM   **PINGUECULA**   **HORDEOLUM**   **CHALAZION**

PAINFUL ABSCESS AT LID MARGIN   NONTENDER LESION UNDER EYELID

GLOBE RUPTURE

- **The outer membranes of the eye are disrupted by <u>blunt or penetrating trauma</u>.**
- **<u>Ophthalmologic emergency</u> — immediate ophthalmologist consult.**

PHYSICAL EXAMINATION
- <u>Visual acuity:</u> markedly reduced (may be light perception only), diplopia. Examination for a relative afferent pupillary defect.
- <u>Orbits:</u> **enophthalmos** or exophthalmos. Foreign bodies may be present. **Severe conjunctival hemorrhage (360° bulbar).**
- <u>Corneal/Sclera:</u> misshapened pupil with prolapse of ocular tissue from the sclera or corneal opening. Prolapse of the iris through the cornea, **positive <u>Seidel's test</u>** = parting of fluorescein dye by a clear stream of aqueous humor from the anterior chamber (not usually performed). Obscured red-reflex, **teardrop or irregularly shaped pupil,** hyphema (blood in anterior eye chamber).

MANAGEMENT
- **Rigid eye shield** protects the eye and avoid any manipulation, pressure, or further eye examination until seen by Ophthalmologist. **Impaled objects should be left undisturbed. IV Antibiotics (eg, Vancomycin + Ceftazidime), analgesia, antiemetics** to prevent increased pressure from vomiting. Tetanus prophylaxis (if needed).
- **Emergent ophthalmology consult.** May need CT scan of the eye without contrast.
- In cases of suspected globe rupture, avoid topical eye solutions and avoid any procedure that may apply pressure to the eyeball (eg, tonometry, eyelid retraction, etc.).

ORBITAL FLOOR "BLOW-OUT" FRACTURES

- Fractures to the orbital floor resulting from blunt trauma, most common at [1] **inferior wall/orbital floor** (maxillary sinus) & [2] **medial wall** (ethmoid sinus through the lamina papyracea).
- May lead to trapping of eye structures (eg, infraorbital nerve, inferior rectus muscle).

Types:
- **Inferior (floor, blowout) fractures are the most common type**. Orbital fat and/or the inferior rectus muscle may prolapse into the maxillary sinus. May cause compartment syndrome of the eye.
- Medial (lamina papyracea): orbital fat & medial rectal muscle may prolapse into the ethmoid air cells.
- Superior (roof) and lateral wall are uncommon types of fractures.

CLINICAL MANIFESTATIONS
- **Eyes:** decreased visual acuity, **restricted eye movement with upward gaze** or diplopia especially with upward gaze (**inferior rectus muscle entrapment**), orbital subcutaneous emphysema from air from the maxillary sinus — eyelid swelling that worsens especially after blowing the nose or with sneezing. **Periorbital ecchymosis.** Chemosis or enophthalmos may be seen.
- **Facial:** epistaxis. Dysesthesias, **hyperalgesia or anesthesia to the anteromedial cheek** due to stretching of the **infraorbital nerve**. Tenderness or step-offs at the infraorbital rim.

DIAGNOSIS
- **CT scan: initial imaging modality of choice** to confirm & localize the fracture:
  "**Teardrop" sign**: inferior herniation of the orbital fat or inferior rectus muscle may be seen.

MANAGEMENT
- **Nasal decongestants** (decreases pain), **avoid blowing nose or sneezing** (worsens edema), corticosteroids reduce edema, **Antibiotics (Cephalexin, Ampicillin-Sulbactam, or Clindamycin).**
- **All blowout fractures should be referred to an ophthalmologist** for dilated examination to rule out unidentified associated retinal tears or detachments & to determine if surgical repair is needed.
- Surgical repair: severe cases, patients with enophthalmos, or for persistent diplopia.

RETINOBLASTOMA

- **Most common pediatric primary intraocular malignancy.**
- **Almost exclusively found in children <5 years of age (most diagnosed before 2 years of age)**
- **Retinoblastoma may be associated with bone neoplasms (eg, Osteosarcoma).**

TYPES
- [1] Non heritable: due to somatic mutations in the RB1 gene in the tumor [RB1 is a tumor suppressor gene on chromosome 13 (13q)]. Associated with unilateral Retinoblastoma.
- [2] Heritable: due to germline mutations in the RB1 gene. May develop bilateral Retinoblastoma.

CLINICAL PRESENTATION
- **Leukocoria: presence of an abnormal white reflex instead of the normal red reflex.**
- May develop Strabismus (crossing of the eyes), Nystagmus, or ocular erythema.

DIAGNOSIS
- Dilated indirect ophthalmoscopic exam: **chalky, off-white retinal mass (soft, friable consistency).**
- Ocular ultrasound — **intraocular calcified mass.** MRI of brain & orbits (preferred imaging of choice), Optical coherence tomography and Ophthalmologic examination under anesthesia.

MANAGEMENT
- First-line therapeutic options include systemic chemotherapy, ophthalmic artery chemosurgery (OAC), cryotherapy, laser photocoagulation, or enucleation, dependent on the extent of the disease.
- Prognosis: Fatal if untreated but survival >95% if treated promptly.

AGE-RELATED MACULAR DEGENERATION (ARMD)

- **Most common cause of permanent legal blindness & vision loss in older adults in the US** (especially >75 years of age). Causes central vision loss (macula normally helps with central vision).
- **>50 years of age, <u>Cigarette smoking</u> most readily modifiable risk factor**, Hypertension, light iris color.

TYPES:
- **<u>Dry (atrophic, geographic, nonexudative):</u> most common type.** Dry is progressive (over decades) and can cause central retinal degeneration due to Drusen body deposition. Atrophy of central retina.
- **<u>Wet (neovascular, exudative):</u> choroidal neovascularization** — abnormal vessels leak blood and fluid into the macula (accumulation of exudative fluid, hemorrhage, and fibrosis) that can lead to sudden vision loss. Not as common as dry but more aggressive (blindness may occur within months).

CLINICAL MANIFESTATIONS
- **<u>Bilateral</u>, progressive (gradual), painless, <u>central vision loss</u> (including detailed & colored vision).** Central scotomas. <u>Micropsia</u>: object seems smaller in the affected eye.
- **Metamorphopsia straight lines appear bent, especially towards the center of vision.** Difficulty adjusting to low light levels and decreased central visual acuity. No ocular pain or redness.
- Wet Macular degeneration may occur more rapidly with acute visual distortion and is more severe (responsible for 90% cases of blindness due to Macular degeneration).

FUNDUSCOPIC EXAMINATION
- **<u>Dry (atrophic):</u> Drusen bodies hallmark — small, round, yellow-white spots on the outer retina** (localized subretinal deposits of extracellular material). Retinal atrophy (depigmentation).
- **<u>Wet (neovascular or exudative):</u> new, abnormal choroidal vessels** that can cause retinal hemorrhaging & scarring. Hemorrhage or fluid in the subretinal space.

DIAGNOSIS
- Funduscopy, Fluorescein retinal angiography. **Amsler grid shows metamorphopsia (line distortion).**

MANAGEMENT OF DRY ARMD
- **<u>Zinc & antioxidant vitamins (C & E)</u> may slow progression** of extensive intermediate-size Drusen but do not reverse changes. Home Amsler grid used to monitor stability over time.
- There is no specific treatment for dry age-related Macular degeneration. **<u>Smoking cessation.</u>**

MANAGEMENT OF WET ARMD
- **<u>Intravitreal VEGF inhibitors</u>** (eg, **Bevacizumab, Ranibizumab, Aflibercept**) decrease new, abnormal vessel formation. Vascular endothelial growth factor inhibitors cause regression of choroidal neovascularization with resorption of subretinal fluid and improvement or stabilization of vision.
- Laser photocoagulation. Antioxidant vitamins.

MACULAR DEGENERATION

Loss of central & detail vision

AMSLER GRID
Metamorphopsia =
Straight lines appear bent in central vision

Age-related Macular Degeneration

MACULAR DEGENERATION

DRUSEN (diffuse)

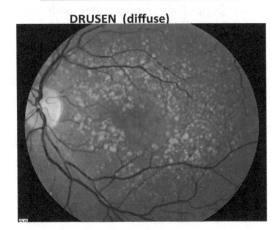

DIABETIC RETINOPATHY

- **Most common cause of new, permanent vision loss in people 25-74 years** (due to maculopathy).
- Diabetic retinopathy affects up to 80% of those who have had diabetes for ≥20 years.

TYPES
- **[1] Nonproliferative (background):** absence of abnormal new blood vessels — **microaneurysms,** cotton wool spots (soft exudates that resemble fluffy gray-white spots due to nerve layer microinfarctions), **hard exudates: yellow spots with sharp margins in a circinate ring** due to lipid or lipoprotein deposits from leaky blood vessels, blot & dot hemorrhages: bleeding into the deep retinal layer; Flame-shaped hemorrhages: nerve fiber layer hemorrhage. May be asymptomatic or may cause distorted vision, blurred vision, floaters, and partial or complete vision loss.
- **[2] Proliferative (neovascularization) — growth of abnormal new blood vessels that can lead to vitreous hemorrhage and vision loss.**
- **[3] Maculopathy: macular edema** or exudates, central retinal swelling &/or thickening, blurred or decreased central vision loss. Can occur at any stage of Diabetic retinopathy. **Vision loss in Nonproliferative often occurs due to macular edema.**

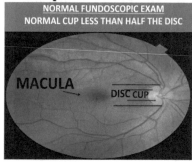 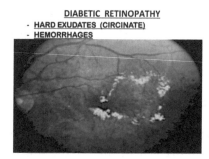 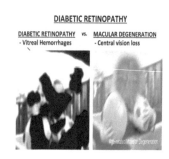

MANAGEMENT
- **Nonproliferative: optimize glucose, lipid, & blood pressure control.** In severe disease, Panretinal laser photocoagulation may reduce the risk of progression to Proliferative diabetic retinopathy.
- **Proliferative: [1] intravitreal VEGF inhibitors (eg, Ranibizumab, Aflibercept, Bevacizumab) with or without [2] laser photocoagulation.** [3] Vitrectomy if refractory to intravitreal anti-VEGF pharmacotherapy and photocoagulation. Optimize glucose, lipid, & blood pressure control.
- PREVENTION: **annual eye exams are performed in diabetics to detect Diabetic retinopathy.** Optimization of glucose, lipid, & blood pressure control & early detection key to avoiding blindness.

HYPERTENSIVE RETINOPATHY

- **Damage to the retinal blood vessels & retina resulting from longstanding high blood pressure.**
- Most patients have no symptoms but may experience decreased or blurred vision or headache.

[1] Mild:
- **Retinal arteriolar narrowing** due to vasospasm resulting in abnormal light reflexes on dilated tortuous arterioles: **Copper wiring** describes moderate narrowing; **Silver wiring** = severe narrowing.
- **Arteriovenous (AV) nicking (nipping)** — venous compression at the arterial-venous junction. Arteriolar wall thickening or opacification.

[2] Moderate:
- Hemorrhages (either flame or dot-shaped) and microaneurysms. Soft exudates: cotton-wool spots.
- Hard exudates: lipid & proteinaceous material leak from the impaired blood–retinal barrier.

[3] Severe (Grade IV):
- **Some or all of the aforementioned + papilledema (blurring of the optic disc/optic disc edema).**
- Considered an **ophthalmologic emergency: requires rapid lowering of the blood pressure.**

MANAGEMENT
- Limit or reverse target organ damage by optimization of blood pressure control.

RETINAL DETACHMENT

- Separation of the retina from the underlying retinal pigment epithelium and choroid.
- **Risk factors: myopia, previous cataract surgery**, advancing age, ocular trauma.

3 TYPES

- **[1] Rhegmatogenous: most common type — <u>full-thickness retinal tear or hole</u>** causes retinal inner sensory layer detachment from the choroid plexus. The tear most commonly begins at the superior temporal retinal area. **Risk factors: Myopia, cataract surgery, & ocular trauma.**
- [2] Tractional: tractional pulling from adhesions separate the retina from its base — eg, proliferative diabetic retinopathy, Sickle cell disease, trauma.
- [3] Exudative (serous): fluid accumulates beneath the retina, causing detachment — eg, Hypertension, Central retinal vein occlusion, papilledema, inflammatory disorders, tumors.

CLINICAL MANIFESTATIONS

- **<u>Photopsia</u> (flashes of lights) with detachment followed by <u>floaters</u>** (spots or "cobwebs" in the visual fields) **followed by <u>progressive rapid unilateral painless peripheral vision loss</u> — shadow or "curtain coming down" in the periphery initially**, spreading to the central visual field (visual loss from the top towards the bottom).
- No ocular pain or redness. There may be a relative afferent pupillary defect.

DIAGNOSIS
Funduscopy (ophthalmoscopy):

- **Retinal tear: detached & elevated tissue "flapping" in the vitreous humor** with irregular ridges.
- **Positive <u>Shafer's sign</u>** = clumping of brown-colored pigment vitreous cells in the anterior vitreous humor resembling tobacco dust.

MANAGEMENT

- **<u>Ophthalmologic emergency</u> — keep patient supine while waiting for ophthalmology consult with the <u>head turned toward the side of the detachment</u>**. Do not use miotic drops as they may cause worsening of the detachment via vitreofoveal traction from pupillary constriction.
- **Laser photocoagulation, cryoretinopexy, or ocular surgery** (eg, retinal repair or reattachment).

AMAUROSIS FUGAX (TRANSIENT MONOCULAR BLINDNESS)

- **<u>Transient monocular vision loss</u> lasting minutes with complete recovery. May be binocular.**

ETIOLOGIES

- <u>Disorders affecting the eye or the optic nerve:</u> **retinal emboli (most common) or ischemia.**
- **Transient ischemic attack (carotid artery disease),** Giant cell arteritis, Central retinal artery occlusion, Migraine (visual aura), Systemic lupus erythematosus, & other vasculitis disorders.

CLINICAL MANIFESTATIONS

- **Vision loss descending over the visual field described as a temporary "curtain or shade" comes down and resolves ("lifts up") usually within 1 hour.** TIA usually lasts 1-15 minutes. Migraine aura usually last 10-30 minutes.

DIAGNOSIS

- Workup determined by the likely cause based on history and physical examination.
- Workup often includes carotid duplex ultrasound and ophthalmologic examination.
- MRI, EEG. ESR & CRP levels if >50 years with transient symptoms (rule out GCA).

MANAGEMENT

- Depends on the underlying etiology.

CENTRAL RETINAL ARTERY OCCLUSION (CRAO)

- Retinal artery thrombus or embolus, resulting in retinal hypoperfusion. Ophthalmologic emergency.
- **Most common 50-80 years. Patients often have a history of atherosclerotic disease.**

ETIOLOGIES
- **Emboli from carotid artery atherosclerosis most common.** DM, Hypertension, Hyperlipidemia.
- **Cardiogenic emboli** — second most common cause overall but most common cause in young patients & patients without atherosclerosis. Thrombotic phenomenon.
- Systemic vasculitis (eg, Giant cell arteritis). Migraine, oral contraceptives, congenital or acquired thrombophilia, and hyperhomocysteinemia are seen especially in young patients.

CLINICAL MANIFESTATIONS
- **Acute, sudden painless monocular vision loss over seconds.** May be preceded by Amaurosis fugax.
- May have an ipsilateral carotid bruit. Branch occlusion may present with incomplete vision loss.
Physical examination:
- Visual acuity is usually reduced to counting fingers or worse, and visual field may be restricted to an island of vision in the temporal field. No ocular pain or redness.
Funduscopy: retinal ischemia:
- **Pale swelling of the retina (diffuse) + a cherry-red macula (central red spot at the fovea).**
- **Boxcar appearance** of the retinal vessels — **segmentation** of blood flow in the arteries & veins.
- Emboli may be seen in the central retinal artery or its branches (Hollenhorst plaques) in 20%.

WORKUP
- To identify carotid and cardiac sources of emboli, obtain duplex ultrasonography of the carotid arteries, ECG, and echocardiography with transesophageal studies, if necessary. ESR & CRP.
- When indicated, obtain CT or MRI studies for internal carotid artery dissection or cerebral infarction.

MANAGEMENT
- No consensus on optimal treatment: may include CO_2 rebreathing (hyperventilation to dilate vessels), 100% oxygen, ocular massage to dilate vessels & attempt to dislodge to clot, intraocular pressure reduction (Acetazolamide, chamber paracentesis), ophthalmology consult, & in-situ fibrinolysis.
Prognosis:
- Poor prognosis even with treatment. No treatment shown to be truly effective but should be attempted.

CENTRAL RETINAL VEIN OCCLUSION (CRVO)

- **Thrombus in the central retinal vein causing retinal venous stasis, edema, & hemorrhage.**
- Risk factors: Atherosclerosis (Hypertension, Diabetes mellitus, Dyslipidemia, smoking, cerebrovascular disease), glaucoma, hypercoagulable states (eg, Polycythemia vera), Multiple myeloma.

CLINICAL MANIFESTATIONS
- **Sudden onset of painless monocular vision loss or blurred vision** (partial if branch occlusion).

DIAGNOSIS
- Funduscopy:
  - **optic disc edema & widespread retinal hemorrhages (blood & thunder appearance).**
  - retinal vein dilation, macular edema, retinal edema, and optic disc swelling may be seen.
- **May have relative afferent pupillary defect (Marcus-Gunn pupil).**

MANAGEMENT
- Ophthalmology consult. No definitive treatment. Options include Anti–VEGF agents, laser-induced chorioretinal anastomosis, Dexamethasone implant, and Intravitreal Triamcinolone.
- Prognosis: vision may be restored with time, at least partially; perform monthly exams initially.

STRABISMUS

- **Misalignment of the visual axis of one or both eyes**.
- Stable ocular alignment is not usually present until age 2-3 months. Acquired strabismus (occurring after the first year of life) may result from a significant visual deficit or CNS disease.

MAJOR TYPES:
- **Esotropia:** convergent Strabismus — **deviated inward (nasally)** "crossed eyed". More serious.
- **Exotropia:** divergent Strabismus — **deviated outward (temporally).** Less serious.

CLINICAL MANIFESTATIONS
- **Diplopia, scotomas.** Amblyopia may be seen, especially if not corrected by 10 years of age.
- Physical examination: Asymmetric corneal light reflex (see below).

DIAGNOSIS
- **[1] Hirschberg corneal light reflex testing often used as initial screening — asymmetric deflection of the corneal light reflex in one eye is seen in Strabismus.** Followed by Cover test.
- **[2] Cover test refixation of the uncovered eye consistent with manifest Strabismus (tropia).**
- **Cover-uncover test** looks for latent Strabismus (phoria) — the misaligned will appear to deviate inward or outward. Convergence testing.

MANAGEMENT OF REFRACTIVE ERROR
- **Patch (occlusive) therapy first-line** — normal eye is covered to stimulate & strengthen the affected eye. Stable Strabismus that persists into childhood is referred nonemergently to an ophthalmologist.
- **Eyeglasses that equalize the vision.** Prism therapy.
- Corrective surgery if severe or unresponsive to conservative therapy.
- **Nonemergent ophthalmology referral for intermittent manifest Strabismus needed if it persists >4-6 months of age to reduce incidence of Amblyopia. Amblyopia = loss of visual acuity not correctable by glasses.**

KERATOCONJUNCTIVITIS SICCA (DRY EYE DISEASE)

- Multifactorial: due to **decreased tear production &/or excessive evaporative loss & hyperosmolarity of the tear film.**
- Causes may include systemic disorders (eg, Sjögren's syndrome, Sarcoidosis); medications (eg, antihistaminic, anticholinergic, and psychotropic medications), Radiation therapy, etc.

CLINICAL MANIFESTATIONS
- **Most patients present with symptoms of chronic eye irritation, such as eye dryness, red eyes (injection), burning, stinging, sandy, or foreign body sensation, photophobia, ocular discomfort.** Decreased production of tears measured by wetting of a filter paper (Schirmer paper).

DIAGNOSIS
- Clinical diagnosis based on patient symptoms and supportive findings of DED from examination.
- Common findings include conjunctival injection and reduced blink rate.

MANAGEMENT
- **Artificial tears first-line management for all patients with dry eye disease.** In addition to symptomatic relief, artificial tears may improve visual acuity & reduce the incidence ocular damage. **Environment modification**: eg, frequent blinking & minimizing exposure to air conditioning or heating; reducing screen time. **Preservative-free ocular lubricants can be tried as next step.**
- Ophthalmologist referral is appropriate for patients in whom the underlying etiology is unknown.
- Other treatment options include topical Cyclosporine, other topical medications (Topical Lifitegrast), Intranasal Varenicline, scleral contact lenses, punctal occlusion (plugs), and surgery.

ORBITAL (POSTSEPTAL) CELLULITIS

- **Serious infection of the orbit (fat & ocular muscles) <u>posterior</u> to the orbital septum.**
- Complications include vision loss, orbital abscess, or intracranial infection.
- <u>Often polymicrobial</u>: *S. aureus* (including MRSA), *streptococci, GABHS, H. influenzae. S pneumoniae.*
- Most common in children especially 7-12 years of age compared to adults.

ETIOLOGIES
- **Most common secondary to sinus infections (especially Ethmoid sinusitis).**
- <u>Less common</u>: untreated Blepharitis, facial trauma, ophthalmic surgery, facial or dental infections.

CLINICAL MANIFESTATIONS
- **Ocular pain especially with eye movements, ophthalmoplegia (extraocular muscle weakness with limitation of eye movements) with diplopia, proptosis (bulging), & visual changes.**
- **Eyelid edema &/or erythema.** Conjunctival chemosis. Fever and leukocytosis may be seen.

DIAGNOSIS
- <u>Clinical diagnosis</u> — Although both can present with eyelid edema &/or erythema, Orbital cellulitis can usually be distinguished from Preseptal cellulitis by its clinical features (pain with eye movements, ophthalmoplegia, and proptosis) and/or by imaging studies (eg, CT scan, MRI) if the diagnosis is not clear clinically. Blood cultures may be obtained.
- **High resolution CT scan** — infection of the fat & ocular muscles behind the septum. MRI.

MANAGEMENT
- **Admission + IV antibiotics: Vancomycin PLUS one of the following — Ceftriaxone or Cefotaxime (Metronidazole or Clindamycin can be added for anaerobic coverage).** If Penicillin allergy, Vancomycin + a Fluoroquinolone (eg, Levofloxacin or Moxifloxacin) with or without Metronidazole. Ampicillin-Sulbactam, Piperacillin-Tazobactam. Symptom improvement often seen in 24-48 hours.
- Prompt surgical drainage of an orbital abscess (especially if >10 cm) or paranasal sinusitis indicated if optic nerve function deteriorates despite antibiotics.

PERIORBITAL (PRESEPTAL) CELLULITIS

- **Less serious infection of the eyelid & periocular tissue <u>anterior</u> to the orbital septum.** Preseptal cellulitis is usually a mild condition that does not commonly result in serious complications.
- Most commonly due to Sinusitis, especially paranasal, or contiguous infection of the soft tissues of the eyelids and face (eg, Hordeolum, Chalazion, trauma, animal or insect bites).
- Most common: *Staphylococcus aureus* (including MRSA), *S. epidermidis, Streptococci,* & anaerobes.

CLINICAL MANIFESTATIONS
- **Unilateral ocular pain, eyelid erythema and edema.** Chemosis is not commonly seen.

DIAGNOSIS
- **Often clinical diagnosis** — Although both can present with eyelid edema &/or erythema, **the absence of proptosis, chemosis, ophthalmoplegia (extraocular muscle weakness), ocular pain with extraocular movements clinically distinguishes Preseptal** from Postseptal Cellulitis.
- **CT or MRI** best tests to distinguish between Preseptal & Postseptal cellulitis if diagnosis is uncertain.

MANAGEMENT
Outpatient management if >1 year of age & mild.
- **Absence of periorbital skin trauma: Amoxicillin-clavulanic acid monotherapy** & warm compresses. <u>Alternatives</u>: Cefdinir, Cefuroxime, Cefpodoxime. <u>Severe Penicillin allergy</u>: Levofloxacin.
- <u>Recent history of periorbital skin trauma</u>: either [1] Linezolid or Vancomycin monotherapy or [2] Trimethoprim-sulfamethoxazole **plus** one of the following agents: Amoxicillin-clavulanic acid, Cefdinir, Cefuroxime, or Cefpodoxime.

CATARACT

- **Lens opacification (thickening).** Usually bilateral. Most common cause of blindness in the world.

RISK FACTORS
- **Increased age**: most common >60 years of age.
- **Cigarette smoking, chronic glucocorticoid use** (systemic & high-dosed inhaled), **Diabetes mellitus,** alcohol consumption, UV light exposure, malnutrition, eye trauma, metabolic syndrome.
- Neonatal cataracts: congenital ToRCH syndrome (Toxoplasmosis, Rubella, CMV HSV); galactosemia.

CLINICAL MANIFESTATIONS
- **Painless blurred vision**: painless, slow, progressive blurred or vision loss over months to years — difficulty with night driving, vision, & reading signs; problems reading fine print, glares or halos around lights, or, in very advanced cases, blindness. There is an increased risk for myopia.

PHYSICAL EXAMINATION
- **Opaque lens, absent red reflex.** Most Cataracts are bilateral, though one eye may be more affected.
- Less mature cataracts may be detected through a dilated pupil with an ophthalmoscope

MANAGEMENT
- Observation if mild.
Cataract surgery
- **Indicated if the visual changes affect activities of daily living.** Performed as an outpatient and improves visual acuity in 95% of cases. Mature cataracts may be removed by **ultrasonic fragmentation (phacoemulsification of the opacified lens) followed by implantation of an artificial intraocular lens most common surgery performed.** Extracapsular cataract extraction. Patients are usually evaluated on the first postoperative day and then 1 week and 1-month post-surgery. Restricted activity for days to weeks.
- Intraoperative floppy iris syndrome: **seen in patients treated with alpha-1 antagonists and some antipsychotics** — loss of muscle tone in the iris with symptom triad of (1) pupil constriction despite pre-operative dilatation with standard mydriatic drugs, (2) fluttering and bellowing of iris stroma, and (3) a marked tendency for the iris to prolapse towards the side port incisions.
- Uncommon complications: Endophthalmitis, Retinal detachment, lens malposition/dislocation.

PRESBYOPIA (AGING SIGHT)

- **Type of refractive error related to loss of accommodation in the aging lens such that it can no longer focus on objects viewed at arm's length or closer.**
- During the natural aging process, the crystalline lens loses its elasticity and becomes less able to increase its refractive power to accommodate on near objects. Patients may use reading glasses.

CLINICAL MANIFESTATIONS
- Presbyopia usually begins after age 40: inability to focus on objects at reading distance (eg, read fine print, dim light). The eye's focusing power for reading is lost progressively and fully by age 65 years.

DIAGNOSIS
- **Standard Snellen chart** to assess visual acuity in can be performed. Patients with visual acuity less than 20/25 in either eye have impaired visual acuity and should be referred to an eye specialist for further assessment.

MANAGEMENT
- **First-line treatments include corrective lenses, such as glasses** (eg, with a plus lens, bifocals, trifocals), **contact lenses, or refractive surgery (eg LASIK).**
- The most common surgical procedure performed to correct refractive errors is Laser in situ keratomileusis (LASIK).

MARCUS GUNN PUPIL [RELATIVE AFFERENT PUPILLARY DEFECT (RAPD)]

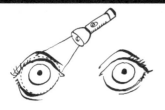

1. **Optic neuritis** most common etiology.
2. <u>Severe retinal disease</u>: eg, CRVO, CRAO, significant retinal detachment.

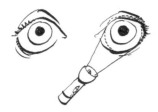

- During swinging-flashlight test into the unaffected eye, both pupils constrict.

- **MARCUS GUNN:** during swinging-flashlight test **from the unaffected eye into the affected eye, the pupils appear to dilate** (due to less than normal constriction).
- **R**elative **A**fferent **P**upillary **D**efect mnemonic = when you shine a
  Ray in the **A**ffected **P**upil it **D**ilates

ARGYLL-ROBERTSON PUPIL

- Near-light dissociation. Pupil **constricts on accommodation but does not react to bright light.**

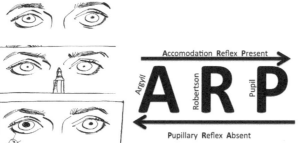

CAUSES OF ARGYLL ROBERTSON PUPIL
- **<u>Neurosyphilis</u> most common**

- Midbrain lesions
  (eg, Parinaud syndrome)

- Diabetic neuropathy

VISUAL PATHWAY DEFECTS

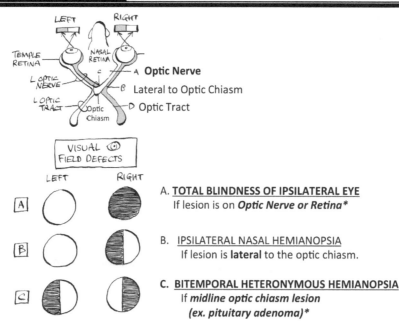

A Optic Nerve
B Lateral to Optic Chiasm
D Optic Tract

VISUAL FIELD DEFECTS

A. <u>TOTAL BLINDNESS OF IPSILATERAL EYE</u>
If lesion is on *Optic Nerve or Retina**

B. <u>IPSILATERAL NASAL HEMIANOPSIA</u>
If lesion is **lateral** to the optic chiasm.

C. <u>BITEMPORAL HETERONYMOUS HEMIANOPSIA</u>
If *midline optic chiasm lesion
(ex. pituitary adenoma)**

D. <u>CONTRALATERAL HOMONYMOUS HEMIANOPSIA</u>
If lesion at *optic tract* or in *occipital lobe stroke*

PAPILLEDEMA

- **Optic nerve (disc) swelling secondary to <u>increased intracranial pressure</u> (usually bilateral).**
- <u>ETIOLOGIES:</u> Idiopathic intracranial hypertension, space-occupying lesion (eg, cerebral tumor, abscess), increased CSF production, cerebral edema, severe hypertensive (Grade IV retinopathy).

CLINICAL MANIFESTATIONS
- **Headache, nausea, vomiting. Transient visual obscurations** may follow abrupt shifts in posture or occur spontaneously. Visual acuity is not affected by Papilledema unless the Papilledema is severe, long-standing, or accompanied by macular edema and hemorrhage.

DIAGNOSIS
- **<u>Funduscopy:</u> swollen optic disc with blurred margins.**
- **<u>Head CT scan or MRI</u> to rule out mass effect, followed by Lumbar puncture — ↑CSF pressure.**

MANAGEMENT
- **<u>Acetazolamide</u> decreases production of aqueous humor & CSF production.** Treat underlying cause.

	PAPILLEDEMA	PAPILLITIS	RETROBULBAR NEURITIS	GLAUCOMA
DEFINITION	Edema of the optic nerve head due to <u>↑ CSF pressure</u>	Edema of optic nerve head <u>in</u> the orbit (eye) - **Optic Neuritis**	Edema of optic nerve <u>behind</u> the eye - **Optic Neuritis**	Edema of the optic nerve from <u>↑intraocular Pressure</u>
LATERALITY	Bilateral usually	Unilateral	Unilateral	<u>Acute:</u> Unilateral <u>Chronic:</u> Bilateral
VISUAL DEFICIT	Not always affected Enlarged blind Spot	Range from central scotoma to complete loss of vision	Range from central scotoma to complete loss of vision	Halos around lights Blindness
FUNDUSCOPIC	Blurred disc-cup	Blurred disc-cup	Normal	Blurred disc-cup
MARCUS GUNN	Negative	**POSITIVE**	**POSITIVE**	Negative
MANAGEMENT	Reduce CSF pressure	Corticosteroids	Corticosteroids	Reduce IOP

OPTIC NEURITIS [OPTIC NERVE (CN II) INFLAMMATION]

- **Acute inflammatory demyelinating injury affecting the optic nerve (cranial nerve II).**
- <u>Risk factors:</u> most common in women and young patients 20-40 years of age.

ETIOLOGIES
- **Multiple sclerosis.** Autoimmune. <u>Medications:</u> **Ethambutol,** Chloramphenicol, PDE5 inhibitors.

CLINICAL MANIFESTATIONS
- **Subacute <u>painful monocular loss of vision</u>, decrease in color vision (<u>color desaturation</u>), <u>visual field defects</u>: central scotoma (blind spot) over hours to a few days. Usually unilateral.**

PHYSICAL EXAMINATION
- **<u>Ocular pain</u> (often behind the eye) that is exacerbated with eye movements.**
- **<u>Marcus-Gunn pupil</u>** (relative afferent pupillary defect) — **during swinging-flashlight test from the unaffected eye into the affected eye, the pupils appear to dilate.**
- <u>Funduscopy:</u> 2/3 normal disc:cup (retrobulbar) or 1/3 optic disc swelling/blurring (papillitis).

DIAGNOSIS
- **<u>MRI brain & orbits with contrast</u>** confirms the diagnosis & also assesses for Multiple sclerosis.

MANAGEMENT
- **<u>IV Methylprednisolone</u> initial management** followed by oral Corticosteroids hastens recovery.
- <u>Newer therapies:</u> Monoclonal antibodies against immune cells and cell-based therapies to deplete or modulate T and B cell responses.

ACUTE ANGLE-CLOSURE GLAUCOMA (NARROW ANGLE)

- **Increased intraocular pressure leading to damage of the optic nerve (cranial nerve 2).**
- Ophthalmologic emergency — leading cause of preventable blindness in the US.
- RISK FACTORS: patients with preexisting narrow angle or large lens — **age >60 years, hyperopes (far-sighted) with a shallow anterior chamber, females**, & Asians.

PATHOPHYSIOLOGY
- Decreased outflow & drainage of aqueous humor via trabecular meshwork & canal of Schlemm through the anterior angle is blocked by anatomic narrowing of the anterior chamber angle. This results in a buildup of fluid, resulting in increased intraocular pressure and optic nerve atrophy.
- Precipitants: **mydriasis (pupillary dilation) further closes the angle [eg, dim lights, sitting in the dark, sympathomimetics (eg, decongestants), anticholinergics].**

CLINICAL MANIFESTATIONS
- **Sudden onset of severe, unilateral ocular pain, nausea, vomiting, severe headache (periorbital).**
- **Vision changes include halos around lights & peripheral vision loss (tunnel vision),** decreased or blurred vision.

ACUTE ANGLE CLOSURE GLAUCOMA
- MID DILATED PUPIL

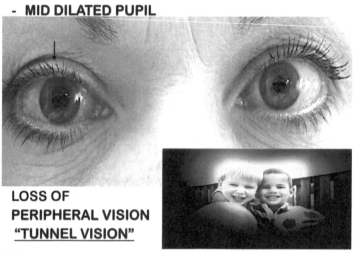

LOSS OF
PERIPHERAL VISION
"TUNNEL VISION"

PHYSICAL EXAMINATION
- **Conjunctival erythema, cloudy "steamy" cornea, mid-dilated fixed pupil (reacts poorly to light).**
- Eye feels hard on palpation due to increased intraocular pressure.
- **Funduscopy: optic disc blurring or "cupping" of optic nerve** (thinning of the outer rim of the optic nerve head).

DIAGNOSIS
- **Tonometry: increased intraocular pressure [IOP] >21 mm Hg (often >30 mm Hg)** or
- **Gonioscopy criterion standard** — allows for observation of a narrow chamber angle.

MANAGEMENT
- **Combination of [1] topical agents to induce reduce intraocular pressure [IOP] (eg, Timolol, Apraclonidine), [2] an agent to induce miosis (eg, Pilocarpine) and [3] a systemic agent to lower intraocular pressure (eg, PO or IV Acetazolamide** or IV Mannitol).
- **Topical Beta-blockers: (eg, Timolol) reduce IOP with no adverse effects on visual acuity.**
- Alpha-2 agonists: Apraclonidine, Brimonidine decrease aqueous humor production & increase drainage.
- Topical miotics/cholinergics: Pilocarpine or Carbachol cause miosis, increasing fluid drainage.
- Prostaglandins: Latanoprost reduces IOP by increasing outflow of aqueous humor.
Definitive:
- **Iridotomy laser (preferred) or surgical** — small hole allows for drainage of aqueous humor.

CHRONIC OPEN-ANGLE GLAUCOMA

- **Slow, progressive <u>painless bilateral</u> peripheral vision loss** (compared to rapid painful unilateral vision in Acute angle-closure glaucoma).
- Usually but not always associated with increased intraocular pressure (IOP).

RISK FACTORS
- Age >40 years, family history, Diabetes Mellitus, Black race.

PATHOPHYSIOLOGY
- In **Chronic open-angle glaucoma**, primary or secondary, intraocular pressure is elevated due to **[1] <u>decreased drainage of aqueous humor fluid</u> through the trabecular meshwork**, which eventually damages the optic nerve. There is a normal anterior chamber but may be associated with **[2] decreased outflow of aqueous humor.**
- In Chronic open-angle glaucoma, optic nerve damage results in a progressive loss of retinal ganglion cell axons, visual field loss and, with time and if left untreated, irreversible blindness.
- Secondary Chronic open-angle glaucoma may result from ocular disease, pigment dispersion, pseudo-exfoliation, uveitis, trauma, or Corticosteroid therapy (eg, intraocular, topical, inhaled, intranasal, or systemic).

CLINICAL MANIFESTATIONS
- **Usually asymptomatic until late in the disease course.** Vision loss is usually the presenting symptom.
- **<u>Vision loss</u>: slow, progressive <u>painless bilateral</u> peripheral vision loss (tunnel vision),** progressing to central vision loss over a period of time.
- Unlike Acute angle-closure glaucoma, Chronic open angle glaucoma is generally not associated with symptoms of acute increased intraocular pressure (eg, ocular pain or conjunctival redness).

PHYSICAL EXAM
- **Abnormal cupping of optic discs**, increased cup to disc ratio, & notching of the disc rim.

MANAGEMENT
- **<u>Reduce intraocular pressure</u>: Prostaglandin analogs first-line (eg, Latanoprost — greater reduction of IOP),** Beta-blockers (Timolol), Alpha-2 adrenergic agonists (Brimonidine), Acetazolamide (carbonic anhydrase inhibitor).
- Laser therapy (trabeculoplasty) if medical therapy fails. Trabeculoplasty increases aqueous outflow by improving drainage of aqueous humor via the trabecular meshwork.
- Surgery last-line treatment.

CHRONIC ANGLE-CLOSURE GLAUCOMA

- In Chronic angle-closure glaucoma, flow of aqueous fluid into the anterior chamber angle is obstructed, resulting in <u>gradual increase in intraocular pressure</u>.

CLINICAL MANIFESTATIONS
- **Similar to Chronic open-angle glaucoma: <u>Vision loss</u>: slow, progressive <u>painless bilateral</u> peripheral vision loss (tunnel vision),** progressing to central vision loss over a period of time.
- <u>Physical examination</u>: elevated intraocular pressure, narrow anterior chamber angles with variable amounts of peripheral anterior synechiae, and optic disc and visual field changes.

MANAGEMENT
- **<u>Laser peripheral iridotomy</u> is the initial step in the management of Chronic angle-closure glaucoma,** to relieve any pupillary block component.
- If the IOP remains elevated, it can be treated medically and surgically much as in Open-angle glaucoma.

EAR DISORDERS

ACUTE OTITIS EXTERNA (AOE)

- Inflammation or infection of the external auditory canal.

RISK FACTORS
- **Water immersion** aka **"swimmer's ear"** — excess moisture raises the pH from the normal acidic pH of the ear, facilitating bacterial overgrowth. ↑risk: age 7-12 years, narrowed ear canals, Psoriasis.
- **Local mechanical trauma** (cotton swabs or hearing aids). Aberrant ear wax (too much or too little).

ETIOLOGIES
- *Pseudomonas aeruginosa* **most common organism associated with AOE (50%).**
- *Staphylococci* (*S. aureus* & *S. epidermidis*), GABHS, Proteus, anaerobes; Aspergillus. Fungi.

CLINICAL MANIFESTATIONS
- **Ear pain (otalgia) & erythema; pruritus in the ear canal** (may have recent activity of swimming).
- **Auricular discharge**, ear pressure or fullness, hearing impairment or loss.
- Physical exam: **edema & pain on traction of the ear canal or tragus, purulent auricular discharge.**
  Otoscopy: External auditory canal erythema of skin, edema, discharge, &/or debris.

MANAGEMENT
- **[1] cleaning the ear canal by clinician + [2] protect the ear against moisture** (drying agents include isopropyl alcohol or acetic acid) **+ [3] topical antibiotics** with coverage against *Pseudomonas* & *Staphylococcus* (**with or without topical glucocorticoids** for inflammation).
  - **Mild external otitis and an intact TM:** **Acetic acid-Hydrocortisone.**
  - **Moderate disease: Ciprofloxacin-Hydrocortisone; Ciprofloxacin-Dexamethasone; Ofloxacin (all 3 are safe if the tympanic membrane cannot be visualized or if it is perforated).**
  - Aminoglycoside combination: Neomycin-Polymyxin-B-Hydrocortisone otic. **Not used if tympanic perforation suspected or if the TM cannot be visualized — Aminoglycosides are ototoxic.**
- If tympanic perforation is suspected or if it cannot be fully visualized, AVOID topical agents that contain [1] Aminoglycosides (eg, Neomycin), [2] alcohol drying agents, & [3] low pH (acidic agents).
- Severe: topical antibiotic with a glucocorticoid, wick placement, & oral antibiotics (Fluoroquinolone).

MALIGNANT (NECROTIZING) OTITIS EXTERNA

- **Invasive infection of the external auditory canal and skull base (temporal bone, soft tissue, and cartilage).** A complication of Acute otitis externa. *Pseudomonas aeruginosa* **>95% of cases.**
- Risk factors: **immunocompromised states — elderly diabetics most common,** high-dose glucocorticoid therapy, chemotherapy, advanced HIV, post-transplant.

CLINICAL MANIFESTATIONS
- **Severe auricular pain, persistent otorrhea. Cranial nerve palsies** (eg, CN 6, 7, 9) if Osteomyelitis.
- May radiate to temporomandibular joint — **pain with chewing.**
- Physical examination: **severe auricular pain on traction of the ear canal or tragus.**

DIAGNOSIS
- Otoscopy: edema of the external auditory canal with erythema, discharge, **granulation tissue at the bony cartilaginous junction of the ear canal floor,** frank necrosis of the ear canal skin.
- **CT or MRI to confirm the diagnosis.** Biopsy is the most accurate test. High ESR & CRP.

MANAGEMENT
- **Admission + IV Antipseudomonal antibiotics — IV Ciprofloxacin first-line antibiotic.**
- Antipseudomonal alternatives include Piperacillin-tazobactam, Ceftazidime, or Cefepime.

EUSTACHIAN TUBE DYSFUNCTION

- Eustachian tube (ET) swelling inhibits the ET ability to autoinsufflate, causing negative pressure.
- **Often follows viral URI or allergic rhinitis;** sinusitis, tumors. **Often precedes Acute otitis media.**

CLINICAL MANIFESTATIONS
- Obstructive dysfunction: **ear fullness, pressure, or pain; popping of the ears with swallowing or yawning, underwater feeling,** disequilibrium, **discomfort with barometric pressure change,** fluctuating conductive hearing loss, tinnitus, delayed speech in children.

Physical examination:
- **Otoscopic findings usually normal but may reveal tympanic membrane retraction or fluid behind the TM** (Serous otitis media).

DIAGNOSIS
- Clinical diagnosis.

MANAGEMENT
- **Treating the underlying cause & symptom management is the mainstay of treatment.**
- **Auto insufflation** — eg, swallowing, yawning, blowing against a slightly-pinched nostril.
- **Decongestants for congestive symptoms:** Pseudoephedrine, Phenylephrine, Oxymetazoline nasal. Patients should be counseled **not to exceed 3 days of nasal decongestant use in order to prevent nasal mucosal dependency and Rhinitis medicamentosa (rebound congestion).**
- Intranasal corticosteroids if sinonasal inflammation is present.
- Refractory: Tympanostomy tube.

BAROTRAUMA

- **Damage to the tympanic membrane** that can occur when pressure differences in the middle ear & the external environment due to sudden pressure changes stretch the tympanic membrane **[eg, flying (most common, especially descent),** rapid descent, diving, decompression, hyperbaric oxygen, blast injuries].
- Stretching of the tympanic membrane TM may case bruising of, bleeding into, or rupture of the TM.
- May be associated with Eustachian tube dysfunction resulting in inability to equalize the barometric pressure on the middle ear; the pressure difference can damage the tympanic membrane.

CLINICAL MANIFESTATIONS
- **Ear pain, aural fullness/pressure; hearing loss that persists after the etiologic event,** dizziness.

PHYSICAL EXAMINATION:
- **Damage to the tympanic membrane: Tympanic membrane visualization may reveal rupture, petechiae, serous or bloody effusion.**
- May have bloody auricular discharge if traumatic.

MANAGEMENT
Avoidance is the best treatment:
- Avoidance of flying with a cold.
- **Auto insufflation eg, swallowing, yawning, chewing gum.**
- **Decongestants,** topical (eg, 1% Phenylephrine or Oxymetazoline nasal spray) or oral (Pseudoephedrine), may be administered prior to descent and before arrival to alleviate or prevent symptoms.
- Myringotomy may be used for severe or refractory cases.

ACUTE MASTOIDITIS

Infection of the mastoid air cells of the temporal bone. Largely a disease of childhood (esp. <2 years).

ETIOLOGIES
- **Usually a <u>complication of Acute otitis media</u>** (accumulation of purulent material in mastoid cavity).
- *Streptococcus pneumoniae* and *Streptococcus pyogenes* common pathogens.

CLINICAL MANIFESTATIONS
- **Deep ear pain (usually worse at night),** fever, fussiness, lethargy, malaise, pulling at ear.

PHYSICAL EXAMINATION
- **Otalgia (ear pain), fever, signs of Otitis media** (bulging & erythematous tympanic membrane).
- **Mastoid (postauricular) tenderness, edema, erythema, &/or fluctuance** (subperiosteal abscess).
- **Protrusion of the auricle.** Narrowed auditory canal. Facial nerve palsy if complicated.

DIAGNOSIS
- **Clinical diagnosis; <u>CT scan with contrast</u> first-line diagnostic test if imaging needed.** MRI.

MANAGEMENT
- **<u>IV antibiotics</u> (eg, IV Ampicillin-sulbactam) + <u>middle ear or mastoid drainage</u> (myringotomy) with or without tympanostomy tube placement. Piperacillin-tazobactam if recent antibiotic use. <u>Severe:</u> IV Vancomycin PLUS either Ceftazidime or Cefepime or Piperacillin-tazobactam.**
- Tympanocentesis can be performed to get cultures. Hospital admission.
- **<u>Refractory or complicated:</u> Mastoidectomy** (surgery).

CHRONIC OTITIS MEDIA

- **Recurrent or persistent infection of the middle ear &/or mastoid cell system in the presence of tympanic membrane perforation >6 weeks.**
- **Complication of recurrent Acute otitis media, trauma, or Cholesteatoma.**

ETIOLOGIES
- ***Pseudomonas* most common,** *S. aureus*, gram-negative rods (eg, *Proteus*), anaerobes, *Mycoplasma*.
- Purulent otorrhea can become worse after a URI or after water enters the ear.

CLINICAL MANIFESTATIONS
- **[1] <u>Perforated tympanic membrane</u> + [2] persistent or <u>recurrent purulent otorrhea</u> (often painless) >6 weeks,** ear fullness, & **[3] varying degrees of conductive hearing loss.**
- May have a primary or secondary Cholesteatoma. Usually no pain, fever, or signs of systemic infection.

MANAGEMENT
- **Removal of infected debris + topical antibiotic drops first-line (eg, Ofloxacin or Ciprofloxacin).**
- **In patients with a tympanic membrane rupture, avoid water, moisture, drying agents (eg, alcohol, acetic acid), & topical aminoglycosides in the ear** (they are ototoxic).
- Systemic antibiotics reserved for severe cases.
- <u>Surgical:</u> tympanic membrane repair or reconstruction.

EXAM TIP

<u>Acute otitis media:</u> **effusion** (decreased mobility & cloudy TM) + <u>**signs or symptoms of inflammation**</u> **(fever, ear pain, bulging &/or marked erythema of the tympanic membrane).**

<u>Serous otitis media</u>: **asymptomatic effusion** (decreased mobility & cloudy TM) + <u>**no signs or symptoms of inflammation**</u> (fever, ear pain, or marked erythema or bulging of the TM) + <u>**flat or retracted TM.**</u>

<u>Chronic otitis media:</u> perforated tympanic membrane + persistent or recurrent purulent otorrhea, otalgia (ear pain), ear fullness, & varying degrees of conductive hearing loss.

ACUTE OTITIS MEDIA (AOM)

- **Infection of middle ear, temporal bone, & mastoid air cells.**
- RISK FACTORS: **peak age 6–24 months** (the Eustachian tube in children is shorter, narrower, & more horizontal), day care, pacifier or bottle use, second-hand smoke, not being breastfed.

MICROBIOLOGY

- *S. pneumoniae*, **nontypeable** *H. influenzae*, **&** *Moraxella catarrhalis* are the most common bacteria isolated from middle ear fluid in children with AOM. Group A Streptococcus.
- **Otitis-conjunctivitis syndrome:** [1] Bacterial conjunctivitis + [2] Acute otitis media commonly **caused by nontypeable** *Haemophilus influenzae*. **Treated with Amoxicillin-clavulanate.**

PATHOPHYSIOLOGY

- **Most commonly preceded by viral URI, which leads to blockage of the Eustachian tube.**

CLINICAL MANIFESTATIONS

- **Fever,** irritability, **otalgia (ear pain), ear tugging in infants,** stuffiness, conductive hearing loss.
- Tympanic membrane rupture: rapid relief of pain + otorrhea (usually heals in 1-2 days).
- **Physical examination:**
- **Bulging & inflamed (erythematous) tympanic membrane (TM) with effusion,** loss of landmarks. In AOM, the tympanic membrane is usually bulging & is typically white or pale yellow & opacified.
- **Pneumatic otoscopy: decreased TM mobility most sensitive.**

DIAGNOSIS

- Clinical. Tympanocentesis for a sample of fluid for culture definitive (eg, in recurrent cases).

MANAGEMENT

- **Observation can be done depending on age and severity; >80% will resolve spontaneously.**
- Initial antibiotic therapy is often given to infants <6 months old and those ≥6 months old with severe symptoms (eg, temperature ≥39°C in the past 48 hours, persistent ear pain for >48 hours, bilateral AOM, otorrhea, uncertain follow-up, immunocompromised, or at risk for severe infection).
- **High-dose Amoxicillin initial antibiotic of choice** for 5-10 days **+ analgesics.**
- **Second line: Amoxicillin-Clavulanic acid, Cefuroxime, Cefdinir, Cefpodoxime, IM Ceftriaxone.**
- Severe Penicillin allergy: Azithromycin, Clarithromycin, Erythromycin-Sulfisoxazole, Trimethoprim–sulfamethoxazole.
- Severe or recurrent cases: myringotomy (surgical drainage) with tympanostomy tube insertion.
- In children with recurrent Otitis media, Iron deficiency anemia workup & CT scan may be needed.

SEROUS OTITIS MEDIA [OTITIS MEDIA WITH EFFUSION (OME)]

- **Middle ear fluid + no signs or symptoms of acute inflammation or infection (no fever, no ear pain, & no marked erythema or bulging of the TM).** Often as a result of a viral URI.
- May be seen after resolution of Acute otitis media or in patients with Eustachian tube dysfunction.
- **Most are asymptomatic. The most common symptoms are decreases in sound conduction & hearing, aural fullness, or a popping sensation.** Tinnitus.
- Children with OME may exhibit impaired language development or communication difficulties.

DIAGNOSIS

- **Otoscopy:** gray, amber, blue, or colorless effusion (air fluid levels or bubbles behind a cloudy membrane), loss of light reflex, **retracted or flat (neutral) tympanic membrane** hypomobile with insufflation.
- Workup may include audiometry, tympanometry, measurement of auditory brainstem responses.

MANAGEMENT

- **Observation (watchful waiting) in most** — usually spontaneously resolves within 4-6 weeks.
- Significant symptoms: antihistamines, oral decongestants, and/or nasal corticosteroids.
- **Persistent or complicated: Myringotomy with tympanostomy tube for drainage** — eg, children with hearing impairment; speech, language, or learning delays; or specific conditions.

FOREIGN BODIES IN THE EXTERNAL AUDITORY CANAL (EAC)

- Can occur at any age but is most common in children ≤6 years of age.
- The most common site of foreign body impaction is the bony cartilaginous junction where the external auditory canal narrows.

CLINICAL MANIFESTATIONS

- **Patients with foreign bodies of the EAC are often asymptomatic or present with ear pain and/or discharge as the ear canal becomes inflamed. Ear fullness or hearing loss may occur.**
- With insects, acute onset of extreme pain may occur, usually with the sensation of something moving in the ear. Nausea or vomiting.
- If the foreign body has been retained for a prolonged period, the patient may present with Acute otitis externa and an auricular discharge (may be foul smelling); EAC erythema &/or edema.

DIAGNOSIS

- **Diagnosis is confirmed by direct visualization with otoscopy.** The other ear and both nostrils should be examined to assess for any additional foreign bodies. In patients with insects in the ear, a thorough examination of the external auditory canal should be performed after insect removal.
- CT scan is not commonly used but may be indicated in patients with Acute otitis externa and Chronic otitis externa if the tympanic membrane cannot be visualized. Plain radiographs not usually helpful.

MANAGEMENT

- Foreign bodies that do not have easily graspable parts but are not deeply embedded can usually be removed with an ear curette, suctioning (makes a lot of noise), or irrigation with warm water.

Instrumentation under direct visualization:

- **Many foreign bodies can simply be grasped and extracted with alligator forceps at the bedside (especially if there are easily graspable parts) or with a right-angle hook.** An otoscope with an operational head through which the instrument can be placed through is helpful to allow direct visualization throughout the procedure. The pinna should be pulled posteriorly and superiorly to straighten the external auditory canal. **Forceps should be used for removing button batteries.**
- Instrumentation can be painful and frequently warrants procedural sedation in young children or other uncooperative patients (eg, Midazolam).
- Soft objects (eg, foam rubber or paper), those with protruding surfaces or irregular edges, and insects may be removed with alligator or bayonet forceps.
- Round or breakable objects can be removed using a right-angle hook, angled wire loop, or angled cerumen curette that is cautiously advanced beyond the object and carefully withdrawn. Freely mobile spherical objects are best removed with suction using a Schuknecht foreign body extractor.
- Wedged smooth or round object: Cyanoacrylate adhesive (eg, Super Glue) can be used to remove wedged, smooth, round foreign bodies. First, petroleum ointment may be carefully applied to the EAC to reduce the risk of gluing the cotton swab to the skin. The glue is applied to the blunt end of cotton swab while the glue dries in 60 seconds. The object is then removed.

Irrigation:

- **Used for small inorganic objects or insects.** Irrigation is often better tolerated than instrumentation and does not require direct visualization. For irrigation, thread a thin catheter attached to a syringe filled with warm water into the ear canal posterior to the foreign body, so that irrigation pushes the foreign body out of the canal. Cold water may induce vertigo.
- **Contraindications** to foreign body removal via irrigation includes **organic objects** (eg, beans, vegetable matter) because they may swell as they absorb water, **button batteries** (increases risk for caustic injury), perforated tympanic membranes, or tympanostomy tubes.
- **Live insects should be killed by instilling mineral oil, 1% Lidocaine, or 2% viscous Lidocaine into the ear canal prior to removal with an alligator forceps or irrigation.**

Other management
- **If there is inflammation is noted after removal of any foreign body, abrasions, or lacerations, a short course of topical antibiotic-corticosteroid otic drops (eg, Ciprofloxacin plus Dexamethasone) may be indicated to reduce the incidence of Otitis externa.**

Otolaryngology consult
- Otolaryngology consult may be indicated if the foreign body is a hazardous material (eg, button battery); if there is concern for associated injury to the canal, tympanic membrane, and/or middle ear; potential penetrating foreign bodies (eg, pencil), marked pain, vestibular symptoms (eg, nausea, vomiting, nystagmus, vertigo, or ataxia), or if the above techniques are not successful.

Complications of foreign body removal:
- **Abrasion or laceration of the EAC is the most common complication (up to 50%).**
- TM perforation, retained parts of the foreign body, bleeding, and infection (Otitis externa), especially with multiple attempts.

AUDITORY EXAMINATION FINDINGS

AC = air conduction. BC = bone conduction.

Assessed with a tuning fork	**WEBER: place on top head**	**RINNE: place on mastoid by ear**
NORMAL	No lateralization	Normal (Positive) AC > BC
SENSORINEURAL LOSS (INNER EAR):	Lateralizes to **NORMAL** ear	**Normal: AC > BC.** Difficulty hearing their own voice & deciphering words.
CONDUCTIVE LOSS (EXT/MIDDLE):	Lateralizes to **AFFECTED** ear	BC ≥ AC (Negative)

SensoriNeural lateralizes to Normal ear + Normal Rinne (think of the **N** for sensori**N**eural).

CONDUCTIVE HEARING LOSS	**SENSORINEURAL HEARING LOSS**
External or middle ear disorders:	**Inner ear disorders:**
• <u>Defect in sound conduction</u> **Cerumen impaction most common cause of conductive hearing loss.** Obstruction from a foreign body in the EAC.	• **<u>Presbycusis</u> most common cause of sensorineural hearing loss (high frequency hearing loss).**
• <u>Damage to ossicles</u>: eg, Otosclerosis, Cholesteatoma	• **<u>Chronic loud noise exposure</u> second most common cause of sensorineural loss.**
• <u>Middle ear disorders</u>: eg, Mastoiditis, Otitis media (Acute otitis media, Serous otitis media).	• **<u>CNS lesions</u>: eg, Acoustic neuroma,** tumors
• Pinna deformity	• **Labyrinthitis**
• Perforated tympanic membrane.	• **Meniere syndrome**
	• Ototoxic medications (see below)
	• Trauma
	• <u>Infection</u>: eg HSV, CMV, Ramsay Hunt syndrome (Herpes zoster oticus), Meningitis. **Rubella is the most common cause of congenital hearing loss.**

OTOTOXIC MEDICATIONS

- <u>Loop diuretics:</u> eg, Furosemide, Bumetanide, Ethacrynic acid (most ototoxic).
- <u>Antibiotics:</u> Vancomycin, Aminoglycosides (eg, Gentamicin, Neomycin), Macrolides (Erythromycin), Tetracyclines.
- <u>Anti-inflammatories:</u> Aspirin and other salicylates, NSAIDs.
- <u>Anti-neoplastics:</u> Cisplatin and other platinum agents, Carboplatin, Cytarabine.
- <u>Anti-malarials:</u> Chloroquine, Hydroxychloroquine, Quinine.
- <u>Phosphodiesterase 5 inhibitors</u>: eg, Sildenafil

Monitoring of hearing acuity, drug levels, or dose adjustments can mitigate risk.

CERUMEN IMPACTION

- External auditory canal wax accumulation that may lead to impaction.
- Cerumen impaction is most often self-induced through incorrect methods to clear the canal of cerumen. Cleaning the external opening only with a washcloth over the finger is recommended.

CLINICAL MANIFESTATIONS
- **Usually asymptomatic but may lead to conductive hearing loss when accumulation blocks the ear canal, ear fullness,** ear pain, itching, cough, dizziness, vertigo, &/or tinnitus.

DIAGNOSIS
- Otoscopy: direct visualization of the impacted cerumen.
- Conductive hearing loss pattern: **lateralization to the affected ear** on Weber testing. Bone conduction > air conduction. **Impaction is the most common cause of conductive hearing loss.**

MANAGEMENT
- **Asymptomatic** cerumen is not usually removed if simple cerumen accumulation.
- **Symptomatic management:**
- **Cerumen softening**: detergent ear drops **(3% Hydrogen peroxide; 6.5% Carbamide peroxide),** **along with aural toilet [eg, mechanical removal (eg, curette), suction, or irrigation].**
- **Aural toilet by clinician: use of curette removal of cerumen (mechanical), suction, or irrigation.**
- Irrigation should (1) only performed when the tympanic membrane is intact (no perforation), (2) performed with water at body temperature to avoid vertigo (vestibular caloric response), and (3) the stream should be directed at the posterior ear canal wall adjacent to the cerumen plug.
- Following irrigation, the ear canal should be dried thoroughly (eg, by the patient using a hair blow-dryer on low-power setting or by the clinician instilling isopropyl alcohol) to reduce the incidence of external otitis from moisture retained in the external auditory canal.

TYMPANIC MEMBRANE (TM) PERFORATION

- Rupture of the tympanic membrane (TM).
- May lead to Cholesteatoma development.

ETIOLOGIES
- Most commonly occurs due to penetrating or noise trauma (most commonly occurs at the pars tensa), Barotrauma, Otitis media. May occur with intense irrigation for Cerumen impaction.

CLINICAL MANIFESTATIONS
- **Acute ear pain & hearing loss with or without bloody otorrhea.**
- **Patients with otalgia prior to rupture may develop sudden pain relief with bloody otorrhea.**
- May experience transient tinnitus or vertigo.

DIAGNOSIS
- **Otoscopic examination: perforated TM.** Do not perform pneumatic otoscopy.
- **May have conductive hearing loss** — Weber: lateralization to the affected ear, Rinne: bone conduction greater than air conduction.

MANAGEMENT
- **Watchful waiting: Most perforated TMs heal spontaneously. Follow up to ensure resolution.**
- Topical antibiotics (eg, Ofloxacin) in some. The canal should be cleaned of blood or debris by clinician.
- **Avoid water, topical agents that contain drying agents (eg, alcohol), low pH (eg, acetic acid), & topical aminoglycosides in the ear with a TM rupture** (Aminoglycosides are ototoxic).
- Prompt evaluation by an otolaryngologist if marked hearing loss or facial nerve injury.

CHOLESTEATOMA

- **Abnormal keratinized collection of desquamated squamous epithelial cells** that may migrate **into the middle ear or mastoid process.** Can lead to bony invasion and erosion of the mastoid.
- Acquired: **most commonly due to chronic middle ear disease or Eustachian tube dysfunction** (often forms as a retraction of the TM). Older age at tympanostomy tube placement.
- Congenital: may be seen with congenital disorders (eg, Trisomy 21, Turner syndrome, cleft palate).

CLINICAL MANIFESTATIONS
- **Painless otorrhea: persistent purulent brown or yellow discharge with a strong odor.**
- **Conductive hearing loss,** tinnitus, dizziness, peripheral vertigo, or cranial nerve palsies (eg, CN VII).

Physical examination:
- **Otoscopy: focal granulation tissue (cellular debris) on TM, white mass behind an intact or perforated TM,** a deep retraction pocket of the TM, especially at the periphery, posterosuperior quadrant, and anterosuperior quadrant. CT scan may be performed if concern for complications.
- **Conductive hearing loss** — lateralization to the affected ear on Weber testing and bone conduction > air conduction in the affected ear on Rinne. May see perforation of the tympanic membrane.

MANAGEMENT
- Surgical excision of the debris & Cholesteatoma, with ossicle reconstruction. Tympanomastoidectomy.

OTOSCLEROSIS

- **Abnormal bony overgrowth of the footplate of the stapes bone, leading to conductive hearing loss.**
- Autosomal dominant disorder (may have **family history** of conductive hearing loss). 85% are bilateral.

CLINICAL MANIFESTATIONS
- **Slowly progressive bilateral conductive hearing loss, especially low-frequencies,** tinnitus.
- Vertigo uncommon.

DIAGNOSIS
- **Conductive hearing loss** — lateralization to the affected ear on Weber testing and bone conduction > air conduction in the affected ear on Rinne. TM is usually normal. Tone audiometry (most useful).

MANAGEMENT
- Observation if mild. Improve hearing loss by either [1] hearing amplification (eg, hearing aid) or [2] surgical replacement of the stapes bone with a prosthesis (stapedectomy).
- Cochlear implantation if severe.

VERTIGO

- **False sense of motion** (or exaggerated sense of motion).   2 types:

	PERIPHERAL VERTIGO		CENTRAL VERTIGO
LOCATION OF PROBLEM	Labyrinth or Vestibular nerve (which is part of CN VIII/8).		**Brainstem or cerebellar**
ETIOLOGIES	1. Benign Positional Vertigo (MC) 2. Meniere: 3. Vestibular neuritis 4. Labyrinthitis: 5. Cholesteatoma	episodic vertigo + no hearing loss episodic vertigo + hearing loss continuous vertigo + no hearing loss continuous vertigo + hearing loss	Cerebellopontine tumors Migraine Cerebral vascular disease Multiple sclerosis Vestibular Neuroma
CLINICAL	• **HORIZONTAL nystagmus** (usually beats away from affected side). **Fatigable.** Gait disturbance with veering towards affected side. • Sudden onset of tinnitus & hearing loss usually associated with peripheral compared to central causes. • Gait disturbance with veering towards affected		• **VERTICAL nystagmus.** **Nonfatigable** (continuous) • Gait issues more severe. • Gradual onset. • **Positive CNS signs.**

MANAGEMENT OF NAUSEA &/or VOMITING IN PATIENTS WITH VERTIGO:

Nausea &/or vomiting caused by sensory conflict **mediated by neurotransmitters GABA, acetylcholine, histamine, dopamine, & serotonin.** Antiemetics block most of these neurotransmitters.

ANTIHISTAMINES & ANTICHOLINERGICS Meclizine Dimenhydrinate Diphenhydramine Scopolamine (anticholinergic)	MOA: acts on the brain's control center for nausea, vomiting, & dizziness. Indication: **first line for vertigo** (nausea/vomiting), **motion sickness.** S/E: **anticholinergic** — dry mouth, blurred vision (dilated pupils), urinary retention, constipation, dry skin, flushing, tachycardia, fever, delirium, sedation. CI/Caution: **acute narrow angle glaucoma, BPH with urinary retention.**
DOPAMINE BLOCKERS Prochlorperazine Promethazine Metoclopramide	MOA: **blocks CNS dopamine receptors ($D_1 D_2$)** in the brain's vomiting center. Indications: nausea, vomiting, motion sickness. S/E: **QT prolongation, sedation,** constipation. **Extrapyramidal Sx (EPS): rigidity, bradykinesia, tremor, akathisia (restlessness).** 3 EPS syndromes include: 1. **Dystonic Reactions (Dyskinesia):** reversible EPS **hours-days after initiation** ⇨ intermittent, spasmodic, sustained involuntary contractions **(trismus, protrusions of tongue, forced jaw opening, difficulty speaking, facial grimacing, torticollis).** **Mgmt: Diphenhydramine IV** or add **anticholinergic agent** (eg, Benztropine). 2. **Tardive Dyskinesia:** repetitive involuntary movements mostly involving extremities & face — lip smacking, teeth grinding, rolling of tongue. Seen with <u>long-term use.</u> 3. **Parkinsonism:** (due to ↓dopamine in nigrostriatal pathways) – rigidity, tremor. **Neuroleptic Malignant Syndrome (NMS):** life threatening disorder due to D_2 inhibition in basal ganglia: **mental status changes, extreme muscle rigidity, tremor, fever, autonomic instability (tachycardia,** blood pressure changes, tachypnea, profuse diaphoresis, incontinence, dyspnea). Management: ice to axilla/groin, ventilatory support; **Dopamine Agonists: Bromocriptine,** Amantadine, Levodopa/Carbidopa.
BENZODIAZEPINES	Lorazepam, Diazepam used in refractory patients (potentiates GABA).
SEROTONIN ANTAGONISTS Ondansetron Granisetron Dolasetron	MOA: **blocks serotonin receptors** (5-HT3) both peripherally & centrally in the chemoreceptor trigger zone of the medulla, suppressing the vomiting center. S/E: neurologic: headache, fatigue, malaise. GI sx: nausea, constipation. Cardiac: prolonged QT interval & cardiac arrhythmias.

BENIGN PAROXYSMAL POSITIONAL VERTIGO (BPPV)

- **A type of peripheral vertigo most commonly due to displaced otolith particles** (calcium carbonate crystals) within the semicircular canals of the inner ear (canalithiasis). When head position changes, gravity causes the debris to move within the canal, producing **vertigo & latent fatigable nystagmus.**
- **BPPV is the most common cause of peripheral vertigo.** Debris in the Posterior canal most common.

CLINICAL MANIFESTATIONS
- **Recurrent episodes of <u>sudden, episodic</u> peripheral vertigo (lasting ≤60 seconds, typically 15-20 seconds) & <u>provoked with certain changes in head position</u>** (eg, rolling over in bed to a lateral position, lying down, rising from a supine position, extending the head to look up).
- May be accompanied by nausea or vomiting. **<u>Not</u> associated with hearing loss,** tinnitus, or ataxia.

DIAGNOSIS
- **Dix-Hallpike (Nylen Barany) test — reproduces vertigo & fatigable nystagmus** if posterior BPPV. The nystagmus is mixed: torsional & vertical [geotropic (downbeating, rotatory nystagmus)].

MANAGEMENT
- **Canalith repositioning: Epley maneuver (treatment of choice) or Semont maneuver** for posterior canal BPPV. Other particle repositioning maneuvers for the other types.
- Because the episodes are so brief, medical therapy is not usually needed.
- Surgical management if not responsive to repositioning maneuvers.

VESTIBULAR NEURONITIS & LABYRINTHITIS

DEFINITIONS
- <u>Vestibular neuronitis:</u> inflammation of only the vestibular portion of cranial nerve VIII (8).
- <u>Labyrinthitis:</u> inflammation of the vestibular AND cochlear portions of cranial nerve VIII (8).
- <u>Etiologies:</u> Idiopathic. **Commonly associated with viral or postviral inflammation** (eg, latent HSV-1).

CLINICAL MANIFESTATIONS
- **<u>Vestibular symptoms</u> (both): <u>continuous</u> peripheral vertigo,** dizziness, nausea, vomiting, gait disturbances (eg, postural instability toward the affected ear but is still able to walk without falling).
- **<u>Nystagmus:</u> usually horizontal, rotary (torsional), & away from the affected side in the fast phase &** suppressed by visual fixation. Not usually associated with headache or other neurological findings.
- <u>Cochlear symptoms (Labyrinthitis only):</u> unilateral hearing loss, tinnitus.
- **<u>Vestibular neuronitis:</u> continuous vertigo + no hearing loss.**
- **<u>Labyrinthitis:</u> continuous vertigo + hearing loss.**

DIAGNOSIS
- Primary a clinical diagnosis; imaging is not usually needed.
- <u>Neuroimaging</u> (MRI preferred > CT) to rule out alternative causes if the symptoms are not fully consistent with a peripheral lesion, prominent risk factors for stroke, focal neurological signs.
- <u>Vestibular testing:</u> reduced caloric response in injured ear with vestibular testing.

MANAGEMENT
- **<u>Glucocorticoids</u> first-line management of Labyrinthitis and Vestibular neuronitis.**
- **<u>Symptomatic relief:</u>** brief use of antihistamines (eg, **Meclizine**) or anticholinergics. Benzodiazepines.
- Both are self-limited — symptoms usually resolve in days to weeks, even without treatment.

MÉNIÈRE'S DISEASE (IDIOPATHIC ENDOLYMPHATIC HYDROPS)

- **Idiopathic distention of the endolymphatic compartment of the inner ear due to excess endolymph fluid in the inner ear (endolymphatic hydrops).**
- Meniere SYNDROME is due to an identifiable cause. Meniere DISEASE is idiopathic.

CLINICAL MANIFESTATIONS
- **<u>Characterized by attacks with 4 findings</u> — [1] <u>episodic</u> peripheral vertigo** (lasting minutes – hours) + **[2] unilateral fluctuating sensorineural hearing loss (low frequencies initially), [3] tinnitus, & [4] ear fullness (aural pressure).** Following the attack, the patient may feel fatigue for days.
- **Horizontal nystagmus,** nausea, &/or vomiting during the attacks.

DIAGNOSIS
- Clinical diagnosis of exclusion; there are no specific test to establish the diagnosis.
- <u>Audiometry</u> during an attack shows a characteristic asymmetric low-frequency hearing loss.
- Transtympanic electrocochleography; loss of nystagmus with caloric testing seen with Meniere.
- Fluorescent treponemal antibody absorption (FTA-ABS) test to rule out Syphilis.

MANAGEMENT
- **<u>Initial:</u> dietary modifications — sodium restriction** (≤2,000 mg/d), **caffeine, nicotine, chocolate, & alcohol reduction** because they increase endolymphatic pressure. Otolaryngologist referral.
- <u>Medical:</u> if no relief with dietary modifications. Antihistamines (**Meclizine,** Dimenhydrinate); Prochlorperazine or Promethazine, benzodiazepines (Diazepam), anticholinergics (Scopolamine), & **Diuretics** (eg, **Hydrochlorothiazide**) are all options to reduce endolymphatic pressure.
- <u>Refractory:</u> surgical decompression (eg, tympanostomy tube), labyrinthectomy, or intraaural Gentamicin (selectively damages the vestibular hair cells relative to the cochlear hair cells).

VESTIBULAR SCHWANNOMA [ACOUSTIC (CN VIII/8) NEUROMA]

- **Benign Schwann cell-derived tumor** often arising from the **vestibular portion of cranial nerve 8**, often in the **cerebellopontine angle**. Can compress structures (eg, **cranial nerves 8, 7, &/or 5**).
- Schwann cells are myelin sheath-producing cells. Median age at diagnosis is ~50 years.

CLINICAL MANIFESTATIONS
- **Slowly progressive unilateral <u>sensorineural hearing loss</u> & vestibular hypofunction (eg, <u>tinnitus</u>).**
- **Ataxia**, unsteadiness with walking, headache, **facial numbness** (CN V), **or facial paresis** (CN VII).

DIAGNOSIS
- **MRI with gadolinium:** imaging test of choice:

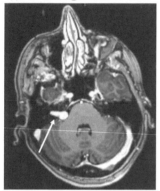

Findings: **well-circumscribed enhancing lesion in the middle ear with extension into the <u>cerebellopontine angle</u> with an "ice cream on cone" appearance** (see arrow).

Unilateral in ~90% of cases.

Bilateral Vestibular schwannomas may be seen with Neurofibromatosis type 2 (NF2).

- **Audiometry screening lab test of choice** — asymmetric sensorineural hearing loss most common.

MANAGEMENT
- Surgery, focused radiation therapy, or observation (depending on age, tumor location, size, etc.).
- Microsurgical excision: larger or rapidly expanding tumors.
- Stereotactic radiotherapy: small tumors or if the patient is not a surgical candidate.

NOSE & SINUS DISORDERS

ACUTE VIRAL RHINOSINUSITIS (COMMON COLD)

- Symptomatic inflammation of the nasal cavity and paranasal sinuses. <u>Acute</u> if <4 weeks of symptoms.
- **The vast majority of cases of acute rhinosinusitis (ARS) are due to viral infection** (common cold) — Rhinovirus, influenza, parainfluenza, & other viruses.

CLINICAL MANIFESTATIONS
- Nasal congestion & obstruction, clear rhinorrhea, hyposmia. <u>Viral symptoms:</u> cough, headache, malaise.
- Eustachian tube dysfunction symptoms: ear pain, fullness or pressure, hearing loss, or tinnitus.
- Acute rhinosinusitis: facial pain, pressure or fullness that is worse or localized with bending down & leaning forward; headache, malaise, purulent nasal discharge, fever, nasal congestion, maxillary tooth discomfort, ear pressure or fullness, halitosis.
Physical examination:
- Erythematous, engorged nasal mucosa without significant intranasal purulence.

MANAGEMENT
- **Supportive management as symptoms are self-limited**, with symptoms resolution usually within 7-10 days. Although symptoms may persist >10 days, there is usually some improvement by day 10. If fever is present, it is usually present early in the illness & disappears within the first 24-48 hours.
- **Sinusitis: symptomatic management — analgesics are considered the mainstay of therapy for Acute sinusitis (eg, Acetaminophen, NSAIDs), nasal lavage (saline irrigation), & intranasal Glucocorticoids.** Decongestants (promote sinus drainage), antihistamines, and mucolytics.

ACUTE BACTERIAL RHINOSINUSITIS (ABRS)

- Bacteria secondarily infect an inflame the sinus cavity, with <4 weeks duration.
- Acute bacterial infection occurs in only 0.5–2% of episodes of ARS (vast majority of sinusitis is viral).

TERMINOLOGY

- <u>Acute rhinosinusitis</u> — symptoms <4 weeks. Symptoms usually resolve of improve within 10 days.
- <u>Subacute rhinosinusitis</u> — symptoms for 4-12 weeks
- <u>Chronic rhinosinusitis</u> — symptoms persist >12 weeks
- <u>Recurrent acute rhinosinusitis</u> — ≥4 episodes of ARS per year, with interim symptom resolution.

PATHOPHYSIOLOGY

- **Impaired sinus drainage:** **ABRS most commonly occurs as a complication of viral infection.** Allergic or nonallergic rhinitis, mechanical obstruction of the nose, dental infections, impaired mucociliary clearance (eg, Cystic fibrosis), or with cigarette smoking.

MICROBIOLOGY

- **The most common bacteria associated with ABRS are** *Streptococcus pneumoniae* & *Haemophilus influenzae* **(both make up ~75%), and** *Moraxella catarrhalis* (organisms similar to Acute otitis media). Microaerophilic & anaerobic bacteria associated with dental root infections.

CLINICAL MANIFESTATIONS

- <u>Acute rhinosinusitis:</u> **facial pain, pressure, or fullness worse with bending down & leaning forward, purulent nasal discharge, nasal congestion or obstruction, headache, fever,** ear pressure/fullness, halitosis, hyposmia **<4 weeks** (symptoms can't distinguish bacterial vs. viral).
- **Suggestive of bacterial cause:** clinical criteria for diagnosis:
- **Persistent symptoms that last ≥10 days <u>without</u> evidence of clinical improvement.**
- **A biphasic pattern: ("double worsening")** — **symptoms initially start to improve but then worsen ~5-6 days later.**

PHYSICAL EXAMINATION

- Erythema/edema over the involved area; watery or purulent drainage in the nose or posterior pharynx.
- **Sinus tenderness to palpation** in order of frequency — Maxillary > ethmoid > frontal > sphenoid.
- **Maxillary: most common** — cheek pain or pressure that can radiate to the upper incisors as well as decreased transillumination of the cheek. <u>Ethmoid:</u> tenderness to the high lateral wall of the nose.
- <u>Frontal:</u> pain around the eyes and the forehead. <u>Sphenoid:</u> mid head tenderness.

DIAGNOSIS

- **Primarily a clinical diagnosis. Imaging is <u>not</u> indicated if classic presentation & uncomplicated.**
- **CT scan is the imaging test of choice if imaging is needed** [eg, signs or symptoms suggesting spread of infection beyond the paranasal sinuses and nasal cavity (CNS, orbit, or surrounding tissues)].
- <u>Sinus radiographs</u> not usually needed. If ordered, Water's view most helpful radiograph view.
- <u>Biopsy or aspirate:</u> definitive diagnosis but usually not needed in most uncomplicated cases.

MANAGEMENT

- **Symptomatic management:** analgesics (eg, NSAIDs), nasal lavage (saline washes), intranasal glucocorticoids. Decongestants may promote sinus drainage, antihistamines, mucolytics.
- **Antibiotics:**
- **Indications: symptoms should be present for an extended period of ≥10-14 days** with worsening of symptoms or earlier if severe.
- **Amoxicillin-clavulanic acid is often the antibiotic of choice.** Amoxicillin.
- <u>Second line:</u> **Doxycycline (can be used first-line if Penicillin allergy).** Third-generation oral Cephalosporin (eg, Cefixime, Cefpodoxime) with or without Clindamycin.
- <u>Respiratory fluoroquinolones</u> (Levofloxacin, Moxifloxacin) usually reserved to prevent resistance.

CHRONIC RHINOSINUSITIS

- Inflammation of the nasal cavity and paranasal sinuses for **≥12 consecutive weeks**.

ETIOLOGIES may include infection (acute, chronic), allergies, & immunological or structural diseases.
- Bacterial: *S. aureus* **most common bacterial cause and anaerobes.** *Pseudomonas aeruginosa.*
- Granulomatosis with polyangiitis [Wegener's granulomatosis] often necrotic.
- Fungal: **Aspergillus most common fungal cause.** Mucormycosis second most common fungal cause.

CLINICAL MANIFESTATIONS
- Similar to Acute sinusitis but duration ≥12 weeks — **[1] nasal obstruction & congestion, [2] facial pain &/or pressure** worse with bending down & leaning forward, **[3] mucopurulent nasal discharge, & [4] decreased olfaction.** Headache, malaise, fever. Cough may be seen in children.

DIAGNOSIS
- Sinus CT imaging or rhinoscopy or nasal endoscopy with decongestion. Allergy evaluation.
- Allergy testing in all patients (often associated with Asthma, Allergic rhinitis, &/or nasal polyps).
- Biopsy or histology allows for identification of the organism & may direct appropriate management.

MANAGEMENT
- Depends on etiology: The goal of therapy is to promote sinus drainage, reduce edema, & eliminate infection [eg, **combination of nasal irrigation, intranasal glucocorticoids (or oral), & ENT follow-up**].
- Antibiotics (if bacterial) with ENT follow up: **Amoxicillin-clavulanate first line.** Alternatives include Clindamycin and combinations of Metronidazole with a second- or third-generation Cephalosporin, Macrolides, or Trimethoprim-sulfamethoxazole.

MUCORMYCOSIS (ZYGOMYCOSIS)

Angioinvasive fungal infection that infiltrates the <u>sinuses, central nervous system, & lungs</u>.
- **Angioinvasion:** the fungus rapidly dissects the nasal canals and eye into the brain. High mortality.

Etiologies:
- **Non-Aspergillus fungal causes:** *Rhizopus* species (eg, *R. oryzae)*, Mucor, & Rhizomucor. *Cunninghamella, Saksenaea,* and *Apophysomyces* may also be causes.

RISK FACTORS
- **Diabetes mellitus [DKA & hyperglycemia (most common)], other immunocompromised states** (eg, post-transplant, chemotherapy, HIV, heme malignancy), Deferoxamine therapy, **iron overload states**.

CLINICAL MANIFESTATIONS
- **Rhino-orbital-cerebral infections:** Sinusitis (facial pain/pressure worse with bending down & leaning forward, **headache, malaise, purulent nasal discharge, fever & nasal congestion) with rapid progression to the orbit & brain. Lung involvement also common.**
- Physical: ± **erythema, swelling, necrosis,** or <u>black eschar</u> on the palate, nasal mucosa, or face.

DIAGNOSIS
- **Biopsy** and histopathologic examination of involved tissue — **non-septate broad hyphae with irregular right-angle (90°) branching.** PCR testing of the blood and tissues obtained.
- MRI & CT are often obtained but show nonspecific findings.

MANAGEMENT
- The standard management of Mucormycosis involves early diagnosis, reversal of risk factors and underlying illness (eg, hyperglycemia, acidosis, cessation of immunosuppressive agents when possible), early aggressive surgical debridement, and prompt administration of IV antifungals.
- **IV Amphotericin B first line + <u>aggressive surgical debridement</u> of necrotic areas.** The lipid formulation of Amphotericin B preferred (allows for higher dose delivery with less nephrotoxicity).
- Second line: Posaconazole or Isavuconazole are alternatives to or in addition to Amphotericin B.

RHINITIS

- **Allergic:** most common type overall — **IgE-mediated** mast cell histamine release due to allergens (eg, pollen, mold, dust, animal dander etc.). Often seen in patients with history of Atopic disease.
- **Infectious: Rhinovirus most common infectious cause (common cold).**
- **Vasomotor:** nonallergic & noninfectious dilation of the blood vessels (eg, temperature change, strong smells, humidity, odors, etc.).
- **Samter's triad:** [1] Asthma, [2] Allergic rhinitis, and [3] Aspirin or NSAID sensitivity.

CLINICAL MANIFESTATIONS

- **Nasal symptoms:** sneezing, nasal congestion (stuffiness), clear watery rhinorrhea (anterior &/or posterior), nasal itching (especially allergic), cough. Eyes, ears, & throat symptoms.

PHYSICAL EXAMINATION

- **Allergic: edematous, pale, or violaceous boggy turbinates, nasal polyps with cobblestone mucosa** of the conjunctiva. May develop an "allergic shiner" — blue/gray to purple discoloration around the eyes. Transverse nasal bridge crease from constant persisting rubbing and pushing up of the nose from itching (allergic salute line).
- **Viral: erythematous (beefy red) turbinates.**
- **Vasomotor:** nasal mucosa bogginess, stuffiness, rhinorrhea after irritant exposure (usually transient).

MANAGEMENT OF ALLERGIC

- **Intranasal corticosteroids most effective pharmacologic therapy for Allergic rhinitis & Nasal polyps** [eg, Mometasone, Fluticasone, Triamcinolone] & are more effective than antihistamines.
- **2nd-generation oral antihistamine** (eg, Loratadine, Cetirizine, Fexofenadine), **antihistamine nasal spray** (eg, Azelastine, Olopatadine), or mast cell stabilizers (Cromolyn nasal spray).
- Short-term decongestants may also be used.
- **Avoidance of allergen and environmental control; exposure reduction.**

Intranasal glucocorticoids:
Mometasone, Fluticasone, Triamcinolone.
- Indications: **most effective medication for Allergic rhinitis** (moderate to severe or persistent) **especially with nasal polyps.**

Decongestants:
- MOA: may improve congestion but have little effect on rhinorrhea, sneezing, or pruritus.
- Intranasal: Oxymetazoline, Phenylephrine, Naphazoline. Oral: Pseudoephedrine.
- **Should not exceed >3-5 days of intranasal decongestant treatment in order to prevent nasal mucosal dependency and Rhinitis medicamentosa (rebound congestion).**

NASAL POLYPS

- **Allergic rhinitis most common cause.** May be seen with Cystic Fibrosis.

CLINICAL MANIFESTATIONS

- **Most are incidental findings but if large, can cause nasal obstruction or anosmia** (decreased smell).

DIAGNOSIS

- Direct visualization: **pale boggy mass on the nasal mucosa.** May have findings associated Allergic rhinitis — eg, pale or violaceous, boggy turbinates & cobblestone mucosa of the conjunctiva.

MANAGEMENT

- **Intranasal corticosteroids most effective pharmacologic therapy for Nasal polyps**
- Functional endoscopic sinus surgery if very large or if medical therapy is unsuccessful.

EPISTAXIS

ANTERIOR EPISTAXIS

- **Kiesselbach venous plexus most common source** (watershed area of the anterior nasal septum).
- Etiologies: most commonly associated with nasal trauma (eg, *nose picking most common in children*, blowing nose forcefully etc.), low humidity, hot environments (dried nasal mucosa), rhinitis, alcohol, cocaine use, antiplatelet meds, foreign body. Hypertension doesn't cause it but may prolong it.

POSTERIOR EPISTAXIS

- Source: **sphenopalatine artery branches & Woodruff's plexus most common sites. May cause bleeding in both nares & the posterior pharynx.**
- Risk factors: Hypertension, older patients, nasal neoplasms, atherosclerosis.

MANAGEMENT OF ANTERIOR EPISTAXIS

- **Direct pressure first-line therapy in most cases. Pressure applied ≥10 minutes with the patient in the seated position, leaning forward** to reduce vessel pressure, ± Oxymetazoline nasal spray. Unremoved septal hematomas can lead to septum destruction if not evacuated.
- Adjunct medications: **topical vasoconstrictors may be adjunctive therapy with direct pressure (eg, Oxymetazoline nasal spray, Phenylephrine,** 4% Cocaine) — cautious use in patients with Hypertension due to increased vasoconstriction.
- **Cauterization: electrocautery or chemical (silver nitrate) if [1] the above measures fail AND [2] the bleeding site can be visualized.**
- **Nasal packing: if direct pressure, vasoconstrictors, & cautery are unsuccessful, if the site cannot be visualized, or in severe bleeding** to tamponade the bleeding [nasal tampon, nasal balloon catheter, gauze packing]. Other options include oxidized Cellulose, thrombogenic foam & absorbable gelatin foam, Tranexamic acid. May consider antibiotic (Cephalexin, Amoxicillin-clavulanate, topical Mupirocin) to prevent Toxic shock syndrome if packed (controversial).
- Septal hematomas are associated with loss of cartilage if the hematoma is not removed.
- Post treatment care: avoid straining or exercise for a few days, avoid hot or spicy foods (they cause vasodilation). Bacitracin, petroleum gauze, & humidifiers helpful to moisten the nasal mucosa.

MANAGEMENT OF POSTERIOR EPISTAXIS

- **Posterior packing: (eg, Balloon catheter) most commonly used initial management.** Monitoring of patients: placed on a monitored bed because posterior packing can cause vagal stimulation with resulting bradycardia and bronchoconstriction. Foley catheter, Cotton packing are other options.

INTRANASAL FOREIGN BODY

- Most commonly seen in young children (eg, beads, paper, toy parts, peas, corn, seeds, nuts).
- **Most are symptomatic. Classically presents with local pain, epistaxis associated with unilateral mucopurulent foul-smelling discharge, & nasal obstruction (mouth breathing).**

DIAGNOSIS

- **Direct visualization (head light & otoscope).** Rigid or flexible fiberoptic endoscopy.
- Radiographs not usually needed; may be helpful if button batteries are suspected & not visualized.

MANAGEMENT

- Removal via positive pressure technique or instrumentation. Button batteries in the nasal cavity and magnets require urgent removal. No irrigation.
- Positive pressure technique: involves having the patient blow his or her nose while occluding the nostril opposite of the foreign body. Oral positive pressure: parent blows into the mouth while occluding the unaffected nostril (used in smaller children).
- Nonocclusive foreign bodies in the anterior portion of the nose: instrumentation rather than positive pressure techniques (eg, hemostat, forceps).
- If a live insect is present, kill with 2% Lidocaine or Mineral oil prior to removal.

THROAT DISORDERS

ORAL HAIRY LEUKOPLAKIA (OHL)

- **Mucocutaneous manifestation of Epstein-Barr virus** (Human herpesvirus-4) due to infection of the lingual squamous epithelium.
- Not considered precancerous.

RISK FACTORS
- **HIV infection: Almost exclusively seen with HIV infection.**
- Other immunocompromised states — post-transplant recipients, chronic corticosteroid therapy (inhaled or systemic), malignancy, chemotherapy.

CLINICAL MANIFESTATIONS
- Most often OHL is asymptomatic.
- **Painless, white smooth or corrugated "hairy" plaque along the lateral tongue borders or buccal mucosa that cannot be scraped off the surface to which they adhere, unlike *Candida*.**
- Rarely, cases it may involve the floor of the mouth, palate, or buccal mucosa.

DIAGNOSIS
- Usually a clinical diagnosis but biopsy can be used for definitive diagnosis.
- If OHL is identified in a patient not known to be HIV infected, risk factors and HIV screening options should be discussed and possibly performed at the patient's discretion.

MANAGEMENT
- **No specific treatment required** may spontaneously resolve & **not considered a premalignant lesion**.
HIV infection:
- **Antiretroviral treatment in patients with HIV infection.**

ACUTE PHARYNGITIS & TONSILLITIS

- **Viral** Respiratory viruses most common **overall** cause of pharyngitis — Adenovirus, Rhinovirus, Enterovirus, Epstein-Barr virus, Respiratory syncytial virus, Influenza A & B, Herpes zoster virus.
- Bacterial: **Group A Streptococcus (*S. pyogenes*) most common bacterial cause of Pharyngitis.**

CLINICAL MANIFESTATIONS
- Sore throat worsens with swallowing, pain on swallowing or with phonation.
- Cervical lymphadenopathy.
- **Viral symptoms: cough (not always), hoarseness, rhinorrhea, coryza, conjunctivitis, diarrhea.**

PHYSICAL EXAMINATION
- May have tonsillar and pharyngeal erythema, edema, with or without exudate, cervical adenopathy.
- Anterior stomatitis: may be associated with discrete ulcers or vesicles; vesicular or petechial pattern on the soft palate and tonsils.

DIAGNOSIS
- Usually clinical. Most cases of viral pharyngitis require no specific diagnostic testing.
- **There are 3 notable exceptions where testing may be indicated: [1] suspected Influenza, [2] Infectious mononucleosis, or [3] Acute retroviral syndrome (HIV).**
- Rapid strep or throat culture may be performed to rule out bacterial cause if suspected.

MANAGEMENT
- **Symptomatic management mainstay of treatment** — oral hydration, warm saline gargles, topical anesthetics, lozenges, NSAIDs. Patients unable to tolerate oral hydration may need IV fluids.

LARYNGITIS

- Acute inflammation of the mucosa of the larynx. Usually self-limited, lasting 3-7 days (≤3 weeks).

ETIOLOGIES
- **Viral upper respiratory tract infection (URI) most common** — Adenovirus, Rhinovirus, Influenza, Respiratory syncytial virus (RSV), Parainfluenza virus.
- Bacterial causes: *Moraxella catarrhalis, Mycoplasma pneumoniae, H. influenzae,* & *S. pneumoniae.*
- **Vocal strain** (eg, screaming or singing). Irritants (eg, acid — GERD), polyps, Asthma, Laryngeal cancer.

CLINICAL MANIFESTATIONS
- **Hoarseness hallmark (raspy or breathy voice), aphonia (loss of voice).** Dry or scratchy throat.
- May have viral (URI) symptoms eg, rhinorrhea, cough, sore throat, anterior stomatitis, diarrhea.

DIAGNOSIS
- **Usually a clinical diagnosis.** Examination with a mirror or flexible laryngoscopy if vocal cord visualization is necessary — erythema and edema of the vocal cords and surrounding structures.

MANAGEMENT
- **Supportive care mainstay — vocal rest is essential, hydration, airway humidification,** warm saline gargles, anesthetics, lozenges, and **reassurance that it is usually self-limited.**
- ENT or GI follow-up if workup needed (eg, GERD, suspected malignancy, >3 weeks).

PERITONSILLAR ABSCESS (QUINSY) AND PERITONSILLAR CELLULITIS

- Abscess between the palatine tonsil & the pharyngeal muscles, resulting from a complication of tonsillitis or pharyngitis. Most common in adolescents & young adults 15-30 years of age.

ETIOLOGIES
- **Often polymicrobial** — the predominant species include **Group A Streptococcus (*S. pyogenes*), Staphylococcus aureus, and respiratory/oral anaerobes (eg, *Fusobacterium necrophorum*).**

CLINICAL MANIFESTATIONS
- Ill-appearing, severe unilateral pharyngitis, dysphagia, odynophagia, high fever, malaise, ear pain.
- **Muffled "hot potato" voice, difficulty handling oral secretions (drooling), trismus** (lockjaw).
Physical examination:
- **Swollen or fluctuant tonsil, causing <u>uvula deviation to the contralateral side</u>,** bulging of the posterior soft palate near the tonsil with fluctuance, inferior and medial displacement of the infected tonsil(s), **asymmetric rise of the uvula,** & tender anterior cervical lymphadenopathy.
- **Peritonsillar Cellulitis: similar symptoms but not associated with fluctuance or deviation.**

DIAGNOSIS
- Primarily a clinical diagnosis without need for imaging or labs if classic. Intraoral ultrasound if unsure.
- CT scan imaging of choice if imaging is needed to differentiate Cellulitis vs. Abscess or complications.

MANAGEMENT
Drainage (Aspiration or I & D or tonsillectomy) + antibiotics. Antibiotics if Cellulitis only.
- Drainage: **needle aspiration (preferred) or incision & drainage (I & D) procedures for most.** A 19-gauge or 21-gauge needle should be passed medial to the molar and no deeper than 1 cm, because the internal carotid artery may lie more medially.
- **Antibiotics: oral (Amoxicillin-clavulanic acid or Clindamycin); Parenteral (Ampicillin-sulbactam or Clindamycin).** MRSA suspected: IV Vancomycin; Linezolid is an alternative.
- Tonsillectomy: usually reserved for patients who fail to respond to drainage, PTA with complications (eg impending airway obstruction), prior episodes of PTA, or recurrent severe pharyngitis.
- PREVENTION: Prompt treatment of Streptococcal infections.

RETROPHARYNGEAL ABSCESS

- Deep neck space infection located in the potential space behind the posterior pharyngeal wall.
- Most common in children 2–4 years. In adults, it is often a result of penetrating trauma (eg, chicken or fish bones, instrumentation, dental procedures, or dental infection).

MICROBIOLOGY:
- **Similar to Peritonsillar abscess — often polymicrobial (eg, Group A *Streptococcus*, *Staphylococcus aureus*, & respiratory anaerobes).**

CLINICAL MANIFESTATIONS
- **Fever, odynophagia**, dysphagia, drooling, sore throat, chest pain, muffled "hot potato" voice, trismus.
- **Neck: neck stiffness especially with neck extension, torticollis (unwilling to move the neck secondary to pain and spasms). Chest pain with mediastinal extension.** Stridor is uncommon.

Physical examination:
- **Midline or unilateral posterior pharyngeal wall edema.** Minimal peritonsillar findings.
- Tender anterior cervical lymphadenopathy. Lateral neck mass or swelling may be seen.

DIAGNOSIS
- **CT scan of neck with IV contrast imaging of choice & preferred imaging if suspicion is high.**
- Lateral neck radiograph: may be performed if low suspicion. Performed during inspiration with slight neck extension — **increased prevertebral space >50% of the width of adjacent vertebral body** (5-7 cm prevertebral widening at the 2nd cervical vertebra).
- In smaller children with respiratory distress, evaluation is often performed in the operating room.

MANAGEMENT
- **Large (≥2.5 cm²) & mature abscess on CT: surgical incision & drainage with antibiotics in the OR.**
- **Small abscesses (<2.5 cm²) & children with no airway compromise may be observed for 24-48 hours with antibiotic therapy and no drainage.** ENT consult for all. Secure the airway if needed.
- **Antibiotics: IV Ampicillin-Sulbactam or Clindamycin (similar to PTA).** IV Vancomycin if no response.

COMPLICATIONS
- Airway obstruction, Mediastinitis (due to spread of the infection), sepsis, atlantoaxial dislocation.

ORAL LICHEN PLANUS

- **Idiopathic cell-mediated autoimmune response affecting the skin & mucous membranes.**
- Most common in middle-aged adults. **Increased incidence with Hepatitis C infection.**

CLINICAL MANIFESTATIONS
- **Reticular: white lines, papules, or plaques in a reticulated or lacy pattern (Wickham striae), especially on the posterior buccal mucosa.** Often painless & asymptomatic. **Most common type.**
- Erythematous (atrophic): red patches that may accompany the reticular lesions. May cause pain, burning, swelling, and mucosal bleeding of the gingiva, palate, floor of the mouth, and labial mucosa.
- Erosive: painful erosions or ulcers covered with a pseudomembrane. Desquamative gingivitis.

DIAGNOSIS
- Mainly clinical. Biopsy often performed in the erythematous & erosive types to rule out malignancy (small ↑ risk of Squamous cell carcinoma). Direct immunofluorescence may also be performed.

MANAGEMENT
- **High-potency topical glucocorticoids initial management of choice** (eg, Clobetasol propionate 0.05%, Betamethasone dipropionate 0.05%, 0.1% Triamcinolone acetonide in Orabase).
- Second line: **Topical Tacrolimus or Pimecrolimus** if no response to topical corticosteroids or topical corticosteroids cannot be tolerated. Cyclosporine or intralesional corticosteroid injections.
- Systemic glucocorticoids if no response to topical therapy.

STREPTOCOCCAL PHARYNGITIS ("STREP THROAT")

- **Group A β-hemolytic Streptococcus (*Streptococcus pyogenes*).** Rare in children <3 years of age.
- **Highest incidence of Rheumatic fever in untreated children 5-15 years of age.**

CLINICAL MANIFESTATIONS
- **Children ≥3 years: abrupt onset of sore throat & odynophagia, which may be accompanied by fever, chills, headache, abdominal pain, nausea, vomiting, poor oral intake.** Myalgias, malaise.
- Not usually associated with symptoms of viral infections: eg, not associated with cough, hoarseness, rhinorrhea, coryza, conjunctivitis, diarrhea, anterior stomatitis, discrete ulcers, nor vesicles.

Physical examination:
- Pharyngeal edema or exudate, tonsillar exudate, and/or petechiae with markedly enlarged erythematous tonsils & tonsillar pillars, palatal petechiae, inflamed uvula (uvulitis).
- **Enlarged tender anterior cervical lymphadenopathy.**
- **Scarlatiniform rash** (erythematous, finely papular rash which characteristically starts in the groin and axilla and then spreads to the trunk and extremities, followed by desquamation) may be seen.

DIAGNOSIS: **Whom NOT to test:**
- **Testing may not be necessary in children & adolescents with manifestations clearly suggestive of viral illness (eg, rhinorrhea, conjunctivitis, cough, hoarseness, anterior stomatitis, discrete ulcerative lesions or vesicles, diarrhea).**
- **In children <3 years of age**, routine testing is not recommended because both GAS pharyngitis and its complication, Acute rheumatic fever, are rare in this age group.

Whom to test
- **Testing for GAS is indicated in children ≥3 years & adolescents with evidence of acute tonsillopharyngitis** (fever, erythema, edema, &/or tonsillar exudates) or scarlatiniform rash on physical examination AND **absence of multiple signs & symptoms of viral infections** (see above).
- **Exposure to an individual with GAS** at home/school or high prevalence of GAS in the community & **symptoms of GAS. If ≥3 Centor criteria [(1) fever ≥38° C, (2) absence of cough, (3) swollen anterior cervical lymph nodes, (4) tonsillar exudates/swelling (1 point for each)].**
- Suspected acute rheumatic fever (ARF) or poststreptococcal glomerulonephritis.

Testing options:
- **Rapid antigen detection test (RADT): best initial test.** 95% specific; only 55-90% sensitive (most useful if positive; **if negative, throat cultures should be obtained, especially in children 5-15y**).
- **Nucleic acid amplification tests** (NAATs) can be used in place of Rapid antigen detection testing.
- **Throat culture: definitive diagnosis (criterion standard).** 90-95% sensitivity; 95-99% specificity.

MANAGEMENT
- **Analgesics** eg, NSAIDs, Acetaminophen, or Aspirin for pain. Anesthetics: Lozenges, throat sprays.
- **Penicillin first-line antibiotic (eg, Penicillin V, Penicillin G, or Amoxicillin) if testing is positive.**

Penicillin allergy:
- **Cephalosporins (eg, Cefuroxime), Azithromycin, Clarithromycin, or Clindamycin are alternatives** for patients who are allergic to Penicillin or who cannot otherwise tolerate Penicillin.
- Mild, non-IgE-mediated reactions to Penicillin (eg, maculopapular rash beginning days into therapy), a **1st-generation Cephalosporin (eg, Cephalexin).**
- Mild, possibly IgE-mediated reactions (eg, urticaria or angioedema but NOT anaphylaxis), 2nd or 3rd generation cephalosporin with a side chain dissimilar to PCN **(Cefdinir, Cefpodoxime, Cefuroxime).**
- Severe angioedema and/or anaphylaxis or with serious delayed reactions or for patients who cannot take cephalosporins, **Macrolides (eg, Azithromycin)** can be used. Clindamycin is an alternative.

COMPLICATIONS
- **Rheumatic fever (preventable with antibiotics). Severe pharyngitis (give IM Dexamethasone).**
- Acute glomerulonephritis (not preventable with antibiotics). Peritonsillar abscess.
- PANDAS: Pediatric autoimmune neuropsychiatric disorders associated with streptococcus.

LUDWIG'S ANGINA

- **Rapidly spreading Cellulitis of the floor of the mouth** (bilateral infection of submandibular space).
- Risk factors: **most commonly due to spread of oral flora secondary to <u>poor dental hygiene & dental infections</u>** (second or third mandibular molars). Increased incidence in Diabetes & HIV.
- Polymicrobial (oral flora): streptococci, staphylococci, *Bacteroides*, and *Fusobacterium*.

CLINICAL MANIFESTATIONS
- Fever, chills, malaise, stiff neck, dysphagia, drooling, muffled voice.
- Late signs: stridor, difficulty managing secretions, & cyanosis (require emergent airway management).

PHYSICAL EXAMINATION
- **Tender, symmetric swelling, "woody" induration, & erythema of the upper neck & under the chin** (may have palpable crepitus), **& floor of the mouth.** Pus on the floor of the mouth.
- Swelling of the tongue *can lead to airway compromise.* No lymphadenopathy or abscess formation.

DIAGNOSIS
- **CT scan initial imaging of choice.** MRI. Definitive airway management if needed most important.

MANAGEMENT IF IMMUNOCOMPETENT
- IV antibiotics: **Ampicillin-sulbactam OR Ceftriaxone plus Metronidazole OR Clindamycin plus Levofloxacin. Add Vancomycin if MRSA suspected.** Secure the airway if needed.

MANAGEMENT IF IMMUNOCOMPROMISED
- IV antibiotics: Cefepime plus Metronidazole OR Imipenem OR Meropenem OR Piperacillin-tazobactam. Add Vancomycin if MRSA is suspected.

OROPHARYNGEAL CANDIDIASIS (THRUSH)

- ***Candida albicans*** is part of the normal flora but can become pathogenic due to local or systemic immunosuppressed states.
- RISK FACTORS: **immunocompromised states** (HIV, chemotherapy, diabetics), **use of inhaled Corticosteroids without a spacer, antibiotic use, xerostomia, or denture use.**

CLINICAL MANIFESTATIONS
- Most individuals are asymptomatic. May be the first manifestation of HIV infection.
- Loss of taste or cotton-like feel in the mouth, loss of taste, throat or mouth discomfort with eating or swallowing. Patients who have denture stomatitis often complain of pain.

PHYSICAL EXAMINATION
- **Pseudomembranous form: white creamy- or curd-like confluent plaques on the buccal mucosa, tongue, palate, &/or the oropharynx that are easily scraped off (may leave behind erythema & friable mucosa when scraped).** Erythema of the oral cavity or oropharynx.
- Atrophic form: erythema only. Atrophic form may be associated with denture Candidiasis.

DIAGNOSIS
- Clinical. **Potassium Hydroxide: budding yeast ± hyphae.** Smear performed on scrapings.
- Fungal culture (rarely done).

MANAGEMENT
- **Topical antifungals: first-line therapy —** Clotrimazole troches, Miconazole mucoadhesive buccal tablets, Nystatin liquid swish and swallow are all options.
- Moderate to severe disease: Systemic antifungals: Oral Fluconazole usually reserved for refractory cases or patients with oropharyngeal AND esophageal Candidiasis.

APHTHOUS ULCERS (CANKER SORE, ULCERATIVE STOMATITIS)

- Unknown cause but may be associated with Human herpes virus 6.
- Recurrent disease seen in patients with Inflammatory bowel disease, acute HIV, Celiac disease, SLE, Methotrexate, Behçet syndrome, & neutropenia.

CLINICAL MANIFESTATIONS
- **Painful, small, shallow round or oval shallow ulcer (yellow, white, or grey central exudate) with an erythematous halo.** Most common on the buccal or labial mucosa (nonkeratinized mucosa).

MANAGEMENT
In immunocompetent patients, **Aphthous ulcers usually resolve without treatment in 10-14 days**.
- **Topical Glucocorticoids first-line management for symptomatic relief** — eg, Clobetasol gel or ointment, Dexamethasone elixir swish & spit, Triamcinolone in Orabase, Fluocinonide ointment 0.05% in adhesive base. Severe: Oral corticosteroids added. Cimetidine for recurrent ulcers.
- **Topical analgesics: 2% viscous Lidocaine**, Topical Diclofenac 3% in hyaluronan 2.5%, Diphenhydramine liquid; Aluminum hydroxide + Magnesium hydroxide + Simethicone.

LEUKOPLAKIA

- Oral potentially malignant disorder characterized by hyperkeratosis due to chronic irritation.
- **Up to 6% are dysplastic or Squamous cell carcinoma**.
- Risk factors: chronic irritation due to tobacco, cigarette smoking, alcohol, dentures, HPV infection.

CLINICAL MANIFESTATIONS
- **Homogenous Leukoplakia: painless uniformly white, thin plaque or patch with well-defined margins that cannot be rubbed or scraped off** (in comparison to Candida).
- Nonhomogeneous leukoplakia: painless speckled (red & white, but predominantly white) lesions; erythroleukoplakia (red and white lesions); granular, nodular, or verrucous white lesions.

DIAGNOSIS
- Biopsy for histopathologic examination to rule out Squamous cell carcinoma — hyperkeratosis.

MANAGEMENT
- Cessation of irritants — eg alcohol, tobacco use (smoked or smokeless).
- **Cryotherapy, laser ablation, and surgical excision are options if increased risk for malignancy or malignant** (eg, clinically nonhomogeneous, are located in high-risk areas, and for those with histopathologic findings of severe dysplasia).

ERYTHROPLAKIA

- Uncommon oral lesion with a high risk of malignant transformation.
- **90% of Erythroplakia cases are either dysplastic or Squamous cell carcinoma.**
- Risk factors: chronic irritation due to tobacco, cigarette smoking, and alcohol. Age > 65 years.

CLINICAL MANIFESTATIONS
- Most are asymptomatic.
- **Painless erythematous (fiery red), soft, velvety, sharply demarcated patch in the oral cavity, most commonly on the mouth floor, soft palate, or ventral aspect of the tongue.**

DIAGNOSIS: **Biopsy** for histopathologic examination to rule out Squamous cell carcinoma.

MANAGEMENT: Complete excision may be needed depending on the biopsy results.

ORAL AND OROPHARYNGEAL CANCER

RISK FACTORS
- **Oral cancer: alcohol and tobacco use (smoked or smokeless)** are major etiologic risk factors.

Oropharyngeal cancer:
- **Alcohol and tobacco use (smoked or smokeless),** oral Lichen planus, Plummer-Vinson syndrome.
- **Human papillomavirus (HPV), the most commonly sexually transmitted infection in the US, [especially types 16 and 18], causes up to 70% of oropharyngeal Squamous cell carcinoma (SCC) & head and neck Squamous cell carcinomas,** as well as anogenital malignancies (cervical, vaginal, vulval, penile, and anal carcinoma).
- **Immunodeficiency** — eg, HIV or solid organ transplantation has been associated with an increased risk of cancer in the head and neck region.

Nasopharyngeal cancer: Epstein-Barr virus (EBV) infection, especially in China.

CLINICAL MANIFESTATIONS

Oral cancer:
- **Raised, firm, white, or erythematous lesions — eg, patch that may progress to a superficial ulcer of mucosal surface, and later develop into an endophytic or exophytic growth. Exquisite pain even on gentle palpation.** Lesions <4 mm in depth have a low propensity to metastasize. **Common areas of Head & neck cancer in order of frequency include the tonsils, base of the tongue, floor of the mouth, and lower lip vermillion border.** May be a solitary lump.
- Larger, advanced cancers may be painful and may erode underlying tissue. Invasion into the tongue may result in a palpable mass that may ulcerate.
- Metastases to submandibular, contralateral or bilateral cervical & submental lymph nodes common.

Oropharyngeal cancer:
- **Mouth pain, unilateral odynophagia, dysphagia, nonhealing oral ulcers, loosening of teeth or dentures, weight loss, bleeding, referred pain to the ear (referred otalgia).**
- Large lesions are often buried within the lymphoid tissue of the palatine or lingual tonsils. **HPV associated tumors often arise in the tonsillar region, the base of the tongue, or lateral soft palate.** Ipsilateral cervical lymphadenopathy.
- Nasopharyngeal carcinoma: the most frequent presenting complaint is a neck mass due to regional lymph node metastasis, which occurs in ~90% of patients.
- **Laryngeal cancer: persistent hoarseness.** Later symptoms may include dysphagia, referred otalgia, chronic cough, hemoptysis, and stridor. Airway obstruction or palpable metastatic lymph nodes.

DIAGNOSIS
- **Biopsy essential for diagnosis — Keratin pearls are pathognomonic, seen in well-differentiated and moderately differentiated Squamous cell cancers.**
- **Confirmation of HPV status:** immunohistochemistry for p16 as a surrogate for HPV status (highly sensitive for HPV associated tumors). In situ hybridization or Polymerase chain reaction (PCR).

MANAGEMENT
- **Non-HPV associated tumors** — Early (stage I and II) non-human papillomavirus (HPV) associated tumors can be effectively treated with either radiation therapy (RT) or minimally invasive transoral surgery. <2 cm: local resection used in most in whom the tumor is detected before it is 2 cm.
- **HPV associated tumors** — For patients with early-stage HPV associated tumors, management may include surgery (eg, resection, neck dissection), external beam radiation (RT), and chemotherapy, either as single modalities or in combination, depending on the extent of the disease.
- Larger tumors of the oral cavity are usually treated with a combination of resection, neck dissection, and external beam radiation. Reconstruction, when needed, is done at the time of initial surgery. Vascularized free flaps, with bone if needed, are commonly used. Myocutaneous flaps often used.
- Tumors of the tonsillar fossa and base of tongue are often treated with radiation, often with concomitant chemotherapy, reserving surgery for salvage.

SIALOLITHIASIS (SALIVARY GLAND STONES)

- Calcium carbonate or Calcium phosphate calculi (stones) within a stagnant salivary gland or duct with no evidence of inflammation.
- **Most common in Wharton's duct (submandibular gland duct) 80-90%; Stensen's duct** (parotid gland duct). Sublingual gland.

RISK FACTORS
- Decreased salivation (eg, dehydration, anticholinergic mediations, diuretics) and trauma.

CLINICAL MANIFESTATIONS
- **Sudden onset of salivary gland pain & swelling with eating or in anticipation of eating that may resemble Parotitis.**

PHYSICAL EXAMINATION
- Stone (small rock-hard mass) may be palpated in the salivary gland or visible at the os.
- If the gland is compressed and no saliva flows, the stone can be obstructive.

DIAGNOSIS
- Usually clinical. Imaging only indicated if the diagnosis is unclear or if a tumor is suspected.
- Intraoral radiographs are more sensitive than extraoral films in identifying salivary calculi. 70% of stones are radiopaque.

MANAGEMENT
- **Conservative management: first-line therapy — sialagogues to increase salivary flow** (eg, **tart, hard candies, lemon drops,** Xylitol-containing gum or candy), increase fluid intake, gland massage, moist heat to affected area, & massage the gland,. Palpable stones may be digitally "milked" from the duct. Avoid anticholinergic medications if possible (anticholinergics decrease salivation).
- Minimally invasive therapy: includes sialoendoscopy, laser lithotripsy, extracorporeal lithotripsy.
- Surgery (eg, sialoadenectomy) reserved for recurrent stone or failure of less invasive techniques.

ACUTE BACTERIAL SIALADENITIS (SUPPURATIVE SIALADENITIS)

- **Bacterial infection of the parotid or submandibular salivary glands.**
- Etiologies: ***S. aureus* most common,** *S. pneumoniae, S. viridans, H. influenzae, Bacteroides.*
- Risk factors: salivary gland obstruction from a stone, dehydration, postop, or chronic illness.

CLINICAL MANIFESTATIONS
- **Sudden onset of very firm and tender gland swelling with purulent discharge** (may be able to express **pus if the duct is massaged), dysphagia, trismus** (reduced opening of the jaw due to spasms of the muscles of mastication). Tender erythematous duct opening.
- **Fever & chills** if severe.

DIAGNOSIS
- **CT scan imaging modality of choice** to assess for associated abscess or extent of tissue involvement.

MANAGEMENT
- **Anti-staphylococcal antibiotics + sialagogues** to increase salivary flow (eg, tart or hard candies), warm compresses, gland massage.
Anti-staphylococcal antibiotics:
- **Dicloxacillin or Nafcillin. Metronidazole may be added for anaerobic coverage.**
- **Clindamycin.**

ACUTE HERPETIC GINGIVOSTOMATITIS

- Inflammation of the gums and the oral mucosa.
- **Most common manifestation of primary Herpes simplex virus type 1 infection in children.** Most commonly occurs between 6 months–5 years.

PATHOPHYSIOLOGY
- **Primary HSV-1 infection in most children is asymptomatic.**
- After primary oral infection, HSV remains latent in the trigeminal ganglion until reactivation as herpes labialis (Cold sore).

CLINICAL MANIFESTATIONS
- **Prodrome:** sudden onset of fever, constitutional symptoms (eg, anorexia, malaise), and refusal to eat and/or drink, followed by the development of oral lesions. May be associated with halitosis.
- **Gingivostomatitis: ulcerative lesions of the gingiva (gum swelling with friability & bleeding) & vesicles on the mucous membranes of the mouth, often with perioral vesicular lesions clustered on an erythematous base** (dew drops on a rose petal). Most lesions are in the anterior two-thirds of the oral cavity.
- **After rupture, the vesicles become ulcerated, yellow, and are surrounded by an erythematous halo.** They may coalesce to form painful ulcers.
- Regional lymphadenopathy eg, submandibular or cervical lymphadenitis.

DIAGNOSIS
- Clinical diagnosis, based upon the classic appearance & location of oral and extraoral lesions.
- Viral Polymerase chain reaction (PCR) for HSV, viral culture, or immunofluorescence.

MANAGEMENT
- **Supportive care: hydration mainstay of treatment (dehydration most common complication),** oral hygiene, oral analgesics/antipyretics, topical analgesics, barrier cream to the lips (eg, petroleum jelly). Lesions usually heal within 1 week.
- **Oral Acyclovir** if within 72-96 hours of disease onset if they are unable to drink or have significant pain.
- Immunocompromised patients: IV Acyclovir.

ACUTE HERPETIC PHARYNGOTONSILLITIS

- **Primary manifestation of Herpes simplex virus-1 (HSV-1) in adults.**

PATHOPHYSIOLOGY
- Primary HSV-1 infection in most adults is asymptomatic.
- After primary oral infection, HSV remains latent in the trigeminal ganglion until reactivation as herpes labialis (Cold sore).

CLINICAL MANIFESTATIONS:
- **Severe mouth pain:** sore throat, fever, malaise, myalgia, headache.

PHYSICAL EXAMINATION:
- **Pharyngeal edema, tonsillar exudate.**
- **Oral & ulcerative lesions: vesicles that rupture, leaving ulcerative lesions with grayish exudates** in the posterior pharyngeal mucosa.
- Cervical lymphadenopathy.

MANAGEMENT:
- **Oral hygiene** — lesions usually resolve within 7-14 days when the ulcers reepithelialize.

PHOTO CREDITS

CHAPTER 6 – REPRODUCTIVE SYSTEM (MALE AND FEMALE)

POOR LATCH ON TECHNIQUE

- A baby must be able to remove enough milk from the breast through correct latch and sucking to gain weight. Poor latch on technique can reduce weight in neonates and cause issues for the mother.

PHYSICAL EXAMINATION
- **May have open, linear bilateral areolar abrasions that cause a bloody-appearing nipple discharge.**
- **Bruising, cracking, and blistering may also be present.**
- Breast engorgement (bilateral, diffusely tender, and engorged breasts). May occur if nipple pain limits the ability to breastfeed.

MANAGEMENT
- **Observation of breastfeeding and patient education** **initial management of choice.**
- Nipple injury is a major risk factor for multiple adverse outcomes (eg, plugged milk ducts, Mastitis, Breast abscess), which often lead to premature discontinuation of breastfeeding.

INFECTIVE LACTATIONAL MASTITIS

- **Infection of the breast; most common in lactating women secondary to nipple trauma in the first 12 weeks postpartum (especially if primigravid in the first 6 weeks postpartum).**
- ***Staphylococcus aureus* most common** (including MRSA). Streptococcus. *Candida albicans.*

CLINICAL MANIFESTATIONS
- **Unilateral localized breast pain, tenderness, warmth, swelling, induration, & skin redness.**
- Systemic symptoms may include fever, chills, myalgias, malaise, and flu-like symptoms.

Physical examination:
- Firm, red, tender, swollen area of one breast. May be associated with fever >38.3°C.
- Sore or cracked nipples; may have visible fissures or purulent nipple discharge.

DIAGNOSIS
- **Clinical diagnosis in most cases — nursing mother with breast pain, redness, & swelling.**
- Culture of breast milk in some cases for culture & sensitivities to guide antibiotic therapy.
- Breast Ultrasound often reserved for cases not responding to empiric antibiotics within 48-72 hours.

MANAGEMENT
- **Supportive — [1] pain control**: warm or cool compresses, NSAIDs, & **[2] emptying of the breasts**.
- **Complete emptying of the breasts**: milk drainage is critical for resolution of infection and for relief of symptoms (continuing breastfeeding, pumping, &/or hand expression), use of a well-fitted bra.

Antibiotic therapy: if accompanied by fever or systemic symptoms or symptoms persist >24-48 hours:
- **Anti-staphylococcal antibiotics — Dicloxacillin, Flucloxacillin, or Cephalexin.**
- **Penicillin-allergic**: Clindamycin or Trimethoprim-sulfamethoxazole. TMP-SMX avoided in the first 2 months of nursing or in G6PD deficiency due to risk to the baby of kernicterus. Erythromycin.
- **MRSA risk factors: Clindamycin or Trimethoprim-sulfamethoxazole. Fungal: Fluconazole.**
- Severe infection (eg, fever, hypotension, tachycardia) — IV Vancomycin + either Ceftriaxone or Piperacillin-tazobactam.
- **Any inflammatory breast in a post-menopausal woman is cancer until proven otherwise.**

BREAST ABSCESS

- Rare complication of progression of Acute mastitis.
- **Most common in lactating women secondary to nipple trauma, especially primigravid women.**
- ETIOLOGIES: ***Staphylococcus aureus* most common.** Streptococcus. *Candida albicans.*

CLINICAL MANIFESTATIONS
- **Symptoms of Acute mastitis** — unilateral breast pain (especially one quadrant) with tenderness, warmth, swelling. May have purulent nipple discharge. Cracked nipples or visible fissures.
- **Abscess: induration & fluctuance** due to pus.

DIAGNOSIS
- Clinical diagnosis based physical examination.
- **Breast Ultrasound may be ordered if there is a question of Cellulitis vs. Abscess — ill-defined mass with septations &/or fluid collection are consistent with a Breast abscess.**

MANAGEMENT
- **Drainage via needle aspiration (lactational abscess) or incision & drainage + antibiotics.**
- **Anti-staphylococcal antibiotics — Dicloxacillin or Cephalexin.**
- **MRSA or Penicillin allergy: Clindamycin or Trimethoprim-sulfamethoxazole.** TMP-SMX avoided in first 2 months of nursing or in G6PD deficiency due to risk of kernicterus.
- Breast infection, including Breast abscess, is not a contraindication to breastfeeding. Milk drainage (eg, breastfeeding, pumping, or hand expression) is important to facilitate resolution of infection.

CONGESTIVE MASTITIS

- **Bilateral breast enlargement 2-3 days postpartum due to <u>milk stasis and congestion</u>.**
- <u>CLINICAL MANIFESTATIONS</u>: **<u>bilateral</u> breast pain & swelling.**

<u>MANAGEMENT</u>
- **<u>Breast drainage</u> mainstay of treatment** — eg, breastfeeding, breast pump use, or hand expression.
- If the woman does not want to breastfeed, treat with ice packs, tight-fitting bras, analgesics, and breast drainage (eg, breast pump use &/or hand expression).
- If breastfeeding is desired, manually empty the breasts completely after baby is done breastfeeding or use breast pump, local heat, analgesics, & continue nursing.

FIBROCYSTIC BREAST CHANGES

- **Noncancerous, fluid-filled breast cysts due to exaggerated response to hormones.**
- Also known as glandular hyperplasia — duct dilation, breast cysts, & stromal fibrosis.
- **Most common benign breast masses in reproductive age women, especially aged 30-50 years.**
- Often regresses after menopause (rare in postmenopausal women).

<u>CLINICAL MANIFESTATIONS</u>
- May cause asymptomatic breast lumps that may be discovered incidentally on palpation.
- **Multiple, painful (or painless) mobile, ill-defined breast masses that may increase or decrease in size with hormonal changes (often occurs or becomes worse in the premenstrual phase of the cycle). <u>Fluctuations in size</u>** & rapid appearance or disappearance of masses can occur.
- There may be a nonbloody, green, or brown discharge from the nipple.
- **<u>Pain, fluctuation in size during the menstrual cycle, and multiplicity of lesions</u> useful to differentiate Fibrocystic changes from Breast carcinoma and Fibroadenoma.**

Physical examination:
- **Usually multiple, nodular, mobile, smooth round or ovoid lumps in both breasts** of varying sizes.
- Often bilateral and not usually associated with axillary lymph node involvement.
- Most commonly found in the upper outer sections of the breast.

<u>DIAGNOSIS</u>
- **<u>Breast Ultrasound</u> initial test of choice** — may be simple, complicated, or complex on imaging.
- <u>Fine needle aspiration</u> not usually performed if simple — straw-colored or green fluid with no blood.
- A Mammogram may be required if lesion is suspicious or persistent after drainage or in older women.

<u>MANAGEMENT</u>
- **<u>Supportive management</u> — observation, reassurance, supportive bra, warm or cool compresses, analgesics** [eg, Acetaminophen, Nonsteroidal anti-inflammatory drugs (NSAIDs) can be used to relieve breast pain]. Oral contraceptives and caffeine reduction may reduce symptoms.
- <u>Fine needle aspiration</u> removal of fluid is diagnostic & therapeutic in complex cases or if inflamed.
- <u>Complex cysts</u> are BI-RADS 4 or 5 and should undergo ultrasound-guided core needle biopsy.

INTRADUCTAL PAPILLOMA

- Tumors involving the lining of the breast duct. Benign but can contain areas of atypia or carcinoma in situ.
- Single or multiple lesions may be identified as a mass on mammography, ultrasound, or MRI.
- **Nipple discharge, especially <u>bloody nipple discharge</u>, is a frequent clinical presentation.**

<u>DIAGNOSIS AND MANAGEMENT</u>
- Individualized decision to excise a papilloma is based on size, symptoms (eg, nipple discharge, palpability), and Breast cancer risk factors. Imaging & follow-up done if excision is not performed. When a core biopsy demonstrates a Papilloma with atypical cells, surgical excision is warranted.
- After excision, if there is no upgrading beyond atypia, a discussion about endocrine therapy for Breast cancer prevention is indicated.

FIBROADENOMA OF THE BREAST

- **Benign solid tumor composed of glandular & fibrous tissue; hormone dependent tumor.**
- Second most common benign breast mass (after Fibrocystic changes) & most common breast tumor in women <30 years. Often occurs at an earlier age in black women than in white women.

CLINICAL MANIFESTATIONS

- Round, firm, discrete, relatively mobile, mass 1-5 cm, usually nontender but may become tender prior to menstruation. Gradually grows over time but may enlarge in pregnancy (hormonal relationship).
- **Does not change significantly in size with menstrual cycle** (unlike Fibrocystic breast changes).

PHYSICAL EXAMINATION

- **Firm, nontender, solitary, smooth, well-circumscribed (discrete), freely mobile, rubbery lump in the breast.** Usually 2-3 cm in diameter (1-5 cm) & without axillary involvement.

DIAGNOSIS

- Clinical diagnosis. **Ultrasound — solid, well-circumscribed, avascular mass with benign features.**
- Fine needle aspiration: definitive diagnosis — **fibrous tissue & collagen arranged in a "swirl".**

MANAGEMENT

- **Conservative: observation, reassurance, and follow-up — most small tumors resorb with time. May [1] repeat the Ultrasound in 3-6 months or [2] manage with core needle biopsy.**
- Local surgical excision: may be needed if enlarging after repeat Ultrasounds or for large masses.
- Cryoablation: alternative to surgery if <4 cm and after a core needle biopsy confirms the adenoma.

GYNECOMASTIA

- **Enlargement of glandular breast tissue & adipose tissue in males due to imbalance of [1] increased effective estrogen (increased production or reduced degradation) &/or [2] decreased androgens.** In some tissues (eg, adipose), aromatase can convert androstenedione into estrogen.
- **Hormonal:** seen in 3 main groups: **[1] infants:** due to high maternal estrogen; **[2] during puberty:** especially 10–14 years (classically may last between 6 months–2 years), & **[3] older males**.
- **Idiopathic**, Male hypogonadism, persistent pubertal gynecomastia.
- **Medications: Spironolactone**, Ketoconazole, Cimetidine, 5-alpha reductase inhibitors, Digoxin, GnRH agonists (eg, Leuprolide), Thiazides, Phenothiazines, Verapamil, & Theophylline.
- Other: malignancies — Large cell lung cancer, renal cell, hepatic, testicular and gastric cancers. Cirrhosis, alcoholism, Hyperthyroidism, Chronic renal disease, Klinefelter syndrome.

CLINICAL MANIFESTATIONS

- **Palpable rubbery or firm mass of tissue, often >2 cm, with 4 classic characteristics: [1] centrally located** (usually underlying the nipple and extending from the nipples), **[2] symmetrical in shape, [3] bilateral in most, and [4] often tender to palpation** in the early phase.

DIAGNOSIS: **Clinical.** Check testosterone levels. Mammogram if Breast cancer is suspected.

MANAGEMENT

- **Supportive: stop offending medications, observation, and reassurance if early in the disease course or physiologic.** If treatment is needed, initiate it within the first 6 months of onset (after 12 months, fibrosis may occur). Evaluation may be considered if it persists >2 years or if >17 years of age.
- **Medical: Tamoxifen** is a Selective estrogen receptor modifier **(estrogen antagonist in the breast). Tamoxifen is often first-line medication in men & boys if medical management indicated (3-month trial).** Androgens (testosterone replacement) in hypogonadal men often improves gynecomastia.

Surgical:
- Reserved for severe disease refractory to medical therapy, large breasts, cosmetically unappealing, fibrosis, longstanding (eg, >12 months), etc.

BREAST CANCER SCREENING

- **Mammogram: best screening in women >40 years of age.** Some Breast cancers may be detected by mammography as early as 2 years before a mass can be palpated clinically.
- Breast self-examination has <u>not</u> been shown to reduce long-term overall mortality.
- Most guideline bodies (eg, American College of Radiology, the American Cancer Society, and the American Medical Association) recommend annual mammograms starting at age 40 years. The American College of Obstetricians and Gynecologists calls for screening mammography every 1–2 years for women ages 40–49 and annually thereafter.
- **USPSTF guidelines** recommends Mammogram once <u>every 2 years</u> beginning at <u>50 years until 74 years</u>. [2023 guidelines draft recommendation (<u>in progress</u>) to start breast cancer screening at age 40 instead of the previously recommended starting age of 50].
- Women with a genetic predisposition to Breast cancer should be screened using MRI beginning at age 25 or the age of earliest onset of Breast cancer in the family, and they should undergo a combination of screening Mammography and MRI beginning after age 30.
- Women with breast implants should undergo the same screening schedule as women without.

CHEMOPREVENTION OF BREAST CANCER

[1] Selective estrogen receptor modulators (SERM):

- **Tamoxifen or Raloxifene: Selective estrogen receptor modulators** that can be used for Breast cancer prevention in high-risk individuals. Also preferred in postmenopausal with Osteoporosis.
- **Tamoxifen or Raloxifene can be used in postmenopausal or in high-risk women >35 years of age.**
- **Treatment usually used for 5 years.**
- Tamoxifen preferred (more effective than Raloxifene but is associated with Endometrial cancer). Tamoxifen is an estrogen antagonist in the breast that upregulates transforming growth factor β, which decreases breast cell proliferation. Tamoxifen also decreases risk of bone fractures.
- **Tamoxifen is associated with increased risk of venous thromboembolism vs. Raloxifene.**
- When using a SERM, Raloxifene may be preferred if patients are more concerned about Uterine cancer and thromboembolic risks than their risk of Breast cancer (Raloxifene is comparable to Tamoxifen in cancer prevention, but without the risk of Endometrial cancer).
- By contrast, for women who are more concerned about Breast cancer prevention or have had a hysterectomy, Tamoxifen may be preferred. Also preferred in **premenopausal** women at high risk.

[2] Aromatase inhibitors (AI): Anastrozole & Exemestane

- For older women (>60 years), especially those with intact uterus, an AI may be more appealing compared with a SERM (slightly superior). Bone mineral density is monitored while on AI.
- <u>Adverse effects:</u> hot flushes, fatigue, arthralgias, insomnia.

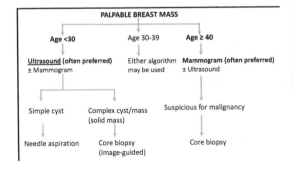

SELECTIVE ESTROGEN RECEPTOR MODULATOR (SERM)		
MECHANISM OF ACTION	**TAMOXIFEN** • <u>Estrogen antagonist</u> in breast • <u>Estrogen agonist</u> in the bone, uterus, and liver **RALOXIFENE** • <u>Estrogen antagonist</u> in breast AND uterus • <u>Estrogen agonist</u> In bone and liver	
INDICATIONS	• <u>Prevention of breast cancer</u> in women >35 years of postmenopausal high-risk patients (eg, Tamoxifen used for 5 years) • <u>Tamoxifen: adjuvant treatment for Breast cancer (more effective)</u> • <u>Raloxifene: Postmenopausal Osteoporosis</u>	
ADVERSE EFFECTS	• **Hot flashes** • **Venous thromboembolism** (Tamoxifen > Raloxifene) **Tamoxifen only:** • **Endometrial hyperplasia & cancer**; Uterine sarcoma	

BREAST CANCER

- **Most common non-skin malignancy in women.** 1 in 8 lifetime incidence.
- Second most commonly diagnosed cancer worldwide & cause of cancer death in women (after lung).

RISK FACTORS
- **Increasing age:** >50% occur >60 years vs. <2% in <30 years of age. Low fiber & high fat diet.
- **Increased number of menstrual cycles**: nulliparity, late first full-term pregnancy >35 years, early onset of menarche (<12 years), late menopause (>50 years of age), never having breastfed.
- **Increased estrogen exposure:** postmenopausal hormonal replacement, prolonged unopposed estrogen, obesity, alcohol use. Endometrial cancer increases Breast cancer risk & vice versa.
- Genetics: **BRCA 1** (chromosome 17) & **BRCA 2** (chromosome 13) — genetic mutations associated with 60-85% lifetime development of Breast cancer & 15-40% development of Ovarian cancer. BRCA positivity seen in 5-10% of cases of Breast cancer. First-degree relative with Breast cancer.
- Obesity, Type 2 Diabetes Mellitus, & Metabolic syndrome.

TYPES
- **Infiltrative ductal carcinoma: most common type of Breast cancer (75%).** Characterized by cords & nests of cells with differing amounts of gland formations. **Associated with lymphatic metastases (especially axillary).**
- Infiltrative lobular carcinoma (8-10% of invasive breast cancers). Characterized by small cells that insidiously infiltrate the mammary stroma & adipose tissue individually and in a single-file pattern.
- **Ductal carcinoma in situ:** confined to breast ducts & lobules; does not penetrate the basement membrane.
- Medullary, mucinoid, tubular, papillary, metastatic, **Inflammatory breast cancers.**
- **Paget disease of the breast**: ductal carcinoma presenting as an eczematous nipple lesion. May have bloody discharge from the nipple. Spreads lymphatically.

Premalignant lesions:
- **Lobular carcinoma in situ considered a premalignant condition associated with increased risk of invasive Breast cancer in either breast.**
- Atypical ductal hyperplasia

CLINICAL MANIFESTATIONS
- **Breast or axillary mass: painless, hard, fixed, immobile breast lump with irregular (ill-defined) borders most common presentation.** May be mobile early on & may be painful in <10%.
- May complain of unilateral nipple discharge (may be bloody).
- **The majority of Breast cancers are diagnosed as a result of an abnormal Mammogram.**

PHYSICAL EXAMINATION
- **Mass most common in the upper outer quadrant** (65%), areola (18%).
- **Skin changes:** asymmetric erythema, discoloration, ulceration, skin retraction (dimpling if Cooper's ligament is involved), changes in breast size & contour, nipple inversion, & skin thickening.
- Early findings: single nontender, firm to hard painless mass, often with ill-defined margins, or picked up as a result of an abnormal Mammogram and, not as common, as a result of a palpable mass.
- **Later findings of locally advanced disease: axillary lymphadenopathy** (locoregional disease) that is matted or fixed; skin or nipple retraction, fixation of the mass to the skin or chest wall.
- Metastatic disease: most common sites are the **bone** (vertebrae, ribs, pelvis, & femur), **lungs** (eg, dyspnea or cough), liver (abdominal pain, nausea, jaundice), or brain. Think 2Bs and 2Ls.
- **Paget disease of the breast:** chronic eczematous itchy scaly rash on the nipples & may spread to the areola (may ooze). **Pain, itching, or burning.** A lump is often present. Seen in <5% of cases.
- **Inflammatory Breast cancer:** rapidly progressing, tender, firm, and enlarged breast with **skin findings [eg, erythema, warmth, itching, thickening, or dimpling of the overlying skin that looks like the peel of an orange (peau d'orange) and itchy breast]** due to **lymphatic obstruction** (associated with **poor prognosis**). Usually without an underlying mass or lump. Often mistaken for Mastitis (biopsy often performed on Mastitis not responsive to 1-2 weeks of an antibiotic course).

BREAST MASS – DIAGNOSIS
A combination of physical exam, Mammography, and core biopsy is highly accurate.
- **Mammography: initial imaging of choice to evaluate breast masses in women >40y** — grouped **microcalcifications & spiculated high-density masses (most specific feature) are highly suspicious for malignancy.** Most effective in older women as early as 40y (less glandular tissue).
- **Ultrasound: recommended initial modality to evaluate breast masses in women <40y** due to high density of breast tissue. May also guide FNA with biopsy or determine if a mass seen on Mammogram is cystic or solid (can also decrease rate of false-negative Mammograms). Sonographic features suggestive of malignancy include hypoechogenicity; internal calcifications; shadowing; a lesion taller than it is wide; and spiculated, indistinct, or angular margins.
- MRI: may be used to screen some women at high risk for Breast cancer. MRI features suggestive of malignancy include rapid uptake of contrast, irregular or spiculated mass margins, heterogeneous internal enhancement, and enhancing internal septa.

BIOPSY OPTIONS
- **Fine needle aspiration:** advantages: removes the least amount of tissue. Disadvantages: **if positive, it doesn't allow for receptor testing** (estrogen, progesterone, HER 2/neu); False negative 10%.
- **Large needle (core biopsy) often with image guidance: has replaced open biopsy.** Advantages — allows for receptor testing if positive (estrogen, progesterone, & HER 2/neu), provides better sampling, & reduces risk of inadequate samples. Disadvantages: can leave greater deformity with the procedure & the needle may miss the lesion. Open biopsy reserved if core biopsy cannot be done.
- Open biopsy: advantages — most accurate diagnostic test, allows for frozen section to be done followed by immediate resection of the cancer & sentinel node biopsy. Removes the most tissue.

BREAST CANCER MANAGEMENT
Treatment based on TNM staging. Metastatic workup recommended for stage III and above.
- **Early-stage cancer: Breast conservation therapy (lumpectomy) with sentinel node biopsy + follow-up postoperative adjuvant radiation usually preferred when possible** to maximize locoregional control. A negative sentinel node eliminates need for axillary lymph node dissection.
- Locally advanced cancer: most patients are treated with neoadjuvant systemic therapy rather than proceeding with primary surgery.
- Modified radical mastectomy may be needed if diffuse, large tumor, prior radiation to the breast, or if radiation post-lumpectomy is contraindicated.
- **Radiation therapy: usually done after lumpectomy or post mastectomy (adjuvant therapy) to destroy residual tumor cells** (eg, external beam radiation or brachytherapy).
- **Anti-estrogen hormonal therapy: if estrogen receptor positive tumors: Tamoxifen is most useful in premenopausal patients.** Estrogen-receptor (ER) positivity associated with a better prognosis. Adverse effect of Tamoxifen: venous thrombosis, hot flushes, uterine bleeding, Endometrial cancer.
- **Aromatase inhibitor hormonal therapy: most useful in postmenopausal ER-positive patients** (eg, **Letrozole, Anastrozole, Exemestane). AIs are slightly more effective than Tamoxifen. AIs are only used in postmenopausal women** because aromatase inhibition can result in paradoxical increase in circulating estrogen levels in women with functioning ovaries (premenopausal women). Adverse effects: **Osteoporosis**, thromboembolism, Myocardial infarction, hot flushes, arthralgias.
- **Anti-HER2/neu Hormonal therapy: Trastuzumab** with or without Pertuzumab added to chemotherapy regimen for HER2 positive tumors. HER2/neu+ is associated with more aggressive tumors. Adverse effects: **cardiotoxicity (reversible dilated cardiomyopathy). Lapatinib.**
- Adjuvant chemotherapy: used to treat any residual disease. Indications include lesions >1 cm, positive axillary lymphadenopathy, breast cancers stage II-IV, & inoperable disease (especially estrogen receptor-negative disease).
  - Options include Doxorubicin or Epirubicin, Cyclophosphamide, Fluorouracil, & Docetaxel.
- **Triple negative [estrogen receptor (ER), progesterone receptor (PR), & HER2-neu-negative) associated with a worse prognosis** because not responsive to hormonal therapies.

CERVICAL INSUFFICIENCY (INCOMPETENT CERVIX)

- **Inability to maintain pregnancy secondary to premature cervical dilation (especially in the second trimester).**
- Short cervical length (≤25 mm) on Transvaginal ultrasound between 16-24 weeks of gestation is associated with an increased risk for spontaneous preterm birth.

RISK FACTORS

- **Previous cervical trauma or procedure** (LEEP or other excisional procedures, cervical conization, D&C etc.), Uterine defects or anomalies, DES exposure.

CLINICAL MANIFESTATIONS

- **Painless cervical dilation in the second trimester:** Usually asymptomatic. May develop pressure, Braxton-Hicks-like contractions, bleeding, or vaginal discharge especially in the 2nd trimester.
- Physical examination: **painless dilation & effacement of the cervix.**

DIAGNOSIS

- Clinical diagnosis
- **Transvaginal ultrasound most accurate & predictive measurement of cervical length.** Findings include wide internal os, shortening of the cervical canal, hourglass appearance, & bulging of the fetal membranes into the os. **Insufficiency present if cervical length ≤25 mm before 24 weeks.**

MANAGEMENT

- **Cervical cerclage (suturing of cervical os) and bed rest, especially if prior history.** If not performed initially, cerclage can also be performed for women who develop a short cervix (≤25 mm) before 24 weeks as determined by ultrasound surveillance.
- **May also use weekly injection of 17 alpha-hydroxyprogesterone** in addition to cerclage in some women with preterm birth history.
- For patients with history-based diagnosis of Cervical insufficiency, history-indicated cerclage at 12 to 14 weeks of gestation rather than Ultrasound monitoring of cervical length.

CERVICAL CANCER SCREENING

- **Screening guidelines recommend regular Pap testing for all women who have reached the <u>age of 21 at 3-year intervals until 30 years of age</u>.** Before this age, even in individuals that have begun sexual activity, screening may cause more harm than benefit.
- **Beginning at age 30, guidelines include co-testing [Pap smear (cervical cytology) + HPV test].** The screening interval for women who test normal using this approach is lengthened to **5 years.**

CERVICAL CANCER SCREENING: ages 21-65 years	
Age <21 years	• **No cervical cancer screening, regardless of sexual activity**
Age 21-29 years	• **Cervical cytology (Pap smear) every 3 years**
Age 30-65 years	• <u>**Co-testing**</u>**: Cervical cytology plus HPV test every 5 years (preferred) OR** • Cervical cytology every 3 years (alternative)
Age >65 years	• **No screening if negative prior screen & low risk**
Hysterectomy (with cervix removed)	• No screening if negative prior screen & low risk
HIV 21-29 years of age	• Onset of sexual intercourse at the time of diagnosis, but no sooner than age 21 years. • **Initial screening colposcopy in addition to cervical cytology at first visit.** If screening with cervical cytology is normal, cervical cytology is performed every 12 months until 3 consecutive normal results (3 years total of negative results), then routine testing every 3 years.
Immunocompromised (eg, organ transplant)	• Women who are immunosuppressed for other reasons should be screened annually.

PAP SMEAR RESULTS				
RESULT	21-24 YEARS OLD	25 – 29 YEARS OLD	≥30 YEARS & HPV NEGATIVE	≥30 YEARS & HPV POSITIVE
Normal	• Pap every 3 years	• Pap every 3 years	• **HPV and Pap cotest every 5 years** (preferred) OR • **Pap every 3 years** (acceptable)	• Co-testing in 1 year or • HPV Genotype testing
ASC-US Atypical squamous cells of undetermined significance	• **Pap test in 1 year (preferred)** OR • Reflex HPV test (acceptable)	• **Reflex HPV testing (preferred)** OR • Pap testing in 1 year (acceptable)	• Repeat co-testing in 3 years	• Colposcopy
LSIL Low-grade squamous intraepithelial lesion	• Repeat pap in 1 year	• Colposcopy	• Repeat pap in 1 year OR • Colposcopy	• Colposcopy
ASC-H Atypical cells can't exclude HSIL	• **Colposcopy**	• **Colposcopy**	• **Colposcopy**	• **Colposcopy**
HSIL High-grade squamous cell intraepithelial lesion	• Colposcopy	• Excisional treatment OR • Colposcopy	• Excisional treatment OR • Colposcopy	• Excisional treatment OR • Colposcopy

Excisional treatment options include:
- Loop electrosurgical excision procedure (LEEP)
- Cold-knife conization
- Laser conization

If **Pap smear test is negative and HPV test is positive**, providers may either:
- **(1) repeat Pap smear and HPV co-testing in 1 year** or
- **(2) order HPV DNA typing** to detect HPV subtypes 16 or 18.
- **Patients positive for HPV 16 or 18 should receive colposcopy**.

Patients with other high-risk HPV types may have repeat HPV-based testing in one year. If the HPV test is again positive, colposcopy should be performed.

ASCUS (Atypical squamous cells of undetermined significance) 21-24 years:
- **Patients <25 years of age have a high rate of spontaneous regression** of human papillomavirus (HPV) and **low risk of developing Cervical cancer**.
- **Because of the lower overall risk of developing Cervical cancer, patients <25 years of age can be cared for more conservatively than patients >25 years of age.** Options include:
  - **[1] Pap test (cervical cytology) in 1 year (preferred)**
  - [2] Reflex HPV testing (acceptable)

ASCUS (Atypical squamous cells of undetermined significance) ≥25 years:

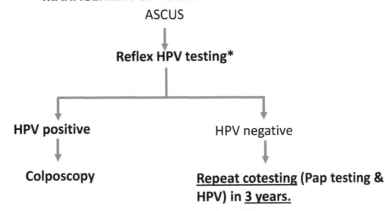

MANAGEMENT OF ASCUS IN WOMEN ≥25 YEARS

ASCUS

Reflex HPV testing*

HPV positive

HPV negative

Colposcopy

Repeat cotesting (Pap testing & HPV) in 3 years.

(ASCUS): Atypical squamous cells of undetermined significance
- **Most common abnormal Pap test result**
- Atypical cells that demonstrate reactive changes but do not meet cytologic criteria for premalignant disease.

Positive HPV 16 or HPV 18 with any cytology result: Colposcopy

ASC-H at any age: Atypical squamous cells, cannot exclude high-grade squamous intraepithelial lesion (ASC-H): **colposcopy**

(HSIL) High-grade squamous intraepithelial lesion at any age: CIN2, CIN3, Cervical cancer
- **(1) Colposcopy or (2) Loop excision.**
- **Endocervical sampling (curettage) if colposcopy results are unsatisfactory.**

Atypical glandular cells of undetermined significance (AGC):
- **Colposcopy AND endocervical sampling**
- **Endometrial biopsy for age ≥35 years**

CERVICAL BIOPSY RESULTS			
PAP SMEAR RESULT	**BIOPSY (HISTOLOGY) RESULTS** CIN = Cervical intraepithelial neoplasia	**DESCRIPTION**	**MANAGEMENT**
LSIL Low-grade squamous intraepithelial lesion	• CIN I	• **Mild dysplasia** contained to basal 1/3 of epithelium. • Cellular changes seen with HPV (often transient in young women)	• For women with **CIN 1 + ASC-US, LSIL or normal cytology** in the presence HPV 16 or 18, **recommended follow-up is cotesting with cytology and an HPV test at one year.** For women with CIN 1 + HSIL or ASC-H either: • Excisional procedure or • Observation with contesting at 12 & 24 months are recommended.
HSIL High-grade squamous cell intraepithelial lesion	• CIN II	• **Moderate dysplasia** including 2/3 thickness of basal epithelium • Usually due to persistent HPV	**For HSIL lesions (CIN I or CIN II) excision or ablation is the mainstay of treatment** (high risk of progression). • **Excision:** LEEP (Loop electrical excisional procedure) or Cold knife conization.
	• CIN III	• **Severe dysplasia** including > 2/3 up to full thickness of the basal epithelium. • **Full thickness = carcinoma in situ** (hasn't invaded basement membrane)	• **Ablation:** cryocautery, laser cautery or electrocautery

HPV VACCINATION

- **HPV types 16 & 18 cause ~70% of all Cervical cancers worldwide & ~90% of anal cancers, as well as a significant proportion of oropharyngeal cancer, vulvar, vaginal cancer, and penile cancer.**
- **HPV types 6 and 11 cause ~90% of genital warts.**
- **Gardasil 9:** targets the same as Gardasil (**6, 11, 16, 18**) as well as HPV types 31, 33, 45, 52, & 58.
- Recombinant 9 valent HPV vaccine (Gardasil 9) can prevent Cervical cancer by targeting the HPV types with greatest risk & protect against low-grade & precancerous lesions caused by other HPV types.

Indications: (ACIP): All females & males:
- Routine vaccination is recommended at 11-12 years & can be administered starting at 9 years of age.
- For adolescents and adults aged 13-26 years who have not been previously vaccinated or who have not completed the vaccine series, catch-up vaccination is recommended.
- For adults 27y-45y and older, catch-up vaccination is not routinely recommended; the ACIP notes that the decision to vaccinate people in this age group should be made on an individual basis.

Dosing:
- **Individuals initiating the vaccine series at 9-15 years of age — Two doses of HPV vaccine** should be given at [1] 0 and [2] at 6-12 months.
- **Individuals initiating the vaccine series at 15 years of age or older — Three doses of HPV vaccine** should be given at 0, 1-2 months (typically 2), and at 6 months. Minimum interval between first 2 doses is 4 weeks, minimum interval between the second & third is 12 weeks.
- **HPV vaccine is contraindicated if pregnant or lactating.**

CERVICAL CANCER

- **3rd most common gynecologic cancer** (#1 = Endometrial cancer; #2 = Ovarian cancer).
- Most commonly metastasize to local areas — vagina, parametrium, & pelvic lymph nodes.

Major types:

- **Squamous cell carcinoma most common** (75%). Adenocarcinoma 25%.
- Adenosquamous carcinoma (3–5%). Clear cell carcinoma is a type linked with DES exposure.

SPREAD

- In order, primary node groups involved in the spread of Cervical cancer include the **paracervical (most common),** parametrial, obturator, hypogastric, external iliac, and sacral nodes.
- It takes on average 2-10 years for carcinoma to penetrate the basement membrane & become invasive.
- SCC appears first in the intraepithelial layers (the preinvasive stage, or carcinoma in situ). Preinvasive cancer (CIN III) is most commonly diagnosed in women 25–35 years of age.

RISK FACTORS

- **Human papilloma virus associated with 99.7%, especially 16 &18 (70%), 31 & 33,** 45, 52, & 58. It is considered a sexually transmitted disease as both squamous cell and adenocarcinoma of the cervix are secondary to infection with HPV, primarily types 16 and 18.
- **Early onset of sexual activity (<18 years), increased number of sexual partners, smoking is a cofactor for Squamous cell carcinoma,** DES exposure, Oral contraceptive use, cervical intraepithelial neoplasia, **immunosuppression (eg, HIV), STIs,** multiparity.
- **40-50 years is the most common age range for diagnosis** (average age at diagnosis is 42 years).

CLINICAL MANIFESTATIONS

- Cervical cancer is usually asymptomatic in the early stages.
- **Post coital bleeding or spotting most common presenting symptom of Cervical cancer.**
- **Abnormal uterine bleeding: irregular or heavy vaginal bleeding or watery vaginal discharge.**
- Advanced disease may present with pelvic or back pain, bladder or rectal dysfunction.
- Physical examination: may have cervical discharge or ulceration if invasive. May be normal early on.

DIAGNOSIS

- **Colposcopy with biopsy** — gross lesions should be evaluated by Colposcopically directed biopsies and not cytology alone. Lesions may appear as **[1] an exophytic, friable lesion (due to tumor growth) or [2] a painless, endophytic ulcerative lesion** (due to tumor necrosis), a polypoid mass, papillary tissue, a cervical ulceration, or necrotic tissue.
- Cervical biopsy & endocervical curettage or conization — performed after a positive Papanicolaou smear to determine the extent and depth of invasion of the cancer. Even if the smear is positive, definitive diagnosis must be established through biopsy before additional treatment is given.
- Staging of invasive Cervical cancer is determined by clinical evaluation, usually conducted under anesthesia. Additional testing, such as ultrasonography, CT, MRI, lymphangiography, laparoscopy, and fine-needle aspiration, are useful for treatment planning.

MANAGEMENT

- **Carcinoma in situ (Stage 0): Excision preferred (Loop electrical excision procedure/LEEP, cold knife conization) or ablation (cryotherapy or laser).** Total abdominal hysterectomy + bilateral salpingo-oophorectomy definitive management if childbearing is not a consideration.
- Microinvasive (stage IA1): total hysterectomy, radical hysterectomy, conization.
- IA2, IB, IIA: combined external beam radiation with brachytherapy OR modified radical hysterectomy with bilateral pelvic lymphadenectomy. Adjuvant chemotherapy or radiation may be used for women with risk factors for recurrence.
- **Locally advanced (IIB, III, IVA): primary radiation therapy (eg, external beam plus brachytherapy) + chemotherapy (Cisplatin-based).**
- Advanced & metastatic: systemic chemotherapy; radiation therapy.

CERVICITIS

- **Cervicitis: inflammation of the uterine cervix** that primarily affects the columnar epithelial cells of the endocervical glands. The squamous epithelium of the ectocervix can also be involved.

ETIOLOGIES
Infectious:
- **Sexually transmitted infections (STIs)** most common causes, with *Chlamydia trachomatis* & *Neisseria gonorrhoeae* being the 2 most common. *Mycoplasma genitalium, T. vaginalis,* HSV.

Noninfectious etiologies (especially if chronic):
- Mechanical or chemical irritation such as from a diaphragm or vaginal douche, respectively.

CLINICAL MANIFESTATIONS
- **Vaginal discharge & cervix friability:**
  - **Gonococcal & Chlamydia:** purulent or mucopurulent (yellow) cervical discharge, edema in the zone of ectopy, &/or easily induced bleeding (friability) from the endocervix on touching it with an endocervical swab.** May progress to pelvic infection (PID) or disseminated infection.
  - Bacterial vaginosis (BV): gray or off-white homogenous malodorous vaginal discharge.
  - Vulvovaginal candidiasis: scant and thick discharge often adherent to the vaginal walls.
  - Trichomoniasis: brownish, yellow-green, or bloody & malodorous discharge; **cervical petechiae.**
  - HSV: diffuse vesicular lesions/ulceration, sloughing of the epithelium; Erosive inflammation.
- Associated symptoms: **abnormal vaginal discharge;** urinary frequency, dysuria.
- **Vaginal bleeding: intermenstrual or postcoital bleeding.**

Pelvic inflammatory disease (PID):
- Cervical motion tenderness, uterine tenderness, or adnexal tenderness in addition to Cervicitis should increase the suspicion for possible PID, which should be treated appropriately.
- Most patients with PID have either mucopurulent cervical discharge or leukorrhea on saline preparation of vaginal fluid.

DIAGNOSIS
- **Clinical diagnosis: Cervicitis is based upon the presence of mucopurulent cervical discharge or friability,** which may be associated with bleeding. **Testing for potential causative organism.**
- **Nucleic acid amplification testing** (NAAT) for *N. gonorrhoeae, C. trachomatis, T. vaginalis, M genitalium.* Performed on a swab of vaginal fluid, an endocervical sample or, if a speculum examination is not possible, on urine.
- Vaginal pH and saline microscopy (wet mount): >10 polymorphonuclear cells/hpf on microscopy suggests chlamydial or gonococcal infection. Motile pear-shaped organisms in Trichomoniasis.
- Testing for Bacterial vaginosis & Trichomoniasis: wet mount prep for microscopy, amine (whiff) test, and vaginal pH — *T. vaginalis* may cause isolated Cervicitis; BV typically affects the vagina.

MANAGEMENT
- For individuals with physical examination findings of Cervicitis, empiric therapy rather than treatment based on risk factors for STI acquisition or targeted test results.
  - **Chlamydia and Gonorrhea infection are the most common infectious etiologies, so empiric treatment often employed [eg, Ceftriaxone 500 mg IM once if <150 kg** (or 1g IM once if ≥150 kg) **+ Doxycycline 100 mg bid for 7 days].** Alternative treatment for Chlamydia is Azithromycin 1 g orally x 1 dose.
  - **Treatment of sexual partners is indicated for patients with Chlamydia, Gonorrhea, or Trichomonas infections.**
  - Individuals who present with recurrent symptoms are reevaluated for possible re-exposure or treatment failure. Patients with persistent Cervicitis for presumed *M. genitalium* are treated if they have not already been treated for this agent and NAAT-based testing has not excluded this.

SEXUALLY TRANSMITTED INFECTION (STI) SCREENING

<u>USPSTF recommendations:</u>
For men & sexually active young women, including pregnant persons, Screen for chlamydia and gonorrhea if:
- **24 years or younger**
- **25 years or older and at increased risk for infection.**

<u>All patients:</u>
- (1) Neisseria gonorrhoeae (via NAAT)
- (2) Chlamydia trachomatis (via NAAT)
- (3) Syphilis (via RPR)
- (4) HIV (4th generation antibody)

<u>Additional testing certain populations:</u>
- <u>Women only:</u> *Trichomonas vaginalis* (wet mount)
- <u>HSV screening</u> (eg, serology) in individuals with characteristic lesions.

INFERTILITY

- **Failure to conceive after 1 year of regular unprotected sexual intercourse.**
- 60% of couples achieve pregnancy in the first 3 years in the absence of a cause for infertility.
- <u>Etiologies in males:</u> 40% of causes — eg, abnormal spermatogenesis.
- <u>Etiologies in females:</u> anovulatory cycles/ovarian dysfunction 30%, congenital or acquired disorders.

<u>DIAGNOSIS:</u>
- **Females:** **Hysterosalpingography** helps evaluate tubal patency or abnormalities.
- **Males:** **evaluate sperm count and motility.**

<u>MANAGEMENT</u>
Letrozole or Clomiphene are first-line medications for ovulation induction.
- **Aromatase inhibitors (eg, Letrozole)** — Anovulatory WHO 2 patients who have a poor outcome with Clomiphene may have a better response with aromatase inhibitors (eg, Letrozole). Advantages of AIs over Clomiphene include [1] production of fewer follicles and lower estradiol levels, decreasing the risk of multiple gestation, and [2] shorter half-life (50 hours versus 5 days), resulting in reduced antiestrogen effects on the endometrium and cervical mucus. **Letrozole may be superior to Clomiphene in inducing ovulation and live birth.**
- **Clomiphene citrate** is a Selective estrogen receptor modulator (SERM) with both estrogen antagonist and agonist effects that increase gonadotropin release. It is an effective method of inducing ovulation and improving fertility of oligoovulatory women in WHO class 2 (normogonadotropic normoestrogenic ovulatory dysfunction). **Second-line to Letrozole for ovulation induction.**

<u>Other options:</u>
- <u>Amenorrhea or Oligomenorrhea:</u> correct endocrine problems; Intrauterine insemination.
- In vitro fertilization (especially if fallopian tube defect is present).
- Surgical reconstruction for young patients with bilateral proximal or distal tubal obstruction and limited access to in vitro fertilization (IVF), with counseling on the success rates of different methods of repair and on the high risk of ectopic pregnancy.

OVARIAN HYPERSTIMULATION SYNDROME (OHSS)

- **Ovarian hyperstimulation syndrome (OHSS) is an exaggerated ovarian response to ovulation induction, particularly in the setting of in vitro fertilization (IVF).**
- Characterized by a shift of serum from the intravascular space to the third space, mainly to the abdominal cavity, in the context of enlarged ovaries due to follicular stimulation.

ETIOLOGIES
- OHSS occurs almost exclusively in the setting of ovarian stimulation with exogenous gonadotropins, and only if human chorionic gonadotropin (hCG) is administered to trigger ovulation.
- Risk factors: Polycystic ovary syndrome (PCOS), luteal phase hCG support, number of follicles, and high serum estradiol concentrations, previous OHSS. Pregnancy increases the risk, severity, and duration of OHSS (as a result of continuous stimulation by endogenous hCG).

CLINICAL MANIFESTATIONS
- OHSS may be classified into mild, moderate, severe, and critical based upon the severity of symptoms, signs, and laboratory findings. Early OHSS begins 4-7 days after dose of hCG. Late if ≥9 days.

Mild OHSS:
- Bilateral ovarian enlargement with multiple follicular and corpus luteum cysts, abdominal distention and discomfort, mild nausea, vomiting and diarrhea. No lab abnormalities.

Moderate OHSS:
- Features of mild OHSS PLUS ultrasonographic evidence of ascites. Ovaries are frequently enlarged ≤12 cm in their longest dimension. Abdominal discomfort and gastrointestinal symptoms (eg, nausea, vomiting, and diarrhea) are more common and intense than in mild OHSS. A sudden increase in weight of >3 kg (6.6 lbs.) may occur.
- Laboratory abnormalities include a hematocrit >41% and white blood cell concentration (WBC) >15,000/microL, with hypoproteinemia.

Severe OHSS
- In addition to the findings of moderate OHSS, severe OHSS is characterized by the presence of clinical evidence of ascites with severe abdominal pain and, in some patients, pleural effusion. Women with severe OHSS may increase as much as 15-20 kg (33-44 lbs.) over a 5-to-10-day period. Ascites and pleural effusion may compromise pulmonary function, resulting in hypoxia.
- Labs: hematocrit >45%, leukocytes >25,000/L, and creatinine >1.6 mg/dL, progressive leukocytosis.

DIAGNOSIS
- The diagnosis of OHSS is based upon [1] clinical history and [2] Transvaginal ultrasound.
- There should be a history of ovarian stimulation followed by ovulation or administration of hCG

MANAGEMENT
Mild OHSS:
- Outpatient management with analgesics (eg, Acetaminophen) and activity modification [eg, avoidance of heavy physical activity and sexual intercourse (which could cause discomfort and increase the risk of ovarian rupture)]. Surveillance of the patient is recommended.

Moderate OHSS:
- Outpatient management that includes avoidance of physical activity, oral hydration (1 to 2 liters per day), and a baseline transvaginal ultrasound (TVUS) and complete blood count (CBC) to assess for ascites and hemoconcentration, respectively.

Severe OHSS:
- Hospitalization and thromboembolism prophylaxis. Prophylaxis also recommended for those managed as outpatients with 2-3 additional risk factors (in addition to OHSS): age >35 years, obesity, immobility, personal or family history of thrombosis, thrombophilias, elevated hematocrit, pregnancy.

MIDCYCLE PAIN (MITTELSCHMERZ)

- **Unilateral abdominal or pelvic pain that <u>occurs at ovulation</u> (10-14 days after initiation of menses).** Pain due to enlargement and rupture of follicular cyst causes irritation to the peritoneum.

CONTRACEPTIVE METHODS

EMERGENCY (POSTCOITAL) CONTRACEPTION

- **In order of maximal to minimal efficacy: Copper TCu380A IUD (<u>most effective</u>) > Levonorgestrel IUD > Ulipristal acetate (UPA) > oral Levonorgestrel.**
- When used for emergency contraception, the copper TCu380A and Levonorgestrel 52 mg IUDs result in pregnancy rates of <1%.
- The oral medication EC methods UPA & oral Levonorgestrel have pregnancy rates of ~1-3%.

COPPER IUD (TCu380A):

- **The most effective method of emergency contraception if inserted within 5-7 days after unprotected intercourse.** Prevents up to 99% of pregnancies.

LEVONORGESTREL IUD (eg, LNG 52 mg IUD)

- **>99% effective (second most effective emergency contraception after the copper IUD).**
- Inserted ideally within 5 days after intercourse.

ULIPRISTAL (UPA):

- Progestin receptor modulator that delays ovulation.
- Must be taken within 5 days (120 hours) after intercourse. **UPA is the most effective <u>oral</u> emergency contraceptive** but requires a prescription and is not stocked by all pharmacies.

ORAL LEVONORGESTREL:

- Levonorgestrel 750 µg twice, 12 hours apart.
- A single dose of 1,500 µg Levonorgestrel may be as effective as the 2-dose regimen.
- **Ideally given within 72 hours after intercourse** but effective up to 5 days (120 hours) after intercourse. <u>Mechanism:</u> inhibits or delays ovulation. Reduces the chance of pregnancy by 75% - 98%. Preferred over the Estrogen-progestin regimen. <u>Adverse effects:</u> nausea & vomiting.

COMBINED ORAL ESTROGEN &/OR LNG CONTRACEPTIVE PILLS (eg, Yuzpe method):

- **Ideally given within 72 hours of unprotected intercourse.**
- 100 µg Ethinyl estradiol & 500–600 µg Levonorgestrel administered twice, 12 hours apart.
- <u>Mechanism:</u> inhibits or delays ovulation. <u>Common adverse effects:</u> nausea & vomiting.

EMERGENCY CONTRACEPTION			
METHOD	**TIMING AFTER INTERCOURSE**	**EFFICACY**	**CONTRAINDICATIONS**
Copper TCu380A IUD	**0-120 hours**	**>99% (most effective emergency contraception)** 0.1% result in pregnancy	• **Wilson disease** • **Active pelvic infection** • Abnormal uterine bleeding • Severe uterine cavity distortion
Levonorgestrel IUD	**0-120 hours**	**>99% (second most effective EC).** 0.3% result in pregnancy	• **Breast cancer** • **Active pelvic infection** • Abnormal uterine bleeding • Severe uterine cavity distortion
Ulipristal acetate	0-120 hours	98-99%	• None significant
Oral Levonorgestrel (Plan B)	**0-72 hours**	92-98%	• Headache, GI symptoms
Oral combined estrogen/progestin pills with Levonorgestrel or Norgestrel	**0-72 hours**	75-89%	• Nausea (50%), vomiting (20%). • An antiemetic (eg, Meclizine) 1 hour before may reduce these effects.

EFFECTIVENESS OF CONTRACEPTION

Most effective (>99% efficacy):

- **Etonogestrel implant (most effective contraceptive) >99% efficacy (0.05% average failure rate)**
- Vasectomy >99% efficacy (0.3% average failure rate)
- **Levonorgestrel IUD >99% efficacy** (0.1-0.4% average failure rate)
- Tubal ligation >99% efficacy (average failure rate 0.5%)
- **Depot medroxyprogesterone acetate injection (DMPA) injection** perfect use failure rate 0.3%, typical use failure rate of 3-5%
- **Copper IUD:** 0.8% average failure rate.

91% efficacy:

- Contraceptive pill
- Hormonal vaginal ring
- Transdermal patch

Lower efficacy:

- Diaphragm
- Male condom (80%): provides highly effective and inexpensive contraception as well as protection against sexually transmitted infections (STIs). When greater contraceptive effectiveness is desired, a second method such as contraceptive vaginal jelly or foam should be used in conjunction with the condom.
- Female condom: advantages: gives more control to the female partner and some protection against STIs. Major disadvantages include the cost and overall bulkiness.
- Withdrawal method (coitus interruptus) (75%)
- Spermicides

COMBINED ESTROGEN + PROGESTERONE ORAL CONTRACEPTIVES

MECHANISM OF ACTION

- Prevents ovulation & implantation by inhibiting midcycle LH surge, thickens cervical mucosa, and thins the endometrium.
- Failure rate: average 9%; 0.3% when used correctly.
- Often started with the onset of menses or within the 5 days after the start of menses. Active pills are taken for 21 days followed by 7 days of no pills or placebos.

ADVANTAGES

- **Protects against Osteoporosis; Ovarian cancer** (40-80%) **& Endometrial cancer** (50%) with >1 year use.
- **Reduces risk of menstrual disorders (including Dysmenorrhea, Abnormal uterine bleeding), Ectopic pregnancy** (90%), **Pelvic inflammatory disease (PID), acne, hirsutism, incidence of Ovarian cysts, incidence of Benign breast disease** (30-50%).

DISADVANTAGES

- **Increased hypercoagulability (DVT & PE),** gallstone formation & gall stasis, increased fluid retention, increased triglycerides, cholestasis, Diabetes mellitus, Myocardial infarction, Stroke.
- Increased risk of hepatic adenoma.
- Cautious use in patients with hepatobiliary disease.

CONTRAINDICATIONS

- History of ischemic heart disease (including MI), Venous thromboembolism (DVT, PE), Stroke.
- **Breast cancer** (prior or current).
- Migraine with aura, pregnancy.
- **Smokers should stop use of OCPs if ≥35 years of age (especially if smoking ≥15 cigarettes a day) due to thrombogenic potential.**
- *Severe* hypertension: eg, systolic ≥160 mmHg &/or diastolic ≥100 mmHg.
- Undiagnosed vaginal bleeding
- Active liver disease

PROGESTERONE-ONLY PILL (NORETHINDRONE "mini pill"); LEVONORGESTREL

MECHANISM OF ACTION

- Thickens the cervical mucus which inhibits the passage of sperm, thins the endometrium, & suppresses ovulation (doesn't prevent ovulation as well as estrogen-containing pills).

INDICATIONS

- **Women in whom an estrogen-containing contraceptive is either contraindicated or causes additional health issues** (eg, Migraine with aura, women ≥35 years of age who smoke ≥15 cigarettes a day, Hypertension, Systemic lupus erythematosus).
- Often initiated on the first day of menses. Back-up contraceptive is not necessary if POPs are started within the first 5 days of the start of menses.
- **Pills must be taken at the same time each day to maximize efficacy** (a delay of 2-3 hours reduces the contraceptive effectiveness for the next 48 hours).

ADVANTAGES

- **No estrogen-related adverse effects** so little effect on coagulation factors, blood pressure, glucose, and lipid levels. Good in patients with Systemic lupus erythematosus, Hypertension, Migraine.
- **Safe during lactation. Reduces the risk of Endometrial cancer**.
- **Less incidence of PID** (due to thicker cervical mucus).

ADVERSE EFFECTS

- **Unscheduled & irregular bleeding** & changes in menses.

PROGESTERONE-ONLY CONTRACEPTIVES

INJECTABLE: Depot Medroxyprogesterone acetate (DMPA).

- Highly efficacious. Perfect use failure rate 0.3%, typical use failure rate 3-5%.
- **Lasts 3 months** usual dose if 150 mg IM deltoid or gluteus maximus every 3 months.
- Mechanism: suppresses pituitary FSH & LH secretion, thickening of cervical mucus, thin endometrium.
- Benefits: **decreased risk of Ectopic pregnancy, Endometrial cancer, reduces Sickle cell crises, reduces Endometriosis symptoms.** Does not increase the risk of arterial or venous disease.
- Adverse effects: menstrual changes (eg, amenorrhea, irregular periods, weight gain, headache, mood changes). **May lead to calcium loss, bone weakness, decreased bone mineral density, & Osteoporosis so not usually used more than 2 years**.
- Return to baseline fertility after discontinuation at an average of 10 months.

PROGESTIN IMPLANTS:

- **Etonogestrel implant most effective contraception** (0.05% average failure rate). **Lasts 3 years**.
- Long-acting, reversible contraceptive, such as the **Levonorgestrel and Copper intrauterine devices (IUDs) and subdermal progestin implant are first-line contraception options for adolescents.**
- Removal is easier than with other implants with the single-rod system.
- Adverse effects include headache, menstrual irregularities, and weight gain.

LEVONORGESTREL INTRAUTERINE DEVICE (IUD):

- **Both LNG 52 mg IUDs are now approved for up to 8 years. IUDs most effective forms of emergency contraception.** LNG-20 IUD reduces menstrual flow, so useful for menorrhagia.
- Mechanism of action: Thickens cervical mucus, impairs plantation. Usually inserted during menses to ensure the patient is not pregnant. Contraindicated if unexplained abnormal vaginal bleeding.
- Long-acting, reversible contraceptive, such as the **Levonorgestrel and Copper intrauterine devices (IUDs) and subdermal progestin implant are first-line contraception options for adolescents.**
- **Levonorgestrel IUD — most effective long-term medical management of heavy bleeding.**
- Adverse effects: uterine perforation, **increased risk of Ectopic pregnancy & Pelvic inflammatory disease, cramping or bleeding with menses**; risk of spontaneous abortion if pregnancy occurs.
- Contraindications: **Breast cancer, Active pelvic infection at time of insertion,** Abnormal uterine bleeding of unknown origin, Severe uterine cavity distortion, Liver tumors, Active liver disease.

COPPER INTRAUTERINE DEVICE (IUD)

MECHANISM OF ACTION:

- Causes inflammation that makes a hostile environment for sperm and ova.
- **Very effective contraceptive method with high efficacy >99% (0.8% average failure rate).**

ADVANTAGES:

- **10-year duration of action, very effective contraceptive method >99% efficacy.**
- **No exogenous hormones:** no effect on Hypertension, no DVT and PE risk, & no effect on future fertility (once removed, immediate return to fertility).
- The copper IUD does not cause anovulation or amenorrhea (patients continue to have cyclic bleeding and less unscheduled bleeding compared to Levonorgestrel IUD).
- **Emergency contraception: Copper IUD is the most effective form of emergency contraception** and can be left in place for ongoing contraception. 0.1% pregnancy rate as emergency contraception.

ADVERSE EFFECTS

- **Increased incidence of Pelvic inflammatory disease (PID) and Ectopic pregnancy; increased menstrual bleed (eg, heavier periods), cramping,** spontaneous abortion, uterine perforation.
- **Contraindications: Wilson disease, Active pelvic infection at the time of insertion,** Abnormal uterine bleeding of unknown origin, Severe uterine cavity distortion.

CLOMIPHENE CITRATE

MECHANISM OF ACTION:

- Partial estrogen receptor agonist that stimulates ovulation via the hypothalamus, leading to increased LH and FSH release.

INDICATIONS:

- **Induces ovulation to enhance fertility, especially in patients with Polycystic ovarian syndrome (second line to the Aromatase inhibitor Letrozole).** Infertility due to anovulation.

ADVERSE EFFECTS:

- **Hot flashes most common,** ovarian enlargement, multiple gestation pregnancy, abdominal discomfort, & visual changes.

LEUPROLIDE

- Mechanism of action: Gonadotropin releasing hormone analog (GnRH).

Indications:

- **Fertility: if given pulsatile** (the natural way the body releases GnRH).
- **Inhibition of estrogen & testosterone: if given continuously** (suppresses LH & FSH with subsequent reduction of estrogen & testosterone via negative feedback). **Most effective medication to shrink Uterine fibroids, advanced Prostate cancer** (decreases testosterone), Abnormal uterine bleeding, & Premenstrual syndrome.

Adverse effects of continuous dosing:

- **Hypoestrogenic effects: Hot flashes,** depression, **osteopenia** ("add-back" Low dose estrogen &/or progesterone can reduce some of these effects). **Anti-androgen adverse effects.**

DANAZOL

Mechanism of action:

- **Hypoestrogenic and hyperandrogenic.**

Indications:

- Endometriosis (suppresses LH & FSH production), Fibrocystic breast disease, Hereditary angioedema. **Limited use due to hyperandrogenic adverse effects.**

Adverse effects:

- **Hyperandrogenic side effects** eg, weight gain, acne, hirsutism, virilization. Hepatic dysfunction.

BASIC PHYSIOLOGY

MENSTRUAL CYCLE OVERVIEW

Understanding the roles of the hormones in the menstrual cycle are critical to understand this chapter.

Follicular phase: during the 1st 14 days (follicular phase), the endometrium thickens under the influence of **estrogen**. In the ovaries, a dominant follicle matures, leading to ovulation.

Luteal phase: after ovulation, the ruptured follicle becomes the corpus luteum, secreting progesterone (& some estrogen). **Progesterone** enhances the lining of the uterus to prepare it for implantation. If there is no implantation, the corpus luteum degenerates, leading to a steep decrease in both estrogen & progesterone. The steep drop in both hormones leads to menstruation.

PHASE 1: FOLLICULAR (Proliferative)

Days 1-12

ESTROGEN PREDOMINATES.

- **Pulsatile GnRH** from the hypothalamus ⇨ ↑FSH & LH from the pituitary gland to stimulate the ovaries.

Ovaries:

- ↑*FSH* causes **follicle & egg maturation in the ovary.**
- ↑*LH* stimulates the maturing follicle to **produce estrogen.**

Endometrium (Uterus)

Estrogen "builds" up the endometrium (proliferative).

Estrogen causes NEGATIVE FEEDBACK in HPO system:

(Hypothalamus-Pituitary-Ovarian)

- The ↑'ing levels of estrogen inhibits hypothalamic GnRH release as well as pituitary release of LH & FSH (so no new follicles start maturing).

OVULATION: Days 12-14

- The ↑estrogen being released from the mature follicle *switches from NEGATIVE TO POSITIVE FEEDBACK* on GnRH, causing mutual ↑'es in estrogen, FSH & LH.
- The sudden **LH surge causes ovulation** (egg release).

PHASE 2: LUTEAL PHASE (Secretory)

Days 14 - 28

PROGESTERONE PREDOMINATES.

- The LH surge also causes the ruptured follicle to become the corpus luteum. The corpus luteum secretes *progesterone* & *estrogen* to maintain the endometrial lining. Estrogen & progesterone switches back to negative feedback.

If pregnancy occurs:

The blastocyst (maturing zygote) keeps the corpus luteum functional (secreting estrogen & progesterone, which keeps the endometrium from sloughing).

MENSTRUAL CYCLE

MENSTRUATION (1st days of Follicular)

If the egg is not fertilized, the corpus luteum soon deteriorates (causing a **fall of progesterone & estrogen levels**). This has 2 effects:

- The endometrium is no longer maintained & sloughs off, leading to **menstruation.**

- The negative feedback on GnRH subsides, causing ↑pulsatile GnRH secretion. This leads to ↑FSH & LH, which starts the follicle maturation process all over again.

GnRH pulses >1 an hour favors LH secretion. Less frequent pulses favor FSH secretion.

MENSTRUAL DISORDERS

ABNORMAL UTERINE BLEEDING (AUB)

- **Unexplained abnormal bleeding in a nonpregnant woman** in regard to quantity, schedule, or duration (formerly Dysfunctional uterine bleeding), other systemic disease, or cancer.
- **Anovulatory (90%):** no ovulation but the ovaries produce estrogen = no corpus luteum formation. **Unopposed estrogen** (not opposed by sufficient progesterone) leads to endometrial growth & proliferation, with unpredictable shedding once the endometrium outgrows its own blood supply.

Structural etiologies: **PALM** — **P**olyp, **A**denomyosis, **L**eiomyoma, **M**alignancy, and hyperplasia.
Nonstructural etiologies: **COEIN** — **C**oagulopathy, **O**vulatory dysfunction, **E**ndometrial, **I**atrogenic, **N**ot otherwise classified. Polycystic ovary syndrome is an example of ovulatory dysfunction.

CLINICAL MANIFESTATIONS
- Abnormal bleeding in regards to volume of flow, frequency, regularity, or duration. Anemia.
- Physical examination: Usually physical examination is relatively normal.

DIAGNOSIS
- Lab workup: there is no specific test for AUB, but **workup may include beta-hCG to rule out pregnancy, CBC, thyroid-stimulating hormone (TSH), & screening for STIs if indicated.** Further testing is directed by the potential etiology. Coagulation studies may be performed.
- **Transvaginal ultrasound: often the initial imaging modality in patients with AUB.** Indicated if a structural etiology is suspected or if symptoms persist despite appropriate initial treatment.
- **Endometrial sampling to rule out Endometrial carcinoma should be done in women with high risk for hyperplasia or malignancy** — eg, all women ≥45 years, <45 years with history of unopposed estrogen exposure (eg, obesity and/or Polycystic ovarian syndrome), hypertension, or Diabetes & all patients with postmenopausal bleeding. Also, if persistent bleeding >6 months.
- Hysteroscopy, Saline infusion sonography & Sonohysterography (TVUS with intrauterine contrast) helpful where Endometrial polyps are noted, images from transvaginal ultrasound are inconclusive, or submucosal leiomyomas are seen. Hysteroscopy and sonohysterography are more invasive.

CHRONIC MANAGEMENT
For most patients with AUB and no known primary etiology, first-line options include [1] Estrogen-progestin contraceptives or [2] Levonorgestrel-releasing IUD (eg, LNG 52 mg IUD).
- **Estrogen-progestin contraceptive oral contraceptive pills (OCPs)** stabilize endometrial proliferation & shedding, suppress endometrial development, reestablish predictable bleeding patterns, decrease menstrual flow, and lower the risk of Iron deficiency anemia.
- Progesterone **Levonorgestrel IUD — most effective long-term medical management of heavy bleeding.** Alternatives if estrogen is contraindicated: oral Progestins, depot Medroxyprogesterone.
- **NSAIDs &/or oral Tranexamic acid in patients unable/unwilling to use hormonal therapy.**
Surgical management:
- Indications: If not responsive to medical treatment or based on patient preference.
- Endometrial ablation or D&C in patients who don't want a hysterectomy. Uterine artery embolization.
- Definitive management: Hysterectomy.

MANAGEMENT OF ACUTE HEMORRHAGE
- **Hormonal therapy (combination oral contraceptives with high-dose estrogen):** [1] high-dose combined oral contraceptives, or [2] IV high-dose conjugated equine estrogen (if unable to tolerate oral therapy, if persistent after oral therapy, or if rapid response needed) or [3] oral Progestins – stabilizes the endometrium.
- IV Tranexamic acid prevents fibrin degradation and can be used to treat acute AUB.
- Uterine tamponade with a Foley bulb is a mechanical option. Uterine artery embolization.
- **Hemodynamically unstable: Dilation & curettage** (removes endometrium) **if unstable or persistent.**

PREMENSTRUAL SYNDROME (PMS)

- **PMS:** cluster of physical, behavioral, & mood changes with cyclical occurrence **during the luteal phase (second half) of the menstrual cycle.**
- **Premenstrual dysphoric disorder (PMDD): severe PMS with functional impairment where anger, irritability, & internal tension are prominent** (DSM V diagnostic criteria).

CLINICAL MANIFESTATIONS
- **Physical: abdominal bloating & fatigue most common**; breast swelling, tenderness, or pain; weight gain, headache, changes in bowel habits or appetite, muscle or joint pain, insomnia, hot flushes.
- **Emotional: irritability most common,** tension, depression, anxiety, hostility, libido changes.
- **Behavioral:** food cravings, poor concentration, noise sensitivity, loss of motor senses.

DIAGNOSIS
- **Symptoms occurring 1-2 weeks before menses (luteal phase), relieved within 2-3 days of the onset of menses,** plus at least 7 symptom-free days during the follicular phase (first half of cycle).
- Recording a diary of symptoms for ≥2 consecutive cycles determines symptom-temporal relationship.

MANAGEMENT
- Lifestyle modifications: stress reduction, relaxation techniques, & exercise most beneficial. Caffeine, alcohol, cigarette, & salt reduction. NSAIDs, vitamins B6 & E. Cognitive behavioral therapy.
- **SSRIs first-line medical therapy for emotional symptoms with dysfunction** (eg, **Fluoxetine, Sertraline**, Citalopram), especially if there is no desire for contraception.
- **Oral contraceptives (especially Drospirenone-containing OCPs for PMDD) in patients who do not want to take SSRIs.** This abolishes the cyclical hormonal changes, preventing symptoms.
- Gonadotropin-releasing hormone (GnRH) agonist therapy (eg, Leuprolide) with low-dose estrogen-progestin "add-back" therapy (to reduce hypoestrogenic symptoms) if no response to SSRIs or OCPs.

DYSMENORRHEA

- **Painful menstruation** that interferes with or prevents normal activities.
- **Primary: due to increased prostaglandins (not due to pelvic pathology).** Prostaglandins cause increased uterine wall contractions. **Usually starts 1-2 years after menarche onset in teenagers.**
- **Secondary: due to pelvis or uterus pathology** (eg, Endometriosis, PID, Adenomyosis, Leiomyoma).

CLINICAL MANIFESTATIONS
- **Recurrent, crampy midline lower abdominal or pelvic pain 1-2 days before or at the onset of menses gradually diminishing over 12-72 hours.** Primary usually develop symptoms before 25y.
- Pain may radiate to the lower back & thighs and may be associated with headache, nausea, or vomiting.
- **Physical exam: normal if Primary dysmenorrhea.** Primary disease often improves with advancing age.
- **Secondary may have signs of the underlying disease** (eg, enlarged uterus, pain with intercourse), **symptom onset >25 years age, unilateral (non-midline) pelvic pain, abnormal uterine bleeding,** worsening over time especially if >30y, or resistance to effective management.

DIAGNOSIS
- Labs & imaging not mandatory to exclude secondary but should be done if pelvic disease is suspected.
- Transvaginal ultrasonography initial imaging choice for patients in whom secondary is suspected.

MANAGEMENT
- **Supportive therapy** includes heat compresses, vitamins B & vitamin E started 2 days prior to and for 3 days into menses, exercise, reassurance. Secondary is treated based on the underlying etiology.
- **NSAIDs or hormonal therapy first-line medical management.** NSAIDs started prior to pain onset & given for 2-3 days. Hormonal therapy: Estrogen-progestin contraceptive pills or Progestin only.
- **Laparoscopy: indicated if unresponsive to 3 cycles of initial therapy to rule out secondary causes** (most common causes of secondary in younger patients are PID & Endometriosis).

LEIOMYOMAS [UTERINE FIBROIDS, FIBROMYOMAS, MYOMAS]

- **Benign uterine smooth muscle tumors that derive from the muscle cells of the myometrium.**
- Most common benign gynecologic tumor. Only 20-25% become symptomatic.
- Types: Intramural, submucosal, subserosal, parasitic. Submucous myomas may become pedunculated and descend through the cervix into the vagina.
- **Growth is estrogen dependent** — may increase in size with relation to the menstrual cycle, anovulatory states, and during pregnancy; may regress after menopause.

RISK FACTORS

- **Increasing age (especially >35 years of age).** Early menarche (<10 years old), late Menopause.
- 5 times more common in black women.
- Nulliparity (1 or more pregnancy decreases risk), obesity, family history, Hypertension, alcohol use.

CLINICAL MANIFESTATIONS

- **[1] Asymptomatic: Most are asymptomatic** & found incidentally, especially if intramural.
- **[2] Abnormal uterine bleeding most common symptom (heavy, prolonged, or irregular). Submucosal myomas** most frequently cause significant heavy menstrual bleeding. Intramural.
- **[3] Pelvic pain/pressure:** lower back pain, pelvic pain, and/or menstrual pain. Pelvic pressure, abdominal bloating. **Menstrual cramps, Dysmenorrhea.** May cause urinary retention.
- **[4] Reproductive dysfunction: may affect fertility** by interfering with implantation (Myomas may significantly distort the uterine cavity), especially if submucosal or intramural. May cause miscarriages, affect pregnancy (eg, may grow), or impair uterine contractility postpartum.

Physical examination:

- Bimanual exam: **Normal or may have palpable discrete, firm, nontender, asymmetric (irregular contour) mobile enlarged mass or masses (heterogeneity) in the abdomen or pelvis.**

DIAGNOSIS

- **Transvaginal ultrasound: most widely used initial imaging test for suspected Fibroids.** Findings on TVUS — **focal heterogenic hypoechoic mass or masses with shadowing.**
- Beta hCG (rule out pregnancy); Iron deficiency anemia if associated with heavy bleeding.
- Hysteroscopy and Hysterosalpingography great at detecting submucosal lesions. MRI in some.

MANAGEMENT

- **Observation: majority don't need treatment, especially is small &/or asymptomatic.** Decision to treat is determined by symptoms, size/rate of tumor growth, & the desire for fertility.

Nonsurgical:

- **Estrogen-progestin oral contraceptives.** Levonorgestrel-releasing IUD (if cavity is not distorted)
- **NSAIDs for dysmenorrhea.** Tranexamic acid &/or NSAIDs may decrease menstrual blood loss.
- **GnRH analogs (Leuprolide, Nafarelin) are the most effective medical treatment but usually used [1] if near menopause or [2] to shrink fibroids 3-4 months prior to hysterectomy or myomectomy.**

SURGICAL MANAGEMENT

- **Myomectomy: surgical treatment of choice for women who wish to preserve fertility.**
- Other: Uterine artery embolization (may preserve fertility if Myomectomy is not an option) or Endometrial ablation; both may affect the ability to conceive. Focused ultrasound surgery.
- **Definitive treatment: Hysterectomy. Fibroids are most common cause for hysterectomy in the US.**

EXAM TIP:
- Asymptomatic women: observation & reassurance.
- **Symptomatic women who desire fertility: nonsurgical treatment or myomectomy.**
- Symptomatic women who do not desire fertility: options include nonsurgical treatment, Myomectomy, Myolysis, Uterine artery embolization, or Endometrial ablation.
- **Symptomatic women desiring definitive treatment: hysterectomy.**

UTERINE ADENOMYOSIS

- **Islands of ectopic endometrial tissue (glands and stroma) within the myometrium** (muscular layer of the uterine wall). May be associated with Endometriosis and Uterine fibroids.
- **Most commonly presents later in the reproductive years (35–50 years).**

PATHOPHYSIOLOGY
- The ectopic endometrial tissue may induce hypertrophy and hyperplasia of the surrounding myometrium, resulting in a diffusely enlarged uterus ("globular" enlargement).

CLINICAL MANIFESTATIONS
- **[1] Asymptomatic: most patients with Adenomyosis are asymptomatic.**
- **[2] Abnormal uterine bleeding: menorrhagia (heavy &/or prolonged)** progressively worsening.
- **[3] Dysmenorrhea:** painful menses (Secondary dysmenorrhea). May cause infertility.
- **[4] Pelvic pain/pressure: Chronic pelvic pain.** Dyspareunia.

Bimanual examination:
- **Symmetrically diffusely enlarged ("globular"), soft (boggy), mobile uterus (may be tender).**

FIBROIDS	**ADENOMYOSIS**
• **Benign uterine smooth muscle tumors of the myometrium**	• **Diffuse infiltration of the myometrium.**

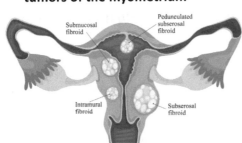
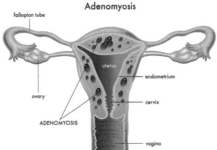

FIBROIDS	**ADENOMYOSIS**
• **Discrete <u>firm, nontender, asymmetric</u> (irregular contour)**	• **<u>Symmetrically</u> diffusely enlarged ("globular")**
• **<u>Firm, nontender</u> mobile** mass or masses	• **<u>Soft (boggy), may be tender</u> mobile.**

DIAGNOSIS
- Clinical diagnosis of exclusion of 2^{ry} amenorrhea (**rule out pregnancy with beta-hCG**, Endometriosis, & Fibroids) in a patient with classic symptoms (eg, heavy menstrual bleeding, dysmenorrhea) with characteristic findings on physical examination (enlarged boggy uterus that may be tender).
- **Transvaginal ultrasound often initial imaging of choice for evaluation of an enlarged uterus, pelvic pain, and/or abnormal bleeding.** Findings — diffusely enlarged heterogenous uterus, asymmetric thickening of the myometrium, poorly visualized endometrial-myometrial junction (JZ), absent vascular flow to the myometrial lesions, and cystic lesions in the myometrium.
- **MRI more accurate & useful when TVUS fails to elucidate a diagnosis.** MRI provides clearer visualization of the transition between endometrium and myometrium if treatment is planned.
- **Definitive diagnosis: Post-total abdominal hysterectomy examination of uterine tissue.**

MANAGEMENT
- **Conservative: used to preserve fertility — NSAIDs, progestins [(eg, Levonorgestrel-releasing intrauterine device (eg, LNG 52)] preferred hormonal treatment** (provides direct action on the uterus, anti-estrogen effect on the implants, and offers long-term effectiveness).
- Alternative hormonal treatment: Combined oral contraceptives, Aromatase inhibitors. GnRH agonists & antagonists have a rapid effect (may need hormonal add back therapy to reduce the hypoestrogenic effects of GnRH medications).
- **Total abdominal hysterectomy is the only effective therapy.** Uterine artery embolization.

ENDOMETRIAL (UTERINE) POLYPS

- **Usually benign focal hyperplastic overgrowth of endometrial glands and stroma that may protrude into the uterine cavity from the endometrium, either in a sessile or pedunculated form with a vascular core.**
- EPs are found in ~25% of the general population; the prevalence of EPs increases with age (peak incidence around the fourth decade of life).

RISK FACTORS
- More common in postmenopausal women. Hypertension and obesity.
- **Hormone dependent: Tissue grows in response to Estrogen.** Tamoxifen is associated with increased occurrence of EPs.

CLINICAL MANIFESTATIONS
- EPs are often asymptomatic and can often be found as an incidental finding on pelvic imaging; they may also be discovered as part of a workup for Abnormal uterine bleeding or infertility.
- **Irregular vaginal bleeding is the most frequent symptom at presentation (intermenstrual bleeding or spotting most common).** May result in postcoital bleeding, heavy menstrual bleeding.
- EPs are associated with decreased reproductive potential. Polypectomy improves pregnancy rates.

DIAGNOSIS
- **Transvaginal ultrasound often initial imaging of choice for evaluation of an enlarged uterus, pelvic pain, and/or abnormal bleeding.** Incidental polyps commonly seen on routine imaging for another reason.
- **Sonohysteroscopy (Saline infusion sonogram [SIS]) has the highest detection rate** or diagnostic hysteroscopy may be used for additional imaging in selected patients with an uncertain finding on TVUS, incomplete visualization of the endometrium, or in whom expectant management is planned.
- A definitive diagnosis of an Endometrial polyp is made based on histologic diagnosis of a specimen, usually collected at time of Polypectomy. Histologic evaluation used to rule out malignancy.

MANAGEMENT
- **Surgical management (eg, transcervical Polypectomy) is often curative** (eg, polyp forceps or with direct visual guidance using hysteroscopy resection).
- Medical treatment has not been shown to be effective for management of Endometrial polyps.

PROGNOSIS
- **Good: very low risk of malignancy (0.5% contain malignant cells), polypectomy is curative.**
- Polyps can rarely undergo hyperplasia and atypia. Endometrial polyps are more likely to be malignant in patients who are postmenopausal and those who present with bleeding.

CERVICAL POLYPS

- Cervical polyps commonly occur during the reproductive years, particularly after age 40 years. The etiology is unknown. **Usually <3 cm in diameter** with a long thin pedicle (may be short and broad).
- Clinical manifestations: most asymptomatic; may cause irregular or postcoital bleeding.
- Physical examination: tear-shaped or lobular structures appear red, purple, or flesh-colored, depending upon the vascularity and congestion, and are often shiny.
- Histologically, Cervical polyps are characterized by vascular connective tissue stroma covered by epithelium, which may be columnar, squamous, or squamocolumnar.

MANAGEMENT
- **Polyps should be removed (Polypectomy) if they are symptomatic (eg, bleeding, excessive discharge), large (≥3 cm), or appear atypical.** Malignancy is rare in a Cervical polyp (0.5%).
- Asymptomatic polyps in women <45 years of age may be left untreated.

ENDOMETRIOSIS

- **Implantation of endometrial tissue (stroma & gland) outside the uterus (ectopic tissue).**
- **Most common gynecologic cause of Secondary dysmenorrhea.**
- Affects up to 10% of women of reproductive age. Peak incidence 25–35 years of age.

LOCATIONS
- **Ovaries are the most common site of Endometriosis (>55%).**
- Anterior cul-de-sac (35%), Posterior broad ligaments (35%), Posterior cul-de-sac (34%), Uterosacral ligaments (28%). Less common sites include the rectosigmoid colon & bladder.

PATHOPHYSIOLOGY
- **The ectopic endometrial tissue responds to cyclical hormonal changes (estrogen-stimulated inflammatory response) — symptoms usually improve during pregnancy and after menopause;** they can recur postpartum or with postmenopausal hormone replacement therapy.

RISK FACTORS
- **Prolonged estrogen exposure** — eg, **nulliparity,** late first pregnancy, early menarche (before 11-13y), short menstrual cycles. Other risks include family history, prolonged or heavy menstruation.
- Reduced risk: Regular exercise (>4 hours per week), higher parity, late menarche (after 14 years), and longer duration of lactation are all associated with a decreased risk for Endometriosis.

CLINICAL MANIFESTATIONS
- **Classic triad: ❶ cyclic premenstrual pelvic pain** (1-2 weeks before menstruation),
  ❷ dysmenorrhea (painful menstruation), and **❸ dyspareunia** (deep thrust painful intercourse).
- **Pelvic or low sacral pain** or pressure both related to menses and at times other than menses. Pain often begins 1-2 weeks prior to menses, peaks 1-2 days before. and relieved soon after flow onset.
- **Abnormal bleeding** (pre- or postmenstrual spotting, heavy menstrual bleeding).
- Bowel or bladder dysfunction: **dyschezia (painful defecation) or dysuria.**
- **May cause infertility** — prevalence of 30–47% among infertile women. Ovarian mass in some.

Physical examination:
- Highly variable: Often normal; may have a fixed tender adnexal mass, fixed retroverted uterus or nodular masses along thick uterosacral ligaments; posterior uterus, or laterally displaced cervix.

DIAGNOSIS: Clinical diagnosis.
- **Pelvic ultrasound initial imaging of choice to rule out other causes** (not to diagnose Endometriosis).
- **Laparoscopy with biopsy definitive diagnosis,** allows for definitive histological examination:
  - Raised, patches of thickened, discolored scarred or "powder burn" appearing implants of tissue.
  - **Endometrioma** — Endometriosis involving the ovaries large enough to be considered a tumor, usually filled with old blood appearing chocolate-colored **("chocolate cyst").**

MEDICAL (CONSERVATIVE) MANAGEMENT:
- **Asymptomatic or mild symptoms: Expectant management.** Pain: **NSAIDs may be used.**
- **Ovulation suppression** — combined oral contraceptive pills first-line in most women; Progestins (eg, pills, Levonorgestrel-releasing IUD, depot MPA) to inhibit endometrial tissue growth.
- **More severe or refractory symptoms: GnRH agonist (eg, Leuprolide) or antagonist (eg, Elagolix).** Add back therapy (eg, Norethindrone acetate) may prevent some of the hypoestrogenic adverse effects of GnRH meds, especially menopause-like symptoms & loss of bone mineral density.
- Aromatase inhibitors (eg, Anastrozole, Letrozole) + Progestins if refractory to GnRH agonist. AIs regulate estrogen formation in the ectopic tissue. Danazol is an androgen that is rarely used.

SURGICAL MANAGEMENT
- **Conservative laparoscopy with ablation of ectopic endometrial tissue used if fertility desired or in severe disease** — preserves the uterus & ovaries and improves pregnancy rates.
- Cystectomy for large Endometriomas often used. Nerve transection procedures for refractory pain.
- Definitive management: Total abdominal hysterectomy and bilateral salpingo-oophorectomy.

MENOPAUSE

- **Cessation of menses >1 year due to loss of ovarian function, leading to decreased estrogen & progesterone production. Average age in the US is 50-52 years.** Premature if it occurs <40 years.
- Perimenopause refers to the time period preceding menopause when fertility wanes and menstrual cycle irregularity increases.

CLINICAL MANIFESTATIONS

- **Estrogen deficiency** — menstrual cycle alterations, vasomotor instability (including **hot flashes most common perimenopausal symptom, night sweats, palpitations), sleep disturbances, mood changes**, skin, nail, & hair changes, increased cardiovascular events, hyperlipidemia, Osteoporosis, dyspareunia (painful intercourse), vaginal atrophy, & urinary incontinence.

Physical examination:
- Decreased bone density; dry & thin skin with decreased elasticity.
- Vaginal atrophy with thin mucosa. Decrease in breast size.

COMPLICATIONS

- Loss of estrogen's protective effects: Osteoporosis, Dyslipidemia, & increased cardiovascular risk.

DIAGNOSIS

- **FSH assay most sensitive initial test** (increased serum FSH >30 IU/mL). Not required for diagnosis.
- **Increased LH; decreased estradiol** <20 pg/mL.
- Androstenedione levels don't change much.
- Estrone is the predominant estrogen after menopause (the adrenal gland is the major source).

MANAGEMENT OF VASOMOTOR INSUFFICIENCY & HOT FLASHES

- Mild symptoms: smoking cessation, dressing in layers, weight loss, alcohol reduction, stress reduction.
- **Hormone replacement therapy:** risks vs. benefits must be considered. **Estrogen only (if no uterus) Estrogen + Progestin (if uterus still present).**
- 2nd-line: SSRIs (eg, Paroxetine), SNRIs, or Gabapentin if contraindication to hormonal therapy.

GENITOURINARY SYNDROME OF MENOPAUSE (VULVOVAGINAL ATROPHY)

- **Seen in hypoestrogenic states (eg, Menopause,** postpartum lactation, and postpartum women, progesterone-only or low-dose oral contraceptives). Hypoestrogenism may cause changes of the labia majora/minora, clitoris, vestibule/introitus, vagina, urethra, and bladder.

CLINICAL MANIFESTATIONS

- **Vulvovaginal dryness, dyspareunia** (decreased lubrication during sex), vaginal inflammation (burning, irritation, pruritus), infection, & recurrent UTIs (urgency, dysuria) with increased pH (loss of lactobacilli which normally converts glucose to lactic acid). Decreased sexual arousal.
- The vaginal rugae progressively flatten and the epithelium thins. Pale dry shiny epithelium. Brownish vaginal discharge may be noted.

MANAGEMENT

- **Vaginal moisturizers: (eg, water soluble lubricants) improves symptoms (eg, dyspareunia, dryness) but have no effect on atrophy.**
- **Topical vaginal estrogens safest, most effective medical therapy** — conjugated Estrogens (cream) and Estradiol (cream, troches, capsule, & ring). Also helpful for recurrent UTIs. Adverse effects: vaginal bleeding, breast pain, nausea, thromboembolism (CVA, DVT, PE) because estrogen increases hepatic production of coagulation factors, but less risk compared to oral (systemic) estrogen.
- Intravaginal dehydroepiandrosterone: improves dyspareunia, vaginal dryness, vaginal pH.
- **Ospemifene:** selective estrogen receptor modulator (SERM) that is an **estrogen agonist in the vagina & bone** and an estrogen antagonist in the breast & uterus. Used in moderate to severe cases.

HORMONAL REPLACEMENT THERAPY (HRT)

- **Estrogen only (if no uterus)**
- **Estrogen + Progestin (if uterus is still present).**

INDICATIONS FOR HRT:

- **Healthy woman <60 years for menopause symptom relief** (eg, vasomotor symptoms, mood changes, vaginal atrophy). **Combination OCPs decrease Endometrial cancer risk.**
- **Decreases Osteoporosis risk** — increases bone mineral density & decreases fracture risk.

RISKS OF HRT:

- Venous thromboembolism: DVT or Pulmonary embolism. Increased risk of gallstones.
- **Endometrial cancer (estrogen only).**
- Increased Breast cancer risk with estrogen-progestin therapy (controversial).
- May increase the risk of coronary artery disease, MI, & stroke.

CONTRAINDICATIONS TO HORMONAL THERAPY:

- Women with increased risk of cardiovascular disease (eg, stroke TIA, CHD), thromboembolic disease (venous or arterial), stroke; Endometrial cancer, Breast cancer, or other estrogen-dependent cancer. Unexplained vaginal bleeding.
- History of liver dysfunction or disease. Untreated Hypertension.

TAMOXIFEN

MECHANISM OF ACTION:

- Selective estrogen receptor modulator (SERM).
- **Tamoxifen is an estrogen antagonist in the breast but an estrogen agonist in the endometrium bone,** liver, & coagulation system.

INDICATIONS:

- **Breast cancer treatment & prevention:** Adjuvant treatment in estrogen & progesterone receptor-positive Breast cancer; Breast cancer prevention.
- **Osteoporosis prevention in postmenopausal women.**

ADVERSE EFFECTS:

- **Increased risk of Endometrial cancer, venous thromboembolism, hot flashes** (induces menopause), & ocular toxicity.

RALOXIFENE

MECHANISM OF ACTION:

- Selective estrogen receptor modulator (SERM).
- **Raloxifene is an estrogen agonist in the bone and liver but an estrogen antagonist in the breast & endometrium.**

INDICATIONS:

- **Breast cancer prevention in high-risk women & Osteoporosis prevention** in postmenopausal women.
- **Because it is an estrogen antagonist in the endometrium, Raloxifene is <u>not</u> associated with increased Endometrial cancer (unlike Tamoxifen, which an estrogen agonist in the uterus)**
  Raloxifene "relaxes" the uterus (no cancer risk); Tamoxifen is "toxic" to the uterus (increased risk).

ADVERSE EFFECTS:

- Weight gain
- Thromboembolic events (less than Tamoxifen)
- Hot flashes (induces Menopause)

MENOPAUSE
Vasomotor symptoms

Mild symptoms:
eg, hot flashes that do not interfere with daily activities

Moderate to severe symptoms

Contraindications to Estrogen?*

Yes   No

Behavioral modifications
- smoking cessation
- dressing in layers
- weight loss
- alcohol reduction
- Stress reduction

Nonhormonal therapy:
- **SSRIs** (eg, Paroxetine)
- Gabapentin, SNRIs

Hormone replacement therapy:
risks vs. benefits must be considered
Intact uterus?

Yes   No

Contraindications to Estrogen*
- Endometrial cancer (estrogen only), Breast cancer
- CVD: heart disease, untreated HTN, TIA, stroke
- Liver disease, Thromboembolism

Estrogen and Progestin   **Estrogen only**

ENDOMETRITIS

- **Infection of the decidua (pregnancy endometrium).**
- **Usually polymicrobial:** often vaginal flora, aerobic, & anaerobic bacteria.

RISK FACTORS
- **Postpartum or postabortal uterine infection — Cesarean section biggest risk factor,** especially when performed after the onset of labor.
- **Prolonged rupture of membranes (>24 hours),** operative vaginal delivery, dilation & curettage (or evacuation), excessive number of digital vaginal examinations, **prolonged labor (>12 hours).**
- Chorioamnionitis (fetal membrane infection). Coitus near term, preexisting Vaginitis or Cervicitis.

DIAGNOSIS
- **Mainly a clinical diagnosis** at least 2 of the following 3 — **[1] fever (>38°C)/100.4°F) often with tachycardia, [2] soft & tender uterus + uterine or lower abdominal pain 2-3 days after C-section, postpartum, or postabortal** (may present later), **& [3] purulent drainage from uterus.**
- May have vaginal bleeding or discharge (**foul-smelling lochia**). Cervical or uterine motion tenderness.
- Laboratory: elevated neutrophil count (leukocytosis). Elevated lactic acid is severe.

MANAGEMENT POST C-SECTION:
- **Clindamycin + Gentamicin first-line** (Clindamycin covers gram + & anaerobes; Gent gram-negatives). **May add Ampicillin** for additional coverage of Group B *Streptococcus* & *Enterococcus spp.*
- **Ampicillin-sulbactam is an alternative to Clindamycin + Gentamicin.**

MANAGEMENT AFTER VAGINAL DELIVERY OR CHORIOAMNIONITIS:
- Ampicillin + Gentamicin.

PREVENTION (PROPHYLAXIS)
- **C-section: First-generation Cephalosporin (eg, Cefazolin) x 1 dose within 60 minutes prior to the skin incision may be given to reduce the incidence of post C-section Endometritis** in addition to vaginal preparation with an antiseptic solution (eg, Povidone-Iodine, Chlorhexidine).

AMENORRHEA

PRIMARY AMENORRHEA

- Failure of menarche onset by age 15 years (in the presence of secondary sex characteristics) OR age 13 years (in the absence of secondary sex characteristics).

WORKUP
- **All women with Primary amenorrhea undergo hCG & FSH testing. TSH & prolactin level.**
- **If increased FSH & little breast development, Karyotyping to rule out Turner's syndrome.**
- **If FSH is normal and the ultrasound indicates that the uterus is absent, the probable diagnosis is Müllerian agenesis or Androgen insensitivity syndrome.** In Müllerian agenesis, the circulating testosterone is in the normal range for women; In Androgen insensitivity, the circulating testosterone is in the male range and testes may be present on exam or on ultrasound.
- If the FSH is normal, breast development is present, and the ultrasound or MRI detects accumulated blood in the uterus (hematometra) or vagina (hematocolpos), an obstructed outflow tract is present.
- If the FSH is low or normal and the uterus is present: delay of puberty, congenital GnRH deficiency, or some of the common causes of secondary amenorrhea that may also cause primary amenorrhea.

	UTERUS PRESENT	UTERUS ABSENT
BREAST PRESENT	**Outflow obstruction:** - Transverse vaginal septum - Imperforate hymen	• Müllerian agenesis (46 XX) • Androgen insensitivity (46 XY)
BREAST ABSENT	• **Elevated: ↑FSH, ↑LH = Ovarian causes** - Premature ovarian failure (46XX) - **Gonadal dysgenesis (eg, Turner's 45XO)** • **Normal or Low ↓FSH, ↓LH** - **Hypothalamus-Pituitary Failure** - Puberty delay: (eg, athletes, illness, anorexia) - Congenital GnRH deficiency	Rare. Usually caused by a defect in testosterone synthesis. Presents like a phenotypic immature girl with primary amenorrhea (will often have intrabdominal testes).

SECONDARY AMENORRHEA

- **Absence of menses for >3 months in a patient with previously normal menstruation**
  or >6 months in a patient who previously had irregular menses.

ETIOLOGIES
- **Pregnancy is the most common cause of Secondary amenorrhea.** Hypo- or Hyperthyroidism.
- **Hypothalamus dysfunction: functional hypothalamic amenorrhea** — puberty delay due (eg, **athletes,** illness, anorexia). **The female athlete triad: [1] hypothalamic amenorrhea, [2] low energy** (with or without an eating disorder), **& [3] decreased bone mineral density** (BMD) due to loss of bone protection by estrogen. FHA can cause primary or secondary amenorrhea.
- **Pituitary dysfunction: Prolactinoma** or Pituitary infarct (Sheehan syndrome).
  Associated with **decreased FSH, LH, & estrogen.**
- **Ovarian dysfunction: decreased estrogen + increased FSH & LH.** Polycystic ovarian syndrome. Premature ovarian failure: follicular failure or follicular resistance to LH or FSH. Turner syndrome. May have symptoms of estrogen deficiency (similar to Menopause).
- **Uterine dysfunction: Asherman's syndrome = acquired endometrial scarring** secondary to postpartum hemorrhage, after dilation & curettage (D & C) or endometrial infection. **Pelvic ultrasound — absence of the normal uterine stripe.** Hysteroscopy.

WORKUP
- **Beta-hCG (to rule out pregnancy) is the best initial test for Amenorrhea.**
- If hCG negative and no evidence of hyperandrogenism, order serum prolactin, FSH, estradiol (E2), & TSH to rule out Hyperprolactinemia, Ovarian failure, and thyroid disease respectively.
- Testosterone measured if evidence of hirsutism or hyperandrogenism.

ENDOMETRIAL HYPERPLASIA

- Endometrial gland proliferation with cytologic atypia. **Precursor to Endometrial carcinoma.**

RISK FACTORS
- **Prolonged unopposed estrogen** (unopposed by progesterone) — chronic anovulation, **estrogen-only therapy,** Polycystic ovary syndrome, **obesity,** perimenopause, early menarche, late menopause, Lynch syndrome, & **Tamoxifen.** Hyperplasia occurs within 3y of estrogen-only therapy.
- **Increasing age: peaks 50-60 years**, perimenopausal, or early postmenopausal women.

CLINICAL MANIFESTATIONS
- **Abnormal uterine bleeding:** menorrhagia, metrorrhagia, postmenopausal, unscheduled (on HRT).
- May be associated with a vaginal discharge. Asymptomatic (may be detected on cervical cytology).

DIAGNOSIS
- **Transvaginal ultrasound** screening test — **thickened endometrial stripe >4 mm.**
  If <4 mm and increased suspicion, endometrial biopsy & sampling may be performed.
- **Endometrial biopsy definitive diagnosis** — indicated if >35y, increased endometrial stripe seen on TVUS, patients on unopposed estrogen therapy, Tamoxifen, persistent bleeding with thick stripe.

MANAGEMENT
- **Hyperplasia without atypia: Progestin (LNG 52 IUD or oral).** Repeat endometrial biopsy in 3-6 months. Progesterone has an antiproliferative effect on the endometrium & can induce endometrial apoptosis.
- **Hyperplasia with atypia** (Endometrial intraepithelial neoplasia [EIN]): **total abdominal hysterectomy. Progestin treatment if not a surgical candidate or if patient wishes to preserve fertility.**

ENDOMETRIAL CANCER

- **Most common gynecologic malignancy in the US** (2 times more common than Cervical cancer).
- **Adenocarcinoma most common type (>80%).** Papillary serous 10%, clear cell 5%, adenosquamous 2% and mucinous 2%.
- **Mainly affects postmenopausal women (75%) — peaks 60-70-years of age.** Perimenopausal 25%.
- Estrogen-dependent cancer in most — associated with antecedent Endometrial hyperplasia.

RISK FACTORS
- **Increased estrogen exposure:** increased ovulatory cycles (eg, nulliparity, early menarche, late Menopause), **chronic anovulation, Polycystic ovary syndrome**, obesity, estrogen-only hormonal therapy, & **Tamoxifen.** Other risks: Diabetes mellitus, Hypertension, & Lynch syndrome (HNPCC).
- **Decreased risk: Combination OCPs (Estrogen + Progesterone) are protective against both Ovarian & Endometrial cancers** (progesterone component prevents unopposed estrogen).

CLINICAL MANIFESTATIONS
- **Abnormal uterine bleeding:** postmenopausal bleeding, pre or perimenopausal bleeding — menorrhagia or metrorrhagia, including prolonged or heavy bleeding.

DIAGNOSIS
- **Transvaginal ultrasound** — thickened endometrial stripe >4 mm. Pap smear also performed.
- **Endometrial biopsy definitive diagnosis.** Hysteroscopy + Endocervical curettage (D&C) alternative.
- Pap smear may show abnormal glandular cells or atypical endometrial cells, needing further evaluation.

MANAGEMENT
- **Stage I: total abdominal hysterectomy with bilateral salpingo-oophorectomy**. May need post-op radiation therapy. Most are well differentiated (one of the most curable gynecologic cancers).
- Stage II, III: TAH-BSO + lymph node excision with or without post-op radiation therapy.
- Stage IV (advanced): systemic chemotherapy. Recurrence: high-dose Progestins or antiestrogens.

POST MENOPAUSAL BLEEDING

ETIOLOGIES
- **Usually benign** (eg, vaginal/endometrial atrophy, cervical polyps, submucosal fibroids).
- **10% due to Endometrial cancer**.
- ANY postmenopausal bleeding in a woman not on HRT (or on HRT with abnormal bleeding) should raise suspicion for Endometrial carcinoma, hyperplasia, or Leiomyosarcoma.

DIAGNOSIS
- **Transvaginal ultrasound usually initial diagnostic test.** If endometrial stripe <4 mm, repeat ultrasound in 4 months. If continued bleeding, biopsy should be performed.
- **Endometrial biopsy if stripe >4 mm.**
- Hysteroscopy may be warranted if focal thickening of endometrium.

UTERINE PROLAPSE

- Uterine herniation into or beyond the vagina.

RISK FACTORS
- **Weakness of pelvic support structures: most common after childbirth** (especially traumatic), increased pelvic floor pressure: multiple vaginal births, obesity, repeated heavy lifting, increased age, constipation.

CLINICAL MANIFESTATIONS
- Pelvic or vaginal fullness, pressure, heaviness, bulging, or "falling out" sensation (eg, protrusion of tissue from the vagina).
- Low back pain, abdominal pain.
- Symptoms may be worse with prolonged standing and relieved with lying down.
- Urinary urgency, frequency, or stress incontinence. Sexual dysfunction.

PHYSICAL EXAMINATION
- Bulging mass especially with increased intrabdominal pressure (eg Valsalva).
- Grades: 0 (no descent) to 4 (through the hymen).
- Grade 0: no descent
- Grade 1: uterus descent into the upper 2/3 of the vagina
- Grade 2: the cervix approaches the introitus
- Grade 3: the cervix is outside the introitus
- Grade 4: entire uterus is outside of the vagina – complete rupture
May be accompanied by
- **Cystocele:** posterior bladder herniating into the **anterior vagina,**
- **Enterocele:** pouch of Douglas – small bowel herniating into the **upper vagina,** or
- **Rectocele:** distal sigmoid colon or rectum herniating into the **posterior distal vagina.**

CONSERVATIVE MANAGEMENT
- **Kegel exercises (pelvic floor muscle exercises),** behavioral modifications, weight control.
- Vaginal pessaries elevate & support the uterus.
- Estrogen treatment may improve atrophy.
- Treatment is generally not indicated for women with asymptomatic prolapse.

SURGICAL MANAGEMENT
- Hysterectomy or uterus-sparing techniques including uterosacral or sacrospinous ligament fixation.
- Vaginal and abdominal approaches (open, laparoscopic, or robotic) and with and without graft materials.

PHYSIOLOGIC (FUNCTIONAL) OVARIAN CYST

- **Fluid-filled sac within the ovaries most commonly related to ovulation** (usually unilateral).
- Common in reproductive years. **Most spontaneously resolve within a few weeks.**

TYPES
- **Follicular cysts most common** — occur when follicles fail to rupture & continue to grow.
- **Corpus luteal cysts:** occur when the corpus luteum fails to degenerate after ovulation.
- Theca Lutein cysts: excess beta-hCG causes hyperplasia of theca interna cells (rare).

CLINICAL MANIFESTATIONS
- **Most are asymptomatic;** Pelvic pain/pressure, abnormal uterine bleeding, dyspareunia, or torsion.
- Physical examination: unilateral pelvic pain or tenderness. ±mobile palpable cystic adnexal mass.

DIAGNOSIS
- **Transvaginal ultrasound: Follicular** — smooth, thin-walled unilocular, anechoic. **Corpus luteal** — complex, thicker-walled with peripheral vascularity seen with Doppler (ring of fire).
  - **Low risk for malignancy: anechoic, unilocular, fluid-filled cysts.**
  - High-risk for malignancy: solid, nodular, thick septations are high-risk for malignancy.
- Order hCG to rule out pregnancy.
- Suspicious for malignancy: tumor markers (eg, CA-125, alpha-fetoprotein, hCG).

- **Management if <8 cm: Supportive & expectant management** — most cysts <8 cm are functional **& usually spontaneously resolve within 60 days without treatment. Rest, NSAIDs, repeat ultrasound after 1-2 cycles.** OCPs may prevent recurrence but don't treat existing ones.
- **Management if >8 cm or persistent: surgical excision** — options include laparoscopy or laparotomy.

Management if postmenopausal:
- Options include laparoscopy or laparotomy if large or if tumor marker CA-125 is elevated.
- Cysts in postmenopausal women are considered to be malignant until proven otherwise.

RUPTURED PHYSIOLOGIC OVARIAN CYST

- **Acute pelvic or abdominal pain** — **abrupt onset of unilateral lower quadrant abdominal pain, often sharp & focal, often occurring during sexual activity or strenuous physical activity.** May be associated with pelvic pain/tenderness or adnexal mass. Pain & abnormal uterine bleeding + adnexal mass may be due to ovarian cyst rupture, adnexal torsion, or ruptured ectopic pregnancy.

DIAGNOSIS
- **Transvaginal ultrasound: initial test** — **adnexal mass + pelvic fluid in patients with symptoms consistent with rupture** (fluid can be a normal finding). Beta-hCG, CBC, & other testing performed.

Differential diagnosis:
- **Adnexal torsion** classically presents with an abrupt onset of severe pelvic pain, often accompanied by **nausea and vomiting.** May have signs of hemodynamic compromise if massive bleeding (rare).
- **Tubo-ovarian abscess: fever, chills, acute lower abdominal pain, vaginal discharge, & adnexal mass.** Pelvic imaging — complex multilocular mass that obliterates normal adnexal architecture.

MANAGEMENT
- **Uncomplicated: expectant management for most ruptured Ovarian cysts** — **observation, analgesics, & rest.** Uncomplicated = absence of all of the following: hemodynamic instability, large volume or ongoing blood loss, fever, leukocytosis, or suspicion of malignancy.
- Stable + significant hemoperitoneum: hospitalization, close observation, & fluid replacement.
- **Hemodynamically unstable or ongoing hemorrhage: laparoscopy usually preferred over laparotomy.** Cystectomy (preservation of tissue) preferred over oophorectomy if premenopausal.
- Prompt intervention for torsion (detorsion if the ovary is still viable) & Tubo-ovarian abscess.

OVARIAN TORSION

- **Complete or partial rotation of the ovary on its ligamental supports [eg, infundibulopelvic (suspensory) ligament], resulting in ischemia that can compromise ovarian blood flow.** Prolonged ischemia may lead to infarction of the affected ovary.

Risk factors:
- **Ovarian mass most common** — usually a mechanical complication of Functional ovarian cysts or Ovarian neoplasm (especially if >5 cm). May occur without a mass, especially in the pediatric population.
- Infertility treatment with ovulation induction.

CLINICAL MANIFESTATIONS
- **Acute pelvic or abdominal pain — abrupt onset of unilateral lower quadrant abdominal pain, often sharp & focal, often accompanied by nausea and/or vomiting.** A history of recent vigorous activity or a sudden increase in abdominal pressure may be an inciting event.

Physical examination:
- **Ovarian enlargement, abdominal tenderness, adnexal mass.** Hemodynamic compromise (severe).

DIAGNOSIS
- **Transvaginal ultrasound with Doppler initial test of choice — decreased ovarian blood flow. Normal flow does not exclude torsion, so definitive diagnosis is made during surgical exploration** & direct visualization of a rotated ovary via laparoscopy. MRI.
- **Definitive diagnosis is made via direct visualization of a rotated ovary via laparoscopy.**

MANAGEMENT
- **Laparoscopy with detorsion, salvage of the involved adnexa,** resection of any associated cyst or tumor, and oophoropexy are treatment goals. Ovarian cystectomy may be needed to remove the causative cyst & preserve the ovary in premenopausal women with benign mass.
- Salpingo-oophorectomy: if necrotic, high suspicion for malignancy, or in postmenopausal women.

BENIGN OVARIAN NEOPLASMS

- 90% of ovarian neoplasms are benign in women of reproductive age. Risk of malignancy ↑'es with age.

TYPES
- Surface epithelial tumors, stromal tumors, and germ cell tumors. Endometriomas in Endometriosis.
- **Dermoid ovarian cyst (mature cystic teratoma) is the most common benign ovarian neoplasm** — may contain tissue derived from all 3 germ cell layers (eg, sebaceous fluid, hair, bone, teeth etc.). Has small malignant potential (0.2–2%).
- Serous or mucinous cystadenoma: They are thin walled, uni- or multilocular, and range in size from 5 cm to <20 cm. Compared with serous cystadenomas, mucinous cystadenomas occur less frequently, are more likely to be multiloculated, are larger, and are less often bilateral (<5% versus 20–25%).

CLINICAL MANIFESTATIONS
- Generally asymptomatic — usually an incidental finding on pelvic examination or imaging.
- May lead to ovarian torsion, rupture, or infection; Teratomas may undergo malignant transformation.

Physical examination:
- Normal or may have adnexal fullness.

DIAGNOSIS
- **Pelvic ultrasound: initial imaging of choice of an adnexal mass** — cystic structure that may contain calcifications & hyperechoic nodules. Mature cystic teratoma: a unilocular cystic mass, which may contain hyperechoic contents, hyperechoic lines or dots, fluid, and acoustic shadowing.

MANAGEMENT
- **Surgical removal (laparoscopic cystectomy preferred)** due to potential risk of torsion or malignant transformation. Salpingo-oophorectomy is another option.

POLYCYSTIC OVARY SYNDROME (PCOS) [STEIN-LEVENTHAL SYNDROME]

- **Characterized by [1] bilateral enlarged cystic ovaries, [2] insulin resistance, [3] hyperandrogenism, & [4] amenorrhea or oligomenorrhea. May cause infertility.**
- Untreated PCOS is associated with **increased risk of metabolic syndrome, Diabetes mellitus,** cardiovascular disease, dyslipidemia, **Endometrial hyperplasia, and Endometrial cancer.**

PATHOPHYSIOLOGY

- Ovarian hormonal dysregulation alters the pulsatile gonadotropin-releasing hormone (GnRH) release, leading to relative increase in LH versus Follicle-stimulating hormone (FSH) production & secretion.
- **Increased LH stimulates excess ovarian androgen production**; relative decrease of FSH prevents adequate stimulation of aromatase activity within granulosa cells, decreasing androgen conversion to potent estrogen estradiol, leading to follicular degeneration & immature follicles (cysts).
- **Functional ovarian hyperandrogenism causes insulin-resistant hyperinsulinism,** which acts on theca cells, increasing steroidogenesis, androgen production, and may cause obesity.

CLINICAL MANIFESTATIONS

- Many patients are asymptomatic. May seek care due to infertility.
- **Menstrual dysfunction: oligomenorrhea or secondary amenorrhea.** Chronic anovulation may result in abnormal uterine bleeding.
- **Increased androgen: hirsutism** (coarse hair on face, neck, & abdomen; acne, male pattern baldness).
- **Insulin resistance: type II Diabetes mellitus, obesity,** & Hypertension.

PHYSICAL EXAMINATION

- Bilateral enlarged, smooth, mobile ovaries on bimanual examination. Acanthosis nigricans.

DIAGNOSIS

- **Rotterdam criteria (2 of 3): ❶ hyperandrogenism:** labs or clinical (eg, hirsutism, male-pattern baldness, acne), **❷ ovulatory dysfunction:** amenorrhea, oligomenorrhea, & **❸ cystic ovaries on Ultrasound.**
- **Labs:** ↑serum total testosterone, ↑LH:FSH ratio ≥3:1. Lipid panel, glucose tolerance test (for DM), estradiol levels, TSH, prolactin, early morning 17-hydroxyprogesterone.
- **Transvaginal ultrasound:** bilateral enlarged ovaries & multiple ovarian cysts with a "string of pearls" appearance.
- GnRH agonist stimulation test: rise in serum hydroxyprogesterone.

MANAGEMENT

- **Lifestyle changes: diet, exercise, and weight reduction** can decrease insulin resistance & regulate the menstrual cycle, promoting ovulation & increasing fertility.
- **Combination oral contraceptives mainstay of treatment in patients not actively trying to get pregnant for the management of menstrual cycle irregularity, hirsutism, & acne.**
- Intermittent or continuous progestins for endometrial protection (eg, Progestin IUD) thins the endometrium.
- Anti-androgenic agents: **Spironolactone (blocks testosterone receptors) may be added if symptoms persist after OCPs.** Leuprolide & Finasteride are other anti-androgenics.

INFERTILITY

- **Letrozole or Clomiphene first-line for ovulation induction.** Letrozole encourages ovaries to ovulate by blocking estrogen production, causing higher FSH release. **Letrozole associated with higher ovulation & effective live birth rates than either Clomiphene or Metformin in PCOS.**
- **Clomiphene: Selective estrogen receptor modulator (SERM) that reestablishes ovulation** in anovulatory women who wish to get pregnant (second-line alternative to Letrozole).
- **Metformin** adjuvant treatment in patients with abnormal LH:FSH ratios may improve menstrual function. After pregnancy is confirmed, it may be discontinued.
- Wedge resection may help to restore ovulation if Clomiphene or Letrozole is ineffective.

OVARIAN CANCER

- 5th most common cancer in American women.
- 2nd most common gynecologic cancer with the **highest mortality of all the gynecologic cancers**.
- **Epithelial cell cancer most common type (>80%)**, seen especially postmenopausal.

RISK FACTORS
- **Increased number of ovulatory cycles** (eg, **nulliparity**, infertility, **>50 years** (40-65y), **early menarche, late menopause)**, family history (7% lifetime risk instead of normal 1-2%), Caucasians.
- Genetic: **BRCA-1 or BRCA-2** (15-40%), Peutz-Jehgers, Turner's syndrome, Lynch syndrome (HNPCC).
- **Decreased risk: Oral contraceptives** (decrease # of ovulatory cycles), breastfeeding, parity, tubal ligation, hysterectomy, bilateral salpingo-oophorectomy.

CLINICAL MANIFESTATIONS
- **Rarely symptomatic until late in the disease course** (extensive METS). Pelvic pressure &/or pain.
- GI/pelvic: abdominal fullness, bloating, or distention; **increasing abdominal girth, back or abdominal pain, early satiety, weight loss**; constipation or bowel obstruction (intestinal compression).
- Urinary urgency or frequency. Irregular menses, menorrhagia, postmenopausal bleeding.

Physical examination:
- **Palpable abdominal or ovarian mass (solid, fixed, irregular).**
- **Ascites,** pleural effusion, Sister Mary Joseph's node (METS to the umbilical lymph nodes).

DIAGNOSIS
- **Pelvic ultrasound initial imaging of choice** — >10 cm complex adnexal mass, irregularity, ascites.
- Additional workups include staging imaging (eg, CT scan of the abdomen & pelvis), baseline CA-125 levels, mammography, chest radiograph, Pap smear, & colonoscopy. MRI used in some.

MANAGEMENT
- **Stage I: surgical removal — Total abdominal hysterectomy + Bilateral salpingo-oophorectomy + selective lymphadenectomy & omentectomy.** Histological diagnosis during surgical removal.
- **Stage II–IV: surgical removal followed by platinum-based chemotherapy — either Cisplatin or Carboplatin + Paclitaxel** (Bevacizumab may be added if high risk). Cisplatin + Cyclophosphamide.
- **Serum CA-125 levels is the tumor biomarker often used to monitor treatment progress.**
- **Poor prognosis:** Ovarian cancer presents late in the disease course and is usually metastatic.

BARTHOLIN ABSCESS & CYST

- Bartholin glands located in the 4 and 8 o'clock positions on each side of the labia minora.

CLINICAL MANIFESTATIONS
- **Noninfected (Cyst): soft, nontender,** unilateral vulvar mass (1-3 cm) at the posterior aspect of the vaginal introitus at the site of the Bartholin gland (blockage leads to mucous-filled cyst formation). **Usually painless; may cause vaginal discomfort with walking, sitting, or sexual intercourse.**
- **Infected gland (Abscess): Localized pain & tenderness, dyspareunia. Unilateral soft, tender, warm, erythematous, edematous, pointing or fluctuant mass** at the location of the Bartholin duct and gland if the cyst becomes infected. *E. coli* **most common pathogen.**

DIAGNOSIS: Clinical; culture of drained fluid if infected. Biopsy if risk for carcinoma (increased age, palpable solid mass, fixation of cyst to surrounding tissue, refractory to treatment.

MANAGEMENT
- **Small cyst: expectant management.** Sitz baths, warm compresses, or analgesics if symptomatic.
- **Small abscess (<3cm): Incision & drainage under local anesthesia.** Antibiotics not needed in most.
- **Large mass (≥3 cm)** — large Bartholin cysts and abscesses should undergo **I&D** to allow evacuation of the mass contents; cultures of the cyst contents if infected + **Word catheter placement** to keep the tract open to allow for continued drainage. Antibiotic therapy if severe infection or if risk factors or for recurrent abscesses. Marsupialization may be needed at a later date.

VULVAR LICHEN SCLEROSUS (LS)

- Benign, chronic, progressive, dermatologic condition characterized by marked inflammation, epithelial thinning, and classic dermal changes that are often accompanied by pruritus and pain.
- **Vulvar LS is the most common nonneoplastic epithelial vulvar disorder, especially in [1] women >60 years & [2] prepubescent children. <u>LS affects the skin in the genital & anal areas</u>.**

CLINICAL MANIFESTATIONS
- **<u>Intense vulvar pruritus</u>** may be so intense it can interfere with sleep. May be asymptomatic.
- Pruritus ani, painful defecation, rectal bleeding, dyspareunia, or dysuria.

Physical examination:
- **The classic finding is <u>thin, white, wrinkled vulvar skin with a cigarette paper appearance</u> localized to the labia minora and/or labia majora. The whitening may extend over the perineum to the perianal area.** Lichenification, hyperkeratosis, hypopigmentation, or atrophy.
- Areas of epithelial hyperplasia, erosions, and ulcerations from chronic rubbing/scratching often seen.
- Fissuring is often present on anogenital skin (perianally, in the interlabial folds, or around the clitoris).
- Agglutination of the anterior parts of the labia minora of both sides to cover the clitoris.

DIAGNOSIS
- The diagnosis of vulvar LS is often made based on the classic clinical manifestations.
- <u>Skin biopsy</u> often performed, especially when the diagnosis is uncertain, to confirm the diagnosis &/or to rule out malignancy. Dermal inflammatory infiltrate is often seen with vulvar LS.
- **<u>Association with malignancy</u>: There is a slightly increased risk of Squamous cell carcinoma (SCC) of the vulva in patients with LS. Adequate treatment of vulvar LS with topical corticosteroids may be associated with a reduced risk of development of neoplasia.**

MANAGEMENT
- **<u>Superpotent topical corticosteroids:</u> initial therapy of choice** (eg, Clobetasol dipropionate 0.05%). Oral antihistamine to stop the itch cycle may be used. Assess the patient in 2-3 months for response.
- **<u>Topical calcineurin inhibitor:</u> (eg, Tacrolimus) if no response to topical corticosteroids &** no other cause is found.
- In persistent or suspicious lesions, biopsy may be indicated.

VULVAR LICHEN SIMPLEX CHRONICUS

- **Thick, indurated skin & hyperkeratosis secondary to chronic, habitual rubbing or scratching.**
- Most commonly seen on the vulva associated with atopic dermatitis, Psoriasis, and Contact dermatitis.

CLINICAL MANIFESTATIONS
- **<u>Itch-scratch cycle</u>: vulvar pruritus, especially at night, often interrupting sleep.** The uncontrollable scratch to soothe the pruritus. Heat, humidity, & sweating exacerbates the itch.

Physical examination:
- **Lichen simplex Chronicus typically presents with a thickened, red epidermis,** similar to Atopic dermatitis, however in **LSC, the plaques may be a deeper red or a red-brown.**
- **<u>Lichenification:</u> the skin is thick and leathery, often with increased skin markings.**

DIAGNOSIS
- The diagnosis is usually clinical. <u>Biopsy</u> may be indicated to rule out malignant conditions. There is no dermal inflammatory infiltrate.

MANAGEMENT
- Vulvar hygiene, Sitz baths, and lubricants can help restore moisture to cells and reconstruct the epithelial barrier. Oral antihistamines may help relieve pruritus. Topical application of medium-potency steroids can decrease the inflammation and pruritus.
- <u>Refractory cases</u>: antidepressants or subcutaneous intralesional injection of steroids.

VAGINAL CANCER

- Rare. 1% of gynecological malignancies. Peak incidence 60-65 years.
- **Squamous cell carcinoma most common primary tumor** (primary tumors are rare). More commonly, Vaginal cancer occurs as a secondary tumor (eg, cervical, vulvar, or distant source).

RISK FACTORS
- Same as in Cervical neoplasia — multiple sexual partners, early age at first intercourse, smoking.
- **HPV types 16 & 18 cause ~70% of all cervical cancers worldwide** and nearly 90% of anal cancers, oropharyngeal cancer, vulvar and vaginal cancer, and penile cancer.

CLINICAL MANIFESTATIONS
- **Abnormal vaginal bleeding most common symptom (postcoital,** intermenstrual or postmenopausal). May be symptomatic.
- Watery vaginal discharge, dyspareunia.

DIAGNOSIS
- On visualization, the lesion may appear as a mass, plaque, or an ulcer that is hyperkeratotic.
- **The posterior wall of the upper one-third of the vagina is the most common site.**
- Biopsy is definitive. If a lesion is not seen, Colposcopy should be performed to determine biopsy site.

MANAGEMENT
- **Stage I: surgical excision or radiation therapy for primary Vaginal cancer.** Up to 15% develop vaginal stenosis or sexual dysfunction after treatment so the use of a vaginal dilator may be needed.
- **Stage II-IV: chemoradiation preferred,** rather than RT. Radiation therapy alone is an alternative.

CANCER OF THE VULVA

- **Squamous cell carcinoma most common type (≥75%).** Malignant melanoma. Clear cell adenocarcinoma is linked to diethylstilbestrol (DES) in utero exposure.
- **Paget disease: vulvar intraepithelial neoplasia** (superficial lesion of the epithelium) that has not invaded the basement membrane [pre-cancer that may progress to carcinoma-in-situ or squamous].

RISK FACTORS
- **HPV types 16 & 18 cause ~70% of all cervical cancers worldwide and nearly 90% of anal cancers,** as well as a significant proportion of oropharyngeal cancer, **vulvar and vaginal cancer,** and penile cancer. Linked to DES exposure, immunosuppression, obesity, cigarette smoking, cervical intraepithelial neoplasia, prior history of Cervical cancer, and Vulvar lichen sclerosus.
- Most commonly seen in postmenopausal women (average age is 68 years).

CLINICAL MANIFESTATIONS
- Vulvar pruritus (itching), irritation, bloody discharge, pain, or discomfort.
- The labia majora are the most common site (50%) followed by the labia minora and rarely the clitoris or Bartholin glands.

PHYSICAL EXAMINATION
- **Vulvar lesion: red or white ulcerative, plaque-like, raised, crusted, or cauliflower-like lesion.**

DIAGNOSIS
- Biopsy — acetic acid or toluidine blue application may help aid biopsy.

MANAGEMENT
- Surgical excision, radiation therapy, chemotherapy (eg, 5-fluorouracil).

BACTERIAL VAGINOSIS (BV)

- **Overgrowth of _Gardnerella vaginalis_** & anaerobes (eg, _Mobiluncus_, _Peptostreptococcus_) **due to altered biome** — decreased _Lactobacillus acidophilus_ (_L. acidophilus_ normally maintains vaginal pH).
- Pregnancy complications include Prelabor rupture of membranes, chorioamnionitis, & preterm labor.

RISK FACTORS
- Although BV is not a sexually transmitted infection, BV is more common in sexually active women with new or multiple partners (new partners alter the vaginal biome).
- Vaginal douching, recent antibiotic use, cigarette smoking, use of an intrauterine device.

CLINICAL MANIFESTATIONS
- ~50–75% of women with BV are asymptomatic.
- **Malodorous vaginal discharge worse after sex & during menses** (↑'ed pH). BV alone typically does NOT cause dysuria, dyspareunia, pruritus, burning, or vaginal inflammation (erythema, edema).

DIAGNOSIS
- **Amsel criteria:** ≥3 of 4: **[1] copious, <u>thin, homogenous, grayish-white vaginal discharge</u>, [2] vaginal pH >4.5, [3] <u>positive whiff-amine test</u>** — amine **(fishy) odor** when 10% KOH is added, **[4] ≥20% clue cells on saline wet mount (epithelial cells covered by adherent coccobacilli)** single most reliable predictor of BV. **Few WBCs** (not inflammatory) & few lactobacilli.
- Microscopy: **few WBCs & polymorphonuclear leukocytes (not inflammatory), few Lactobacilli.**

MANAGEMENT
Metronidazole or Clindamycin first line management if symptomatic (both safe in pregnancy).
- **Metronidazole** 500 mg twice daily orally for 7 days or gel 0.75% once daily vaginally for 5 days.
- **Clindamycin:** intravaginal 2% cream daily for 7 days; Pregnancy: 300 mg PO twice daily for 7 days.
- **Partners do not need treatment.** Treatment for asymptomatic nonpregnant women not indicated.

TRICHOMONAS VAGINITIS (TRICHOMONIASIS)

- **_Trichomonas vaginalis_ is a flagellated pear-shaped protozoan that is <u>transmitted sexually</u>.**
- Complications: increased risk of HIV transmission & complications during pregnancy.

CLINICAL MANIFESTATIONS
- **Women: vaginitis, cystitis, or cervicitis** — copious malodorous vaginal discharge worse with menses, postcoital bleeding, dyspareunia, dysuria, & frequency. Vaginal pruritus or erythema.
- Men: most men are asymptomatic but may develop urethritis or pruritis after intercourse.

PHYSICAL EXAMINATION
- **Copious frothy yellow-green vaginal discharge, vaginal inflammation** (pruritus, erythema, edema).
- **Cervical petechiae punctate hemorrhages (red macular lesions) visible on the vagina and cervix (strawberry cervix).**

DIAGNOSIS
- Microscopic examination (saline wet mount) — **motile protozoan trophozoites with a single flagellum, vaginal pH >4.5 (usually 5.0-6.0),** increased WBCs (PMNs) > epithelial cells.
- Nucleic acid amplification test (NAAT) or culture should be performed if wet mount is negative.

MANAGEMENT
- **Metronidazole 2 g oral dose x 1 dose or 500 mg bid x 7 days. Tinidazole alternative.** Treatment is indicated for both symptomatic & asymptomatic men & women. **Partners must be treated.**
- Follow up: because of high reinfection rate, NAAT retesting performed within 3 months of treatment.
- Reinfection: Metronidazole 500mg orally bid x 7 days (single-dose therapy avoided if recurrent).

	BACTERIAL VAGINOSIS	TRICHOMONIASIS	CANDIDA	CYTOLYTIC VAGINITIS
PATHO PHYSIOLOGY	• Decreased Lactobacilli acidophilus (normally maintains vaginal pH) ⇨ overgrowth of normal flora ex *GARDNERELLA VAGINALIS*, *anaerobes* (Mobiluncus, Peptostreptococcus) • *MC cause of vaginitis**	• *TRICHOMONAS VAGINALIS:* pear shaped flagellated protozoa • Sexually transmitted	• *Candida albicans overgrowth* (part of the normal flora due to change in normal vaginal environment (ex. use of abx) • ↑c DM, steroid, pregnancy	• *Overgrowth of LACTOBACILLI*
CLINICAL MANIFESTATIONS	• Vaginal odor worse after sex • ± Pruritus • >50% asymptomatic	• Vulvar pruritus, erythema, dysuria • Dyspareunia	• Vaginal & vulvar erythema, swelling, burning, pruritus • Burning when urine touches skin, Dysuria, Dyspareunia	• Vaginal or vulvar pruritus & burning • Dysuria
VAGINAL DISCHARGE	• Copious discharge • *Thin, homogenous, watery* <u>*GREY-WHITE "FISH ROTTEN"* smell</u>	• Copious malodorous discharge • *FROTHY YELLOW GREEN DISCHARGE**worse c menses • *STRAWBERRY CERVIX*: (cervical petechiae)*	• *THICK CURD-LIKE/COTTAGE CHEESE DISCHARGE**	Nonodorous discharge white to opaque
VAGINAL pH	>5	>5	Normal (3.8- 4.2)	Normal (3.8- 4.2)
WHIFF TEST	Positive: *FISHY ODOR** with *10% KOH Prep*	May be present	Negative	Copious lactobacilli Large # of epithelial cells
MICROSCOPIC	• *CLUE CELLS:** epithelial cells covered by bacteria. • *Few WBC's*, few lactobacilli	• Mobile protozoa (wet mount) • WBC's	• *HYPHAE, YEAST** & spores on KOH prep	
MANAGEMENT	• *METRONIDAZOLE* (Flagyl) *x 7 days* - Safe in pregnancy - May use gel or PO • *CLINDAMYCIN* - May use gel or PO	• *METRONIDAZOLE* [Flagyl] - *2g oral x 1 dose* OR - 500mg bid oral x 7days - Safe in pregnancy - *Oral preferred* • *TINIDAZOLE*	• *FLUCONAZOLE* (PO x 1 dose) • *Intravaginal antifungals* - Clotrimazole, Nystatin - Butoconazole - Miconazole	• *Discontinue tampon usage* (to decrease vaginal acidity) • *Sodium Bicarbonate* - Sitz bath with NaHCO3 - Douche with NaHCO3
PREVENTION	• *Avoid douching* - Douching promotes loss of Lactobacilli • *Treating partner unnecessary* - Unclear if sexually transmitted. - But reduced recurrence if male uses condoms	• *Spermicidal agents:* ex. nonoxynol 9 reduces transmission <u>*MUST TREAT PARTNER*</u>	• Keep vagina dry, 100% cotton underwear, avoid tight-fitting clothes, avoid use of feminine deodorants & bubble baths	
COMPLICATIONS	Pregnancy- PROM, preterm labor, chorioamnionitis.	Perinatal complications, ↑HIV transmission		

PELVIC INFLAMMATORY DISEASE (PID)

- **Ascending acute or subclinical infection of the <u>upper female reproductive tract</u>.**
- <u>Risk factors</u>: Multiple sexual partners, unprotected sex, prior PID, age 15-25 years, nulliparous, IUD.
- **Usually polymicrobial** — *Chlamydia trachomatis* **(most common),** *Neisseria gonorrhoeae*, M. *genitalium*, **anaerobes** (*Gardnerella vaginalis*, *Peptostreptococcus* species, *Bacteroides* species), enteric or respiratory pathogens etc. Gonococcal PID often more severe than other causes.

CLINICAL MANIFESTATIONS

- **<u>Pelvic or lower abdominal pain</u> cardinal symptom (often bilateral),** recent onset of pain that worsens during coitus (**dyspareunia**) or with jarring movements. The onset of pain during or shortly after menses is very suggestive. May be accompanied by nausea &/or vomiting.
- <u>Abnormal uterine bleeding:</u> eg, post-coital bleeding, inter-menstrual bleeding, menorrhagia.
- <u>Genital symptoms:</u> urinary frequency, dysuria, abnormal vaginal discharge.
- Some are asymptomatic but are later suspected to have had it due to tubal factor infertility or scarring.
- <u>Physical examination:</u> **Pelvic organ tenderness: uterine, cervical, and/or adnexal tenderness is the defining characteristic of acute symptomatic PID. Cervical motion tenderness (chandelier sign** = pelvic exam elicits pain, causing the patient to reach up towards the ceiling for relief). **Purulent cervical discharge.**

DIAGNOSIS

- **<u>Primarily clinical</u> — ❶ abdominal tenderness + ❷ cervical motion tenderness + ❸ adnexal tenderness plus at least 1 of the following:** oral temperature >101°F (>38.3°C), WBC >10,000, pelvic abnormality on bimanual exam or ultrasound, ↑ESR or CRP, abnormal cervical or vaginal mucopurulent discharge or cervical friability, ↑ white blood cells on saline microscopy of vaginal secretions (eg, >15-20 WBCs/hpf or more WBCs than epithelial cells), documentation of cervical infection with *N. gonorrhoeae, C. trachomatis,* or *M. genitalium,* pus on culdocentesis or laparoscopy.
- **Workup includes pregnancy test (rule out Ectopic pregnancy)** & nucleic acid amplification test (for Gonorrhea & Chlamydia). Pelvic US first-line imaging for tubo-ovarian abscess (CT may be used).
- <u>Laparoscopy</u> is the most accurate test for PID (rarely performed) — may be done in uncertain cases, severe disease, or if no improvement with antibiotics.

OUTPATIENT MANAGEMENT

- **<u>Ceftriaxone</u>** (500 mg for individuals <150 kg or 1 g for individuals ≥150 kg, intramuscularly in a single dose) **PLUS <u>Doxycycline</u>** (100mg bid x 14 days). **Metronidazole 500mg bid x 14 days often added to cover anaerobic bacteria** (eg, *Gardnerella vaginalis*).
- Levofloxacin + Metronidazole alternative if true Penicillin allergy.

INPATIENT MANAGEMENT

- **<u>Second generation Cephalosporin</u> (eg, Cefoxitin or Cefotetan) PLUS <u>IV Doxycycline.</u>**
- **<u>Pregnancy or true Penicillin allergy:</u> Clindamycin + Gentamicin.**
- **<u>Indications for hospitalization:</u> <u>severe clinical illness:</u> fever ≥38.5°C [101°F], nausea and vomiting,** Complicated PID with pelvic abscess, inability to tolerate oral medications, **pregnancy.**
- Tubo-ovarian abscesses may require surgical excision or transcutaneous or transvaginal aspiration.

FITZ HUGH-CURTIS SYNDROME

- **<u>Perihepatitis</u>** with hepatic fibrosis, scarring & peritoneal surface of the anterior right upper quadrant **in the setting of Pelvic inflammatory disease (PID).** Seen in 10% of women with PID.

CLINICAL MANIFESTATIONS

- **RUQ pain** due to perihepatitis (liver capsule involvement). May radiate to the right shoulder.
- <u>Physical examination:</u> marked RUQ tenderness.

DIAGNOSIS

- **<u>Laparoscopy</u> — "violin-string" adhesions** on the anterior liver surface. Normal or slight ↑LFTs.

STAPHYLOCOCCAL TOXIC SHOCK SYNDROME (TSS)

- **Staphylococcal toxic shock syndrome (TSS) is a clinical illness characterized by rapid onset of fever, rash, hypotension, and multiorgan system involvement due to exotoxins produced by *Staphylococcus aureus.***
- *S aureus* produces toxins that cause 3 important conditions: [1] "Scalded skin syndrome" in children, [2] Toxic shock syndrome in adults, and [3] Enterotoxin food poisoning.

PATHOPHYSIOLOGY
- Preformed toxins are superantigens that activate a large number of T cells, which releases various inflammatory mediators (IL-2, IL-1, TNF).
- The inflammatory response causes capillary leakage, circulatory collapse, and multi-organ failure.

RISK FACTORS
- **Menstrual: 50% associated with high absorbency tampon use.**
- **Nonmenstrual: recent surgery or infection** — surgical & postpartum wound infections (involving skin or soft tissue or other site), burns, & contraceptive sponge use.

CLINICAL MANIFESTATIONS
- **Sudden onset of high fever (≥39°C/102.2°F),** chills, tachycardia, nausea, vomiting, diarrhea, pharyngitis. These symptoms develop rapidly (within 48 hours) in a previously healthy individual.
- Sore throat, myalgias, malaise, fatigue and headache are common. **Nonpurulent conjunctivitis.**
- **Skin: diffuse erythematous macular rash (erythroderma) resembles sunburn — includes the palms & soles,** followed by desquamation 1-2 weeks after onset of illness.
- Multisystemic involvement ≥3 organ systems (GI, mucous membrane, renal, muscular, hematologic, CNS) — **Hypotension (may include orthostasis or syncope),** abdominal tenderness or pain, severe watery diarrhea, decreased urine output, headache, somnolence, lethargy, confusion.

DIAGNOSIS
- **Clinical diagnosis — Staphylococcal TSS should be suspected in patients with rapid onset of high fever, vomiting, rash, watery diarrhea, hypotension, and multiorgan system involvement;** relevant risk factors include recent tampon use, recent surgery, and recent infection (involving skin or soft tissue or another site).
- Cultures including blood cultures and cultures from mucosal sites [including the vaginal canal in cases of suspected menstrual TSS], wound sites, and nares should be obtained.
- Detection of *Staphylococcus aureus* in culture is **not** required for the diagnosis of staphylococcal TSS. Classically, blood cultures are negative because symptoms are due to the effects of the toxin & not systemic infection (positive in ~5% of cases). Recovered from wound or mucosal sites in 80–90%.

MANAGEMENT
- **Aggressive supportive therapy: hospital admission, removal of offending object (if still present), management of shock, aggressive IV fluid replacement, & antibiotics.**
Removal of offending objects:
- Wound exploration (with debridement if warranted) should be performed in patients with TSS in the setting of recent surgery, and any packing should be removed if present.
- Any foreign material in the vaginal canal (eg, tampon, contraceptive sponge, or intrauterine device) should be removed if present.
Antibiotic coverage:
- For patients with sepsis of unknown cause that might represent staphylococcal TSS, Vancomycin, Clindamycin, AND either a combination medications containing a penicillin plus beta-lactamase inhibitor or a Carbapenem. **Clindamycin suppresses toxin synthesis.**
- **TSS due to Methicillin-resistant *S. aureus* or Empiric: Clindamycin plus Vancomycin.**
- **TSS due to Methicillin-susceptible *S. aureus*: Clindamycin PLUS EITHER Oxacillin, Nafcillin, or Cefazolin.**

SPONTANEOUS ABORTION

- **A pregnancy that ends before 20 weeks gestation.** Almost 80% occur prior to 12 weeks.
- Includes threatened, inevitable, incomplete, complete, missed, & septic abortions.
- **Threatened is the only spontaneous abortion that is potentially viable.**

ETIOLOGIES
- **Chromosomal abnormalities most common cause of Spontaneous abortions (60-80%).**
- Maternal factors include STIs, antiphospholipid syndrome, trauma, Rh isoimmunization, malnutrition, and anatomic abnormalities.

CLINICAL MANIFESTATIONS
- Crampy abdominal pain & vaginal bleeding.

DIAGNOSIS
- Ultrasound, CBC, blood type and Rh screen, serial hCG titers, & progesterone levels.

TYPE OF ABORTION	ULTRASOUND & CERVICAL FINDINGS	MANAGEMENT
THREATENED	• **Products of conception (POC) intact** • **Cervical os closed**	• **Supportive: observation at home,** bedrest and **close follow up** to see if either symptoms resolve or progress to abortion. • Serial beta-hCG to see if doubling to see if viable.
INEVITABLE	• **POC intact** • **Cervical os DILATED**	Options include: • **Surgical evacuation:** dilation & curettage <16 weeks or dilation & evacuation ≥ 16 weeks. • Medical: **Misoprostol** • Expectant management
INCOMPLETE	• **Some POC expelled from the uterus** • **Cervical os DILATED**	Options include: • **Expectant** – allow POC to fully pass with serial beta-hCG & transvaginal US to determine when complete. • **Surgical evacuation:** dilation & curettage <16 weeks or dilation & evacuation ≥ 16 weeks. • Medical: **Misoprostol**
COMPLETE	• **All POC expelled from the uterus** • Cervical os usually closed	• RhoGAM if indicated, follow up beta-hCG
MISSED	• **POC intact** • **Cervical os closed.**	• **Surgical evacuation:** dilation & curettage <16 weeks or dilation & evacuation ≥ 16 weeks. • Medical: **Misoprostol**
SEPTIC	• Some POC retained • Cervical os closed. **Cervical motion tenderness.** • Foul brown discharge, fever, chills	• **D & E to remove products of conception + broad spectrum antibiotics** (e.g., Levofloxacin + Metronidazole)

All women who are Rh-negative should also receive anti-D Rh immunoglobulin at this time for all abortions.

MANAGEMENT OPTIONS
- **[1] Expectant management: consists of watchful waiting for pregnancy tissue to pass.** Patient must follow up to confirm an empty uterus. If not, a different treatment option should be considered.
- **[2] Medical: Combined treatment with Mifepristone and Misoprostol** results in higher rates of emptying the uterus compared with Misoprostol alone. **Misoprostol alone is another option.**
- **[3] Uterine aspiration** during the first trimester [eg, Dilation and Curettage (D & C)] can safely and acceptably occur in an outpatient or emergency department setting if <16 weeks, while second-trimester uterine aspiration [dilation and evacuation (D & E) more often occurs in an operative setting if ≥16 weeks.

ELECTIVE (INDUCED) ABORTION

MEDICAL

- **Mifepristone followed by Misoprostol 24-48 hours afterwards.** FDA-approved for up to 70 days (≤10 weeks of gestation).
  - Mifepristone is a progesterone receptor antagonist that leads to dilation and softening of the cervix, as well as placental separation.
  - Misoprostol is a prostaglandin E1 analog that causes uterine contractions. Patients must return 7-14 days after Mifepristone to confirm complete termination of pregnancy.

- **Methotrexate followed by Misoprostol 3-7 days later (safe up to 7 weeks).**
  - Methotrexate is a folic antagonist. This regimen is less effective.

SURGICAL

Can be performed up to 24 weeks from LMP

- Dilation and Curettage (D & C): includes usage of a curette or suction curettage (manual or electric vacuum aspiration). Used most commonly during the first 4-12 weeks of gestation.

- Dilation and Evacuation (D & E): Initial use of vacuum aspiration followed by use of forceps after cervical dilation used more commonly >12 weeks gestation

PLACENTAL INSUFFICIENCY

- Impairment or inability of the placenta to provide oxygen & nutrients to the fetus.
- Etiologies: placenta previa or abruption, post-term pregnancy, intrauterine growth restriction.

DIAGNOSIS

- **Fetal heart monitoring — late decelerations** (gradual decrease in fetal heart rate initiating at the peak of contraction and into the second half of the contraction) due to mechanical compression of maternal vessels traversing the uterine wall during uterine contractions. May be associated with gradual return of heart rate to baseline.

INITIAL MANAGEMENT

- Placing the mother on her side, administering oxygen by mask, and correcting hypotension.

PHYSIOLOGIC LEUKORRHEA

- **White, odorless mucoid cervical discharge composed of cervical mucus, normal vaginal flora, and vaginal squamous epithelium.**
- **Increasing amounts of this normal vaginal discharge typically occurs midcycle** (eg, 10-14 days after previous menses as estrogen levels increase prior to ovulation, and then regresses).

CLINICAL MANIFESTATIONS

- **Physiologic leukorrhea presents without manifestations of infection such as pruritus, erythema, pain, or a malodorous discharge.**
- Prior to the diagnosis of physiologic leukorrhea, other causes of increased vaginal discharge must be excluded.

DIAGNOSIS

- Microscopic examination of the discharge **reveals no evidence of inflammation or infection (eg, rare polymorphonuclear leukocytes).** Normally, increased PMNs are evidence of a local response (eg, inflammation).
- Rare polymorphonuclear leukocytes on microscopy, helps to rule out infectious etiologies as the cause of the discharge.

UNCOMPLICATED PREGNANCY

PREGNANCY TESTS
- Serum hCG: detected within 5–7 days after conception or at menstrual age of 20–22 days' gestation (after the LMP). hCG levels peak at 10–12 weeks gestation and decrease afterward.
- Urine hCG: can detect pregnancy 14 days after conception; ↑serum progesterone.

PHYSICAL EXAMINATION
- **Uterus changes**
  - **Ladin's sign:** uterus softening after 6 weeks.
  - **Hegar's sign:** uterine isthmus widening & softening after 6-8 weeks of gestation.
  - **Piskacek's sign:** palpable lateral bulge or softening of uterine cornus at 7-8 weeks gestation.
- **Vaginal changes: leukorrhea** — increased vaginal discharge containing epithelial cells & cervical mucus.
- **Cervix changes**
  - **Goodell's sign:** cervical softening due to increased vascularization ~4-5 weeks gestation.
  - **Chadwick's sign: bluish coloration of the cervix & vulva** ~8-12 weeks.
- **Fetal heart tones are detectable by handheld Doppler by 10-12 weeks gestation** or by fetoscope (after 18–20 weeks gestation). The normal heart rate is 110–160 beats per minute, with a higher fetal heart rate often noted during early pregnancy.
- **Ultrasound** is the most useful technical aid in diagnosing and monitoring pregnancy. Cardiac activity is detectable at 6 weeks via transvaginal sonography, limb buds at 7–8 weeks, and finger and limb movements at 9–10 weeks. At the termination of the embryonic period (10 weeks by LMP), the embryo has a human appearance. The gestational age can be ascertained by the crown rump length between 6-13 weeks gestation, with a margin of error of ~8% or 5 days.
- Fetal movement: 16-20 weeks (quickening), depend on initial vs. subsequent pregnancies.

GPA CLASSIFICATION

- **Gravida:** # of times pregnant (regardless of if carried to term).
- **Para:** # of births (>20 weeks) including viable or nonviable births (ex. stillbirth). Multiple gestations (eg, twins) count as 1 for notation.
- **Abortus:** # of pregnancies lost for whatever reason (miscarriages, abortions).

Ex: G_3P_3 = 3 pregnancies 3 births. $G_4P_3A_1$ = 4 pregnancies, 3 births, 1 miscarriage (or abortion).

FUNDAL HEIGHT MEASUREMENT

12 weeks	At or above the pubic symphysis
16 weeks	Midway between the pubis & umbilicus
20-22 weeks	**At the level of the umbilicus**
20-32 weeks	Height (cm) above symphysis = gestational age (weeks)
36 weeks	**At the xyphoid process** (highest it will reach before regression)
38 weeks	2-3 cm below the xiphoid process

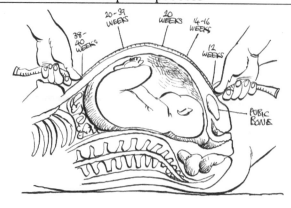

NORMAL PHYSIOLOGIC CHANGES DURING PREGNANCY

Normal Pregnancy

Increased
- **Blood volume** (10-15% as early as 6 weeks), **cardiac output, stroke volume,** RBC mass.
- **Increased tidal volume** to meet the increased oxygen demand. Hypercoagulable state.
- Heart rate increases 10–15 bpm; increased intensity of S1, exaggerated splitting of S2.

Decreased:
- Functional residual capacity by 20%, decreased exercise capacity for some. Hemoglobin.
- **Systemic vascular resistance (peripheral vasodilation),** which is compensated for by the increased stroke volume & cardiac output.
- **Blood pressure decreases in the second trimester** (decreases of 5-7 mm Hg of both SBP & DBP). Blood pressure normalizes in the third trimester. Decreased GI motility (may lead to GERD).

Other:
- Respiratory alkalosis: third trimester.

NORMAL FINDINGS DURING PREGNANCY
- Fetal heart tones usually heard around 10-12 weeks by Doppler.
- Serum hCG: doubles roughly every 2 days in early pregnancy.

Transvaginal ultrasound:
- **Intrauterine pregnancy (IUP) visualized as early as when serum hCG >1,500 IU/L**

Transabdominal ultrasound:
- IUP visualized when serum hCG >4,000 IU/L

Weight gain:
- Weight gain of 25-35 lbs. for women of healthy BMI pre-pregnancy.

ESTIMATED DATE OF DELIVERY (EDD)
- Human pregnancy duration is 280 days or 40 weeks (9 calendar months or 10 lunar months) from the LMP.
- The EDD can be determined mathematically using Naegele's rule: subtract 3 months from the month of the LMP and add 7 to the first day of the LMP.
- The EDD may also be calculated as 266 days or 38 weeks from the last ovulation (if known).
- The easiest method of determining gestational age is with a pregnancy calendar or calculator; smartphone apps are readily available.

MULTIPLE GESTATIONS
- Associated with rapid maternal weight gain and growth of the uterus.
- **Dizygotic (fraternal):** due to fertilization of 2 ova by 2 different sperm (66%).
- **Monozygotic (identical):** formed from the fertilization of 1 ovum that splits. Increased risk of fetal transfusion syndrome and discordant fetal growth.

DIAGNOSIS
- Ultrasound to visualize the fetuses.
- **Elevated levels of beta-hCG & maternal serum alpha-fetoprotein higher than normal.**

MATERNAL COMPLICATIONS
- Preterm labor, spontaneous abortion, preeclampsia, anemia.

FETAL COMPLICATIONS
- Intrauterine growth restrictions, placental abnormalities, breech presentation, umbilical cord prolapse, preeclampsia.
- Multiple gestations considered a high-risk pregnancy.

PRENATAL CARE

ROUTINE TESTS DURING FIRST PRENATAL VISIT

- Blood pressure, random glucose, screening for Sickle cell, & Cystic fibrosis.

ROUTINE LABORATORY TESTS	
Initial prenatal visit	• **Blood group, RhD type, and red blood cell antibody screen** • <u>CBC & iron studies</u>: hemoglobin, hematocrit, MCV, ferritin • HIV, Syphilis (VDRL or RPR), anti-HCV Ab, Hep B serologies (HBsAg) • Detection of immunity to Rubella & Varicella zoster • <u>Urine studies</u>: Urine culture (assess for asymptomatic bacteriuria); Urine dipstick for protein, UA to assess for glucose & protein. • Pap test (if screening is indicated) • Chlamydia PCR (if risk factors are present)
24-28 weeks	• **Gestational Diabetes mellitus: 1-hr 50-g glucose tolerance test** • Hemoglobin/hematocrit • **Rh antibody screen at 28-29 weeks if Rh(D)-negative**
36 0/7-37 6/7 weeks	• **Group B Streptococcus screening via rectovaginal culture**

FIRST TRIMESTER SCREENINGS & TESTS

Weeks 1–12 of pregnancy

<u>Testing for chromosomal abnormalities (eg, aneuploidy):</u>

- **[1] Biochemical screening** combination tests may be performed:
  - **Free or total beta-hCG:** abnormally high or low may be indicative of chromosomal abnormalities (eg, Trisomies 13, 18, and 21).
  - **PAPP-A (serum pregnancy-associated plasma protein-A): usually low with fetal Down syndrome**
- **[2] Fetal nuchal translucency ultrasound at 10-13 weeks.** Screens for trisomies 13, 18, & 21 (Down syndrome). Increased thickness is considered abnormal.
  - **If increased thickness, Chorionic villous sampling or Amniocentesis may be offered.**
- <u>Combined testing</u> [eg, Maternal serum total beta-hCG or free beta-hCG subunit, Maternal serum pregnancy-associated plasma protein A (PAPP-A), and Ultrasound measurement of nuchal translucency (NT)] may be used if a high value is placed on detecting Down syndrome in the first trimester.

<u>Other tests</u>

- **Ultrasound:** fetal heart tones usually heard around 10-12 weeks by Doppler. Transvaginal ultrasound can detect fetal heart activity as early as 5-6 weeks after LMP.**
- <u>Uterine size & gestation</u>: if abnormal, Chorionic villus sampling (CVS) or Amniocentesis can be offered at around 10-13 weeks.
- Individuals who receive a screen-positive result for any of the screening tests discussed should be offered the choice of an invasive test for definitive diagnosis (CVS through 14 weeks, amniocentesis at ≥15 weeks) or a secondary screening test based on cell-free DNA.

<u>Invasive diagnostic testing for aneuploidy:</u>

- **Chorionic villus sampling (CVS): may be performed ~10-13 weeks (preferred technique before 15 weeks). May be offered to women with increased risk of chromosomal abnormalities,** including those with a prior child with a chromosomal abnormality, maternal age >35 years, abnormal first or second trimester maternal screening tests, abnormal nuchal translucency & prior pregnancy losses. The detection rate for aneuploidy is almost 100%.
  - <u>Advantage</u>: allows for the option of early termination of the pregnancy if abnormalities are found.
  - <u>Disadvantages</u>: Complication rates 0.1-0.3% — performing it increases the risk of spontaneous abortion, increased infection, or fluid leak. Cannot be used in alpha-fetoprotein testing for neural tube defects.

SECOND TRIMESTER SCREENINGS & TESTS (WEEKS 13-27 OF PREGNANCY)

- <u>Screen for anemia</u> with a CBC at 24-28 weeks gestation.

Screening for Chromosomal abnormalities:

- **Triple screening: alpha-fetoprotein, unconjugated estriol, & β-hCG testing** usually offered at 15-20 weeks (ideally @ 16-18 weeks) if they desire screening & did not receive it in the first trimester.
- **Quadruple screening adds Inhibin A.** High levels of inhibin A indicate chromosomal abnormalities.

α-FP	β-hCG	Unconjugated Estriol (uE3)	Diagnosis
Low	High	Low	**Down Syndrome (Trisomy 21)**
High			• **Open neural tube defects** eg, **Spina bifida** OR • **Multiple gestation.**
Low	Low	Low	**Trisomy 18:** often born stillborn or die within the 1st year of life.

The detection rate of a quad screen is between 65% and 75% for trisomy 21, 18, and 13 and between 80% and 85% for open neural tube defects. The false-positive rate is ~5%.

Gestational diabetes screening:

- **Gestational diabetes screening: at 24–28 weeks with a 50-g glucose load.**
- Earlier screening should be considered in women with significant risk factors — eg, gestational diabetes in a prior pregnancy, family history of diabetes in a first-degree relative.

Invasive testing for aneuploidy (if desired):

- **Amniocentesis:** may be offered to women including those with a prior child with a chromosomal abnormality, maternal age >35 years, abnormal 1st or 2nd trimester maternal screening tests, abnormal ultrasound, prior pregnancy losses. **Usually performed ~15-20 weeks gestation.**
- Amniocentesis complication rate is ~0.1–0.3%, and the detection rate for aneuploidy is almost 100%.

NEURAL TUBE DEFECTS

- Birth defects of the brain, spine, or spinal cord.
- **The two most common types are [1] Spina bifida and [2] Anencephaly.**
- **Increased incidence with maternal folate deficiency.**

PATHOPHYSIOLOGY

- <u>Spina bifida:</u> incomplete closure of the embryonic neural tubule leads to non-fusion of some of the vertebrae overlying the spinal cords. This may lead to protrusion of the spinal cord through the opening. Most commonly seen at the lumbar and sacral areas of the spine.
- <u>Anencephaly:</u> failure of closure of the portion of the neural tube that becomes the cerebrum.

TYPES OF SPINA BIFIDA

- **Spina bifida with myelomeningocele: most common type.** Meninges and spinal cord herniates thought the gap in the vertebrae. Often leads to disability.
- <u>Spina bifida occulta:</u> mildest form. No herniation of the spinal cord. The overlying skin may be normal or have some hair growing over it, dimpling of the skin or birthmark over the affected area.
- <u>Spina bifida with meningocele:</u> only the meninges herniate through the gap in the vertebrae.

CLINICAL MANIFESTATIONS

- Sensory deficits, paralysis, hydrocephalus, hypotonia.

SCREENING

- **[1] <u>Increased maternal serum alpha-fetoprotein</u>** often performed at 15-20 weeks (ideally at 16-18 weeks), **followed by**
- **[2] <u>Amniocentesis</u> showing increased alpha-fetoprotein & increased acetylcholinesterase.**

THIRD TRIMESTER SCREENINGS & TESTS (WEEK 28 UNTIL BIRTH)

- **Gestational diabetes screening: at 24–28 weeks.**
  Earlier screening should be considered in women with significant risk factors (eg, gestational diabetes in a prior pregnancy, family history of diabetes in a first-degree relative).
- **Repeat antibody titers: in Rh(D)-negative, antibody-negative (unsensitized) women:**
  Anti-D Rh immunoglobulin: RhoGAM (300 micrograms of anti-D immune globulin) given at 28-29 weeks gestation in unsensitized, D-negative patients.
- **CBC to screen for anemia** — The hemoglobin or hematocrit should be checked early in the third trimester to screen for anemia. Can also be done at 35 weeks.
- **Screen for sexually transmitted infections** — The CDC recommends testing for STIs (eg, HIV, syphilis, chlamydia, gonorrhea) in the third trimester (28 to 36 weeks) in women at increased risk.
- Biophysical profile: looks at 5 variables including: fetal breathing, fetal tones, amniotic fluid levels, NST, & gross fetal movements. 2 points each (maximum score of 10 points).
- **Non-Stress Testing:** Category I FHR tracings are **normal tracings which are not associated with fetal asphyxia — eg, baseline heart rate between 110-160, moderate variability** defined as "fluctuations in the baseline heart rate that are irregular in amplitude and frequency of 6-25 bpm", no late or variable decelerations, possible early decelerations, and possible accelerations.

	DEFINITION	PROGNOSIS	MANAGEMENT
REACTIVE NST	• **≥2 accelerations of fetal heart rate ≥15 bpm** from baseline lasting at least 15 seconds over a 20-minute period. • Detection of two fetal movements	• **Fetal well being**	• Repeat weekly or biweekly
NONREACTIVE	• *No fetal heart rate accelerations or* ≤15bpm lasting ≤15 seconds	• Sleeping, immature or compromised fetus	• Vibratory stimulation to wake fetus up • May try contraction stress

CONTRACTION STRESS TEST (CST): measures fetal response to stress at times of uterine contraction.

	DEFINITION	PROGNOSIS	MANAGEMENT
NEGATIVE CST	• **No late decelerations** in the presence of 3 contractions in 10 minutes	• **Fetal well being**	• Repeat CST as needed
POSITIVE CST	• **Repetitive late decelerations** following ≥50% of contractions	• Worrisome especially if nonreactive NST	• **Hospitalize for prolonged fetal monitoring or delivery.**

GROUP B STREPTOCOCCUS (GBS) COLONIZATION SCREENING

- Group B *Streptococcus* (*S. agalactiae*) [GBS] frequently colonizes the female reproductive tract and the upper respiratory tract of young infants.
- Vertical transmission of Group B *Streptococcus* infection during labor is the leading cause of neonatal infection and the major cause of sepsis in newborns.

Complications of GBS infection:
- Maternal: chorioamnionitis, preterm labor, asymptomatic bacteriuria, cystitis, and pyelonephritis.
- **Neonates: early postpartum infection** (eg, Meningitis, Septic arthritis, Osteomyelitis, sepsis).

GBS Screening:
- **Rectovaginal screening culture: ACOG guidelines recommend screening at 36+0/7 to 37+6/7 weeks of gestation** with the following 2 exceptions:
  Exceptions to screening:
  - (1) women with bacteriuria during the current pregnancy and
  - (2) women who previously gave birth to an infant with invasive GBS disease.
  Women who fit exception criteria should receive intrapartum antibiotic prophylaxis.

Intrapartum prophylaxis against GBS:
- **If positive screening or one of the 2 exceptions, prophylactic antibiotics given during labor (most effective if administered at least 4 hours before delivery) — IV Penicillin G first-line agent** (5 million units followed by 2.5 million units every 4 hours until delivery).
- **Second line: Ampicillin,** extended-spectrum Penicillins, Cephalosporins (eg, Cefazolin), Clindamycin, and IV Vancomycin.

FETAL HEART RATE PATTERNS

	FHR pattern (VEAL)		ETIOLOGIES (CHOP)		INTERVENTIONS (MINE)
V	Variable decelerations	C	Cord compression	M	Maternal repositioning
E	Early decelerations	H	Head compression	I	Identify labor progress
A	Accelerations	O	Okay baby!	N	No interventions
L	Late decelerations	P	Placental insufficiency	E	Employ interventions

[1] VARIABLE DECELERATIONS:

- Defined as a change in the FHR from baseline by >15 beats per minute (BPM), lasting between 15 seconds and 2 minutes. **Characterized by a sharp drop with relatively quick recovery**.
- Variable decelerations typically occur during the onset of a contraction and reach its lowest BPM (eg, nadir) in <30 seconds. However, they can also be episodic and unrelated to contractions.

Etiologies:
- **Cord compression: Variable decelerations occur due to fetal baroreceptor response to umbilical cord compression**, often after acute loss of amniotic fluid from rupture of membranes.
- However, Variable decelerations also occur in patients with oligohydramnios and intact membranes.
- **Variable decelerations are usually transient**; however, persistent or worsening decelerations can lead to adverse fetal outcomes (eg, hypoxia, acidemia).

Management includes
- **[1] Maternal repositioning in the right or left lateral decubitus (knee chest) position to relieve umbilical cord compression** or Trendelenburg position.
- [2] if decelerations do not improve with conservative management, the next step is intrauterine pressure catheter placement and administration of an amnioinfusion (eg, if oligohydramnios).
- [3] C-section if Late decelerations or significant Variable decelerations unresponsive to above.

[2] EARLY DECELERATIONS:

- **Early decelerations are fetal heart rate decelerations that occur during a contraction** [the nadir corresponds to the peak of the uterine contraction (**flipped mirror image of the contraction**)]. Most often, there is a **gradual decrease in fetal heart rate which then returns to baseline within 30 seconds of the conclusion of the contraction.**
- **Etiology: Fetal head compression:** Early decelerations are due to a **parasympathetic (vagal) response from fetal head compression** (typically caused by descent through the vaginal canal).
- **Management: identify labor progress. These decelerations are often considered benign** (eg, no threat to the fetus).

[3] ACCELERATIONS:
Oxygen is okay!
- Accelerations often last >15 seconds (sustained) but <2 minutes. They may peak ≥15 BPM higher than the fetal baseline heart rate.
- **Common reassuring finding:** Fetal heart rate accelerations are often due to fetal movement, scalp stimulation, stimulation by contractions, or acoustic stimulation.
- **Management: No intervention needed — These patterns on the fetal monitor are common and reassuring** (accelerations often happen in response to fetal movement).

[4] LATE DECELERATIONS:
- Late decelerations are a gradual decrease in the FHR that **reaches a nadir after the peak of a contraction** (FHR slightly offset from the contractions), often with a prolonged return to baseline.
- Etiologies: **poor fetal oxygenation during uterine contractions** and are associated with **uteroplacental insufficiency, fetal growth restriction,** inadequate uterine perfusion, excessive uterine activity, maternal hypotension, and fetal hypoxia
- **Management: Employ interventions** — eg, place mom in left lying position, IV fluids, oxygen, discontinue Oxytocin, notify the provider, & prep for possible surgery if unresolved (eg, C-section).

ECTOPIC PREGNANCY

- Fertilized ovum implantation outside of the uterine cavity. Typically presents 6-8 weeks after LMP.
- **Locations: ampulla of the fallopian tube most common (70%),** isthmus of fallopian tube (12%), fimbral (11.1%); abdomen (1.4%), ovary & cervix (0.15% each), interstitial (2.4%).
- **Occlusion of the fallopian tube secondary to adhesions is the most common cause.**

RISK FACTORS

- **High risk: Previous ectopic strongest risk factor, history of Pelvic inflammatory disease (one of the most common causes), IUD use,** previous abdominal or tubal surgery (due to adhesions), history of tubal ligation, Endometriosis, assisted reproduction (eg, IVF).
- Intermediate: infertility, history of genital infections, multiple partners, & cigarette smoking.

CLINICAL MANIFESTATIONS

- **Classic Triad: [1] unilateral pelvic or lower abdominal pain, [2] vaginal bleeding or spotting, & [3] amenorrhea (pregnancy) — triad may also be seen with Threatened abortion, which is more common.**
- Atypical: vague symptoms, menstrual irregularities.
- **Ruptured: severe abdominal, left shoulder pain (Kehr sign),** dizziness, nausea, vomiting. Peritonitis (guarding, rigidity, or rebound tenderness). Signs of shock (from hemorrhage): **syncope,** tachycardia, **hypotension, or the presence of free fluid in the pelvis on TVUS.**

Physical examination:

- **Adnexal mass. Cervical motion tenderness.** May have blood in the vaginal vault.

DIAGNOSIS

- **Quantitative hCG:** confirms pregnancy; hCG should increase 35-50% every 48-72 hours. **Serial hCG that fails to rise as expected, decreases, or plateaus may indicate Ectopic or nonviable pregnancy (distinguished by TVUS). If initial value <1,500 IU/L, repeat every 2-3 days.** Discriminatory zone is often defined as hCG 1,500-2,000 mIU/mL.
- **Transvaginal ultrasound: recommended imaging technique for most patients with suspected Ectopic pregnancy. The absence of an intrauterine gestational sac with hCG levels >2,000 IU/L strongly suggests Ectopic pregnancy.** By 5-6 weeks gestation, an intrauterine pregnancy should be identifiable by ultrasonography as a gestational sac containing a yolk sac.
- Other: culdocentesis — nonclotted blood present (not done often). Laparoscopy is not used often.

MANAGEMENT OF **STABLE/UNRUPTURED**:

- **Methotrexate** destroys rapidly proliferating trophoblastic tissue.
  Indications for Methotrexate: [1] hemodynamically stable patients with [2] early gestation (≤3.5 cm, hCG ≤5,000, no embryonic cardiac activity), & no evidence of rupture, who will be compliant to follow-up, are immunocompetent, & have normal liver and renal function tests.
- Laparoscopic Salpingostomy or Salpingectomy are alternatives.
- Anti-D immune globulin 300 mcg should be given to Rh-negative unsensitized women.

MANAGEMENT OF **UNSTABLE/RUPTURED**:

- **Laparoscopic salpingostomy (with Ectopic pregnancy removal) often surgical procedure of choice *when possible*** (may need reparative procedure to save reproductive organs) + IV fluids.
- Salpingectomy if salpingostomy cannot be performed.
- Anti-D immune globulin 300 mcg should be given to Rh-negative unsensitized women.

FOLLOW UP:

- **Serial hCG measurements to see if there is at least 15% decrease from day 4 to day 7 after injection of Methotrexate.** hCG then followed weekly until 0 (often takes ~5-7 weeks).
- If Methotrexate was given and there is no significant decrease, a second dose can be given. If no response to the second dose, surgery should be performed for definitive management.
- Contraception should be used for at least 2 months after an Ectopic pregnancy.

GESTATIONAL TROPHOBLASTIC DISEASE [HYDATIDIFORM MOLE (MOLAR PREGNANCY)]

- **Neoplasm due to abnormal placental development with trophoblastic tissue proliferation (chorionic villi)** arising from gestational tissue rather than maternal tissue. 80% benign.

[1] COMPLETE Molar pregnancy:
- **Diploid (46XX 90%; 46XY 10%) most common type** — empty (enucleated) egg with no DNA fertilized by 1 or 2 sperm. **All paternal chromosomes lead to the absence of fetal tissue.** Associated with theca lutein cysts & higher risk of malignant development into Choriocarcinoma (20%).

[2] PARTIAL Molar pregnancy:
- **Triploid (69XXX or 69XXY)** — an egg is fertilized by 2 sperm (or 1 sperm that duplicates its chromosomes). **Fetal tissue may be seen but it is always abnormal and not viable.**

RISK FACTORS
- **[1] Prior Molar pregnancy & [2] extremes of maternal age** <20 years or >35 years. Asians.

CLINICAL MANIFESTATIONS
- **Painless vaginal bleeding (often in the first trimester), Preeclampsia early onset [6-16 weeks (before 20 weeks)], Hyperemesis gravidarum** (due to elevated hCG levels), & pelvic pain.

Physical examination:
- **Uterine size & date discrepancies** (larger or smaller than expected). Often, the uterus is enlarged.

DIAGNOSIS
Initial evaluation includes [1] quantitative serum hCG and [2] Pelvic ultrasound examination.
- **[1] Quantitative serum hCG markedly elevated** — eg, >100,000 mIU/mL in ~40% of complete & 6% of partial moles (complete moles often produce higher levels of hCG compared to partial moles).
- **[2] Pelvic ultrasound:**
  Complete — central heterogenous mass with multiple discrete hypoechoic and anechoic spaces **("snowstorm" or "cluster of grapes" appearance), absence of fetal parts & fetal heart tones.**
  Partial — gestational sac & fetal heart tones may be present plus abnormal tissue (eg, enlarged cystic spaces, often described as a "Swiss cheese" appearance) or indeterminate.
- Blood type, CBC, thyroid, liver, & renal function tests. Diagnosis based on tissue from evacuation.
- **Obtain chest radiograph to look for METS (Choriocarcinoma) — lungs is the most common site.**

MANAGEMENT
- **Complete surgical uterine evacuation mainstay of treatment as soon as possible to avoid risk of Choriocarcinoma development** — Suction curettage under general anesthesia commonly used.
- Patients are followed weekly until quantitative hCG levels fall to an undetectable level.
- If malignant tissue is discovered at surgery, chemotherapy (eg, Methotrexate) is indicated.
- Hysterectomy also an option for definitive management of a Molar pregnancy.

PRURITIC URTICARIAL PAPULES & PLAQUES OF PREGNANCY [PUPPP]

- Common benign, self-limiting rash in pregnancy. Also known as Polymorphic eruption of pregnancy.
- Most commonly occurs in the first pregnancy in the third trimester ≥35 weeks or postpartum and completely disappears within 2 weeks after delivery.

CLINICAL MANIFESTATIONS
- **Extremely pruritic erythematous papules within the striae gravidarum that spread outward & coalesce to form urticarial plaques;** spares periumbilical region (white halo), face, palms, & soles.

MANAGEMENT
- **Topical corticosteroids to decrease pruritus.** Antihistamines are usually helpful.
- Usually resolves spontaneously by 15 days postpartum.

PLACENTA PREVIA

- **Abnormal placenta placement over or close to the internal cervical os.**
- <u>Complete:</u> complete coverage of the cervical os by the placenta.
- <u>Partial:</u> partial coverage of the cervical os by the placenta.
- <u>Marginal:</u> adjacent to the internal os (leading edge of the placenta is <2 cm from the internal os).

<u>Photo credit:</u>
Shutterstock (used with permission)

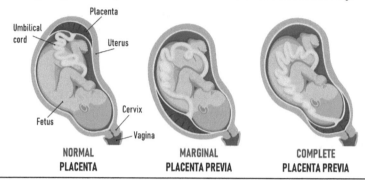

RISK FACTORS
- <u>**Major:**</u> **previous placenta previa, previous C-section, multiparity, and multiple gestations.**
- Advanced maternal age (>35 years), previous uterine surgery or scarring (eg, curettage), smoking.

CLINICAL MANIFESTATIONS
- **Sudden onset of <u>painless</u> vaginal bleeding (may be bright red) in the third trimester after 24 weeks** (one-third of patients with Placenta previa will present with bleeding before 30 weeks, one-third will present between 30 and 36 weeks, and one-third will present after 36 weeks).
- **Absence of abdominal pain or uterine tenderness** usually.
- Most common presentation is asymptomatic finding on routine ultrasound at 16-20 weeks gestation.

<u>Physical examination:</u>
- **Soft, nontender uterus.** Usually no fetal distress (in contrast with Vasa previa).
- ***Do not perform digital vaginal or speculum exam* if Placenta previa is suspected** (may cause increased separation, resulting in severe hemorrhage).

DIAGNOSIS
- <u>**Transabdominal ultrasound**</u> **often performed initially (screening) followed by confirmation on Transvaginal ultrasound** (TVUS is more sensitive & helps monitor placement of the placenta).
- A <u>Kleihauer-Betke test</u> should be sent for all women who are Rh negative. CBC & blood typing.
- Ultrasound may also rule out Placenta accreta, where the placenta invades the uterine wall and does not separate after delivery, which may lead to postpartum bleeding.

MANAGEMENT
- <u>Stabilization with preterm fetus:</u> watchful waiting if the patient is stable. Pelvic rest (no vaginal intercourse/excess physical activity). Hemodynamic stabilization. Rhogam in RhD-negative women.
- <u>**Conservative expectant management**</u> **often indicated between 24-36 weeks, if maternal & fetal stability and well-being are assured** — Hydration & blood transfusion as needed, bed rest with bathroom privileges, pelvic rest (no vaginal intercourse), stool softeners, iron supplementation, and steroids to promote fetal lung maturity if the gestational age is <34 weeks. <u>**Scheduled cesarean birth at 36+0 to 37+6 weeks**</u> **(Vaginal delivery contraindicated if <2 cm from the cervical os).**
- <u>**Delivery when stable**</u> **if L:S ratio >2:1, ≥36 weeks, blood loss >500 mL, persistent bleeding, coagulation defects, or persistent labor. <u>C-section usually preferred</u> in complete, major degrees, & with fetal distress.** Vaginal delivery may be an option if the margins are at least 2 cm away from internal os, mild degrees, & no fetal distress.
- <u>Delivery</u> is always indicated if there is a nonreassuring fetal heart rate pattern despite resuscitation efforts, including maternal supplemental oxygen, left-side positioning, or intravascular volume replacement; if there is life-threatening maternal hemorrhage; or if the gestational age is >34 weeks and there is known fetal lung maturity.

ABRUPTIO PLACENTAE (PLACENTAL ABRUPTION)

- **Partial or complete premature separation of the placenta from the uterine wall after 20 weeks gestation but prior to delivery of the fetus.**
- The blood may be concealed (within the uterine cavity) or external (blood drains through the cervix).
- **Due to rupture of maternal blood vessels in the decidua basalis,** leading to bleeding into the separated space. Subsequent release of tissue factor & thrombin generation lead to other findings.

RISK FACTORS
- **Maternal hypertension most common** (eg, chronic, Preeclampsia, Eclampsia). African Americans.
- **Prior abruption, cigarette smoking,** alcohol use, **cocaine,** folate deficiency, advanced maternal age, blunt abdominal trauma, multiple gestation, increasing parity, PPROM, & Chorioamnionitis.

CLINICAL MANIFESTATIONS
- **Sudden onset of [1] <u>uterine bleeding</u> — <u>painful</u> third-trimester vaginal bleeding (often dark red)** [either external or concealed], & **[2] severe abdominal/back pain (uterine contractions).**

Physical examination:
- **Tender, firm, and rigid (hypertonic) uterus. Do not perform a digital pelvic examination.**
- **Fetal distress may occur** — bradycardia, nonreassuring fetal heart rate tracing, or poor biophysical profile score may indicate fetal compromise.

DIAGNOSIS
- **Primarily a clinical diagnosis. <u>Transabdominal ultrasound</u>** may show a retroplacental clot (but not reliable). May be helpful to distinguish between abruptio and previa. Labs ± show ↓ fibrinogen.

MANAGEMENT
- **If nonreassuring heart tracing (category III) or mother is hemodynamically unstable, expeditious delivery is indicated (Cesarean delivery is preferred route);** if vaginal delivery is imminent, spontaneous or instrument-assisted vaginal birth is preferable.
- When the fetus & mother are both stable options include **[1] delivery indicated for most pregnancies at 34+0-36+6 weeks (eg, C-section);** [2] expectant management is an option as long as the patient remains asymptomatic; or **[3] delivery for all pregnancies ≥36 weeks of gestation.**
- **For pregnancies <34+0 weeks of gestation with no evidence of ongoing major blood loss or coagulopathy, conservative management until 37+0 to 38+0 weeks** with administration of a course of antenatal corticosteroids to promote fetal lung maturity is indicated.

> **EXAM TIP:**
> - **Placenta previa vs. Abruptio placentae**
> - Both are common causes of third trimester bleeding.
> - **Previa: painless vaginal bleeding + soft, nontender uterus**
> - **Abruptio: painful vaginal bleeding + abdominal pain + firm tender uterus.**
> - Think **P**revia is **P**ainless whereas **Ab**ruptio is associated with **Ab**dominal pain.

VASA PREVIA

- Fetal vessels are present over the cervical os, crossing over the os in front of the fetal presenting part.
- Fetal mortality approaches 60% if not detected before delivery due to fetal exsanguination.

CLINICAL MANIFESTATIONS
- **Triad of [1] rupture of membranes followed by [2] painless vaginal bleeding, and [3] fetal distress (eg, bradycardia & changes in the fetal heart tracing)** due to compression of umbilical vessels.

DIAGNOSIS: may be seen on Ultrasound prior to delivery as the vessels crossing the os.

MANAGEMENT: **deliver immediately via Cesarean section to prevent impending fetal demise.**

RH ALLOIMMUNIZATION

PATHOPHYSIOLOGY

- **Occurs when Rh(D)-negative women carry a Rh(D)-positive fetus** with exposure to fetal blood mixing of D-positive RBCs (eg, during C-section, spontaneous abortion, abruptio placentae, placenta previa, amniocentesis, vaginal delivery etc.).
- The mixing causes maternal alloimmunization & maternal anti-Rh(D) IgG antibodies (sensitization).

- **During subsequent pregnancies, if she carries another Rh(D)-positive fetus**, the antibodies may cross the placenta & attack the fetal RBCs, **leading to hemolysis of the fetal RBCs** (hemolytic disease of the fetus or newborn).
- If the mother of the fetus is Rh(D)-negative & father of the fetus is Rh(D)-positive, there's a 50% chance baby will be positive.
- At-risk pregnancy: **Rh(D)-negative mother and Rh(D)-positive father (or unknown Rh).**

WORKUP

- **Antibody screen:** RhD typing and an antibody screen at the first prenatal visit **to see if mother is Rh(D)- or Rh(D)+.**
- **In Rh(D)-negative women, the antibody screen may be repeated at 28 weeks of gestation and at delivery.**
- **Antibody titers: performed in Rh(D)-negative women. Unsensitized = no Rh(D) antibodies present.** If sensitized (Rh antibodies present), titers are performed via indirect antiglobulin test.
    - **The patient is considered Rh sensitized if positive titer level >1:4.**
    - If titer is <1:16, no further treatment is necessary.

If antibody titer ≥1:16, perform an initial amniocentesis at 16-20 weeks. If fetal cells are Rh(D)-negative, treat like normal pregnancy. If fetal cells are Rh(D)-positive and bilirubin is:
- Low — repeat amniocentesis in 2-3 weeks.
- Medium — repeat amniocentesis in 1-2 weeks.
- High — perform a percutaneous umbilical blood sample (fetal hematocrit). If fetal hematocrit is low, perform an intrauterine umbilical vein infusion.

PREVENTION

In Rh(D)-negative, antibody-negative women:
- **Anti-D immune globulin** given in **3 instances:**
    (1) given at 28 weeks gestation [300 µg of anti-D immunoglobulin (Rh IgG)] AND
    (2) within 72h of delivery of a Rh(D)-positive baby AND
    (3) after any potential mixing of blood (eg, spontaneous abortion, ectopic pregnancy, amniocentesis).

VACCINES DURING PREGNANCY	
SAFE (IF indicated)	**CONTRAINDICATED**
Mom is in her	(or safety not established)
Third Trimester – Mnemonic	**Live vaccines:**
	• **Varicella (Chickenpox)**
• **M**eningococcal	• **MMR**
• **T**etanus (eg, Td, Tdap)	• **Polio**
• **H**epatitis B,	• **BCG**
• **I**nactivated influenza	
• **R**abies	• Inactivated **HPV vaccine**
• **D**iphtheria	• **Intranasal influenza**
	• Yellow fever (in most), Smallpox

- Pregnant women with prior complete Td immunization should receive single dose of Tdap ideally during early part of 27-36 weeks of gestational age in each pregnancy.
- Ideally, all women who get pregnant or will get pregnant during flu season should get the inactivated Influenza vaccine. SARS-CoV-2 is safe in pregnancy.

MORNING SICKNESS & HYPEREMESIS GRAVIDARUM (HEG)

- Morning sickness: nausea &/or vomiting **up until 16 weeks (most common in the first trimester).**
- Hyperemesis gravidarum: **severe, excessive form of morning sickness (nausea, intractable vomiting) associated with weight loss** (>5% of pre-pregnancy body weight) **& electrolyte imbalance.** Develops during 1st or 2nd trimester and may persist >16 but <20 weeks of gestation.
- Risk factors: primigravida, previous hyperemesis in past pregnancy, multiple gestations, molar pregnancy.

PATHOPHYSIOLOGY
- **Vomiting center oversensitivity to hormones of pregnancy (eg, hCG).**
- Some degree of nausea with or without vomiting occurs in ≤90% of pregnancies, typically with **onset at 5-6 weeks of gestation, peaks 9 weeks, & usually improves by 16-18 weeks of gestation.**

CLINICAL MANIFESTATIONS
- Nausea and or vomiting. **Hyperemesis gravidarum is associated with more severe symptoms, weight loss of >5% of pre-pregnant weight,** & acidosis or **dehydration (from starvation).**
- Electrolyte imbalance from vomiting: **hypokalemia, hypochloremic metabolic alkalosis,** ketones.

MANAGEMENT
- **Lifestyle modifications: initial management of choice** — **ginger**, dietary changes (eg, high protein foods, small & frequent meals, avoiding trigger foods, such as spicy or fatty foods), increase fluids.
- **Pyridoxine (vitamin B$_6$) first-line medical management. Doxylamine may be added if persistent.**
- **Second line: substitute with another antihistamine [eg, Diphenhydramine, Dimenhydrinate, Meclizine]** if nausea continues, accompanied by vomiting but without hypovolemia.
- **Third line: add a dopamine antagonist — Metoclopramide, Promethazine, or Prochlorperazine.**
- **Fourth line: oral or intravenous Ondansetron.** Used on case-by-case basis in patients <10 weeks of gestation, after discussion of effectiveness & potential risks (small risk of congenital anomalies).
- If no response to Ondansetron, add glucocorticoids.
- **Hypovolemia: IV rehydration, electrolyte repletion, IV Thiamine.** Dimenhydrinate, Meclizine, or Diphenhydramine. **Ondansetron if severe vomiting.** Total parenteral nutrition if severe.

UTERINE RUPTURE

- **Complete transection of the uterus from the endometrium to the serosa.** If the peritoneum remains intact, it is known as uterine dehiscence. Most occur during labor at the site of a prior C-section.
- **Life-threatening to the mother and fetus.**

RISK FACTORS
- **Previous uterine rupture, prior Cesarean section (eg, fundal or vertical),** induction of labor (especially with Misoprostol), trauma (especially MVA), **uterine myomectomy** (patients with prior myomectomy require scheduled C-section at 36-37 weeks to prevent risk of uterine rupture), uterine overdistention (eg, multiple gestation, polyhydramnios), placenta percreta, abdominal trauma.

DECREASED RISK
- **A prior vaginal delivery** either before or after the prior C-section significantly reduces rupture risk.

CLINICAL MANIFESTATIONS
- **Sudden onset of extreme abdominal pain, decreased or absent uterine contractions,** abnormal bump in the abdomen, & possible regression of fetal parts. Vaginal hemorrhaging.
- The most common fetal heart rate pattern is fetal bradycardia, but No FHR pattern is pathognomonic.

MANAGEMENT
- **Immediate laparotomy & delivery of the fetus to reduce fetal and maternal mortality, followed by either (1) repair of the uterus or (2) hysterectomy (definitive management).**
- If repair is performed, all subsequent pregnancies will be delivered via Cesarean at 36 weeks.
- High fetal mortality rate (50-75%) depending on if the placenta remains attached to the uterine wall.

CHRONIC (PREEXISTING) HYPERTENSION

- **Hypertension [systolic BP ≥140 mm Hg &/or diastolic BP ≥90 mm Hg] present on 2 occasions (1) before pregnancy or (2) BEFORE 20 weeks gestation** OR persistence >12 weeks postpartum.
- Usually asymptomatic but headache or visual symptoms may be seen if severe (>160/110 mm Hg).
- Severity: Mild: ≥140/90 mm Hg. Moderate: ≥150/100 mm Hg. **Severe: ≥160/110 mm Hg.**

MANAGEMENT OF **MILD CHRONIC HYPERTENSION**

- In pregnant women with mild Hypertension and no evidence of renal disease, serious medical complications are rare so **antihypertensive medication is not usually necessary.**
- Monitor every 2-4 weeks, weekly between 34-36 weeks, and weekly thereafter. **Delivery should be initiated between 38 0/7 and 39 6/7 weeks.**
- At each visit, blood pressure, urine protein, & fundal height are evaluated. Patients are questioned regarding signs/symptoms of Preeclampsia (eg, headache, abdominal pain, blurred vision).

MANAGEMENT OF **SEVERE HYPERTENSION**

- **Antihypertensive agents may be indicated in women with severe Hypertension (systolic blood pressure ≥160 mm Hg or diastolic blood pressure ≥105-110 mm Hg)** due to higher risk for serious complications, such as heart attack, stroke, or progression of renal disease. A lower threshold for initiation of medications (≥150/100 mm Hg) may be recommended for women with end-organ involvement (eg, cardiac or renal disease).
- **Medications — Labetalol, long-acting Calcium channel blockers (eg, Nifedipine), or Methyldopa are first-line agents** to reduce maternal &/or fetal complications. **Hydralazine is an alternative.**
- **Contraindicated in pregnancy: ACE inhibitors & Angiotensin receptor blockers.** Spironolactone.
- Frequent prenatal visits may be needed to check the effectiveness of the medication. Fetal growth, blood pressure, and proteinuria are assessed during every visit.
- **Low-dose Aspirin prophylaxis — recommended after 12 weeks of gestation for prevention of Preeclampsia** as these patients are at high risk of developing the disease (eg, previous pregnancy with Preeclampsia, Diabetes mellitus, Multifetal gestation, Kidney disease, SLE).

TRANSITIONAL (GESTATIONAL, PREGNANCY-INDUCED) HYPERTENSION

- **NEW onset of Hypertension [systolic BP ≥140 mm Hg &/or diastolic BP ≥90 mm Hg] present on 2 occasions 4 hours apart** in a previously normotensive woman **AFTER 20 weeks gestation + no proteinuria or new signs of end-organ dysfunction.** Returns to normal by 12 weeks postpartum.
- These patients are usually asymptomatic.

DIAGNOSTIC WORKUP

- Measure blood pressure once or twice weekly and measure urine protein, platelets, and liver enzymes weekly used to distinguish Gestational from Preeclampsia.

MANAGEMENT
Mild Hypertension:

- **Fetal surveillance** with ultrasound for fetal growth every 3 weeks, daily fetal kick counts, and weekly NSTs and amniotic fluid volume measurement (with BPPs being reserved for a nonreactive NST) can assess fetal well-being. **Maternal surveillance** includes twice-weekly blood pressure measurements, evaluation of proteinuria, at each prenatal visit. **Delivery at 37 weeks gestation.**
- Antihypertensive drugs are not prescribed unless Hypertension is severe or approaching the severe range or the patient has preexisting end organ dysfunction (eg, renal, cardiac disease).

Severe Hypertension:

- **Antihypertensive agents may be indicated if severe (systolic blood pressure ≥160 mm Hg or diastolic blood pressure ≥105-110 mm Hg)** due to higher risk for serious complications (eg, cardiac or renal disease). **Nifedipine, Labetalol, or Methyldopa are first-line agents.**
- When antihypertensive treatment is initiated, the blood pressure goal is 130-150 mm Hg systolic and 80-100 mm Hg diastolic, similar to that in Preeclampsia.

ECLAMPSIA

- The occurrence of <u>new-onset of generalized tonic-clonic seizures</u> in the absence of other causative conditions in a patient with a hypertensive disorder of Pregnancy [Preeclampsia almost always precedes Eclampsia (even if unnoticed)], Gestational hypertension, HELLP syndrome [hemolysis, elevated liver enzymes, low platelets].
- In patients not receiving antiseizure prophylaxis, an eclamptic seizure occurs in 2-3% of patients with severe features of Preeclampsia and in 0-0.6% of those with Preeclampsia without severe features.
- <u>Gestational age at occurrence</u> — Eclampsia occurs before term in ~50% of patients. 35-55% of Eclampsia occurs antepartum, 15-35% percent occurs intrapartum, 5-40% occurs ≤48 hours postpartum, and 5-15% occurs >48 hours postpartum. ~90% of postpartum seizures occur within one week of delivery.

CLINICAL MANIFESTATIONS

- **Maternal signs/symptoms** — **Eclampsia is manifested by a generalized tonic-clonic seizure with either a postictal phase or coma after convulsion.** Individuals may experience prodromal signs/symptoms hours prior to development of the first seizure (eg, headache, visual disturbances, right upper quadrant, or epigastric pain) or signs (eg, Hypertension) or proteinuria. **In most cases, eclamptic seizures are self-limited, lasting 1–2 minutes. The initial objective is to protect the mother by ensuring the airway is clear & to prevent injury and aspiration of gastric contents.**
- **Fetal heart rate** — Fetal bradycardia lasting at least 3-5 minutes is a frequent occurrence during & immediately after an eclamptic seizure (due to maternal hypoxemia and lactic acidemia due to seizures). If the fetal heart rate tracing does not improve within 10 to 15 minutes of maternal and fetal resuscitative interventions, emergency cesarean birth should be considered.

MANAGEMENT

- The primary goals of management are to prevent maternal hypoxia and trauma, blood pressure stabilization (treat severe hypertension if present), prevent recurrent seizures with Magnesium sulfate, followed by prompt delivery (once the mother is stabilized).
- **Magnesium sulfate** — **IV Magnesium is the first-line management of seizures due to Eclampsia over other anticonvulsants (eg, Lorazepam)** due to reduced rate of recurrent seizures and reduced rate of maternal mortality. A regimen used is a 6-gram loading dose over 15 to 20 minutes, followed by 2 grams/hour as a continuous intravenous infusion. Loading doses of 4 or 5 grams may also be used & a lower or higher maintenance dose (1 or 3 g/hour) may also be considered. The maintenance phase is given only if a patellar reflex is present (**loss of deep tendon reflexes is the earliest manifestation of symptomatic hypermagnesemia**), respirations are >12 per minute, and urine output is >100 mL in 4 hours. **Once the patient is stabilized, delivery is usually indicated.**
- **Refractory cases** — If the patient is actively seizing for >5 minutes after Magnesium sulfate, consider Lorazepam. If ongoing seizures, patients who do not improve within 10 to 20 minutes following control of hypertension and seizures, and those with neurologic deficits should be evaluated by a neurologist and options include **sodium Amobarbital**, Thiopental, or Phenytoin.
- **Antihypertensive therapy** — **A common threshold for initiating antihypertensive therapy is sustained diastolic pressures >105-110 mm Hg or systolic blood pressures ≥160 mm Hg. Labetalol or Hydralazine are the preferred drugs for urgent blood pressure reduction in pregnancy. Nicardipine (parenteral) or Nifedipine are also options.**
- **Delivery** — **Delivery is the only curative treatment** (eg, induction of labor). Cesarean delivery is a reasonable option for women <32-34 weeks of gestation with an unfavorable cervix. After a seizure, in the absence of fetal bradycardia, waiting 15 to 20 minutes and until the mother and fetus show signs of recovery (control of seizures; mother oriented to name, time, and place; fetal heart rate reassuring) before proceeding to surgery, if possible.
- **Postpartum care** — Seizures due to Eclampsia always resolve in the postpartum period, generally within a few hours to days. When administered prior delivery, Magnesium sulfate is often given for 24 to 48 hours postpartum.

PREECLAMPSIA

- **[1] NEW onset of Hypertension [systolic BP ≥140 mm Hg &/or diastolic BP ≥90 mm Hg] present on 2 occasions 4 hours apart** in a previously normotensive woman **AFTER 20 weeks' gestation + [2] proteinuria or end-organ dysfunction.**
- Impaired vasodilation of spiral arteries & increase in thromboxane A2 cause placental ischemia, increased vascular tone, increased vasoconstriction, decreased vasodilation, & platelet aggregation.

RISK FACTORS:
- Preexisting Hypertension, nulliparity, primiparity, maternal age of <20 years or >35 years, diabetes, chronic renal disease, or autoimmune disorders.

PREECLAMPSIA WITHOUT SEVERE FEATURES
- **Blood pressure ≥140/90 mm Hg + proteinuria (≥300 mg in a 24-hour urine specimen or a spot urine protein/creatinine ratio ≥0.3).** Protein ≥2+ on dipstick = 100 to 300 mg/dL.

PREECLAMPSIA WITH SEVERE FEATURES: Any of the following:
- **[1] systolic blood pressure ≥160 mm Hg &/or diastolic blood pressure ≥110 mm Hg + proteinuria at least 5 grams in a 24-hour urine specimen** (or dipstick ≥3+).

Symptoms of end-organ damage
- **[2] thrombocytopenia** platelet count <100,000/μL. Disseminated intravascular coagulation (DIC).
- **[3] impaired liver function**: (1) elevated liver transaminases to twice normal concentration or (2) **severe or persistent epigastric or right upper quadrant pain** with no other cause.
- **[4] Progressive renal insufficiency:** serum creatinine >1.1 mg/dL or oliguria (<500 ml of urine in 24 hours or 30 cc/hour), or a doubling of the serum creatinine in the absence of other renal disease.
- **[5] pulmonary edema or peripheral edema.**
- **[6] cerebral or visual disturbances** — eg, new-onset or persistent headaches, flashing lights, blurred vision, altered mental status changes.
- **HELLP syndrome: Hemolytic anemia, Elevated Liver enzymes, & Low Platelets.**

MANAGEMENT OF PREECLAMPSIA WITHOUT SEVERE FEATURES
- **≥37+0 weeks gestation or greater hospitalized for initial evaluation & managed with delivery.**
- **34+0 to 36+6 weeks: expectant management until 37+0 weeks is reasonable** if fully informed of the risks and benefits, because the absolute maternal risk of a serious adverse outcome is low, and there are modest neonatal benefits from delivery at 37+0 weeks rather than earlier. Planned late preterm delivery (34+0 to 36+6 weeks) versus planned early term delivery at or shortly after 37+0 weeks can be decided by the patient and the medical team.
- **Before 34+0 weeks: expectant management is used for most,** given the high risk of neonatal complications from preterm birth.

Expectant management:
- **Laboratory follow-up** — Laboratory evaluation should include CBC (platelet count), serum creatinine, and liver enzymes. These tests should be repeated at least twice weekly in patients with Preeclampsia without severe features to assess for disease progression, and more frequently if clinical signs and symptoms indicate progressive or worsening disease.
- **Monitoring blood pressure and treatment of Hypertension** — Blood pressure measured twice daily at home & at least twice weekly in the office when the patient presents for laboratory and fetal evaluation. Evaluation of signs & symptoms consistent with Preeclampsia with severe features.
- Initial fetal evaluation consists of obtaining an ultrasonographic estimated fetal weight and amniotic fluid index as well as an NST with a BPP only if the NST is nonreactive.
- Fetal surveillance: An ultrasound for fetal growth every 3 weeks, daily fetal movement counts and twice weekly nonstress testing (NST) plus assessment of amniotic fluid volume, or twice weekly biophysical profiles, beginning at the time of diagnosis of preeclampsia.
- **Antihypertensives, bed rest, & Magnesium sulfate (seizure prevention) are not recommended as they have not been shown to improve outcomes, & bed rest may also increase harm.**
- Prior to 34 weeks, the administration of corticosteroids for fetal lung maturity is recommended.

MANAGEMENT OF PREECLAMPSIA WITH SEVERE FEATURES

- The primary components in managing patients with Preeclampsia are management of severe Hypertension, prevention of seizures, optimal timing of delivery, and postpartum surveillance.
- **The definitive treatment of Preeclampsia is delivery** to prevent development of maternal or fetal complications from disease progression.
- **Preeclampsia with features of severe disease is generally an indication for delivery**, regardless of gestational age, due to increased risk of serious maternal morbidity. However, prolonged antepartum management in a tertiary care setting or in consultation with a maternal-fetal medicine specialist is an option for selected patients remote from term (<34 weeks of gestation).
- **Antihypertensive therapy is indicated for treatment of severe Hypertension (defined as systolic blood pressure ≥160 mm Hg and/or diastolic blood pressure ≥110 mm Hg)** to prevent stroke (eg, **Hydralazine, Labetalol, or long-acting Nifedipine**); it does not prevent Eclampsia. The goal of antihypertensive therapy is to achieve a systolic blood pressure <160 mm Hg and a diastolic blood pressure <110 mm Hg.

TIMING OF DELIVERY

- **Diagnosis at term — For patients at term (≥37+0 weeks) with Preeclampsia without features of severe disease, delivery is often preferred** rather than expectant management.
- **Diagnosis preterm** — For patients with early preterm (<34 weeks) and late preterm (34+0 to 36+6 weeks) Preeclampsia without features of severe disease, expectant management with delivery when the pregnancy has reached 37+0 weeks of gestation is often recommended. Earlier delivery is indicated for standard obstetric indications (eg, nonreassuring fetal testing, preterm premature rupture of membranes).

EXPECTANT MANAGEMENT:

- **Close monitoring during expectant management of Preterm preeclampsia without features of severe disease consists of**:
- Maternal surveillance: blood pressure measurements at least twice daily, laboratory monitoring (platelet count, liver and renal function tests) at least twice weekly, blood pressure measurement at least twice daily, ongoing assessment and report of symptoms.
- Fetal surveillance: evaluation of fetal growth at diagnosis, repeat ultrasound in three to four weeks if the fetus is appropriate weight for gestational age Evaluation of fetal well-being with daily fetal movement counts and twice weekly nonstress testing plus assessment of amniotic fluid volume, or twice weekly biophysical profiles.
- In most patients with nonsevere Hypertension (systolic blood pressure <160 mmHg or diastolic blood pressure <110 mm Hg), antihypertensive therapy is **not** indicated.

ANTENATAL CORTICOSTEROIDS:

- **<34+0 weeks: for patients with a viable fetus & Preeclampsia <34+0 weeks of gestation, administration of a course of antenatal corticosteroids to promote fetal lung maturity.**
- Use of steroids at 34 to 36 weeks is controversial.

SEIZURE PROPHYLAXIS:

- **For patients with Preeclampsia with features of severe disease, intrapartum and postpartum seizure prophylaxis with Magnesium sulfate is indicated.**
- **Monitor for signs of Magnesium toxicity — although uncommon, signs of toxicity include loss of deep tendon reflex, such as the patellar reflex (often the earliest sign),** respiratory paralysis, & cardiac arrhythmias.

    Calcium gluconate is the antidote for cardiac toxicity due to Hypermagnesemia.

PREVENTION OF PREECLAMPSIA

- **Low-dose Aspirin prophylaxis: The USPSTF recommends the use of low-dose Aspirin** (eg, 81 mg/day) **as preventive medication after 12 weeks of gestation** (12-28 weeks) **in patients at high risk for Preeclampsia** (prevents platelet aggregation & helps prevent placental ischemia).

GESTATIONAL DIABETES MELLITUS (GDM)

- **Glucose intolerance or Diabetes mellitus with onset or first recognition during pregnancy.**

RISK FACTORS:

- Family or prior history of Gestational diabetes, spontaneous abortion, history of infant >4,000g at birth, multiple gestations, **Obesity,** BMI ≥25 kg/m², >25 years of age.
- Non-Caucasians: African American (highest), Hispanic, Asian or Pacific Islander, & Native American.

PATHOPHYSIOLOGY

- **<u>Maternal insulin resistance</u> in women with undiagnosed beta cell dysfunction** exacerbated by placental release diabetogenic hormones: **human placental lactogen** (also known as human somatomammotropin), growth hormone, & corticotropin-releasing hormone.
- Maternal insulin resistance allows for increased glucose availability for the growing fetus.

Fetal complications of GDM:

- **Fetal hyperinsulinemia leads to <u>fetal macrosomia (most common)</u>,** birth injuries from macrosomia (shoulder dystocia), **preterm labor,** delayed fetal lung maturity, fetal hyperglycemia but **neonatal hypoglycemia** (high fetal insulin levels + abrupt removal of maternal glucose after delivery), **neonatal hypocalcemia,** hypomagnesemia, hyperbilirubinemia, and stillbirth.
- Unlike progeny of women with pregestational Diabetes, congenital malformations (cardiac, musculoskeletal, and CNS) occur less in GDM because GDM occurs later in the pregnancy course.

<u>Maternal complications of GDM:</u>

- **>50% chance of developing type 2 Diabetes mellitus after pregnancy later in life.**
- >50% chance of recurrence with subsequent pregnancies. Preeclampsia, Abruptio placentae.

<u>SCREENING (two-step approach):</u>

- **<u>Step 1:</u> 1-hour 50-gram glucose challenge test (GCT), usually at 24–28 weeks gestation.** Screen-positive patients (glucose >130–140 mg/dL) should go on to a 3-hour oral glucose tolerance test.
- **<u>Step 2:</u> 3-hour oral 100-gram glucose tolerance test [OGTT] (diagnostic criterion standard).** The threshold for glucose levels on a 3-hour glucose tolerance test are 2 of the 4: fasting >95 mg/dL, 1 hour >180 mg/dL, 2 hour >155 mg/dL, or **3 hour >140 mg/dL.**

SCREENING (alternative one-step approach): 75g 2-hour oral glucose tolerance test (more sensitive).

MANAGEMENT

- Lifestyle modifications: **diabetic diet & exercise (eg, walking) initial treatment of choice.** *Pregnant patients are <u>not</u> told to lose weight.* Glucose levels are monitored several times daily in patients with GDM — self-monitoring before breakfast & at 1 or 2 hours after the beginning of each meal
- Optimal glucose levels during pregnancy are fasting levels of 70–95 mg/dL and 1-hour postprandial values <130–140 mg/dL or 2-hour postprandial values <120 mg/dL.

Medical management: Indications: if fasting glucose >95 mg/dL or greater and 1-hour postprandial glucose >130-140 mg/dL **after a trial of diet & exercise.**

- **Insulin often the first-line medication of choice** because it doesn't cross the placenta, is effective, easily adjustable based on glucose levels, and safe for the fetus.
- **Glyburide or Metformin are the only oral antihyperglycemic drugs used in pregnancy in women who are unable to comply with or refuse Insulin therapy.**

Labor induction:

- **GDM with good glucose control — scheduling induction 39+0 to 41+0 weeks of gestation.**
- **Patients well controlled with nutritional medical therapy alone** & candidates for vaginal birth, offer induction at 39+0 weeks of gestation & suggest performing induction by 41+0 weeks.
- GDM medically managed with insulin or oral agents and those with managed with nutrition with **<u>suboptimal glucose control</u> — induction of labor at 39+0 to 39+6 weeks of gestation.**
- If a concomitant medical condition (eg, Hypertension) is present, birth should be undertaken as clinically indicated prior to 39+0 weeks of gestation. **Scheduled cesarean birth at 39+0 weeks as the method of delivery if macrosomic (eg, fetal weight ≥4,500 grams) to avoid birth trauma.**

PREGESTATIONAL DIABETES MELLITUS

* Preexisting type I or type II Diabetes mellitus prior to pregnancy.

Maternal complications:
* Preeclampsia, spontaneous abortion, postpartum hemorrhage.

Fetal complications:
* **Congenital anomalies** (eg, cardiac and neural tube defects), Macrosomia, and Preterm labor.

SHOULDER DYSTOCIA

* **Failure of the shoulders to spontaneously traverse the pelvis after delivery of the fetal head due to impaction** (anterior shoulder is stuck behind the mother's pubic bone).
* Considered an obstetric emergency.
* During delivery, the turtle sign may occur (retraction of the baby's head, similar to a turtle retracting into its shell) or red, puffy face.

RISK FACTORS
* **Macrosomic infants of diabetics (most common),** post-term pregnancy, multiparity, prolonged second stage of labor, forceps delivery, maternal obesity, advanced maternal age, epidural anesthesia.

FETAL COMPLICATIONS
* **Brachial plexus injuries** due to traction during shoulder dystocia, **Erb's palsy,** Klumpke paralysis, Cerebral palsy.
* **Erb-Duchenne palsy** is a lesion in the upper trunk (root) injury (C5-C6 with or without C7) of the brachial plexus, leading to the characteristic "waiter's tip" deformity (arm in adduction with elbow extension, forearm pronation, and wrist flexion with the fingers curled up).
* **Clavicular fractures,** long bone fractures, fetal asphyxia, anoxic brain injury, death.

MATERNAL COMPLICATIONS:
* Perineal or vaginal tears, Postpartum hemorrhage, Uterine rupture.

MANAGEMENT
Nonmanipulative:
* Initial steps in management include having the patient stop pushing, ensuring proper patient position, convene essential personnel, and draining of a distended bladder.
* **[1] McRoberts maneuver without and then with suprapubic pressure as the initial approach for releasing the impacted shoulder,** as it is less invasive than other maneuvers. McRoberts maneuver: hyperflexion and abduction of the mother's hips towards the abdomen without and then with suprapubic pressure. An extending episiotomy may need to be performed.

Manipulative
* **[2] Delivery of the posterior arm if the McRoberts maneuver with suprapubic pressure is unsuccessful.**
* **[3] Axillary traction for delivery of the posterior arm** to attempt to deliver the shoulder if it is not possible to reach elbow or forearm (pull on the axilla to bring it down into posterior pelvic space).
* **[4] Rotational maneuver** if the above maneuvers are unsuccessful (eg, Woods corkscrew, Rubin) may be performed. **Woods corkscrew maneuver:** rotation of the fetal shoulders 180°.
* **The Gaskin all-fours maneuver** may be a good initial choice for the mother in a birthing bed with no or only local or pudendal anesthesia.
* Zavanelli maneuver: push the fetal head back into the vaginal canal followed to cesarean section.

PREVENTION:
* **Scheduled cesarean birth at 39+0 weeks as the method of delivery if macrosomic (eg, fetal weight ≥4,500 grams)** in weight in a diabetic mother or >5,000 grams in a nondiabetic mother.

BREECH PRESENTATION

- **The fetus whose presenting part is the buttocks and/or feet.**
- Spontaneous version may occur at any time prior to delivery.

EPIDEMIOLOGY
- Occurs in 3-5% of fetuses at term (37-40 weeks).

TYPES
- Frank: both hips are flexed and both knees are extended (the feet are adjacent to the fetal head). **Frank breech is the Most common type of breech presentation at term (50-70%).**
- Complete: both hips and both knees are flexed (5-10% at term).
- Incomplete: one or both of the hips are not completely flexed (10-40%).

Complete breech   Frank breech   Incomplete breech

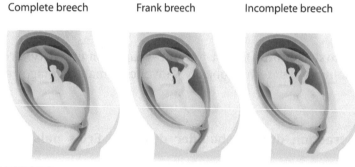

Photo credit:
Shutterstock (used with permission)

RISK FACTORS
- Underlying conditions associated with Breech presentation include congenital anomalies, fetal growth restriction, preterm birth) and, in part, to birth trauma, often not associated to vaginal breech birth.

Complications:
- Complications of Breech presentation include developmental dysplasia of the hip, torticollis, and mild deformations (eg, frontal bossing, low set ears, prominent occiput).

DIAGNOSIS
- Physical examination — a soft mass (eg, buttocks) instead of the normal hard surface of the skull. Leopold maneuvers are a set of 4 maneuvers that can determine the estimated fetal weight and presenting part of the fetus.
- Ultrasound can be used to confirm if the diagnosis is uncertain.

MANAGEMENT
Choice of delivery route includes patient preference, expertise of the provider, etc.
Options include:
- External cephalic version before labor, followed by a trial of labor (if the version is successful) & cesarean delivery if version is unsuccessful is an option for women at or near term at a low risk of labor and delivery-related complications. Planned Cesarean delivery of the breech fetus if the breech persists reduces maternal and perinatal death.

- External cephalic version before labor, followed by a trial of labor if the version is successful. If the version is unsuccessful, a trial of labor and vaginal breech birth are offered to patients at low risk of labor and delivery-related complications. Cesarean delivery is offered to patients at increased risk or if patient does not want to attempt a vaginal breech birth.

- Planned cesarean delivery for Breech presentation, without a trial of external cephalic version.

- A trial of labor and vaginal breech birth for patients thought to be at a low risk of labor and delivery-related complications, without a trial of external cephalic version.

UMBILICAL CORD PROLAPSE

- **Occurs when the cord extends past the presenting part of the fetus and protrudes into the vagina.**
- A prolapsed cord can lead to reduced fetal oxygenation as a result of umbilical artery vasospasm and/or umbilical vein occlusion.

RISK FACTORS

- Fetal and maternal factors include low birth weight, malpresentation, long umbilical cord, pelvic deformities, low-lying placentation, polyhydramnios, prematurity, etc.

CLINICAL MANIFESTATIONS

- **Sudden onset of (1) severe, prolonged fetal bradycardia or (2) moderate to severe Variable decelerations** after a previously normal tracing. The prolapse may be overt or nonovert (occult).
- The cord may be palpable on vaginal examination.

MANAGEMENT

- **Emergent Cesarean section to avoid fetal compromise or death from cord compression.**
  - Preoperative intrauterine resuscitation aims at increasing oxygen delivery to the placenta and umbilical blood flow — eg, manual elevation of the fetal presenting part to prevent compression, **placing the patient in Trendelenburg or knee-chest position,** tocolytics, etc.
- **Vaginal delivery is an option when delivery is impending and can be securely assisted.**

CESAREAN DELIVERY

- The use of surgery for delivery of the fetus.

INDICATIONS

- **Conditions where vaginal delivery would put the fetus &/or mother at risk** — examples include **failure of labor progression (most common), nonreassuring fetal status, fetal malpresentation,** problems with the placenta or the umbilical cord, multiple gestations, maternal hypertension, maternal infection with significant risk of perinatal transmission via vaginal birth, suspected macrosomia, uterine rupture.

TIMING

- **Scheduled primary Cesarean deliveries at term is often performed at 39th or 40th week of gestation.**
- Obstetrically & medically indicated Cesarean deliveries are performed as necessary.
- The timing of elective repeat Cesarean delivery is dependent on a many factors.

ANTIBIOTIC PROPHYLAXIS

- **Preoperative: up to 60 minutes prior to making the initial incision.**
- **IV Cefazolin to prevent Endometritis.** Azithromycin may be added if the Cesarean delivery is performed after rupture of membranes or intrapartum.
- Clindamycin and Gentamicin if Penicillin-allergic.
- For women in labor & women with ruptured membranes, vaginal cleansing before cesarean delivery (eg, Povidone-iodine vaginal scrub for 30 seconds) reduces the frequency of postpartum Endometritis.

THROMBOPROPHYLAXIS

- For all women undergoing Cesarean delivery, mechanical thromboprophylaxis is suggested.
- Women at high risk of venous thromboembolism should receive mechanical thromboprophylaxis plus pharmacologic thromboprophylaxis.
- Pharmacologic prophylaxis is initiated 6-12 hours postoperatively, after concerns for hemorrhage have diminished and continued until the woman is fully ambulating.

PRELABOR RUPTURE OF THE MEMBRANES (PROM) AT TERM

- **Amniotic membrane rupture ≥37+0 weeks prior to the onset of labor or regular uterine contractions.** Preterm prelabor rupture of membranes (PPROM) occurs prior to 37+0 weeks.

RISK FACTORS
- STIs, UTIs, prior preterm delivery, multiple gestations, antepartum bleeding, smoking, cerclage.

CLINICAL MANIFESTATIONS
- **Vaginal discharge: "gush" of clear or pale to yellow fluid or persistent leakage of fluid in the absence of regular uterine contractions.**

Complications:
- **Chorioamnionitis or Endometritis if prolonged (>24 hours).** Cord prolapse, placental abruption.

DIAGNOSIS
- Evaluation includes confirmation of membrane rupture, assessment of maternal & fetal well-being (nonstress testing), & assessment of need for Group B streptococcal chemoprophylaxis.

Sterile speculum exam:
- Sterile speculum examination to assess for cervical dilatation & effacement. Assess for any signs of vaginal bleeding, cervicitis, or umbilical cord prolapse. Obtain fluid for cultures.
- **Visualization of amniotic fluid passing from the cervical os into the canal and pooling of secretions in the posterior fornix of the vagina with inspection often confirms a diagnosis of membrane rupture.** If the diagnosis is uncertain, perform Fern or Nitrazine testing of the fluid.
- **Nitrazine paper test: turns blue if pH >6.5 — PROM is likely** because normal amniotic fluid pH is ~7 compared to vaginal pH, which is usually ~4.
- **Fern test: amniotic fluid dries in a fern pattern (crystallization of estrogen & amniotic fluid).**
- **Avoid digital cervicovaginal examination before labor in most cases** unless the patient is in active labor or delivery is imminent to avoid introduction of infection.

Other testing
- Ultrasound to check the amniotic fluid index.
- Fetal well-being is evaluated with a Nonstress test.
- Fetal position is determined by Transabdominal ultrasound &/or physical examination (Leopold's maneuvers).
- Maternal evaluation includes assessment for contractions, signs of infection (eg, fever, fetal tachycardia, maternal leukocytosis), and oligohydramnios (either single deepest pocket <2 cm or amniotic fluid index ≤5 cm).
- Baseline Complete blood count: leukocytosis is a nonspecific finding and can be associated with inflammation asides from infection. A marked elevation in the white blood count (>20,000/mm^3) or a significant left shift suggest Chorioamnionitis.

MANAGEMENT
- **Prompt delivery: induction of labor** (if it does not occur spontaneously within 6 hours of rupture) **in patients with term PROM unless there are contraindications to labor or vaginal delivery, in those instances, prompt Cesarean delivery is performed.** Compared with expectant management, induction of labor is associated with a reduction in maternal and neonatal complications, reduced treatment costs, and no increased need for Cesarean delivery. **Labor induction with Oxytocin** without preinduction cervical ripening is as effective as Prostaglandin cervical gel, easier to titrate, and may be cheaper. **Group B Streptococcus prophylaxis should be administered if indicated.** Misoprostol or Prostaglandin E2 cervical gel for cervical ripening used in some patients with an unfavorable cervix.
- **Expectant management: to wait for spontaneous labor in patients who choose this option.** >50% of expectantly managed patients go into active labor within 1 day & 95% will be in active labor within 3 days, but with **higher risk for developing maternal or neonatal infection than those in whom labor are induced. GBS prophylaxis should be administered as indicated.**

PRETERM PRELABOR RUPTURE OF MEMBRANES (PPROM)

- **Rupture of the amniotic membranes before the onset of labor occurring <u>prior to 37+0 weeks</u>.**
- <u>**Complications:**</u> **Chorioamnionitis & Endometritis are major complications of PROM & PPROM.**
- <u>Risk factors</u>: Genital tract infection, a history of PPROM in a previous pregnancy, antepartum bleeding, and cigarette smoking.

CLINICAL MANIFESTATIONS
- **"Gush" of clear or pale-yellow fluid** or persistent leakage of fluid from the vagina, vaginal discharge.

DIAGNOSIS
- The initial evaluation when PPROM is suspected should include confirmation of membrane rupture, assessment of maternal & fetal well-being (nonstress testing), & Group B streptococcal screening.
- <u>**Sterile speculum exam:**</u> **pooling of secretions in posterior fornix with inspection.** Obtain fluid for cultures, Nitrazine paper or Fern test if diagnosis is uncertain. <u>**Nitrazine paper test**</u>: **turns blue if pH >6.5** (PROM is likely because normal amniotic fluid pH is ~7 compared to vaginal pH usually ~4). <u>**Fern test**</u>: amniotic fluid dries in a fern pattern (crystallization of estrogen & amniotic fluid).
- <u>Ultrasound</u> to check amniotic fluid index.
- Avoid digital vaginal exam unless delivery is imminent in most cases (to avoid introduction of infection).

MANAGEMENT
[1] Stable patients (mother & fetus) <34 weeks:
<u>**Expectant management**</u> **rather than delivery.** In addition:
- **(1) <u>administer antenatal corticosteroids</u> (eg, Betamethasone) to enhance fetal lung maturity,**
- **(2) <u>prophylactic antibiotics</u> IV Ampicillin + Azithromycin once, followed by oral Amoxicillin,**
- **(3) <u>hospitalization</u>** during the entire period of expectant management to wait for spontaneous labor (diagnosis of PPROM to delivery).
- Tocolytics may be given to delay delivery up to 48 hours in some patients to allow the effect of administration of glucocorticoids on fetal lung maturity. Tocolytics should not be used in patients in advanced labor (>4 cm dilation), signs of chorioamnionitis, if nonreassuring fetal testing (eg, nonreactive nonstress test [NST]), abruptio placentae, or if significant risk of cord prolapse (eg, dilated cervix and fetal malpresentation).

[2] Stable patients (mother & fetus) in Late preterm (34-36 weeks):
- <u>**Delivery**</u> **rather than expectant management if optimal gestational dating.** If gestational dating is suboptimal, expectant management with delivery when the best estimate of gestational age is 36 to 37 weeks. GBS prophylaxis (eg, Penicillin G) if needed. Corticosteroids if L:3S <2.0.

[3] Infection or instability (fetal &/or maternal) & <34 weeks:
- <u>**Prompt delivery**</u> **indicated if there are signs of maternal or fetal infection or distress.**
- <u>**Intraamniotic infection treatment:**</u> **eg, Ampicillin + Gentamicin.**
- <u>Antenatal corticosteroids</u> (eg, Betamethasone) to enhance fetal lung maturity. Tocolytics in some.
- <u>Magnesium sulfate</u> if between 24+0 to <32+0 weeks gestation for fetal neuroprotection.

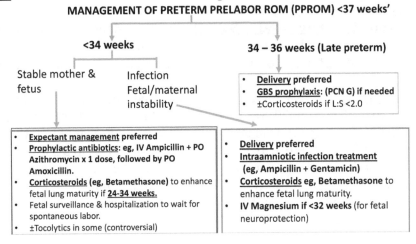

MANAGEMENT OF PRETERM PRELABOR ROM (PPROM) <37 weeks'

PRETERM LABOR

- **[1]** <u>Labor</u> = regular painful uterine contractions (≥6 in 60 minutes) + progressive cervical effacement & dilation ≥3-4 cm + **[2]** <u>preterm</u>: between 20-36 weeks gestation (<37 weeks).

ETIOLOGIES
- **Maternal infection most common cause** (eg, UTI, vaginal group B streptococci), cigarette smoking, cocaine use, cervical incompetence, low prepregnancy weight, uterine abnormalities, idiopathic.

CLINICAL MANIFESTATIONS
- <u>Nonspecific:</u> painful or painless uterine contractions (eg, menstrual-like cramping; mild, irregular contractions); low back pain; pressure sensation in the vagina; water or bloody discharge [vaginal discharge of mucus which may be clear, pink, or slightly bloody (eg, mucus plug, bloody show)].

PHYSICAL EXAMINATION
- **Speculum examination** performed using a wet non-lubricated speculum (lubricants may interfere with tests performed on vaginal specimens). Examination for (1) cervical dilation estimation — **cervical dilation ≥3 cm supports the diagnosis of Preterm labor**; (2) assessment of the presence and amount of uterine bleeding (bleeding from placental abruption or placenta previa can trigger Preterm labor); (3) assessment of fetal membrane status (intact or ruptured). Usage of a swab to obtain a cervicovaginal fluid specimen in case fetal fibronectin (fFN) testing is necessary after transabdominal ultrasound examination.
- **Digital cervical examination** — In most patients, cervical dilation & effacement are assessed by digital examination after placenta previa and rupture of membranes have been excluded by history and physical, laboratory, and ultrasound examinations, as appropriate. **Cervical dilation ≥3 cm in the presence of regular painful uterine contractions at 20+0 to 36+6 weeks and >80% effacement supports the diagnosis of Preterm labor.**

Transvaginal ultrasound examination:
- TVUS measurement of cervical length is useful for supporting or excluding the diagnosis of Preterm labor when the diagnosis is unclear. Normal cervical length is 4 cm.
- **A short cervix (<30 mm) before 34 weeks of gestation is predictive of an increased risk for Preterm birth in all populations.** A length of 2 cm at 24 weeks increases risk of delivery.
- A long cervix (≥30 mm) has a high negative predictive value for preterm birth.

Obstetric ultrasound examination:
- Obstetric ultrasound examination provides useful information in addition to cervical length, including presence/absence of fetal, placental, and maternal anatomic abnormalities; confirmation of fetal presentation; assessment of amniotic fluid volume; and estimated fetal weight.
- The information obtained in Ultrasound is beneficial to advise patients about the potential causes and outcomes of Preterm birth and determining the best option for birth.

Laboratory evaluation:
- **Rectovaginal group B streptococcal (GBS) culture**, if not done within the previous 5 weeks; GBS antibiotic prophylaxis administration is dependent on the results.
- **Urine culture** since asymptomatic bacteriuria is associated with an increased risk of Preterm labor and birth.
- **Fetal fibronectin (fFN)** in pregnancies <34 weeks of gestation with cervical dilation <3 cm and cervical length 20 to 30 mm on TVUS examination. Useful marker of predicting spontaneous Preterm birth and to distinguish true preterm labor from false labor. **Cervical length & fFN abnormalities = 50% chance of delivery before 30 weeks. Absence of fFN means a low risk of delivery within 2 weeks.** Identification of true preterm labor allows for interventions as needed.
- Testing for sexually transmitted infections (eg, chlamydia, gonorrhea), based on the patient's risk factors for these infections and, if indicated, whether antepartum testing was recently done.

DIAGNOSIS OF PRETERM LABOR IN SINGLETON PREGNANCIES

- **The diagnosis of Preterm labor (20-36 weeks of gestation) is based on presence of [1] <u>regular painful uterine contractions</u> (≥4 every 20 minutes or ≥6 in 60 minutes) accompanied by [2] cervical dilation ≥3 cm and/or effacement.**
- **Cervical dilation ≥3 cm OR** Cervical length <20 mm on transvaginal ultrasound **OR** Cervical length 20 to <30 mm on transvaginal ultrasound AND positive fetal fibronectin.
- <u>PTL likely</u>: cervical dilation 2-3 cm with <80% effacement or if >1cm cervical dilation on serial exams.

MANAGEMENT

≥34 to 37+0 weeks of gestation:

- **Patients ≥34 weeks without progressive cervical dilation and effacement after an observation period of 4-6 hours can be discharged to home**, provided that fetal well-being is confirmed and obstetric complications associated with Preterm labor (eg, Chorioamnionitis, membrane rupture, abruption) have been excluded. **Patients in Preterm labor are admitted proceeding with birth.**

<34 weeks + cervical dilation ≥3 cm:

- **(1) delay delivery with tocolytic administration (eg, Nifedipine if 32-34 weeks) for up to 48h.**
- **(2) antibiotics for group B streptococcal chemoprophylaxis (when appropriate),** and
- **(3) antenatal corticosteroid (eg Betamethasone)** to enhance fetal lung maturity. Effects begin at 24 hours, peak at 48 hours, and last 7 days.
- If <32 weeks of gestation, Magnesium sulfate is administered for fetal neuroprotection.

<34 weeks of gestation + cervical dilation <3 cm:

- Transvaginal ultrasound measurement of cervical length and laboratory analysis of cervicovaginal fetal fibronectin (fFN) level help to support or exclude the diagnosis of Preterm labor. For patients diagnosed with Preterm labor, administer tocolytic drugs for up to 48 hours, antibiotics for group B streptococcal chemoprophylaxis (when appropriate), and antenatal corticosteroids (eg, Betamethasone). Magnesium sulfate for neuroprotection for pregnancies <32 weeks of gestation.

24 weeks but <32 weeks (very preterm)

- **Antenatal corticosteroids (eg, Betamethasone)** to enhance fetal lung maturity.
- **Tocolysis: eg, Indomethacin.**
- <u>GBS prophylaxis</u>: Penicillin G if GBS+ or unknown.
- **Magnesium sulfate is administered for neuroprotection to pregnancies <32 weeks** of gestation (protects against severe motor dysfunction & cerebral palsy).

PRETERM LABOR MANAGEMENT

<u>Preterm labor</u>: regular contractions causing cervical change at <37 weeks' with intact membranes.

- Maternal instability
- Intrauterine infection → **Yes** → **Immediate delivery**
- Fetal distress/demise

No

24 but <32 weeks (very preterm)	32-34 weeks (moderate preterm)	34-37 weeks (late preterm)
• **Antenatal corticosteroids**	• **Antenatal corticosteroids**	• **Antenatal Corticosteroids**
• **Tocolysis**: eg, **Indomethacin**	• **Tocolysis**: eg, **Nifedipine**	• **GBS prophylaxis**: **Penicillin G** if GBS+ or unknown
• **GBS prophylaxis**: **Penicillin G** if GBS+ or unknown	• **GBS prophylaxis**: **Penicillin G** if GBS+ or unknown	
• **Magnesium sulfate for neuroprotection**		

Antenatal corticosteroids (eg, Betamethasone) to enhance fetal lung maturity.

Magnesium sulfate if <32 weeks for neuroprotection against motor dysfunction & cerebral palsy.

TOCOLYTICS

- Tocolytics are medications used to suppress uterine contractions.

Indications:
- **Patients with Preterm labor ≤34+0 weeks of gestation:** if the cervix is dilated <5 cm, tocolytics **allow for delay in delivery for 48 hours for administration of Antenatal corticosteroids (ACS) to enhance fetal lung maturity to prevent Neonatal respiratory distress syndrome.** This allows for ACS to achieve the maximal effect (effects begin at 24 hours, peak at 48 hours, and last 7 days) and allows for maternal transport to facility for special neonatal care if deemed necessary.
- **Tocolytics are usually discontinued 48 hours after administration of the first ACS.**

CHOICE OF TOCOLYTIC DRUG
First-line therapy ≤32+0 weeks:
- **Indomethacin is usually used first-line for labor inhibition if ≤32+0 weeks** because of a relatively favorable maternal & fetal adverse effect profile & compatibility with concomitant neuroprotective administration of Magnesium sulfate. Indomethacin inhibits prostaglandin-mediated uterine contractions. Contraindications include maternal bleeding disorder, platelet dysfunction, gastrointestinal ulcerative disease, renal dysfunction, hepatic dysfunction, or Aspirin hypersensitivity. **Because of potential premature narrowing or closure of the ductus arteriosus, Indomethacin is not usually used in gestations >32+0 weeks or for >72 hours.**
- **Nifedipine alternative in patients ≤32+0 weeks who have a contraindication to Indomethacin.** If the patient received Nifedipine as a first-line agent, Terbutaline may be used.

First-line therapy >32+0-≤34+0 weeks:
- **Nifedipine is the first-line therapy for patients who are candidates for Tocolysis >32+0 and ≤34+0 weeks of gestation.** Nifedipine inhibits calcium influx, leading to myometrial relaxation. Adverse effects include nausea, flushing, headache, dizziness, maternal hypotension, & tachycardia.
- **Terbutaline is a second-line agent infrequently used for patients at >32+0 and ≤34+0 weeks.** Terbutaline is a beta-2 receptor agonist that cause myometrial (uterine muscle) relaxation. Maternal adverse effects are due to beta-1 adrenergic receptor stimulation (eg, increase maternal heart rate and stroke volume), beta-2-adrenergic receptor stimulation (peripheral vasodilation, diastolic hypotension, and bronchial relaxation). May cause hyperglycemia or myocardial ischemia. Pulmonary edema is a rare adverse effect.

Other tocolytics
- Magnesium sulfate: The American College of Obstetricians and Gynecologists (ACOG) and the Society for Maternal-Fetal Medicine consider Magnesium sulfate an option for short-term prolongation of pregnancy (up to 48 hours) to allow administration of ACS to patients at risk for preterm birth within 7 days. Adverse effects: diaphoresis & flushing, muscle weakness, hyporeflexia.

PITUITARY INFARCTION (SHEEHAN SYNDROME)

- **Postpartum pituitary gland infarction & necrosis in the setting of obstetric hemorrhage (eg, postpartum hemorrhage) complicated by hypotension.**

CLINICAL MANIFESTATIONS:
Anterior pituitary hormone deficiency:
- **Decreased prolactin: lactation failure soon after delivery.**
- Decreased LH & FSH: amenorrhea, hot flashes, vaginal atrophy.
- **Decreased ACTH (Secondary Adrenal insufficiency): hypotension, anorexia, weight loss (low ACTH & low cortisol).** Decreased TSH: fatigue, dry skin, constipation, and weight gain.
- Decreased growth hormone: decreased lean body mass.

MANAGEMENT: replacement of deficient hormones.

LABOR & DELIVERY

INTRAPARTUM

- **Ruptured Membranes:** sudden gush of liquid or constant leakage of fluid.
- **Bloody show:** passage of blood-tinged cervical mucus late in pregnancy. Occurs when the cervix begins thinning (effacement).
- **Braxton-Hicks contractions (False labor):** spontaneous uterine contractions late in pregnancy **not associated with cervical changes or dilation & wane over time. Managed with reassurance.**
- **True labor:** contractions of the uterine fundus with radiation to lower back & abdomen. **Regular & painful contractions of the uterus that causes cervical dilation & progress over time.**
- **Lightening:** fetal head descending into the pelvis causing a change in the abdomen's shape and sensation that the baby has "become lighter".

7 CARDINAL MOVEMENTS OF LABOR

1. **Engagement:** when the fetal presenting part enters the pelvic inlet. In primigravida, often occurs in the last 2 weeks; in multiparous women, often occurs at the onset of labor.
2. **Descent:** passage of the presenting part (eg, head) into the pelvis (commonly called "lightening"). The remaining movements occur superimposed with descent.
3. **Flexion:** flexion of the head to allow the smallest diameter to present to the pelvis. Flexion is essential for both engagement and descent.
4. **Internal Rotation:** fetal vertex moves from occiput transverse position to a position where the sagittal suture is parallel to the anteroposterior diameter of the pelvis.
5. **Extension:** vertex extends as it passes beneath the pubic symphysis and descends into the introitus. At this point, spontaneous delivery is imminent.
6. **External rotation (restitution):** fetus passively externally rotates the fetal head back to the anatomical position of the fetal body after the head is delivered so that the shoulder can be delivered. During this movement, the anterior shoulder rotates under the symphysis pubis.
7. **Expulsion:** delivery of the entire fetus.

STAGES OF LABOR

3 STAGES OF LABOR

STAGE I:	**Onset of labor (true regular contractions) to <u>full dilation of cervix (10 cm).</u>** - **Latent phase:** cervix effacement with gradual (slow) cervical dilation. - **Active phase:** rapid cervical dilation, usually beginning at 3-4 cm.
STAGE II:	**Time from full cervical dilation until <u>delivery of the fetus</u> (expulsion).** - **Passive phase:** complete cervical dilation to active maternal expulsive efforts. - **Active phase:** from active maternal expulsive efforts to delivery of the fetus. Often lasts 30 minutes to 3 hours in primigravid women and from 5–30 minutes in multigravid women.
STAGE III:	**Postpartum until <u>delivery of the placenta</u>. 0-30 minutes usually (average 5).** **3 signs of placental separation:** **(1) fresh gush of blood** appears from the vagina. **(2) lengthening of the umbilical cord** outside the vagina. **(3) anterior-cephalad movement of the uterine fundus (becomes globular and firmer)** after the placenta detaches. Gentle controlled contraction may facilitate delivery of the placenta if needed. Placental expulsion: due to downward pressure of the retroplacental hematoma, uterine contractions.

The period 1-2 hours after delivery after placental expulsion when the uterus regains its tone and begins the process of involution where the mother is assessed for complications is sometimes called the 4th stage.

INDUCTION & AUGMENTATION OF LABOR

- **Induction of labor**: stimulation of uterine contractions to initiate labor prior to the onset of spontaneous labor. <u>Augmentation:</u> artificial stimulation of labor that has begun spontaneously.

INDICATIONS:
- **Labor induction via vaginal delivery is indicated when maternal and/or fetal risks associated with expectant management or continuation of the pregnancy outweigh the risk associated with delivery & there are no contraindications to vaginal birth.**
- <u>Maternal indications:</u> Preeclampsia, eclampsia, HELLP (hemolysis, elevated liver enzymes, low platelet count), diabetes (pregestational or gestational), chronic hypertension, and heart disease.
- <u>Fetal indications:</u> Late-term or post-term pregnancy, fetal abnormality, chorioamnionitis, premature rupture of membranes, prelabor rupture of membranes, placental insufficiency, oligohydramnios, suspected intrauterine growth restriction, fetal demise, and multiple gestation.
- Elective Induction may be offered to low-risk women without other medical indication at 39 weeks of gestation (well dated). It not usually performed electively prior to 39 weeks of gestational age.

CONTRAINDICATIONS
Situations in which the risks of induction of vaginal delivery is greater than cesarean delivery.
- **Absolute contraindications: transmural myomectomy, placenta previa, prolapsed cord, active genital herpes, transverse fetal lie, uterine scar from previous <u>classical</u> cesarean section incision, & cephalopelvic disproportion, contracted pelvis.**
- <u>Relative contraindications:</u> breech presentation, multiple gestation, prematurity, & previous C-section with low transverse scar.

The Bishop score is the best available tool for assessing cervical status.
- Most consider a Bishop score ≥6 as favorable & a score ≤3 as unfavorable; <u>Gray zone:</u> scores of 4 or 5.

A. Favorable cervixes (eg, Bishop score ≥6):
- For women with favorable cervixes undergoing induction, administration of Oxytocin with amniotomy (preferably "early" rather than "late" in timing) rather than amniotomy alone may be more efficacious.
- **(1) IV Oxytocin is a uterotonic agent & the most effective medical means to induce labor.** Monitor uterine activity & fetal heart rate.
- **(2) Amniotomy** artificially rupturing the membranes with a small hook. May be performed if the cervix is partially dilated & there is effacement of the cervix. Monitor fetal heart rate.

B. Unfavorable cervix (eg, Bishop score ≤3):
- **Preinduction cervical ripening**: For women scheduled for labor induction with an unfavorable cervix (eg, low Bishop score), preinduction cervical ripening **increases the likelihood of a successful induction** (progression of labor, vaginal delivery, especially in primigravid patients). **Both pharmacologic (eg, Prostaglandins) and mechanical approaches (balloon catheter or laminaria) are reasonable choices unless a patient has a contraindication.** Oxytocin can be initiated 30 minutes after Prostaglandin insert is removed in patients with an unfavorable cervix.
- **(1) Prostaglandin gel or vaginal insert: [eg, Dinoprostone (PGE$_2$)]** placed directly on the cervix. Promotes cervical ripening and may lead to uterine contractions and improve the Bishop score. Prostaglandins are contraindicated for cervical ripening or labor induction in term pregnancies with a prior cesarean birth or other prior major uterine surgery. Preexisting regular painful uterine activity is a relative contraindication. **Misoprostol intravaginally (PGE$_1$) is an alternative.** <u>Adverse effects</u> include fetal heart deceleration, fetal distress, emergency C-section, uterine hypertonicity, nausea, vomiting, fever, and peripartum infection.
- **(2) Transcervical balloon catheter or laminaria** (dilates the cervix). There are no absolute contraindications to mechanical methods of cervical ripening in women who are candidates for labor and vaginal delivery. A low-lying placenta is a relative contraindication since the edge of the placenta may be disrupted by manipulation during device placement.

POSTPARTUM (PUERPERIUM) 6-week period after delivery

- **Uterus:** at the level of the umbilicus after delivery, involution (shrinks) after 2 days, descends into the pelvic cavity ~2 weeks. Normal size around 6 weeks postpartum.
- **Lochia serosa:** pinkish/brown vaginal bleeding especially postpartum days 4-10 (from the decidual tissue). Usually resolves by 3-4 weeks postpartum.
- **Breasts/menstruation:** breast milk in postpartum days 3-5 bluish-white. If lactating, mothers may remain anovulatory during that time. If not breastfeeding, menses may return after 6-8 weeks.

POSTPARTUM HEMORRHAGE

- **Greater than expected bleeding [eg, >500 ml if vaginal delivery is performed or >1,000 ml if cesarean section is performed].** Loss requiring transfusion or a 10% decrease in hematocrit.
- Common cause of maternal death within 24 hours of delivery.
- Early: blood loss within 24 hours postpartum; delayed >24 hours up to 8 weeks postpartum.
- Pathophysiology: After delivery of the placenta, myometrial contraction compresses the blood vessels supplying the placental bed local clotting factor release results in hemostasis. PPH occurs due to disruption of 1 or both of these mechanisms.

ETIOLOGIES: **4 Ts:**
- **Tone uterine atony most common cause** (80%) — uterus unable to contract to stop the bleeding. Risk factors for uterine atony: **prior PPH, prolonged labor,** rapid labor, overdistended uterus (eg, multiple gestation), multiparity, C-section, general anesthesia, retained placenta.
- **Tissue:** retained placental or fetal tissue, blood clots, or placenta accreta spectrum (5-10%).
- **Trauma** to the cervix, perineum or vagina, Uterine rupture, obstetric lacerations, surgical incision.
- **Thrombin:** coagulopathy (7%) — Hemophilia A, von Willebrand disease, ITP, DIC, thrombocytopenia.

CLINICAL MANIFESTATIONS
- **Prolonged bleeding. May have signs & symptoms of hypovolemia.**
- Hypovolemic shock — hypotension, tachycardia, pale or clammy skin, decreased capillary refill.
- Examination: **Soft flaccid boggy enlarged uterus if uterine atony is the cause; dilated cervix.**

WORKUP
- CBC to evaluate hemoglobin & hematocrit (poor indicators of acute blood loss). IV access.
- Low fibrinogen level (<200 mg/dL) is predictive of severe PPH & need for transfusions.
- Ultrasound may detect bleeding source or retained products of conception (echogenic uterine mass).

MANAGEMENT
- Treatment goals are to restore or maintain adequate circulatory volume to prevent hypoperfusion of vital organs (eg, IV fluids, blood products if indicated), restore or maintain adequate tissue oxygenation, reverse or prevent coagulopathy, and manage the obstetric cause of PPH.

Management of Uterine atony:
- **Bimanual uterine massage & compression first-line treatment ± utetoronics (eg, Oxytocin).**
- **Uterotonic agents: IV Oxytocin first-line medical treatment to increase uterine contractions. If Oxytocin ineffective, Methylergonovine (if no hypertension, coronary or cerebral artery disease) or Prostaglandin analogs:** IM Carboprost tromethamine (if no Asthma), Misoprostol.
- Minimally invasive procedures (eg, intrauterine balloon tamponade) & progress to more invasive procedures (eg, uterine artery embolization, surgical ligation of the uterine artery, hysterectomy) until hemorrhage is controlled.

Management due to retained products: compression & massage. Curettage may be needed in some.
Management of Uterine inversion: manual reposition of the uterus: elevate the posterior fornix as initial management + discontinuation of uterotonic agents. Suspect if a red mass protrudes from the vagina.
- Uterine relaxing agent: Nitroglycerin, Terbutaline, Magnesium sulfate.
Management of coagulopathy: transfusion of blood products and/or clotting factors.

APGAR SCORE

Usually done at 1 & 5 minutes after birth. Repeated at 10 minutes if abnormal.

Score from 1-10: **7-10 = excellent condition;** 4-6 fairly low; ≤3 critically low.

- **Neonates with an APGAR score of <7 require active resuscitation** and should have sequential APGARs assessed every 5 minutes until the score is ≥7.

	0	1	2
Appearance Skin color changes	Cyanotic (blue-gray) or pale all over	• <u>**Pink with acrocyanosis:**</u> body pink but blue extremities	• **Pink baby (no cyanosis)**
Pulse	0 (absent)	• <100 beats/minute	• ≥ 100 beats/minute
Grimace (Reflex irritability)	<u>No response</u> to stimulation	<u>Minimal response:</u> • Grimaces feebly on suction or aggressive stimulation	<u>Prompt response:</u> • Pulls away, sneezes, or coughs • Cries on stimulation.
Activity (Muscle tone)	None (absent) Limp/flaccid	<u>Some flexion:</u> • arms and legs flexed	<u>Active movement:</u> • Well flexion of arm & legs • Resists extension
Respiration	Absent (apneic)	• Weak, gasping • Slow, irregular breathing	• Strong, vigorous cry • Normal respirations (30-60/min)

Screen using the Edinburgh Postnatal Depression Scale (EPDS).

	POSTPARTUM BLUES	POSTPARTUM DEPRESSION	POSTPARTUM PSYCHOSIS
ONSET	• **2-3 days,** peaking over the next few days.	• **Typically within 4-6 weeks** (can be up to 1 year).	• Days to weeks
CLINICAL MANIFESTATIONS	• <u>**Mild & self-limited:**</u> tearfulness, irritability, anhedonia, fatigue, depressed mood. • Concern if she is a good mother • **No thoughts of harming the baby**	• **≥5 Major depression symptoms,** anhedonia. • Functional impairment • Crying most days of the week • May have thoughts of harming baby.	• **delusions,** • **hallucinations,** • **thought disorganization,** • **bizarre behavior.** • **Thoughts of harming the baby.**
DURATION	• **Resolves within 14 days of onset**	• Resolves within 3-14 months	
MANAGEMENT	• **Reassurance, support, & monitoring** • Cognitive behavioral therapy.	• <u>**Antidepressants**</u> **(eg, SSRIs)** • **Cognitive behavioral therapy.**	• **Antipsychotics, antidepressants. Mood stabilizers,** <u>**hospitalization.**</u> • **Do not leave mother alone with infant (risk of infanticide**

PHOTO CREDITS

INDEX

PANCE PREP APP

TRY OUR SWEET APP :)

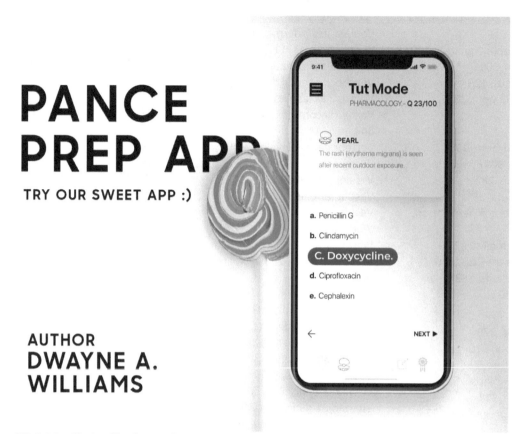

AUTHOR
DWAYNE A. WILLIAMS

Over 15,000 clinically-based practice examination questions specifically formulated to enhance clinical skills and improve performance on examinations, such as the PANCE, PANRE, OSCES, USMLE, end of rotation examinations and comprehensive medical examinations.

Special clinical pearls, disease review, explanation of the answers, test taking strategies and much more.

3 modes,
Timed mode to simulate the exams
Tutor mode that allows you to review the disease states in addition to the questions and **improve mode** to enhance your weak areas.

For every question in tutor mode, there is a feature for a hint to see if you are going in the right direction, answer explanation, a clinical pearl, and a bonus questions. Create your own examination based on organ systems or task areas. The ultimate study and exam preparation app!

PANCE PREP QUESTION APP
EARN 20 CATEGORY 1 SELF-ASSESSMENT CME CREDITS

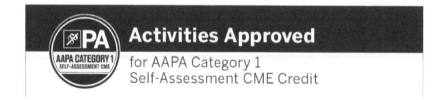

CYTOCHROME P450 INDUCERS

John was **wor**thy when referred & <u>**inducted**</u> into sainthood for giving up **chronic alcohol** use & placing himself **on a real** fast, **fend**ing off **greasy carbs**, leading to **less warfare** with **theo**logians.

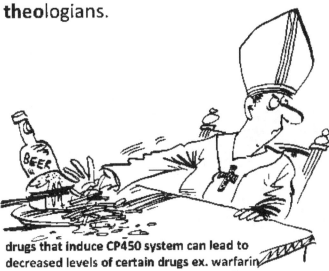

drugs that induce CP450 system can lead to decreased levels of certain drugs ex. warfarin (less warfare), theophylline (theologians) and phenytoin

INDUCERS OF THE P450

- **St. Johns Wort**
- **rifampin** (referred)
- **chronic alcohol use**
- **sulfonylureas**
  (self on a real)
- **Phenytoin**
- **Phenobarbital** (fend)
- **Griseofulvin** (greasy)
- **Carbamazepine**
  (carbs)

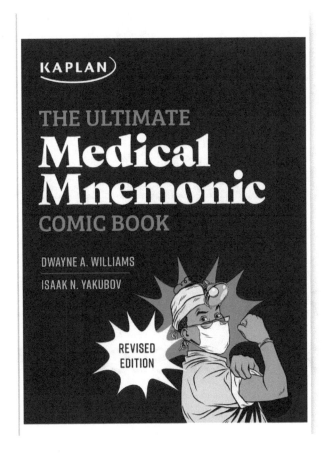

EARN 20 CATEGORY 1 SELF-ASSESSMENT CME CREDITS

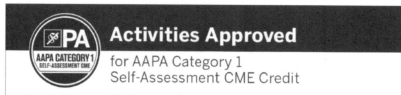

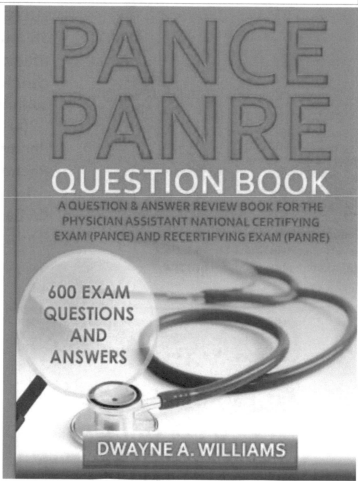

COMING SOON IN 2024: PANCE PREP QUESTION BOOK SECOND EDITION!

Made in United States
Troutdale, OR
01/16/2025